vn below.

OXFORD MEDICAL PUBLICATIONS

Oxford Handbook of
Public Health
Practice

Oxford Handbook of Clinical Medicine 6/e (also available for PDAs and in a Mini Edition)
Oxford Handbook of Clinical Specialties 7/e
Oxford Handbook of Acute Medicine 2/e
Oxford Handbook of Anaesthesia 2/e
Oxford Handbook of Applied Dental Sciences
Oxford Handbook of Cardiology
Oxford Handbook of Clinical Dentistry 4/e
Oxford Handbook of Clinical and Laboratory Investigation 2/e
Oxford Handbook of Clinical Diagnosis
Oxford Handbook of Clinical Haematology 2/e
Oxford Handbook of Clinical Immunology and Allergy 2/e
Oxford Handbook of Clinical Pharmacy
Oxford Handbook of Clinical Surgery 2/e
Oxford Handbook of Critical Care 2/e
Oxford Handbook of Dental Patient Care 2/e
Oxford Handbook of Dialysis 2/e
Oxford Handbook of Emergency Medicine 3/e
Oxford Handbook of Endocrinology and Diabetes
Oxford Handbook of ENT and Head and Neck Surgery
Oxford Handbook for the Foundation Programme
Oxford Handbook of Gastroenterology and Hepatology
Oxford Handbook of General Practice 2/e
Oxford Handbook of Genitourinary Medicine, HIV and AIDS
Oxford Handbook of Geriatric Medicine
Oxford Handbook of Medical Sciences
Oxford Handbook of Nephrology and Hypertension
Oxford Handbook of Neurology
Oxford Handbook of Obstetrics and Gynaecology
Oxford Handbook of Oncology 2/e
Oxford Handbook of Ophthalmology
Oxford Handbook of Palliative Care
Oxford Handbook of Practical Drug Therapy
Oxford Handbook of Psychiatry
Oxford Handbook of Public Health Practice 2/e
Oxford Handbook of Rehabilitation Medicine
Oxford Handbook of Respiratory Medicine
Oxford Handbook of Rheumatology
Oxford Handbook of Tropical Medicine 2/e
Oxford Handbook of Urology

Oxford Handbook of
Public Health
Practice

Second edition

Edited by

David Pencheon

Charles Guest

David Melzer

J.A. Muir Gray

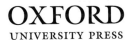

OXFORD
UNIVERSITY PRESS

OXFORD
UNIVERSITY PRESS

Great Clarendon Street, Oxford OX2 6DP

Oxford University Press is a department of the University of Oxford.
It furthers the University's objective of excellence in research, scholarship,
and education by publishing worldwide in

Oxford New York

Auckland Cape Town Dar es Salaam Hong Kong Karachi
Kuala Lumpur Madrid Melbourne Mexico City Nairobi
New Delhi Shanghai Taipei Toronto

With offices in

Argentina Austria Brazil Chile Czech Republic France Greece
Guatemala Hungary Italy Japan Poland Portugal Singapore
South Korea Switzerland Thailand Turkey Ukraine Vietnam

Oxford is a registered trade mark of Oxford University Press
in the UK and in certain other countries

Published in the United States
by Oxford University Press Inc., New York

British Library Cataloguing in Publication Data
Data available

Library of Congress Cataloging in Publication Data
Data available

Typeset by Newgen Imaging Systems (P) Ltd., Chennai, India
Printed in Italy
on acid-free paper by
LegoPrint S.p.A.

ISBN 0–19–856655–7 (flexicover: alk.paper)
      978–0–19–856655–7 (flexicover: alk.paper)

10 9 8 7 6 5 4 3 2 1

Editors' dedication

The junior editors of the *Oxford Handbook of Public Health Practice* thank Muir Gray, knighted for services to the UK National Health Service as this text went to press, for his inspiration over many years. The second edition is dedicated to him, with the hope of contributing to improvements in public health practice around the world, as Muir has.

DP
CSG
DM

Foreword to the second edition

At some point in their lives, readers of this handbook have no doubt confronted the same dilemmas that I faced when I chose to retire from clinical practice to embark on a career in public health. At the time I made my choice, my senior colleagues alerted me to the strict hierarchy that exists across the diverse branches of the health sciences. They cautioned that the prestige of any given specialty within the house of medicine is inversely proportional to the size of the object it addresses. Hence if your chosen field of specialty happens to deal with microscopic objects like chromosomes and genes, you can be assured of high prestige as well as unlimited access to funding. If, on the other hand, your chosen field happens to deal with the opposite end of the spectrum from genes—that is, the health of entire populations—then you had better resign yourself to a life of chronic under-funding, low prestige, and being ignored by the rest of the world. Treating individual patients (as in clinical practice) lies somewhere between these two extremes. Clinical practice may not be as 'sexy' as genetics, but at least you can be assured of a steady income as well as the satisfaction of seeing the fruits of your labor on a daily basis. By contrast, the translation of public health knowledge into practice often seems excruciatingly slow, and the results of our interventions are seldom directly observable at the individual level.

Nowadays we are constantly reminded of the achievements of the genetic revolution. Barely 50 years have elapsed since Watson and Crick discovered the structure of DNA. Yet within that short span of time, remarkable progress has been made in understanding the molecular basis of life and disease. The human genome has been mapped out in its entirety, and our newspapers trumpet the latest breakthroughs in genetic science on a daily basis. By contrast, we have understood the major population threats to health for what seems like aeons. For instance, we have known for over 150 years that poverty causes illness. Yet progress in solving the problems of health disparities seems painfully, if not embarrassingly, slow. Even today, some 40 per cent of humanity subsists on a meager standard of living of less than $2 a day, and millions of people perish worldwide from diseases caused by extreme poverty. Does this mean that we should all give up what we are doing and become molecular scientists? Of course not.

As this handbook illustrates, the public health approach has at its disposal a powerful set of practices that can transform the health of populations. Indeed, public health can lay claim to a number of significant victories that have improved the lives of millions. Thomas McKeown considered that the major improvements in mortality from infectious diseases during the last century occurred not through medical advances but through public health measures, specifically improvements in sanitation and nutrition. The earliest convincing evidence of cigarette smoking as a cause of cancer was published by Ernest Wynder in 1953—the same year as the discovery of the genetic code. Armed with this knowledge (as well as subsequent epidemiological evidence), public health practitioners have helped millions of smokers to quit their habit, as well as prevented millions more from initiating, with the result that countless lives have been saved. It represents a victory on a scale that few in the molecular field could lay claim to—at least so far.

As Geoffrey Rose pointed out, the public health approach to prevention is about shifting the population distribution of risk (the so-called 'population strategy of prevention'). In contrast to the high-risk strategy which characterizes the clinician's approach to prevention, the public health approach yields small individual benefit—hence accounting for its lack of public visibility—but large and often radical population benefit. For example, mandatory seat belt laws are unlikely to protect any given individual. After all, most drivers are unlikely to ever be involved in a car crash in which wearing a seat belt would have saved their life. On the other hand, applying this small statistical benefit to the population level results in a substantial health gain, measured by the number of lives saved. [Editor's note: When Dr Kawachi was invited to write the foreword, he immediately identified the omission of the term prevention paradox from the index in the first edition of this book. We thank him for explaining the concept here, which also now appears now in the glossary. CSG] The lives saved by public health practice are statistical ones. Public health practitioners cannot derive the same satisfaction in their daily practice as clinicians who can often observe their patients revive on the end of a hypodermic needle or the scalpel. As frustrating as this may seem, the public health practitioners also understand that the population impact of their practices are often directly proportional to the size of the object that they tackle.

A further type of artificial hierarchy that occurs within professions is the distinction between researchers and practitioners. The world is divided into those who seek to understand society versus those who seek to change it. Within public health, higher prestige is often bestowed upon researchers, compared with those who toil at the 'coal face' of practice. This is an unwarranted distinction, as the section on personal effectiveness in this handbook demonstrates. The mission of public health is to protect and promote the health of populations. No public health researcher can hope to accomplish this mission without mastery of the skills of public health practice, as exemplified by effective communication, working in teams, and advocating for change. It has been lamented that in many professional schools of public health today a student can graduate without learning the basic principles of public health practice. By the end of their training, they may know all about how to calculate a p value, but little about how to translate public health knowledge into effective advocacy, policies, and practical action. There are dozens of textbooks dealing with advanced epidemiological methods but precious few that focus on the skills needed to practice the art of public health. This handbook provides a valuable antidote to that imbalance. In our daily practice, we should all carry the handbook with us in the pockets of our invisible white coats.

Ichiro Kawachi
Professor of Social Epidemiology
Harvard School of Public Health
Boston, USA

Foreword to the first edition

Originality, practical focus and comprehensive coverage are not qualities normally found together in textbooks in the field of medicine and health care. In public health, the field, at least in Britain is even thinner.

The editors have pulled off a remarkable feat—meeting these challenges and drawing together a team of diverse talents to do the thinking and writing. From values to decision-making, from organizations to people, from strategy to team-working, the whole of public health practice is conceptualized in a fresh imaginative way.

Readers will see, described in this book, the skills they use day-to-day but will seldom recognize themselves, they will identify needs and knowledge gaps which they had not previously acknowledged, and they will find inspiration in the examples of good practice.

Simon Chapman's short chapter on using media advocacy to shape policy, Edmund Jessop's guide on writing to effect change and Alison Hill's road map to find evidence are just a small number of examples of areas which would not be covered in other books yet are the very stuff of modern public health practice.

Osler who graced Oxford with his inspirational presence nearly a century ago once said 'No bubble is so iridescent or floats longer than that blown by the successful teacher'.

Oxford, with Muir Gray as its guiding light, is once again a metaphorical meeting place for ideas, inspiration and great teaching.

Just as Laurent Blanc kissed the bald pate of Fabien Barthez before each game in France's glorious World Cup winning run, kiss the cover of the *Oxford Guide to Public Health Practice* before you open it. You will have found a true soul mate.

Liam Donaldson
Chief Medical Officer
Department of Health
February 2001

Editors' lament

Editing a book is no easy task. If we don't include every reference, people say we are superficial. If we do include every reference, people will say it is too dense. If we include every perspective, people will say we are too discursive. If we don't, people will say we are being too simplistic. If we are occasionally light-hearted, people say we are flippant. If we are not, people say we are too serious. If we invite too many contributing authors, people say we are too lazy to write ourselves. If we don't, we are accused of being too confident in our own abilities. If we don't include everyone's contribution, we fail to appreciate true genius. If we do include them, the book is full of rubbish. Now, most likely, someone will say we took this from another book. We did.

DP
CSG
DM
JAMG

Acknowledgements

Not every idea in this or any book can be traced to its source. We apologize for any omission here, and would be grateful to hear from readers with amendments, corrections, or other suggestions, using the evaluation card enclosed. Alternatively, we would welcome direct contact by mail.

We would like to thank the following people without whom this book would not be what it is: Harry Rutter, Brian Ferguson, Iain Lang, Joan Self, Kate Smith, Rosemary Lees, Ruairidh Milne, June Crown, Jill Meara, Helen Liepman, Eve Allsopp, Nic Williams, and Tania Pickering. As in the first edition, you would not be seeing this book if it were not for the dedicated and unstinting perseverance, cool head, and grace under pressure demonstrated to all the editors and many of the authors by Brenda McWilliams (publishing editor). We are heavily indebted.

DP
CSG
DM
JAMG

Contents

Detailed contents

Contributors

Ibrahim Abubakar
Clinical Senior Lecturer/Consultant
Epidemiologist,
University of East Anglia
School of Medicine,
Health Policy and Practice,
Norwich, UK

Jenny Amery
Senior Health and Population
Adviser,
Department for International
Development,
London, UK

Gerard Anderson
Professor of Health Policy,
Department of Health Policy
and Management,
Johns Hopkins Bloomberg School
of Public Health, Baltimore, MD,
USA

John Appleby
Director,
Health Systems Programme,
King's Fund, London, UK

Kate Ardern
Head of Public Health,
Cheshire and Merseyside Strategic
Health Authority, UK

Tar-Ching Aw
Professor and Head,
Division of Occupational Health,
Kent Institute of Medicine
& Health Sciences,
University of Kent, UK

Gabriele Bammer
Professorial Fellow
National Centre for Epidemiology
and Population Health,
College of Medicine and Health
Sciences, The Australian National
University, Canberra ACT,
Australia

Nicholas Banatvala
Senior Health and Population
Adviser,
Department for International
Development,
London, UK

Alex Barratt
Associate Professor of
Epidemiology,
Department of Public Health and
Community Medicine School of
Public Health, University of Sydney,
Sydney, Australia

John Battersby
Director of Public Health,
Southern Norfolk Primary Care
Trust, UK

Martin Birley
Lead Consultant
BirleyHIA, UK

Paul Bolton
Associate Professor,
Center for International Health and
Development,
Boston University School of
Public Health,
Boston, MA, USA

Peter Brambleby
Director of Public Health,
Norwich City Primary Care Trust
Norwich, UK

Anne Brice
Head of Service,
National Library for Health
Oxford, UK

Amanda Burls
Senior Clinical Lecturer in Public
Health and Epidemiology,
Department of Public Health and
Epidemiology,
University of Birmingham,
Birmingham, UK

Sir Kenneth Calman
Vice Chancellor and Warden,
University of Durham,
UK

Martin Caraher
Reader in Food and Health
Policy Centre for Food Policy,
Department of Health
Management and Food Policy,
City University, London, UK

Julia Carr
General Practitioner and Public
Health Practitioner,
Wellington, New Zealand

Simon Chapman
Professor,
School of Public Health,
University of Sydney,
Sydney, Australia

Ronald Davis
Director,
Center for Health Promotion and
Disease Prevention,
Henry Ford Health System,
Detroit, MI, USA

Angus Dawson
Centre Director and Senior
Lecturer in Ethics & Philosophy,
Centre for Professional Ethics,
Keele University, UK

Don Detmer
Professor Emeritus and Professor
of Medical Education,
Department of Public Health
Sciences, University of Virginia
School of Medicine, Charlottesville,
VA, USA

Anna Dixon
Lecturer in European Health Policy,
London School of Economics,
London, UK

Anna Donald
Chief Executive, Bazian, and
Honorary Fellow,
Department of Public Health and
Epidemiology,
London, UK

Martin Eccles
Professor of Clinical Effectiveness
and The William Leech Professor
of Primary Care Research Centre
for Health Services Research,
University of Newcastle Upon
Tyne, Newcastle upon Tyne,
UK

Vikki Entwistle
Reader,
Social Dimensions of Health
Institute, University of Dundee
Dundee, UK

Gene Feder
Professor of Primary Care
Research and Development,
Centre for Health Sciences,
Barts and the London,
Queen Mary's School of
Medicine and Dentistry,
London, UK

Julian Flowers
Scientific and Technical Director,
Eastern Region Public Health
Observatory, Institute of Public
Health, Cambridge,
UK

Michael Frommer
Adjunct Professor and Director
Sydney Health Projects Group,
The University of Sydney
Sydney, Australia

Peter Gentle
Freelance Consultant in Public
Health, Sidmouth, UK

Steve Gillam
Public Health Teaching
Specialist/GP,
Department of Public Health and
Primary Care Institute of
Public Health,
Cambridge, UK

Lawrence Gostin
Associate Dean,
Professor of Law, and Director,
Center for Law & the Public's
Health, Georgetown and Johns
Hopkins Universities,
Washington, DC, USA

Caron Grainger
Director of Public Health
Redditch and Bromsgrove Primary
Care Trust, UK

Sir JA Muir Gray
Programme Director,
UK National Screening Committee
and Director of Clinical
Knowledge and Safety,
Department of Health, UK

Sian Griffiths
Professor of Public Health,
The Chinese University of Hong
Kong, School of Public Health,
Prince of Wales Hospital
Shatin N.T., Hong Kong

Chris Griffiths
Professor of Primary Care
Centre for Health Sciences,
Barts and the London, Queen
Mary's School of Medicine and
Dentistry, London, UK

Jeremy Grimshaw
Director,
Clinical Epidemiology Programme,
Ottawa Health Research Institute,
Ottawa, Canada

Charles Guest
Senior Specialist,
Australian Capital Territory
Department of Health and
Australian National University,
Canberra, Australia

Pamela Hall
Deputy Medical Director,
Essex Strategic Health Authority,
Chelmsford, UK

Bec Hanley
Director,
TwoCan Associates, UK

Malcolm Harrington
Emeritus Professor of Occupational
Health, UK

Ian Harvey
Professor of Epidemiology
and Public Health,
School of Medicine,
Health Policy and Practice,
University of East Anglia,
Norwich, UK

Nick Hicks
Director of Public Health,
Milton Keynes Primary Care Trust
and Milton Keynes Council,
Milton Keynes, UK

Alison Hill
Director,
South East Public Health
Observatory, Oxford, UK

Tony Hope
Director of the Ethox Centre
Division of Public Health &
Primary Care, Oxford, UK

Richard Hopkins
Medical Epidemiologist,
Acute Disease Epidemiology
Section, Bureau of Epidemiology,
Florida Department of Health,
Tallahassee, FL, USA

Peter Sotir Hussey
Research Associate,
Department of Health Policy and
Management, Johns Hopkins School
of Hygiene and Public Health,
Baltimore, MD, USA

Rebekah Jenkin
Senior Associate,
Sydney Health Projects Group
School of Public Health,
The University of Sydney,
Sydney, Australia

Edmund Jessop
Medical Adviser,
National Specialist Commissioning
Advisory Group,
UK Department of Health, UK

Tony Jewell
Director of Clinical Quality and
Health Improvement,
NSC Strategic Health Authority
Cambridge, UK

Mike Jones
Visiting Professor, and Director,
Pi Associates,
Middlesex University, UK

Ichiro Kawachi
Professor of Social Epidemiology,
Department of Society, Human
Development and Health, Harvard
School of Public Health,
Boston, MA, USA

Andrew Kibble
Honorary Lecturer,
Division of Environmental Health
and Risk Management,
School of Geography,
University of Birmingham,
Birmingham, UK

Yi Mien Koh
Professor,
Director of Public Health and
Performance Management,
NW London SHA,
London, UK

Dee Kyle
Director of Public Health
Bradford South & West Primary
Care Trust, Bradford, UK

Tim Lang
Professor of Food Policy,
Centre for Food Policy, Dept
Health Management & Food Policy
Institute of Health Sciences,
City University, London, UK

David Lawrence
Specialist in Public Health Planning
Information,
London School of Hygiene and
Tropical Medicine, UK

Tom Ling
Professor of Public Policy,
RAND Europe and Anglia Ruskin
University, Cambridge, UK

Georgios Lyratzopoulos
Consultant in Public Health
NSC Strategic Health Authority
Cambridge, UK

Katherine Mackay
Research Associate,
Australian Capital Territory
Department of Health and
Australian National University
Medical School,
Canberra, Australia

Annabelle Mark
Professor of Healthcare
Organisation,
Middlesex University Business
School, UK

Alan Maryon-Davis
Director of Public Health,
Southwark Primary Care Trust,
London, UK

Mohammed Rashad Massoud
Senior Vice President,
Institute for Healthcare
Improvement,
Cambridge, MA, USA

Don Matheson
Deputy Director General,
General Practitioner and Public
Health Physician,
Wellington, New Zealand

Martin McKee
Professor of European Public
Health, European Centre on Health
of Societies in Transition,
London School of Hygiene and
Tropical Medicine, London, UK

Brenda McWilliams
Publishing Editor/Research
Associate,
Institute of Public Health,
Cambridge, UK

David Melzer
Professor of Epidemiology and
Public Health,
Peninsula Medical School,
University of Exeter,
Exeter, UK

Anjum Memon
Senior Lecturer and Honorary
Consultant in Public Health,
Department of Public Health and
Primary Care, Cambridge, UK

Ruairidh Milne
Consultant in Public Health,
Wessex Institute of Public Health
National Coordinating Centre
for Health Technology Assessment,
University of Southampton,
Southampton, UK

John Newton
Professor of Public Health and
Epidemiology,
University of Manchester, UK

Don Nutbeam
Pro-Vice-Chancellor and Head,
College of Health Sciences,
University of Sydney
Sydney, Australia

Sarah O'Brien
Professor of Health Sciences and
Epidemiology,
University of Manchester, UK

David Pencheon
Director,
Eastern Region Public Health
Observatory, Institute of Public
Health, Cambridge, UK

Angela Raffle
Consultant in Public Health,
Bristol North Primary Care Trust,
Bristol, UK

Jem Rashbass
Director,
Eastern Cancer Registry and
Intelligence Centre,
Clinical and Biomedical Computing
Unit, Addenbrooke's Hospital,
Cambridge, UK

Richard Richards
Director of Public Health,
Newark and Sherwood Primary
Care Trust,
Newark, UK

Jean-Marie Robine
INSERM
Equipe démographie et santé
Centre Val d'Aurelle Parc
Euromédecine, Centre Val
d'Aurelle, Parc Euromédecine
Montpellier, France

George Rubin
Professor of Public Health and
Director, Centre for Health
Services Research,
University of Sydney School of
Public Health, Sydney
Australia

Patrick Saunders
Honorary Senior Lecturer
Department of Public Health and
Epidemiology,
Birmingham, UK

Gabriel Scally
Regional Director of Public
Health, Government Office for the
South West, Bristol, UK

Alex Scott-Samuel
Senior Lecturer in Public Health
Director, Liverpool PHO,
Department of Public Health,
University of Liverpool,
Liverpool, UK

Paul Shekelle
Staff Physician, West Los Angeles
Veterans Affairs Medical Center,
Consultant, RAND Health,
CA, USA

Fiona Sim
Public Health Consultant
Radlett, UK

Daniel Sosin
Captain, US Public Health Service,
Senior Advisor for Science and
Public Health Practice,
Coordinating Office of Terrorism
Preparedness and Emergency
Response, Centers for Disease
Control and Prevention,
Atlanta, GA, USA

Chris Spencer Jones
Director of Public Health
Birmingham South Primary Care
Trust, Birmingham, UK

Nick Steel
Senior Lecturer in Primary Care
School of Medicine,
Health Policy and Practice,
University of East Anglia,
Norwich, UK

Andrew Stevens
Professor of Public Health,
Department of Public Health &
Epidemiology, University of
Birmingham, UK

Alison Stewart
Chief Knowledge Officer,
Public Health Genetics Unit,
Strangeways Research Laboratory,
Cambridge, UK

Roscoe Taylor
Director of Public Health and
Director, Population Health,
Department of Health and Human
Services, Hobart, Tasmania
Australia.

Barry Tennison
Honorary Professor of Public
Health and Policy,
London School of Hygiene and
Tropical Medicine,
London, UK

David Tipene-Leach
General Practitioner,
Gisborne, New Zealand

Michelle Tjhin
Research Officer,
Australian Network for Effective
Healthcare, Department of Public
Health & Community Medicine,
University of Sydney, Sydney
Australia

Charlie Tomson
Health Foundation Fellow
Institute for Healthcare
Improvement,
Cambridge, MA, USA

Jeanette Ward
Director and Professor in
Public Health,
Institute of Population Health,
University of Ottawa, Ottawa
Ontario, Canada

Paul Watson
Medical Director,
Essex Strategic Health Authority
Chelmsford, UK

Julius Weinberg
Director,
Institute of Health Sciences,
City University, London, UK

Stuart Whitaker
Senior Lecturer in Occupational
Health, St Martin's College,
Lancaster, UK

Peter Wightman
Director of Modernisation,
Huntingdonshire Primary Care
Trust, UK

John Wilkinson
Director,
North East Public Health
Observatory, University of Durham
Stockton Campus, UK

John Wright
Consultant in Epidemiology
and Public Health,
Bradford Teaching Hospitals
NHS Trust, UK

Ron Zimmern
Director,
Public Health Genetics Unit
Strangeways Research Laboratory,
Cambridge, UK

Introduction

The last two decades of the 20th century saw a renewal of interest in the eternal verities of public health, in disease prevention, communicable disease control, health protection, and health promotion. This was partly due to the realization that continued investment in clinical care brings diminishing returns, and partly because of the recognition that the problems tackled so successfully by public health actions in the last half of the 19th century and the first half of the 20th century have not disappeared. In some cases, they are re-emerging as bacteria develop resistance to antibiotics and as new threats to health develop in the physical environment, both locally and globally.

Public health practice therefore continues to be a major force in the 21st century: there will be a need for guides such as this for those who make decisions and who face both the traditional and the newer challenges that threaten the public health. If clinicians spend their time discovering new ways of managing old diseases, public health practitioners are constantly relearning the old ways of managing newer patterns of disease.

The role of public health is to contribute 'to the health of the public through assessment of health and health needs, policy formulation, and assurance of the availability of services'.[1] As this guide will show, many public health practitioners and teams make their biggest contribution through the development of health systems. A health system, in its broadest sense, is composed of 'personal health care, public health services and other inter-sectoral initiatives'.[2] It is rarely helpful to claim one part of such a system contributes more than another. A balanced view—and a balanced health system—should contribute to a fair and healthy society.

Many problems can be classified as public health problems, and public health problems and challenges can be classified in many ways. The contents page illustrates one such way of classifying the public health world. Significantly it begins with the task of sorting out what the actual issues, questions, and challenges are before too much effort is spent solving the wrong problem. The challenge for public health practitioners is to cope with conflicting priorities for improving the health of populations, and the increasing need to show that potential solutions are not just effective, but are also cost-effective.[3] As the scope of the public health challenge broadens, for example with the development of the new genetics and the renaissance of infectious diseases, it becomes impossible for any one individual to have a complete grasp of the knowledge needed to identify, analyze, and tackle the problems that influence their population's health. Public health practitioners therefore need a broad range of skills and selective depth in specialist knowledge areas. In particular, public health practitioners need to be skilled at finding and appraising sources of knowledge. The focus of public health practitioners on a population and its health needs should persist, even while other professional groups are specializing and subspecializing to cope with the exponential growth of knowledge.

When public health is defined as the science and art of improving the population's health through the organized efforts of society,[4,5] using the techniques of disease prevention, health protection, and health promotion, these words are chosen carefully. This guide outlines the important tasks and skills needed by today's public health practitioners to ensure these efforts are well directed and well made.

The guide is structured around identifying and clarifying public health problems and the practical tasks needed to address them. It is designed to help new public health practitioners appreciate the scope, frameworks, and techniques in public health. In addition, it is a constant refresher and reference guide for the more experienced practitioner.

We do not intend this book to be the last word in any area; rather, we have tried to present what might be considered the first words and the most important concepts in the essential activities of public health practice.

***

We assume that users of this book already have a basic understanding of epidemiology and statistics (although we provide a brief chapter on the former to remind people of the basic techniques) in the same way as a textbook of medicine assumes the reader has a knowledge of anatomy and physiology. This guide book covers the building blocks of public health practice. Those seeking more detailed guidance concerning epidemiology, statistics, and research methods will need to turn to other texts.[6–9]

An under-rated task of public health practitioners is that of turning complex and seemingly messy issues into solvable problems. Skills to find and assess the knowledge that underpins problem-solving are carefully examined. Deciding on the most appropriate public health action almost always involves difficult, but important, choices. These choices are rarely simple, technical issues with quantitative answers. In Part 1 we therefore examine the approaches used in addressing the values and ethics in public health that cannot, and should not, be avoided in such decision-making. Part 2 outlines the principles and practice of using data and evidence.

After applying these techniques, the issues may eventually become clearer, the options more obvious, and the decisions that need to be taken more apparent. Only then should the most appropriate methods of public health action be chosen and applied.

This handbook also presents the diversity and appropriateness of methods of taking direct action on the immediate determinants of public health. Part 3 covers examples of the specific tasks facing public health: protecting and promoting health, and preventing disease through different techniques for different challenges, in different places, and for different populations, around the globe.

The influencing, making, and implementing of policy (whether by governments or by large multinational organizations) is a fundamental part of public health practice. Part 4 of the handbook shows how science and rationality need to be combined with emotion and power (e.g. though the media) to achieve public health gains, not only through the *formulation* of policy but also in its *implementation*.

We do not wish to pursue the false dichotomy concerning the influence of health care versus other public health activities on the population's health. However, the organization and delivery of health care is an area where many public health practitioners have the opportunity to play a significant role. In Parts 5 and 6, we present the tasks and skills needed to assess and assure the important dimensions of quality in health-care organization and delivery. In addition, many of the principles outlined in this section are transferable to other services that influence the public's health.

The art of public health refers to the interpersonal and organizational skills needed to effect real change. Without these personal and organizational skills, the best evidence and the best intentions amount to nothing. The last parts of the handbook cover the personal and organizational skills needed to create effective change in collaboration with other individuals and teams throughout the health system.

***

The guide is not intended to be read from start to finish. The order of the parts and chapters may imply that decisions and action do not take place until a complete assessment of the health of the population is performed. Life is rarely that simple. Most public health action around the world involves simultaneous firefighting of multiple real and perceived threats to (and opportunities for) public health. Many professionals therefore begin tasks with the scoping of apparent problems, rather than with the prior and more theoretical assessment of real ones.

Throughout this guide, we have tried to address, where possible, the 10 core activities of Public Health as outlined by the US Health and Human Services Public Health Service:[10]

1. preventing epidemics
2. protecting the environment, workplaces, food, and water
3. promoting healthy behavior
4. monitoring the health status of the population
5. mobilizing community action
6. responding to disasters
7. assuring the quality, accessibility, and accountability of medical care
8. reaching out to link high-risk and hard-to-reach people to needed services
9. researching to develop new insights and innovative solutions
10. leading the development of sound health policy and planning.

Public health is centrally concerned with the pursuit of social justice and efficiency. Such achievements have sometimes only been possible because of opportunism, serendipity, and charisma. Nonetheless, learning and improvement are never complete for any of us. Like any of the big tasks facing us today, we need clarity of purpose and attention to detail. The leaders in public health have always needed the skills of data, evidence, and communication. The processes outlined in this guide should enable public health practitioners to improve old skills and learn new skills, all of which are needed to address the big public health challenges, both local and global, in the 21st century.

DP
CSG
DM
JAMG

July 2005

References

1 Institute of Medicine (1988). *The future of public health*. Institute of Medicine, Washington, DC. Available at: http://fermat.nap.edu/catalog/1091.html (accessed 20 May 2006).

2 World Health Organization (2000). *World health report 2000. Health systems: improving performance*. World Health Organization, Geneva. Available at: http://www.who.int/whr/en/ (accessed 5 October 2005).

3 Wanless D (2004). *Securing good health for the whole population*. HM Treasury, London. Available at: http://www.hm-treasury.gov.uk/consultations_and_legislation/wanless/consult_wanless04_final.cfm (accessed 5 October 2005).

4 Acheson D (1988). *Public health in England*. HMSO, London.

5 Last JM (ed.) (2001). *A dictionary of epidemiology*, 4th edn. Oxford University Press, Oxford.

6 Maxcy KF, Rosenau MJ, Last JM (eds) (1988). *Public health and preventive medicine*, 13th edn. Appleton & Lange, Norwalk, CT.

7 Detels R, McEwen J, Beaglehole R, Tanaka H (eds) (2004). *Oxford textbook of public health*, 4th edn. Oxford University Press, Oxford.

8 Kerr C, Taylor R, Heard G (eds) (1998). *Handbook of public health methods*. McGraw-Hill, Sydney.

9 Donaldson LJ, Donaldson RJ (2000). *Essential public health*, 2nd edn. Petroc Press, Newbury.

10 US Health and Human Services Public Health Service (1995). *For a healthy nation: returns on investment in public health*. US Government Printing Office, Washington, DC.

Options and decisions

Introduction

People who dislike decisions should not become public health practitioners. Sometimes there appears to be only one option—a single case of meningitis necessitates some action, but what action? Even when the initial decision is easy to take, others follow which are more subtle and challenging. The first decision is whether or not there is a public health problem to be tackled. Not all problems that affect populations are appropriate for public health practitioners or departments alone. Often the issue has to be examined from different perspectives to understand what is actually going on. Trouble on a housing estate, for example, high levels of crime, violence, and environmental decay, combined with social deprivation, flares up one hot summer's day and makes local and national headlines. Obviously the health of that population is affected both in the long term and in the short term. Is this a public health problem, an economic problem, or a political problem? Or, to be more precise, what should a public health practitioner or department do?

Public health options have to take into account a wide range of different types of factor such as:

- the needs of the population and the relative importance of different problems
- the evidence about the cost-effectiveness of different options
- the values of the population and the ethical basis of those values.

Choices in public health therefore have to be based upon the integration of economics, evidence, and ethics, and they are rarely easy or clear-cut, particularly because public health so often has to manage a mess.

Many of the great achievements of nineteenth-century public health were made on the principle that disorder and mess were the causes of disease, and anything that was offensive to the senses, to the eyes or the nose or the taste buds, was *ipso facto* harmful to health; the word 'nuisance', which we use to refer to a relatively trivial problem today, derives from the Old French 'nuire', to harm, and the concept of the nuisance was at the heart of the nineteenth-century public health revolution. Today, public health is also involved in what management theorists call 'messes'—highly complex problems with two managerial characteristics:

- there is no ideal solution and
- every solution creates further problems.

For example, increasing the price of cigarettes reduces consumption but also increases smuggling; the pedestrianization of a city centre may cause problems for people with disabilities; partnerships with major supermarket chains to improve the diet may widen the health gap between rich and poor.

Decisions, decisions, decisions

The public health professional, therefore, faces issues and problems every day, some of which are possible to scope (Chapter 1.1) and turn into answerable questions (Chapter 1.2). These two chapters identify the steps needed for turning messy issues into answerable questions.

Becoming more specific, one then needs to be able to understand, quantify, and address the needs of the population, especially those in greatest need (Chapter 1.3). Even when needs are well identified and quantified, it may still be difficult to actually invest in an area or a service where the priority is seemingly obvious (Chapter 1.4). Nowadays we need to justify everything and demonstrate that the overall impact of any intervention will be positive (Chapter 1.5). Many of these seemingly intractable problems now need to be assessed, not just from a practical and financial perspective but also through the perspective of people's values and ethics (Chapters 1.6 and 1.7). Finally, one can stare problems in the face, but nothing is going to change unless the public health practitioner has the competence and confidence to innovate (Chapter 1.8).

There has been a large literature on clinical decision-making in the last decade; in this section of the book we focus on public health decision-making to help the reader make better choices.

DP

1.1 Scoping public health problems

Gabriele Bammer

Objectives

This chapter aims to help you figure out what you can most effectively do, within the constraints of the resources you have, to address the public health problem you are concerned with.

What does scoping mean?

Scoping is the preparatory stage of a project where we systematically think about what we can best do with the time, money, and people we have at our disposal in order to use those resources most effectively. It involves considering:
- what we want to achieve and who will be affected
- who needs to be on-side
- what needs to be done to get there
- what the likely blocks are and how they can be overcome.

Why is scoping an important public health skill?

There are four reasons why scoping is particularly important. It helps us:
- set boundaries
- broaden our view of the problem beyond what we know and understand, recognizing and respecting different point of view
- decide if we want to challenge the way in which the problem is generally viewed, by paying more attention to something society sees as marginal or excluded
- work out who we need to have on-side to give the project legitimacy.

Essentially, scoping is the process of setting the boundaries around how we will address the problem. There is always a limit to what anyone can do and think about, but we often think of these boundaries as being natural, rather than something we construct. Scoping makes us consciously think about what we, and society generally, include, exclude, and marginalize. In other words, whenever we address a public health problem some considerations will be central (included), some will be peripheral (marginalized), and some will be excluded.

It may seem odd, but an important boundary-setting process is to start by broadening the view of the problem, to move us beyond our own outlook and to help us see the problem through the eyes of others. The approach taken to the problem is then not limited to what we know and understand, but incorporates the knowledge and understanding of others. The problem then becomes central, rather than our own expertise.

This process involves recognizing and respecting different points of view, especially in controversial areas. Paying attention to the range of arguments usually smooths the path to compromise. Views will often soften once people feel they have been respectfully heard. In addition, if people know that all reasonable alternatives are being considered, they will usually be more satisfied with the choice that is made. Therefore, starting off with a broad approach can help get people on-side for the action that is eventually decided upon.

In addition, there will be a way in which the public health problem being considered is already viewed in society. Scoping helps us decide if we want to work within that view or if there are aspects of the problem that are currently not thought about, or on the periphery, that should be more central.

Regardless of whether we work within an accepted social view or challenge it, the way in which we tackle the project needs to have legitimacy and effective alliances. The bona fides of the project come through the funding sources and the standing of the organization and people involved and of those who support the project.

Even if the resources are very limited, scoping can show us a helpful first step that may lead to more resources later. It stops us from putting a lot of time and effort into issues that are peripheral and helps us focus on what's most important. It stops us from reinventing the wheel and helps us cast new light on the problem. It also helps us plan ahead, so that we can finish the project rather than running out of resources half-way through.

Eight questions useful for scoping

- What do we know about the problem?
- What can different interest groups and academic disciplines contribute to addressing this problem?
- What areas are contentious?
- What are the big-picture issues? In other words, what are the political, social, and cultural aspects of the problem?

and

- Why is this problem on the agenda now?
- What support and resources are likely to be available for tackling the problem?
- What parts of the problem are already well covered and where are the areas of greatest need?
- Where can the most strategic interventions be made?

The first four questions help identify the dimensions of the problem, while the last four help set priorities.

Ways of addressing the scoping questions

Finding out what we know about the problem

Chapter 2.1 provides a good guide here, not only to sources of information but also to how we can evaluate the quality of what we find in libraries, on the Internet, and through personal contact with experts.

Working with interest groups and disciplines

Key steps include:
- identifying which interest groups and disciplines are relevant
- finding appropriate representatives
- getting their input
- rewarding them.

Chapter 8.4 takes you through these steps for identifying and involving consumers. Think about which other stakeholders are relevant—perhaps service providers, police, business people, or policy makers. Who in your networks can help you understand their point of view or identify someone who can? Many of the steps for involving consumers are also relevant for other stakeholders—it has to be made clear that they can make a meaningful contribution, that they will be listened to respectfully, and that what they say will be taken into account.

It is also worth thinking about what research can contribute, what sort of research has been conducted, and what sort of previously ignored research might cast a new light (see Chapters 1.8, 2.9, and 2.10).

Dealing with areas of contention

While it can be tempting to avoid areas of contention, it is generally advisable to deal with them explicitly and early. It helps greatly if you can be dispassionate and genuinely open to hearing all arguments. Try to identify the basis of the controversy—is it a clash of egos, a misunderstanding resulting from poor communication, a conflict of interests, or a difference in values (see Chapter 1.6)? This will help you think about how you want to position your approach to the health problem and if you want to try to resolve the disagreement. There are a number of participatory and soft systems methods that can help people understand why others think differently. In general, people respond positively if they feel confident that their views are being heard and taken seriously. Then even if they disagree with the final approach that is taken they will often think it is fair.

Tackling big-picture issues

The influence of government policy, advertising, and business practice on public health issues deserves the same level of attention as individual behaviour, and changes here can be more far-reaching and effective. On the one hand, you should view these perspectives as you would those of any other interest group, i.e. something that you need to respectfully take into account. On the other hand you need to recognize the power imbalance and that the key players may not see the problem under consideration as being of any consequence or may not wish to legitimize your activity by participating in it, especially if it threatens their interests.

Find out who the key actors are, if there is any formal level of coordination and what level of authority the actors and the coordinating group carry. Attempt to involve players who can represent big-picture issues and do not just assume that they will not be interested. They may well be aware of the problem and welcome an opportunity to be involved in dealing with it. But you do need to exercise extra caution, so that they do not hijack the agenda or find ways in which to bog the process down.

Setting priorities

Reflection and discussion with key players about the context of the problem (why it is on the agenda now), the resources you have, what is already well covered, the areas of greatest need, and the points of strategic intervention can help you decide on priorities.

An iterative, rather than a linear, process in addressing the eight scoping questions will most probably work best and reduces the danger of getting bogged down, especially when charting unfamiliar territory. The judicious use of experts is crucial in saving time and maintaining momentum. The challenge is to figure out what is needed to put together an understanding of the problem, what you know and don't know, and who to bring in to fill the gaps. As new players are brought into the picture, their contributions may lead you to revisit your understandings of what is known or the areas of disagreement or the priorities. You must be open to this, but you also need a clear sense of direction so that you are not diverted by less relevant agendas which other players may have.

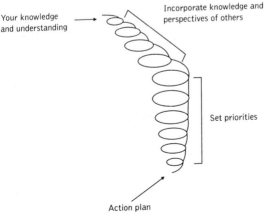

Figure 1.1.1 Broadening, aligning, and focusing perspectives

Back-to-back spirals are illustrative of the process—the outward expansion of the top spiral indicates the build up of knowledge and perspectives, whereas the inward direction of the second shows the knowledge and perspectives being used to set priorities (Figure 1.1.1). The loops illustrate revisiting what is known, bringing in other people who might have a useful perspective, and so on. As the figure illustrates, the starting point may be somewhat off centre, in other words, your own knowledge and expertise may be limited but the action plan should address central issues.

'Reality testing' can profitably be undertaken at several points. The aim here is to find holes in the knowledge base or the arguments on which priorities are based and, from this, to highlight where further data gathering or consultation is required. This is where advisory and reference groups can be invaluable, as they can be asked to comment along the way.

What are the competencies needed for effective scoping?

Key competencies include:

- integrity
- credibility and a dispassionate approach
- possession of a wide-ranging network of contacts, so that you know the key players or an intermediary
- skill in facilitating meetings and interactions, including encouraging open debate and the challenging of ideas, handling negotiations and conflict, and creating a positive atmosphere
- management skills
- an open mind to ideas from others, as well as the ability to come up with original ideas
- understanding of the 'cultures' of different interest groups and the ability to empathize with different concerns
- the ability to identify which disciplines are relevant and enough knowledge about the disciplines to know what they can offer, to identify experts, and to involve experts in the problem
- an understanding of relevant policies and other big-picture issues, their history, the key players, and the political sensitivities
- the ability to integrate a range of knowledge and expertise, to cut through to the essentials, and to lead a priority-setting process
- an ability to build alliances with those you need to have on-side in order to move forward.

What are the potential pitfalls in the scoping process?

Potential pitfalls include:

- Not having enough resources to undertake an adequate process.
- No real political commitment to understand and deal with the problem. For example a process can be set in train for reasons of political expediency and the plug may be pulled as soon as the political heat dies down.
- Not being the right person for the job—for example, if you are not interested in this process, not experienced enough to keep control, or if you hold a strong view about the problem and cannot deal with opposition respectfully.
- Getting bogged down. Losing momentum and timeliness can be fatal. Beware of wallowing in factual detail, meetings without a clear purpose, and red herrings. Don't feel that you have to be on top of all the material—rely on experts who understand the interest group or disciplinary perspective.
- Choosing inappropriate representatives of interest groups. Involving people in a process helps legitimize their point of view and you should think carefully about including fringe groups. If people who are not respected are included in the process, respected players may pull out or not participate fully.
- An inappropriate balance. The problem has to be seen in perspective, so that the process involves an appropriate mix of interest groups and academic disciplines, the powerful and the powerless, and, for contentious issues, different points of view.
- Avoiding the contentious issues. Ignoring particular groups in an attempt to avoid contentious issues will often backfire, with their exclusion providing them with an additional opportunity to further their cause and even undermining the outcomes of the process.
- Exhausting key players. Interest group representatives and experts from particular disciplines usually have a substantive job to do and they may get no recognition or credit for being involved in the scoping process. Use their time wisely, sparingly, and efficiently.
- Promoting conflict. Scoping processes that involve contentious issues usually seek to find compromise, but if the players are not chosen carefully and the process is not handled appropriately, conflict can be escalated rather than reduced.
- Not showing leadership. If those in charge of the scoping process do not show leadership, the process is open to being hijacked by the more powerful participants. This can also be a factor in the promotion of conflict.
- Avoiding decisions. Never underestimate the temptation not to make a decision when the problem is difficult or contentious. Yield not to temptation!
- Not being prepared to combat the wrath of the powerful. When scoping processes involve challenging entrenched power bases,

provoking a reaction could well be a measure of success. Don't be naïve and do be prepared to counter these forces.
- Not learning from your mistakes.
- Inexperience. Find mentors, powerful allies, and supportive colleagues.

How will you know when you have been successful?

The key markers of success are problem definition that has:
- broad-based support
- clear and implementable steps for solution
- commitment from the key players and the interest groups they represent to stay involved in seeking a solution
- respect between opponents

For issues where a major power base has been challenged and where the power base is seeking to protect its interests, measures of success include:
- a coalition, which includes people of influence, that will stand up to the power base and continue to fight for the solution
- openings for negotiation.

A successful scoping process lays a strong foundation for effectively tackling a problem and increases the chances of developing a solution on budget and on time.

Further resources

Scoping and rapid assessment

Executive Office of the President, Council on Environmental Quality (30 April, 1981). *Memorandum for general counsels, NEPA liaisons and participants in scoping*. Available at: http://ceq.eh.doe.gov/nepa/regs/scope/scoping.htm (accessed 5 November 2004).

Longhurst R (1987). Rapid rural appraisal: an improved means of information-gathering for rural development and nutrition projects. *Food Nutr*, **13**, 44–7.

Melville B (1993). Rapid rural appraisal: its role in health planning in developing countries. *Trop Doct*, **23**, 55–8.

Purdue University. *Environmental Assessment Resource Guide*. http://pasture.ecn.purdue.edu/~agenhtml/agen521/epadir/earg/start.html (accessed 5 November 2004).

Stimson G, Fitch C, Rhodes T, Ball A (1999). Rapid assessment and response: methods for developing public health responses to drug problems. *Drug Alcohol Rev*, **18**, 317–25.

Toth FL (1988). Policy exercises: procedures and implementation. *Simulat Games*, **19**, 256–76.

Boundary work and participatory systems methods

Flood RL and Jackson MC (1991). *Creative problem solving: total systems intervention.* Wiley, Chichester.

Midgley G (2000). *Systemic intervention: philosophy, methodology, and practice.* Kluwer Academic/Plenum, New York.

1.2 Turning public health problems into answerable questions

Georgios Lyratzopoulos and
Ian Harvey

> 'Far better an approximate answer to the right question…
> than an exact answer to the wrong question' [4]

The scope of public health

Although public health is defined as 'the science and art of preventing disease, prolonging life and promoting health through the organised efforts of society'[1] this science and art can only be effected if the principles underpinning it are appreciated and understood:

- the emphasis on collective responsibility for health and the major role of the state in protecting and promoting the public's health
- a focus on whole populations
- an emphasis upon prevention, especially primary prevention
- a concern for the underlying socio-economic determinants of health and disease, as well as more proximal determinants, such as health care
- a multidisciplinary basis which incorporates quantitative and qualitative methods as appropriate
- partnership with the populations served.

(adapted from Beaglehole and Bonita[2]).

The breadth of public health is both its strength and its potential weakness. It grapples with the 'big issues' in a way that is quite different in approach and methods from individually based health care. However the 'big issues' are often so large and complex that focus can be easily lost. Public health practitioners are sometimes guilty of posing, and attempting to answer, virtually unanswerable questions.[3] This problem can usually be overcome by breaking down the large questions into smaller sub-questions.

How to avoid making issues more complex: general principles

Clear thinking is critical in public health. There are several vital steps to be taken in proceeding from the general awareness of public health problems through to taking well-targeted action:

- Be aware that different groups will often identify public health problems affecting a given population in different ways. Local communities, patient groups, managers, and health-care professionals may have different views on priorities and required actions. It will not be easy, or even possible, for the public health professional to 'satisfy' everybody, but engagement with diverse views and a synthesis of diverging accounts is necessary. Explore ways of collecting and prioritizing these diverse views.[5]
- One of the most difficult steps in turning many public health problems into answerable questions is clearly defining the perceived problem. There will often be many different perceptions of this, depending on who is asking and who is asked.
- Public health practitioners should never be afraid to use the challenging words 'why' and 'what'—both to themselves and others. 'Why do you feel this is important?' 'What do you understand by this concept?' It can be helpful to try and write down in a few sentences the key questions that need to be addressed.
- Use a lateral thinking approach to properly explore what is really meant by apparently simple terms, such as 'deprivation', 'poverty', or 'prioritize'.
- Before suddenly collecting or presenting data (whether quantitative or qualitative), ensure that the data will help you answer one or more of the questions you have posed. Avoid collecting 'orphan data' (i.e. data that have been collected without a clear idea of how they will be used), while remembering that on occasion the act of collecting even orphan data may serve a useful wider purpose of allaying public concern.
- Pursue the questions that you have identified as important—avoid distracting side-issues.
- Remember the basic rules of traditional planning (see Chapter 5.2): where are we now? where do we want to get to? how do we get there? (both in terms of what action to take and how to get support for that action).
- Remember that 'unless data are turned into stories that can be understood by all, they are not effective in any process of change'.[6] Explore every opportunity to use figures, diagrams, and, when appropriate, geographic mapping, to communicate 'sterile' data tables and text-based information.

Key steps in formulating answerable questions

Be realistic and pragmatic:

Box 1.2.1

'As pure scientists, epidemiologists can remain tentative about the nature of associations. As public health specialists, however, judgements must be made in the absence of final proof in order to reduce the health risks to the public.'[2]

- Think broadly. Recognize at the outset that intervening to modify the determinants of public health potentially embraces social, political, and environmental factors, lifestyle factors, issues of clinical effectiveness, access to clinical services, and genetics. All are legitimate areas of concern for public health.
- Decide first if there is a 'real' public health problem present at all. On occasion there may be an apparent rather than a real increase in disease occurrence. The most common reasons for this are:
  - statistically non-significant temporary increase in cases, due to chance
  - pseudo-epidemics, due to increased ascertainment, or to changes in disease definition, and/or coding practices
  - identification of at risk populations post hoc, after inspecting the data[7]
  - heightened awareness of otherwise stable disease activity, due to media publicity (see Chapters 2.5 and 2.6).
- In some instances mass sociogenic illness can result as a spin-off of real public health problems (such as an 'epidemic' of illness in Belgium after drinking Coca-Cola believed at the time to be contaminated with dioxin).[8] Even artefactual public health problems need to be managed rigorously and account taken of differences between professional and lay approaches to risk.[9]
- What approach does the problem require?—a mainly data based/empiric approach or a predominantly organizational/social psychology approach? (An example of the latter would be a campaign to increase the proportion of children registered with a dentist.)
- If an empiric element is helpful, should this involve quantitative data, qualitative data, or a mixture of the two? The best approach is to select methods solely on the basis of whether they are likely to produce the most valid and useful answer.
- Can already published data be used, or routinely available data? Will a rapid ethnographic approach (an approach designed to understand the behaviour of particular communities) be useful to describe the size of the problem, for example in needs assessment?[10] Is *ad hoc* data collection necessary, and if so what resources are required?
- Questionnaire-based studies are often used to collect data rapidly, often as an interim solution.[11] If you are to conduct a questionnaire survey, make every effort to use an instrument that has been already validated, especially if you are measuring complex attributes such as quality of life (see Chapter 2.2). Developing you own valid instrument from scratch takes time and effort. The administrative burden of surveys is considerable, especially when the necessary effort is invested. This burden has to be appreciated in your decision-making. The most common and most important risk with any questionnaire study among general population samples is that the response rate will be too low to elicit meaningful results.

An example of turning an issue into a question

Obesity, particularly in early life, has been identified as a growing public health problem in many, if not most, industrialized countries. The public health questions include:

Descriptive questions—to quantify the problem ('what is the size and nature of the issue?'):

● How large is the problem currently?

● How large will the problem be in the future?

● What is the pattern of growth in rates of overweight and obesity subdivided by time, place, and personal characteristics, e.g. are individuals living in some areas (or of a certain age and social class) affected differentially?

● What proportion of overweight and obese individuals could benefit from health promotion interventions specific to a particular setting, e.g. at community level or within schools and workplaces?

Analytic questions—to identify options ('understanding what leads to this problem in order to appreciate what could be done': although it is tempting to believe that every problem has a solution, there are many examples in public health of 'success without interventions' and 'interventions without success'):

● To what degree is overweight in early life associated with morbid obesity in later life?

● To what extent are unemployment and poor social support risk factors for overweight and obesity?

● What overweight and obesity interventions, both preventative and curative, have been shown (in the published literature) to be effective?

● What plausible overweight and obesity measures have yet to be evaluated, at both an individual and at a community level, and how should they be evaluated? (See 'What is causing this public health problem?' below.)

Managerial questions to plan the intervention ('getting the right people involved to implement the right things in the right way'):

● Which agencies need to be included in any systematic efforts to reduce overweight and obesity, e.g. by enabling an increase in population levels of physical exercise?

● Which agencies will tend to be enthusiastic about such an initiative and which not?

● How can such skepticism be overcome?

Specific public health questions

● '*What is* causing *this public health problem*?' The focus should be on identifying the mechanism via which the problem is caused. A classic example is an outbreak of infectious disease, the archetypal vehicle for applied epidemiology. Such epidemiologic detective work requires hypotheses to be developed. This needs descriptive data (e.g. time, place, and person breakdown) from the history taken from patients and generated by the investigator in the light of prior knowledge. These hypotheses can then be tested, typically using either a case–control or cohort study approach (see Chapter 2.3). Finally, practical action needs to be taken—such as the closure of a food outlet in the case of food-borne disease. Perhaps the best recent examples of this detective work have been the identification of the causes of such conditions as AIDS and toxic shock syndrome.

- '*How do we alleviate this problem?*' '*What effective action can be taken?*' A good example is the case of social class inequalities in health, which are by common consent viewed as unjust. Much energy has been devoted to describing the extent of these, and many reports have been produced at local, national, and international level, but less is known about how to address these inequalities. What is required to begin to answer this question is generation and assimilation of high-quality research. As soon as the specific research questions are clarified, systematic reviews of the published literature (to summarize what we already know) supplemented with further evaluative research (to fill in the many gaps) are needed. Systematic reviews are now being produced and are beginning to provide a stronger evidential basis for public health activities aimed at reducing inequalities.[12] Among the interventions identified as effective are those aimed at reducing unwanted pregnancy among teenage girls and mentoring of disadvantaged first-time mothers by experienced mothers to improve uptake of immunization and enhance the mothers' self-esteem. Modelling studies, based on published evidence of effectiveness of interventions (from primary studies or meta-analyses), particularly if using local demographic and health-care utilization data, can greatly help in decision-making.[13]

Public health questions—scientific and socio-political

The most effective public health practitioners are both scientists and agents of change. Turning issues into questions that lead to a combination of data and oratory is a key skill in public health practice; hence the importance of where these two areas overlap—the science and evidence base of communication and behaviour change at all levels, individual, organizational, and political. Every public health problem should therefore lead to both:

- scientific/technical questions (what causes lung cancer?) and
- socio-political questions (who are the key people who will need persuading?).

The latter can involve such techniques as SWOT analysis (Strengths, Weaknesses, Opportunities, Threats)[14] and stakeholder analysis.[15] These techniques are aimed at identifying the significant individuals and groups whose views should be taken into account and whose support should, if possible, be gained.

Being opportunistic and realistic

As a public health practitioner you must be both scientifically astute and politically adept.

Box 1.2.2

'Problem solvers often complain that they have worked out ideal solutions but that no one will use them…Real problems include not only the specified problem situation but also the "person situation", which includes the people who have to accept and act on the solution'[3]

A solution is not a solution if it is not possible to implement it. The same is true, albeit at a different level, for a policy (see Chapter 4.1).

You must keep abreast of developments at international, national, and local levels, embracing statutory and voluntary organizations as well as the views of the media and local communities. Newly produced policies and reports often provide an opportunity to bring a favoured public health issue to the fore. Every public health problem requires some sort of analysis of the key people or groups to involve or inform, so that successful public health action will happen. Public health specialists almost always need to work with, and enlist the support of, others such as local government, non-statutory organizations, and the private sector, as well as health services. They also need to work with other professionals, including health professionals, statisticians, economists, behavioural scientists, and policy analysts.

Public health practitioners should be realistic enough to practice 'the art of the possible', whilst remaining imbued with a realistic optimism about possible progress. In other words, public health practitioners need passion as well as knowledge and skills.[16].

There are clear examples of effective public health action where perceived public health problems have been successfully translated into answerable questions. They also exemplify that effective action can sometimes occur for the wrong reasons, and often needs luck. For example, Edwin Chadwick, a lawyer by training, produced his 'Report on the sanitary conditions of the labouring population of Great Britain' (1842) mainly in response to concern that ill-health was putting upward financial pressure on the cost of Poor Law relief. The Public Health Act that resulted (1848) was a landmark in the development of clean water and effective sewage disposal, though it was vigorously opposed in some quarters. Chadwick did not, however, subscribe to the modern view that poverty can cause ill-health—he maintained that the reverse applied.[17] He also supported the 'miasma' (bad smells) theory rather than the germ theory of transmission of infection, a belief which directed his efforts—beneficially as it happens, but for the wrong reasons—towards improved hygiene. Concerns in government about the hazards posed by cholera outbreaks gave much needed additional impetus to his controversial reforms.

Remember finally that public health action taken in response to the answer to a public health question can sometimes have counterintuitive and unintended harmful results. This can be minimized by:
- considering the complexity of and the relationships between social factors
- being as inclusive as possible when measuring the outcome of public health interventions
- mastering the art of seeing the big picture as well as the detail, and crucially, not getting the two perspectives confused.

In 1927 in Stockton-on-Tees, northeast England a natural experiment occurred in which the occupants of one area of poor housing were re-housed in modern accommodation whilst a control group remained in slum dwellings. Age/sex standardized death rates *increased* sharply among those rehoused. This unexpected finding was eventually traced back to a deterioration in diet among those rehoused, resulting from a reduction in disposable income caused by the higher rental costs of the newer housing.[18]

Further resources

A wide range of public health problems and the approaches used to answer them are available in a database of abstracts from the reports submitted as part of the Part II examination for membership of the UK Faculty of Public Health at: http://www.fph.org.uk (accessed December 2004).

Handy CB (1985). *Understanding organisations.* Penguin Books, London.

References

1 Acheson ED (1988). *Public health in England. Report of the Committee of Inquiry into the future development of the public health function.* HMSO, London.
2 Beaglehole R, Bonita R (1997). *Public health at the crossroads.* Cambridge University Press, Cambridge.
3 de Bono E (1971). *Lateral thinking for management.* McGraw-Hill, Maidenhead.
4 Tukey JW (1962). The future of data analysis. *Ann Math Stat,* **33**, 1–67.
5 Baum F (1995). Researching public health: behind the qualitative-quantitative methodological debate. *Soc Sci Med,* **40**, 459–68.
6 Duhl L, Hancock T (1988). *A guide to assessing healthy cities.* WHO Healthy Cities, Paper No 3. FADL Publishers, Copenhagen.
7 Harvey I (1994). How can we determine if living close to industry harms your health? *BMJ,* **309**, 425–6.
8 Nemery B, Fischler B, Boogaerts M, Lison D (1999). Dioxins, Coca-Cola, and mass sociogenic illness in Belgium. *Lancet,* **354**, 77.
9 Department of Health. *Communicating about risks to public health: pointers to good practice.* Available at: http://www.dh.gov.uk/assetRoot/04/03/96/70/04039670.pdf (accessed 14 January 2006).
10 Savage J (2000). Ethnography and health care. *BMJ,* **321**, 1400–2. Available at: http://bmj.bmjjournals.com/cgi/content/full/321/7273/1400 (accessed 14 January 2006).

11 Boynton PM, Greenhalgh T (2004). Selecting, designing and developing your questionnaire. *BMJ*, **328**, 1312–15. Available at: http://bmj.bmjjournals. com/cgi/content/full/328/7451/1312 (accessed 14 January 2006).

12 Arblaster L, Entwistle V, Lambert M, Forster M, Sheldon T, Watt I (1995). *Review of the research on the effectiveness of health service interventions to reduce variations in health*, CRD Report 3. NHS Centre for Reviews and Dissemination, York.

13 Critchley JA, Capewell S (2002). Why model coronary heart disease? *Eur Heart J*, **23**, 110–16.

14 Casebeer A (1993). Application of SWOT analysis. *Br J Hosp Med*, **49**, 430–1.

15 Evans DA (1996). Stakeholder analysis of developments at the primary and secondary care interface. *Br J Gen Pract*, **46**, 675–7.

16 Horton R (1998). The *new* new public health of risk and radical engagement. *Lancet*, **352**, 251–2.

17 Hamlin C, Sheard S (1998). Revolutions in public health: 1848 and 1998? *BMJ*, **317**, 587–91.

18 Holland WW, Stewart S (1998). *Public health: the vision and the challenge*. The Nuffield Trust, London.

1.3 Assessing health needs

John Wright and Dee Kyle

Objectives of this chapter

Health needs assessment is a systematic method of identifying the unmet health and health-care needs of a population and making changes to meet these unmet needs. Health needs assessment is used to improve health and other service planning, priority setting, and policy development.

This chapter will describe why health needs assessment is important and what it means in practice. Most clinical health professionals are familiar with assessing the health needs of individual patients. Professional training and clinical experience teaches a systematic approach to this assessment before starting treatment that the health professional believes to be effective. Such a systematic approach has often been missing in assessing the health needs of local or practice populations.

The following example (Box 1.3.1) shows what happens when you do a health needs assessment systematically. Both health outcomes and service delivery were improved.

Box 1.3.1 Example 1: TB service in a rural African hospital[1]

Setting: A rural district hospital in South Africa.

Problem: Increasing overcrowding in the hospital due to the rising incidence of TB resulting from HIV/AIDS. Concerns by staff about high levels of treatment failure.

Methods: Review of TB register information on detection rates and outcomes. Review of current clinical practices. Interviews with health professional and patients to determine views of TB care.

Results: Case detection rate of TB had increased by 90% over a period of 4 yr. Patients were admitted to hospital for the 2-month intensive phase of treatment creating major problems of overcrowding. Haphazard follow-up in any local clinic led to poor data on outcomes. Outcome data indicated only 27% ($n = 66$) of patients were cured or completed treatment and 43% ($n = 160$) were lost to follow-up. Major gaps in patients' understanding about TB and its relationship to HIV/AIDS were identified.

Action: New guidelines were developed for the region to allow home-based treatment. A community-based treatment service was established using village health workers to support treatment in patients' own homes. An outreach team was set up to coordinate care, promote community awareness, and train and support village and clinic health workers. Within 12 months care and completion rates had improved to 86% with patients having to stay for days rather than months in hospital.

Defining need

An understanding of health needs assessment requires a clear definition of need. Need, in the sense used in this chapter, implies the capacity to benefit from an intervention. 'To speak of a need is to imply a goal, a measurable deficiency from the goal and a means of achieving the goal'.[2]

Health needs assessment is *not* the same as population health status assessment (see Chapters 2.8 and 2.9). Health needs assessment incorporates the concept of a capacity to benefit from an intervention. It therefore introduces an assessment of the effectiveness of relevant interventions to supplement the identification of health problems. Health needs assessment should also make explicit what benefits are being pursued by identifying particular interventions.

Economists argue that the capacity to benefit is always greater than available resources and that health needs assessment should also incorporate questions of priority setting through considering the cost-effectiveness of the available interventions (see Chapters 1.4 and 5.4).[3]

Approaches to needs assessment

A number of approaches to needs assessment have been suggested,[4] including:

- 'epidemiologically based' needs assessment—combining epidemiologic approaches (specific health status assessments) with assessment of the effectiveness and possibly the cost-effectiveness of the potential interventions
- comparative—comparing levels of service receipt between different populations
- corporate—canvassing the demands and wishes of professionals, patients, politicians, and other interested parties.

In this chapter an epidemiologic and qualitative approach to determining priorities is explored. This incorporates clinical effectiveness, cost-effectiveness, and patients' perspectives.[5] While comparisons of health service usage are commonly used as indicators of need, population-based usage rates typically vary markedly between areas, often for unexplained reasons. In addition, the link between usage rates and improved health outcomes is often hard to demonstrate.

The distinction between individual needs and the wider needs of the community is important to consider when assessing needs. If individual needs are ignored then there is a danger of a top-down approach to providing health and other services, reflecting what a few people perceive to be the needs of the population, rather than what they actually are.

It is important to appreciate that health needs assessment involves the active, explicit, and systematic identification of needs rather than a passive, *ad hoc*, implicit response to demand. The assessment of health needs can be made clearer by differentiating the issues into needs, demands, and supply, remembering that health needs are not restricted to health-*care* needs. Health needs include wider social and environmental determinants of health such as deprivation, housing, diet, education, and employment. Health needs should ideally be appropriately addressed ('met'), but these needs are too often unmet (e.g. waiting lists, undiagnosed hypertension, ignored moderate depression) or 'overmet' (e.g. prescribing antibiotics for sore throats).

Box 1.3.2 Different aspects of health needs

Felt needs: what people consider and/or say they need.

Expressed needs: needs expressed by action, e.g. visiting a doctor.

Normative needs: what health professionals define as need.

Assessing health needs provides the opportunity for:
- assessing the population's health status (see Chapters 2.8. and 2.9), describing the patterns of disease in the local population and the differences from district, regional, or national disease patterns
- learning more about the needs and priorities of patients and the local population
- highlighting areas of unmet need and providing a clear set of objectives to work towards to meet these needs
- deciding rationally how to use resources to improve the health of the local population in the most effective and efficient way
- influencing policy, interagency collaboration, or research and development priorities.

Importantly, it also provides a method of monitoring and promoting equity in the provision and use of health services and addressing inequalities in health (see Chapters 2.10 and 5.5).[6]

The use of health needs assessment as part of the health equity audit cycle enables the tackling of health inequalities to be integrated into mainstream planning and service delivery.[7]

Health equity audits focus on how fairly resources are distributed in relation to the health needs of different groups and are cyclic processes. Box 1.3.4 shows how an epidemiologic health needs assessment demonstrated inequity in service access which needed to be addressed by completing the health equity audit cycle.[8]

Box 1.3.3

Health equity audit is a process by which partners systematically review inequities in the causes of ill health and access to effective services and their outcomes for a defined population, and ensure that further action is agreed and incorporated into policy, plans, and practice. Finally, actions taken are reviewed to assess whether inequities have been reduced.[7]

Box 1.3.4 Example 2: Epidemiologic health needs
assessment—coronary heart disease[9]

Objective: To assess whether the use of health services by people with
coronary heart disease reflected need.

Setting: A health district with a population of 530,000.

Methods: The prevalence of angina was determined by a validated
postal questionnaire. Routine health data were collected on
standardized mortality ratios, admission rates for coronary heart
disease, and operation rates for angiography, angioplasty, and coronary
heart disease. Census data were used to calculate Townsend scores to
describe deprivation for electoral wards. The prevalence of angina and
use of services were then compared with deprivation scores for each
ward.

Results: Angina and mortality from heart disease were more common
in wards with high deprivation scores. However, treatment by
revascularization procedures was more common in more affluent
wards.

Conclusion: The use of revascularization services was not commensurate
withneed. Steps should be taken to ensure that health care is targeted
to those who most need it.

A framework for assessing the health needs of a population

Box 1.3.5 summarizes the questions or steps involved in a formal health
needs assessment project. The process seldom follows a simple linear
progress through the steps—needs assessments often develop from
several steps concurrently. Health needs assessment can be approached
in much the same way as doing a jigsaw, so that different pieces are put
together to give a complete picture of local health.

Box 1.3.5 Questions to be answered in a formal health needs assessment project

1. *What is the problem?* Identify the health problem to be addressed in the defined population.
2. *What is the size and nature of the problem?* Carry out a health status assessment for the population, covering the relevant areas of ill-health and/or potential health gain.
3. *What are the current services?* Identify the existing services and interventions being delivered, including, where relevant, the service targeting, quality, effectiveness, and efficiency.
4. Identify interventions by asking what patients, professionals, and other stakeholders want. Consult.
5. Identify interventions by reviewing the scientific knowledge. What are the most appropriate and cost-effective solutions? Find and appraise.
6. *What are the resource implications?* Choose between competing ways of meeting needs (competing interventions) and decide on competing priorities—resources are always limited.
7. *What are the recommendations and the plan for implementation?*
8. *Is assessing need likely to lead to appropriate change?* Identify expected health gains.

Needs assessment requires careful preparation

Undertaking needs assessment involves identifying the right issue, using the right technical methods, and managing the process effectively. Start with attention to defining the task. Objectives should be clarified and should be as simple and focused as possible. Care should be taken not to raise over-ambitious expectations. The right project team should be convened, with all relevant stakeholders, including (as relevant to the issue) the service funders, the clinicians, and the users (public involvement) (see Chapter 8.4). Good leadership is important (see Chapter 7.1), as is clear and effective communication during the project, especially if there is multiagency involvement. Access to relevant information and informants should be sought at an early stage.

What is the health issue?

The health problem on which to focus the needs assessment exercise should be clearly identified. A health problem may come to attention from many sources, including the results of a population health status assessment, input from patients or stakeholders, government priority setting, or the scientific and professional literature.

An initial clarification of the issues can be valuable. A first step in clarifying the definition of the needs problem is a search of the health and social science databases for the topic. A review of the published health literature will provide a national and international perspective about the health topic and provide methods and results (for example case definitions, disease incidence and prevalence, current provision of health services) that may be applicable to the local population.[4,6] A search of grey literature sources (for example public health professional bodies and government health department databases) can also provide useful models and information.

After initial clarification, it should become apparent whether the problem justifies a full and systematic needs assessment.

What is the size and nature of the problem?

With a working definition of the health problems in mind, relevant health status data can then be collected. This should aim to establish:

- how many people in the studied population are likely to be suffering from the target condition or conditions
- what their characteristics are
- to what extent they are already receiving appropriate interventions.

Accurately estimating how many people would benefit from each of the potential interventions is desirable but often difficult. Previous chapters provide a guide to sources of information.

What are the current services?

There are several sources of data on health care in a locality. Hospital activity data can provide information on hospital admissions, diagnoses, length of stay, operations performed, and patient characteristics. Clinical indicators can provide information on the comparative performance of hospitals and health authorities.

Health-care provision (e.g. numbers of family doctors per capita, number of operations per capita) is often compared with national or international norms, although there is rarely evidence of a link between provision and health outcome.

What do professionals, patients, and other stakeholders want?

Consult a wide range of stakeholders to describe local health needs. Local health professionals in primary and secondary care will have valuable contributions to make about the health needs of their local community. Other stakeholders such as health authorities, local government agencies, and voluntary groups are also important contributors, not only for their knowledge and beliefs but also so as to engage them in the assessment and encourage ownership and eventual implementation of the results.

Consult users, carers, and the public (see Chapter 8.4). Health services have been historically weak at involving users and the public in decision-making about local health care. With increasing recognition of the importance of obtaining greater public involvement, various methods have been used, including:[10]

- *Citizens' juries*: local people who are representative of the population are selected to sit on a jury for a specified period of time. Members are presented with information from different experts on health topics and debate the issues surrounding them.
- *Health panels*: standing panels of local people representative of population. These can be large (more than 1000 people) panels which are surveyed at regular intervals about key health issues, or smaller panels where the members meet and discuss different topics. Members are replaced at regular intervals.
- *Focus groups*: groups of 6–12 participants with a facilitator who encourages discussion about health topics, which is recorded on tape or by an observer.
- *Interviews*: interviews with randomly or purposefully selected individuals to canvass their views and opinions. Users, carers, or other stakeholders (e.g. community leaders) can all be valuable contributors.
- *Questionnaires*: these allow structured information to be collected from a large sample of local people on one or more health topics. Such surveys can provide information on user satisfaction, perceived needs, and use of health services. Other generic health measures such as quality of life scores,[11] or disease-specific measures can also be included.
- *Specific planning methodologies*: for example, meta-planning, 'Planning for Real®', 'open space' events. These are all approaches to planning which use specific techniques to promote the involvement of local communities and stakeholders.

What are the most appropriate and cost-effective interventions?

An essential part of a health needs assessment is the review of the clinical effectiveness and cost-effectiveness of interventions that can address the identified health needs. Evidence about the effectiveness of health interventions or services can be found in databases of good-quality systematic reviews such as the Cochrane Library,[12] or publications such as the *Effective Health Care Bulletins*.[13] The United States Agency for Healthcare Research and Quality[14] and the UK National Institute of Health and Clinical Effectiveness[15] can also be good source of information on effectiveness and on professional consensus on treatment. Where there is limited evidence of effectiveness of interventions then professional consensus about best practice may have to be relied on.

What are the resource implications?

If needs are to be matched to limited available resources so that as much need as possible is met, then economic appraisal, including cost-effectiveness information, must be considered. At a practical level this involves:[16]

- determining how resources are currently spent (programme budgeting—see Chapter 2.6)
- defining options for change (marginal analysis) by specifying alternatives:
  - (a) identify potential services requiring more resources
  - (b) identify services which could be provided at the same level of effectiveness but at reduced cost, releasing resources for (a)
  - (c) identify services which are less cost-effective than those identified in (a)
- assessing the costs and benefits of the principal options
- decide on the best option, aiming to increase investment in (a) and reduce investment in services identified in (b) and (c).

The third example in this chapter (see Box 1.3.6) shows how the needs assessment process can help plan services, using generalizable research and local surveys involving users.

Implementation

In drawing a needs assessment together, the collected information should be collated, analyzed, and presented, usually in report form. A summary of key findings is very useful in communicating the results to the decision-makers and those who will be affected by the decisions.

Reporting results, however, is not an end in itself. This is where too many health needs assessments end, when they should only just be beginning. Building agreement to a practical implementation plan for meeting the unmet needs is an essential part of needs assessment.

Does assessing need create change?

Factors that will increase the likelihood of needs assessment leading to change are:

- consideration of the potential resource implications of the assessment from the beginning (discussion between commissioners and assessors)
- methodological rigor to ensure that the results are valid and believed
- ownership of the project by relevant stakeholders from the start and effective involvement during the work
- effective dissemination of the results (see Chapters 6.7 and 6.8)
- the existence of a practical plan for implementing the necessary actions to partly or fully meet the identified unmet needs.

Box 1.3.6 Example 3: Needs-based services for people with multiple sclerosis[17]

Background: With rising health-care costs, limited resources, and the move to a needs-led health-care system it has become increasingly important to purchase and plan health services that match resources to patients' needs. The aim of this study was to assess the health needs of a community-based cohort of people with multiple sclerosis (MS) in the metropolitan city of Leeds, UK and to define the current service provision.

Methods: Work undertaken included a systematic review of the literature; focus groups with people with MS and their carers; in-depth interviews with representatives of service providers, purchasers, and voluntary organizations; and in-depth interviews with 30 people with MS randomly selected from the Leeds population-based register and stratified according to age, gender, household, duration of MS, and disease course.

Results: Five major themes emerged: information needs, emotional support for people with MS and their families, access to services (particularly respite care and rehabilitation services), increasing public awareness of MS, and maintaining independence.

Outcome: This health needs assessment provided a framework for reorganization of the services provided for people with MS in Leeds. A patient information group was established for new diagnoses. An information resource centre was set up for patients and carers. Patient-held records are being piloted. A dedicated MS clinic with multidisciplinary input is now operational.

Health needs assessment starts from the health of a defined population and results in proposals (for policy, programmes, strategy, plans, or other developments). Health impact assessments (HIAs) (see Chapter 1.5) and integrated impact assessment (IIA) start from proposals and compare how they may impact on health. Table 1.3.1, adapted from Quigley *et al.,*[18] compares these three approaches.

Table 1.3.1 Comparison of health needs assessment with health impact assessment (HIA) and integrated impact assessment (IIA)[18]

	Health needs assessment	Health impact assessment	Integrated impact assessment
Starting point	Population	Proposal	Proposal
Primary output recommendations	Inform decisions about strategies, service priorities, commissioning, and local delivery plans, and inform future HIAs and IIAs	Suggest how to maximize benefits and minimize negatives of a proposal to inform decision-making; and improve joined-up working	Suggest how to maximize benefits and minimize negatives of a proposal to inform decision-making; and improve joined-up working
Aims to take account of inequalities, help improve health, and reduce health inequalities	Describe health needs and health assets of different groups in local population	Compare how proposals may impact on most vulnerable groups in population	Compare how proposals may impact on most vulnerable groups in population
Involvement of stakeholders	Always	Always	Always
Involvement of community	Always	Ideally (dependent on resources)	Ideally (dependent on resources)
Involvement from many sectors	Sometimes	Usually	Always
Base on determinants of health	Usually	Ideally	Always
Best available evidence is used	Always	Always	Always

Conclusion

Health needs are not static, and any assessment will only provide a snapshot of the needs of the local population. These needs and the health and social care services that try to address them are always changing and it is important to return to the assessment work, to review it and update it, and to evaluate the impact it has had.

Further resources

Hooper J, Longworth P (2002). *Health needs assessment workbook*. HDA, London.

Murray SA (1999). Experiences with 'rapid appraisal' in primary care: involving the public in assessing health needs, orientating staff, and educating medical students. *BMJ*, **3**(18), 440–4.

National Health Service Management Executive (1991). *Assessing health care need*. Department of Health, London.

Wright J (1998). *Health needs assessment in practice*. BMJ Books, London.

References

1 Wright J, Walley J, Philip A et al.(2004). Direct observation for tuber-culosis: a randomised controlled trial of community health workers versus family members. *Trop Med Int Health* **9**, 559–65.

2 Wilkin D, Hallam L, Dogget M (1992). *Measures of need and outcomes in primary health care.* Oxford Medical Publications, Oxford.

3 Donaldson C, Mooney G (1991). Needs assessment, priority setting, and contracts for healthcare: an economic view. *BMJ*, **303**, 1529–30.

4 Stevens A, Raftery J (eds) (1997). *Health care needs assessment*, 2nd series. Radcliffe Medical Press, Oxford.

5 Wright J, Williams DRR, Wilkinson J (1998). The development of health needs assessment. In: *Health needs assessment in practice* (ed. J Wright), pp. 1–11. BMJ Books, London.

6 Rawaf S, Bahl V (1998). *Assessing health needs of people from minority ethnic groups.* Royal College of Physicians, London.

7 Hamer L, Jacobson B, Flowers J, Johnstone F (January 2003). *Health equity audit made simple: a briefing for Primary Care Trusts and local strategic partnerships working document.* Available at: http://www.publichealth.nice.org.uk/page.aspx?o=502511 (accessed 14 January 2006).

8 Jacobson B (2002). Delaying tactics. *Health Service J*, **112**(5793), 22.

9 Payne N, Saul C (1997). Variations in use of cardiology services in a health authority: comparison of coronary artery revascularisation rates with prevalence of angina and coronary mortality. *BMJ*, **314**, 256–61.

10 Jordan J, Dowswell T, Harrison S, Lilford R, Mort M (1998). Whose priorities? Listening to users and the public. *BMJ*, **316**(7145), 1668–70.

11 Bowling A (1997). *Measuring health: a review of quality of life meas-urement scales*, 2nd edn. Open University Press, Buckingham.

12 Cochrane Library. Available at: http://www.cochrane.org/reviews/clibintro.htm (accessed 14 January 2006).

13 Royal Society of Medicine Press. *Effective health care bulletins*. Available at: http:// www.york.ac.uk/inst/crd/ehcb.htm (accessed 30 June 2005). [Effective Health Care Bulletins are bimonthly publications for deci-sion-makers which examine the effectiveness of a variety of health-care interventions. They are based on a systematic review and synthesis of research on the clinical effectiveness, cost-effectiveness, and accept-ability of health service interventions. This is carried out by a research team using established methodological guidelines, with advice from expert consultants for each topic. The bulletins are subject to exten-sive and rigorous peer review.]

14 The United States Agency for Healthcare Research and Quality. Available at: http://www.ahrq.gov/ (accessed 30 June 2005).

15 National Institute of Health and Clinical Effectiveness. Available at: http://www.nice.org.uk (accessed 14 January 2006).

16 Scott A, Donaldson C (1998). Clinical and cost effectiveness issues in health needs assessment. In: *Health needs assessment in practice* (ed. J Wright), pp. 84–94. BMJ Books, London.

17 Ford HL, Gerry EM (1999). Needs based services for people with MS. *Multiple Sclerosis*, **5**, S48.

18 Quigley R, Cavanagh S, Harrison D, Taylor L (2004). Clarifying approaches to: health needs assessment, health impact assessment, integrated impact assessment, health equity audit, and race equality impact assessment. Available at: http://www.publichealth.nice.org.uk/page.aspx?o=505665 (accessed 14 January 2006).

1.4 Economic evaluation—the science behind the art of making choices

Peter Brambleby and John Appleby

Introduction

All professional activity involves making choices. This can be particularly challenging in protecting and promoting health and preventing disease since:

- the outcome is quality of life, or life itself
- the resources are limited
- the evidence base on outcomes and resources is seldom perfect.

Objectives

This chapter explains a way of thinking about outcomes and costs and describes some of the more frequently used techniques of health economics and when to apply them. It will help the reader to:

- understand the language of health economics
- apply the concepts of health economics when they appear in management situations
- pose better questions when important choices are apparent and when the help of a professional health economist is involved.

What is health economics?

The practitioner often has to make, or advise others on making, choices such as:

- deciding whether or not to introduce a new intervention or service
- deciding how one could go about comparing many bids for new money when only a few of the bids could be funded
- deciding the best way to find how to take money out of a service.

Whether one is involved with the planning or the delivery of health care, the job involves many complex choices. In predominantly publicly funded systems (such as the UK's National Health Service (NHS)), or public/private mixed economies (such as most of continental Europe), there is the added dimension of having to be publicly accountable for stewardship of scarce resources. The techniques of health economics help to expose the trade-offs between the options and make the decision-taking process open to scrutiny and participation.

Box 1.4.1

Health economics is a discipline that brings a systematic approach to the management of issues of scarcity and choice in health care.

Despite its name, economics is not primarily about 'making economies' nor even about money. Money is just one type of resource. Other resources include people, time, and buildings. Costs can be tangible and easy to ascribe a monetary value to, such as medicines, staff, or journeys to hospital, or they can be intangible, such as pain. All types of cost are relevant. Economic appraisal is about relating outcomes to costs. It is just as concerned with effectiveness as it is with resources.

Since economic appraisal is usually concerned with the relationship between costs and outcomes, the steps often follow this sequence:
- What are we trying to achieve?
- What are the different ways of achieving this (options)?
- Do these options work at all?
- If so, how do they compare with each other, taking adverse effects into account as well as benefits?
- What costs are involved for each option, taking not only health-care factors and tangible costs into consideration, but other factors such as costs to social services or to the patient?

Similarly, if a service might be stopped, the considerations are:
- What are we trying to achieve?
- What are the different ways of achieving this (options)?
- What benefits will be lost with each option?
- What resources will be released with each option?
- How might these resources be used, and the outcomes realized, in comparison with the outcomes of the original service?

Health economics provides a means of handling these decisions. It can be regarded as an overall way of thinking (a shared perspective on problem solving that decision-makers find useful) and as a particular set of techniques.

Health economics as a way of thinking

Health economics is not a substitute for thought, but a way of organizing it.[1] Nor is it a technical fix that tells you precisely what to do.[2] The approach is
- *utilitarian*—trying to get the greatest good for the greatest number, and concerned with
- *efficiency*—getting the greatest outcome from a fixed amount of resource.

Although these are the health economist's starting points, they need not necessarily be adopted as the deciding criteria when decisions are taken. The gulf between what is possible and what can be afforded (by the individual or the state), and the inevitability of having to choose, is the starting point for economic appraisal. Health economics recognizes the existence of trade-offs inherent in any system. Choice involves sacrifice. It is perfectly legitimate to trade off some efficiency for the sake of other considerations such as equity. Equity can be described as the willingness to give a protected 'fair share' to a particular group in society in need, even if that does not maximize total outcomes from the available resources for the population as a whole. It serves to emphasize that choices are not free—there is an *opportunity cost* (benefit foregone) once resources are committed. In other words, once resources have been committed, the real cost is not the monetary value but the best alternative use to which that resource could have been put. Just like many other disciplines that contribute to the practice of public health (e.g. epidemiology and sociology) it is concerned with whole populations and not just individuals.

Economic evaluations

Economic evaluations deal with the relationships between costs and outcomes when choices have to be made between competing options. Sometimes the outcomes are the same and the issue is simply 'which option consumes least resources, taking all costs into consideration?' In this situation the appropriate tool is *cost minimization analysis*.

More often, the costs and outcomes are both different, but the units in which the outcomes are measured are the same (typically 'natural units', like years of life added for choices between cancer treatments, peak expiratory flow rates for choices between asthma treatments, or successful live births in choices between infertility treatments). In such cases the appropriate tool is *cost-effectiveness analysis*.

Sometimes the choice is between very different types of outcome, measured in very different units, and with very different costs. An example would be deciding whether to put some additional resources into cancer care, orthopaedics, or diabetes. The issue is one of finding a common set of units such as quality-adjusted life years (QALYs) or disability-adjusted life years (DALYs) to allow a 'cost per QALY' or 'cost per DALY' comparison on a like-for-like basis. The term given to appraisals that convert different sorts of outcome into these common 'utility' units is *cost–utility analysis*.

Sometimes it is simply a question of weighing up whether the costs of a new intervention outweigh the benefits or not, and whether it should go ahead at all. Costs and benefits are both ascribed a monetary value in order to make the comparison. This is called 'cost–benefit analysis'. (Note that 'cost–benefit analysis' has a precise meaning and is not a blanket term for all comparisons of costs and outcomes—a better phrase to describe these techniques collectively is 'economic appraisal'.)

The tools for addressing these situations are shown in Box 1.4.2.

Box 1.4.2 Forms of economic evaluation

Cost minimization analysis: When the outcomes (the benefits) of alternative interventions are the same in terms of volume and type, the cheapest programme should be chosen on the grounds of efficiency, for example choosing between a branded and a generic antibiotic to treat a streptococcal infection.

Cost-effectiveness analysis: When the number (but not the type) of outcomes of alternative programmes are *different*, then the efficient choice is that programme which costs least to produce a unit of outcome (such as a life saved), for example choosing between two interventions of different cost and effectiveness which both lower blood pressure in people with hypertension.

Cost–utility analysis: When the type (and perhaps the number) of outcomes from alternate programmes are *not* the same, then a 'common outcome currency' (such as a quality-adjusted life year (QALY)) is used as a measure of benefit and to enable comparisons to be made between programmes. Choice of programme will then depend on the cost of producing a unit of the chosen currency (e.g. the cost per QALY), for example choosing between hip replacements, coronary artery bypass grafts, and haemodialysis for the next time period's investment.

Cost–benefit analysis: The preceding evaluative methods all leave the outcome/benefit side of the equation in 'natural' units (clearing infection, lowering blood pressure, QALYs, etc.). Cost–benefit analysis places monetary values on these benefits (to enable comparison with the monetary units used to measure costs). This analysis compares 'doing something' with 'doing nothing' (as opposed to 'doing something' versus 'doing something else'), for example advising the highways authorities on whether or not to invest in crash barriers along a 10 mile stretch of road to avoid road traffic deaths and injuries.

Additional concepts

The appraisal tools described above are a simplification of the decision-guiding process. A health economist will also apply an annual percentage 'discounting' to costs and benefits which fall at some time in the future to give them all a present-day value (this could be of the order of, for instance, 6% per annum). A benefit in the future is valued less highly than a benefit today (hence the value of a benefit only available at some time in the future is 'discounted').

A 'sensitivity analysis' would also be done to *several* values rather than single point estimates, since data on costs and outcomes are seldom precise. This yields a range of estimates to assist decision-makers.

Priority setting through programme budgeting and marginal analysis (PBMA)

Table 1.4.1 Programme budgeting and marginal analysis (adapted from Mooney et al.[6])

Action	Comment
Define health-care programmes	Break down the priority setting process into more manageable programmes (e.g. client groups, specialties, disease groups) and define health-care objectives and outputs for each programme
Establish programme management groups	Management groups (clinicians, managers, user representatives) are responsible for priority setting within their programme
Estimate programme budgets	Identify current spending on, and broad outputs from, each programme. Often we know how much is spent on, say, nurses, but not on hip replacements
Define subprogrammes of care	Identify further breakdowns in programmes, with estimates of spending and defined objectives and outputs
Focus on marginal change	Most priority setting concerns changes to existing services (i.e. changes at the margin). Therefore, most attention can be paid to changes within rather than between programmes. However, do not be afraid to look horizontally at the entire programme for a district, spread across several hospitals, and examine marginal changes in the whole programme
Identify incremental (and decremental) 'wish lists'	Given extra (fewer) resources, what services should be expanded (reduced) for the greatest benefit of (causing least distress to) patients?
Cost the wish lists	How much would it cost to health services and patients to implement incremental and decremental wish lists?
Examine relative benefits generated by changes in spending	What would be implemented from the wish lists if specific amounts of money were made available or taken away?
Consider equity implications	The steps above focus on efficiency—getting more health care/healthiness for each unit of resource—but who is to benefit?
Consult	Out of necessity 'point estimates' of cost and outcome are used, but in reality confidence limits are wide and overlapping. Do not let the veneer of scientific precision blind you to the underlying value judgements. The process to this point is about clarifying and organizing thought. It is imperative to check the assumptions with those most affected
Choose where to invest and where to disinvest, and evaluate afterwards	Having identified new patterns of spending based on clinical and economic evidence, decisions need to be taken to implement changes—and evaluate them too

A pioneer of this technique was Professor Alain Enthoven, who took it from its application to the American armed forces and applied it to health-care planning (or purchasing) at the population level. He endorsed its use in the UK NHS in his 1999 Rock Carling Fellowship review.[3] An entire issue of *Health Policy*[4] was devoted to articles on this topic. Table 1.4.1 gives an outline of PBMA.

The UK Department of Health, with parallels in other parts of the UK NHS, has been exploring PBMA. This was promised by the 1997 Labour government in its first major policy document on health *The New NHS: Modern, Dependable* (London, 1997):

- Para 6.22: 'Partnerships between secondary and primary care physicians and with social services will provide the necessary basis for the establishment of "programmes of care", which will allow planning and resource management across organisational boundaries.'
- Para 9.18: 'Efficient use of resources will be critical to delivering the best for patients. It is important that managers and clinicians alike have a proper understanding of the costs of local services, so that they can make appropriate local decisions on the best use of resources.'

An even more significant strand of policy was the creation of the National Institute for Health and Clinical Excellence (NICE), now emulated in many other countries around the world, which appraises evidence of effectiveness and cost-effectiveness and publishes technology appraisals and clinical guidance (see http://www.nice.org.uk/).

Is *health* economics different from conventional economics?

From the conventional point of view of economics, health care is unusual.[5] Standard economic ideas of supply and demand are often difficult to square with the reality of how health-care systems actually function. In virtually all countries demand for health care is mediated through a medical professional—consumers are not sovereign as in a typical market model. Patients need the help of a clinician to identify what their state of health really is, what their health-care needs are, and what interventions are appropriate to address them. This is known as the *agency role* of the health professions.

Both supply and demand for health care, especially secondary health care, are heavily regulated and managed. Complex insurance markets—run by the state, the independent sector, or a mixture of the two—have grown up in response to the inherent uncertainties of illness and the costs of treatment. Governments can play a significant part in health-care regulation, from setting rules about practitioner qualifications through to resource allocation, standard setting, and direct control of provision.

The importance of the margin

Another important concept in health economics is that of the '*margin*'—the cost of the *next* (or one additional) unit of input or the benefit of the *next* unit of output. The importance of this is that in health care many choices are made about relatively small incremental changes in service (either to increase or decrease) rather than whole-scale strategic shifts. The issue is often described thus: 'What is the extra cost over and above what we pay now, and what is the extra benefit?' (The reverse applies for disinvestment decisions: 'What resources do we release and what benefits do we lose?')

A related concept is the '*stepped cost*'.

Examples

Suppose a cardiac surgery unit is built, staffed, and equipped to deal with 900 patients a year and funded accordingly. This would mean all the costs—'fixed costs' (like buildings), 'semi-fixed costs' (like staff salaries), and 'variable costs' (like medicines)—were covered. Suppose that with this complement of buildings, the staff and equipment could actually cope with a further 50 patients. The additional (marginal) cost of each extra patient up to 50 would be relatively small, and chiefly reflect the 'variable costs'. But a point would come when, to accommodate just one more patient, extra staff would have to be taken on or a new ward built—that would be a substantial 'stepped cost'.

To see the relevance of this, imagine you are a health-care purchaser with 200 extra patients requiring cardiac surgery and three cardiac centres within reasonable travel distance for your population. It would be in everyone's interest to try and spread that additional workload between all three centres if that would enable them all to work closer to capacity, but if that were not possible, then it might be better to make a single strategic investment (stepped development) at just one.

The same applies to benefits. Suppose an immunization programme reaches only 80% of the child population. An additional £50,000 might enable a further 10% to be reached, but the addition of a yet another £50,000 on top of that might only enable a further 5% to be reached. In common parlance this is 'the law of diminishing returns'; to the economist it is known as 'diminishing marginal benefit'.

The important points to remember are that *average* cost and benefit (*total* cost divided by *total* benefit) can differ substantially from *marginal* cost and benefit. Marginal cost and marginal benefit do not increase (or decrease) in a smooth linear fashion, they tend to go in steps.

Ethics and equity

The ethical stance of health economics is sometimes questioned by clinicians because the utilitarian approach can be at odds with the 'Hippocratic' ethic of doing the very best for the individual in a trusting doctor–patient relationship. (Economics is not known as the 'dismal science' for nothing!) But an economist would justify the pursuit of efficiency on the grounds that the true cost of inefficiency is borne in terms of pain, disability, and premature death by those waiting for treatment. In a publicly funded health-care system, where policy-making, funding, and provision are all controlled largely by the state, the primary objective of trying to ensure the greatest good for the greatest number is legitimate. One could extend this and argue that it is better to have a system where everyone gets access to a service which meets basic standards, even if those are not the very best possible, if the alternative means that some should go without altogether (see Chapter 1.7).

Efficiency (technical versus allocative)

In general terms, health-care policy-makers and those who 'commission' are primarily concerned with *allocative efficiency*—trying to maximize the population health gain from a fixed allocation of resources. (One is trying to reach a position where no one waiting for treatment has a greater ability to benefit than anyone who is already being treated.)

Health-care 'providers' are more often concerned with *technical efficiency*—achieving a desired objective at the least cost. Many of the objectives are set for them: numbers to be treated, waiting times, and so on.

In the 1990s, in an attempt to address both types of efficiency, the UK NHS experimented with a market model whereby the funds are held by 'purchasers' and devolved, ostensibly according to population need, to 'providers' who deliver the care. This was an attempt to harness 'market forces' to drive up quality and drive out inefficiency. Although introduced by a Conservative administration, the Labour administration which followed it in 1997 perpetuated many elements of the model, especially the separation of purchasing and providing roles. For a lucid analysis of the strengths and weaknesses of the market models in the NHS see Enthoven.[3]

Conclusions

Everyone concerned with health care can benefit from a familiarity with health economists' ways of thinking, language, and some of the tools in their toolkit. Health economics gives a structured approach to decision-making in health care where resources are always scarce, need appears almost limitless, and choices are inevitable. It is not a formulaic approach that bypasses critical appraisal, but it can greatly improve the rigor and transparency of the decision-making process.

Further resources

Mitton C, Donaldson D (2001). Twenty-five years of programme budgeting and marginal analysis in the health sector, 1974–1999. *J Health Serv Res Policy*, **6**, 239–48.

Ruta D, Mitton C, Bate A, Donaldson C (2005). Programme budgeting and marginal analysis: bridging the divide between doctors and managers. *BMJ*, **330**, 1501–3.

Samuelson PA (1980). *Economics*, 11th edn. McGraw-Hill, London.

UK Department of Health. National Programme Budget Project—publications and resourcesguidance manual, spreadsheets, case studies, discussion forum and contacts. Avaliable at : http://www.dh.gov.uk/programmebudgeting (accessed 15 January 2006).

References
1 Drummond MF, O'Brien BJ, Stoddard GL Torrance GW (1997). *Methods for the economic evaluation of health care programmes*, 2nd edn. Oxford University Press, Oxford.
2 Robinson R (1993). Economic evaluation and health care (a series of six articles in the BMJ). What does it mean? *BMJ*, **307**, 670–3. Costs and cost minimisation analysis. *BMJ*, **307**, 726–8. Cost effectiveness analysis. *BMJ*, **307**, 793–5. Cost utility analysis. *BMJ*, **307**, 859–62. Cost benefit analysis. *BMJ*, **307**, 924–6. The policy context. *BMJ*, **307**, 994–6.
3 Enthoven A (1999). *Rock Carling Fellowship 1999. In pursuit of an improving National Health Service*. The Nuffield Trust, London.
4 *Health Policy* (1995) **33**. Special issue devoted to programme budgeting and marginal analysis.
5 McGuire A, Henderson J, Mooney G (1988). *The economics of health care: an introductory text*. Routledge, London.
6 Mooney G, Gerard K, Donaldson C, Farrar S (1992). *Priority setting in purchasing: some practical guidelines*, Research Paper 6. National Association of Health Authorities and Trusts (NAHAT), Birmingham.

1.5 Assessing health impacts on a population

Alex Scott-Samuel, Kate Ardern, and Martin Birley

Objectives

By reading this chapter you will become familiar with:
- the background and policy context of health impact assessment (HIA)
- current and emerging concepts and methods of HIA
- the impact of HIA
- an approach to conducting rapid and comprehensive prospective HIAs on major public policies, programmes, and projects.

Definition and scope

Health impact assessment is 'a combination of procedures, methods and tools by which a policy, programme or project may be judged as to its potential effects on the health of a population, and the distribution of those effects within the population'.[1] Health impact assessment may focus on projects such as a new factory, housing development or health centre, programmes such as crime reduction or urban regeneration, or policies such as an integrated transport strategy or a youth unemployment policy. On a broader scale, HIA can be employed to assess global public policies in areas such as international trade, war, and human rights. (Compare HIA as a method with health *needs* assessment by referring to Table 1.3.1.)

Health impact assessment builds on the fact that a wide range of economic, social, psychological, environmental, and organizational influences determines a community's health. It is important to try to estimate these influences on health *prospectively* and so HIA should precede the start of the project, programme, or policy concerned.

The aims of prospective HIA are:
- to systematically assess the potential health impacts, both positive and negative, of projects, programmes, and policies
- to improve the quality of public policy decisions by making recommendations that are likely to enhance predicted positive health impacts and minimize negative ones.

The key output of an HIA is a set of recommendations for beneficially modifying a proposal so that its overall health impacts are enhanced and any potential health inequalities are minimized.

The importance of health impact assessment

Health impact assessment is an important public health method because it:

- promotes equity, sustainability, and healthy public policy in an unequal and frequently unhealthy world
- improves the quality of decision-making in health and partner organizations by incorporating into planning and policy-making the need to address health issues
- emphasizes social and environmental justice (it is usually the already disadvantaged who suffer most from negative health impacts)
- involves a multidisciplinary approach
- encourages public participation in debates about public health, planning, and other public policy issues
- gives equal status to qualitative and quantitative assessment methods
- makes values and politics explicit and opens issues to public scrutiny
- demonstrates that health is far broader than health-care issues.

Health impact assessment is used in public policy decision-making in a wide and rapidly increasing range of 'developed' and 'less developed' countries throughout the world. Health impact assessment has had a high profile in countries of the South since the 1980s.[2] The remainder of this section documents more recent developments in the North.

Europe

The UK,[3,4] The Netherlands, and Sweden were the first countries in Europe to establish HIA programmes. In The Netherlands, HIA became government policy in 1995, following which a screening programme on new policy and legislation was introduced. In Sweden, HIA has been used since 1998 at local government level to assist in achieving local public health targets. The World Health Organization's (WHO) European Centre for Health Policy, together with other European partners, initiated a project in 1999 to bring together available experience and try to reach a degree of consensus on how HIA can best be used to improve health policy development. The most important outputs of this project have been the Gothenburg consensus statement[1] and the generally raised levels of awareness of HIA both in European countries and in the European Commission (EC).

There has been considerable interest in the European Union (EU) in incorporating HIA into the development of all EU policy. In 2001 the EC Directorate General for Health and Consumer Protection (DG Sanco) commissioned the development and piloting of a methodology for HIA of European policy. The resulting European Policy Health Impact Assessment (EPHIA) guide was published in 2004.[5]

The EC has also published and implemented proposals for the integrated impact assessment (IIA) of all EU policy.[6] Integrated impact assessment implies the relatively superficial impact assessment of policies on a number of different dimensions. This was partly a response to the range of assessments, for example environmental, health, gender, economic, being carried out on new European policies.

United Kingdom

The UK government is strongly committed to the principle of HIA. Most recently, the 2004 English public health White Paper *Choosing Health* reiterated the importance of HIA for assessing national and local policies, programmes, and projects. The devolved governments in Scotland and Wales have commissioned substantial programmes of HIA, and the Greater London Assembly has carried out HIAs on London's culture, urban renewal, transport, energy, housing, and waste management strategies. The establishment in England in 2002 of Primary Care Trusts, whose directors of public health are responsible for undertaking HIAs, has led to HIAs being undertaken as part of the capital planning process within the NHS. The UK Faculty of Public Health has included HIA as a core competency for all public health professionals.

The UK's National Institute for Health and Clinical Excellence (NICE) HIA Gateway (http://www.publichealth.nice.org.uk/page.aspx?o=HIAGateway) has enabled HIA practitioners to share good practice and lessons learned from undertaking HIA as well as acting as an evidence base for HIA practice and evaluation. The former Health Development Agency has also commissioned work on the development of rapid appraisal and integrated impact assessment methods.[7]

North America

In Canada, health has featured within environmental impact assessments (EIAs) since the 1980s. Health impact assessment as a separate procedure was first incorporated into the legislative framework of British Columbia in 1993, though this pioneering initiative subsequently lapsed. Health impact assessment has since been introduced in a number of Canadian provinces, including Nova Scotia and Quebec.

In the USA, while health considerations have similarly played a role within EIA, HIA has been slow to emerge. Pioneering projects have been undertaken in California (San Francisco and Los Angeles) and in Minnesota. In 2002 a meeting was organized at the Harvard School of Public Health to assess the possibilities for HIA within the USA.[8] In 2004 the Centres for Disease Control and the Robert Wood Johnson Foundation held a further meeting to consider the potential for HIA in local public health and planning departments.

Australasia

Both Australia and New Zealand developed health-focused EIA in the 1990s. More recently, in 2004, the New Zealand government launched a policy tool for HIA.[9] In the same year an Australian–New Zealand collaborative project developed and piloted an equity-focused HIA approach.[10]

Globally

At a global level, the WHO has appointed a HIA adviser at its Geneva headquarters, and has published a special issue of its *Bulletin*[11] on HIA. The WHO has also played a major role in promoting the consideration of health within strategic environmental assessment (SEA). Strategic environmental assessment is concerned with the strategic impact of policies and has been the subject of recent policy and legislation by the EC and by the UN Economic Commission for Europe.

Health impact assessment is increasingly used by global agencies such as the World Bank and by transnational corporations like Shell, which recently appointed a global HIA adviser. Its potentially important role in global public policy is beginning to be recognized.[12,13]

The HIA process

Advantages

As the number of HIA studies grows, accumulating evidence shows that HIA can draw attention to potential health impacts in a way which permits constructive changes to be made to project or policy proposals. This has potentially enormous benefits for major developments which are costly or which propose significant change to existing service provision or organization.

Disadvantages

However, potential drawbacks to the adoption of HIA as a routine part of planning include the limited capacity and capability to undertake HIA. Therefore, whilst this chapter describes a comprehensive approach to HIA, we appreciate that time and resources may dictate a more condensed approach. There has been considerable interest in the development of rapid HIA among a number of researchers including Ison[14] who has described participatory and non-participatory techniques, Milner[15] who has developed a screening tool for rapid HIA and Ardern,[16] who has developed a rapid HIA tool which has been used on a major housing programme and on NHS capital schemes.

In both comprehensive and rapid HIA, it is important to distinguish between *procedures* and *methods* for health impact assessment (see Figure 1.5.1):

- procedures are frameworks for commissioning and implementing HIAs
- methods are the systems for carrying them out.

Procedures   **Methods**

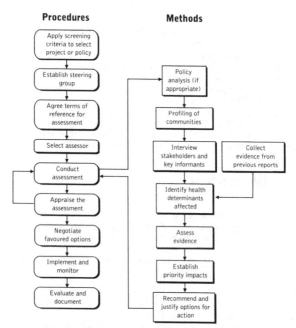

Figure 1.5.1 Stages in the HIA process

Managing an HIA: procedures

There are four procedures in the HIA process
- screening
- steering group, terms of reference, and scope of HIA
- negotiation of favoured options
- implementation, monitoring, and evaluation.

Screening

The issues on which the selection of candidates for HIA is based are listed below. Potential projects, programmes, or policies should be rapidly assessed with regard to their likely performance in relation to each of these issues. While the procedure is necessarily crude, it can give a useful indication of how resources for HIA can be most effectively deployed. For the remainder of the sections describing procedures and methods, the term 'project' is used to refer to projects, programmes, or policies.

Health impact assessment screening procedure:
- *Economic issues*
  - the size of the project and of the population(s) affected
  - the costs of the project, and their distribution.

- *Outcome issues*
  - the nature of potential health impacts of the project
  - the likely nature and extent of disruption caused to communities by the project
  - the existence of potentially cumulative impacts.
- *Epidemiologic issues*
  - the degree of certainty (risk) of health impacts
  - the likely frequency (incidence/prevalence rates) of potential health impacts
  - the likely severity of potential health impacts
  - the size of any probable health service impacts
  - the likely consistency of 'expert' and 'community' perceptions of probability (i.e. risk), frequency and severity of important impacts. The greater the agreement between expert and lay perceptions of important impacts: the greater the need for a HIA.

During HIA screening, there is a general need to give greater priority to policies than to programmes, and to programmes than to projects, all other things being equal. This is due to the broader scope—and hence potential impact—of policies as compared with programmes and to projects. Another strategic consideration is that HIA should be prospective wherever possible. Timing may be affected by planning regulations and other statutory frameworks, such as whether the project requires an environmental impact assessment. The relevance of the HIA to local decision-making is another key concern.

Steering group, terms of reference, and scope

Following screening and project selection, a multidisciplinary steering group should be established to agree the terms of reference (ToR) of the HIA and to provide advice and support as it develops. Its membership should include representatives of the commissioners of the HIA, the assessors carrying it out, the project's proponents, affected communities, and other stakeholders as appropriate. Members should ideally be able to take decisions on behalf of those they represent.

The ToR provide a quality assurance procedure for the HIA. They are project specific, but should always include:

- steering group members' roles, including those of chair and secretary
- the nature and frequency of feedback to the steering group
- the HIA methods to be used
- the form of the project's outputs and any associated issues, e.g. ownership, confidentiality, and copyright
- the scope of the HIA—what is to be included and excluded, and the boundaries of the HIA in time and space
- an outline programme, including any deadlines
- the budget and source(s) of funding.

Negotiation of favoured options

The consideration of alternative options does not conclude the process. Even when there appear to be clear messages regarding the best way forward it cannot be assumed that these will automatically be adopted. Achieving agreement on options for mitigating or enhancing predicted health impacts may require skillful negotiation on the part of those involved.

Implementation, monitoring, and evaluation

To some extent, a HIA is analogous to an audit cycle in which the results of subsequent monitoring and evaluation in turn influence the continuing operation of the project. The indicators and methods proposed for monitoring will depend on the nature and content of the project, and also on the perceived importance of this stage of the assessment. A tool which can be used for monitoring the distribution of impacts on a given population is *health equity audit*, with its local indicators of health inequalities. The former Health Development Agency has published a helpful guide to evaluation of HIAs.[17]

In HIA, outcome evaluation is constrained by the fact that negative impacts which have been successfully avoided (or weakly positive ones which have been successfully enhanced) due to the modification of the project will clearly not be identifiable. In practice, things are rarely this perfect and it may be possible to construct and compare notional and actual outcomes relating to the originally proposed and actual post-HIA projects. Multimethod assessments of specified outcomes (*triangulation*) should be undertaken where feasible, in order to increase validity.

Process evaluation involves the assessment of HIA procedures and methods against the terms of reference initially agreed by the steering group; impact evaluation involves the assessment of the extent to which the agreed recommendations of the HIA were successfully implemented.

A consistent finding of a number of studies is that undertaking HIA has produced unpredicted beneficial outcomes such as improved local partnerships, raising the profile of health issues on the political agenda, reducing social exclusion, empowering and engaging local communities, and improving and informing the quality of local decision-making. For example, the HIA of the New Home Energy Efficiency Scheme in Wales[18] demonstrated the programme's relevance to other key health determinants such as crime and disorder and accidents and injuries. These unexpected outcomes require systematic recording and follow-up. Evaluation of a HIA needs ideally to incorporate methods that can capture this, such as film and photography. The HIA of the New Deal for Communities programme in Huyton, Merseyside, UK[19] is an example of the use of these techniques in HIA evaluation.

Methods for assessing health impacts

The range of methods used for HIAs should reflect the nature and complexity of the subject matter. It is important to use all methods and involve all disciplines that may contribute to the overall task. Commonly used methods include:
- policy analysis
- profiling of affected areas/populations
- identification of potential positive and negative health impacts
- assessment of perceived health risks
- quantification and valuation of health impacts
- ranking the most important impacts

- consideration of alternate options and recommendations for management of priority impacts.

Before looking at these methods, we will discuss the key area of participation.

Participation in HIAs

The process of HIA requires broad participation if a comprehensive picture of potential health impacts is to be established. Public participation throughout the HIA is essential, both to ensure that local concerns are addressed and for ethical reasons of social justice. The cooperation and expertise of a wide range of stakeholders and key informants will be needed, including:

- those involved at all levels in the project
- those likely to be directly affected by the project
- others who have knowledge or information of relevance to the project and its outcomes, e.g. local shopkeepers or service providers, community groups
- local or outside experts whose knowledge is relevant to the project
- relevant professionals, e.g. general practitioners, health visitors, social or community workers
- voluntary organizations.

Barnes[20] has identified the importance of using robust and well-planned methods of community participation in adding value and credibility to HIA recommendations. She also highlights the need for HIA practitioners to understand and record people's health experiences which underlie routinely collected statistics. Exclusive reliance on quantitative methods may oversimplify the complexity of real life situations.

Policy analysis

Health impact assessments of policies will require initial policy analysis to determine key aspects that the HIA will need to address; this may build on or use material already available from earlier policy development work.[5] Key aspects include:

- content and dimensions of the policy
- socio-political and policy context
- policy objectives, priorities, and intended outputs
- trade-offs and critical socio-cultural impacts which may affect its implementation.

Profiling of affected areas/populations

A profile of the areas and populations likely to be affected by the project is compiled using available socio-demographic and health data and information from key informants across the public and non-statutory sectors. The profile should cover groups whose health could be enhanced or placed at risk by the project's effects. Vulnerable and disadvantaged groups require special consideration.

Identification of potential positive and negative
health impacts

Table 1.5.1 Health determinants encountered in health impact
assessment

Categories of influences on health	Examples of specific health determinants
Biological factors	Age, sex, genetic factors
Personal and family environment	Family structure and functioning, primary/secondary/adult education, occupation, unemployment, income, risk-taking behaviour, diet, smoking, alcohol, substance misuse, exercise, recreation, means of transport (cycle/car ownership)
Social environment	Culture, peer pressures, discrimination, social support (neighbourliness, social networks, isolation), community/cultural/spiritual participation, crime
Physical environment	Air/water quality, noise, smell, view, housing conditions, working conditions, public safety, civic design, shops (location/range/quality), communications (road/rail), land use, waste disposal, energy, local environmental features
Public services and public policy	Access to (location/disabled access/costs), quality of primary/community/secondary health care, child care, social (security) services, housing, leisure amenities, employment, public transport, law and order, other health-relevant public services, non-statutory agencies and services, equity/democracy in public policy.

The range of potential health impacts identified in a HIA depends on the
definition of health that is employed. Like most governments and the
World Health Organization, we recommend using a socio-environmental
model which features a wide range of linkages by which projects can
impact upon health, and a causal model of health impact in which a project changes the prevalence of health determinants and this, in turn, may
change the health status of the affected population groups. Table 1.5.1
presents the health determinants most often encountered in HIA.

Methods for identifying the potential health impacts of a project will
vary according to the human and financial resources available. Clearly, a
short workshop discussion involving a group of stakeholders around a
table will employ different methods from a comprehensive assessment.
Ideally, impact identification should involve qualitative fieldwork (typically
interviews, focus groups, and sometimes Delphi studies or scenarios) and
quantitative studies such as mathematic modelling of project outcomes,
surveys, and economic analysis.

Respondents will include relevant experts and purposive samples of key informants, including affected subpopulations. Literature searches are also employed in impact identification. The essential aim, whichever methods are used, is to systematically consider the range of potential changes to health determinants and outcomes likely to result from the operation of the project.

Assessment of perceived health risks

Perceptions of risk are, when possible, recorded at the time of identification of potential impacts. In some instances existing evidence will permit precise assessment of risk. In many cases, however, risk assessment will be based on subjective perceptions. Assuming adequate sampling, such subjective risk data are arguably no less valid or important than are more precise technical data—particularly where sensory perceptions (such as increased noise or smell, or deterioration of outlook) are concerned. Petts et al.[21] have produced a useful guide to understanding what influences people's assessment of risk.

Risk perceptions can be recorded using simple three-point scales of measurability (potential impacts are characterized as qualitative, estimable, or calculable) and of likelihood of occurrence (definite, probable, or speculative). The temptation to quantify such scales should be resisted—such numbers could not be compared or manipulated with validity and would carry a spurious authority.

Quantification and valuation of health impacts

It may prove possible to assess the size of quantifiable impacts at the time they are identified by informants; in other cases this will need to be done separately, e.g. through reviews of previously published evidence. The same applies to valuation—though evidence on the resource implications and opportunity costs of potential impacts will often prove hard to come by. However, such data can in principle be made comparable using quality-adjusted life years (QALYs) or disability-adjusted life years (DALYs), or other such cost–utility measures. Some authors have described mathematic modelling methods used to quantify health impacts, particularly in relation to environmental impacts on health such as air pollution, road accidents, and methods of waste disposal. The Foresight Vehicle Initiative HIA undertaken for the UK's Department of Trade and Industry[22] used modelling and health and transport economic forecasting to quantify the health impacts of innovations in road transport technology.

Ranking the most important impacts

Informants should be encouraged to prioritize or rank those potential impacts that they identify. Once all the initial evidence has been collected, a priority-setting exercise should be carried out. Because of differential perceptions of risk there will rarely be complete consensus; criteria may need to be agreed so that the views of all informants are adequately reflected and valued. Such criteria are likely to include the frequency with which potential impacts are identified, the probability of occurrence, severity/importance, and public and political opinion.

Consideration of alternative options and recommendations for management of priority impacts

Unless there is total consensus, a series of options for providing the optimum health impact of the project being assessed should be defined and presented. The ultimate result will be an agreed set of recommendations for modifying the project such that its health impacts are optimized—in the context of the many and complex constraints which invariably constitute the social, material, and political environment in which it will be undertaken.

Communicating with key stakeholders is critical to the success or otherwise of an HIA. There are often political and organizational systems that require formal feedback such as local authority committees, health service boards, and local strategic partnerships. An HIA which is submitted to a planning enquiry will sometimes require a nominated senior officer to give evidence.

Recommendations

If HIA is going to be a worthwhile exercise it is crucial that it is able to demonstrate both effectiveness and efficient use of resources. Therefore it follows that any recommendations resulting from HIA studies should:

- be practical
- aim to maximize health gain and minimize health loss
- be socially acceptable (a degree of pragmatism may be inevitable)
- consider the cost of implementation
- consider the opportunity cost
- include preventive as well as curative measures
- be prioritized in terms of short-, medium-, and long-term objectives
- identify a lead agency or individual
- identify the drivers and barriers to change
- be acceptable to the lead agency
- be capable of being monitored and evaluated.

The list given above is, of course, not definitive and as HIA develops other criteria will be added. Too often, however, recommendations are of a general rather than a specific nature which makes monitoring difficult if not impossible. Also, if there was poor teamwork the recommendations may only reflect one person's viewpoint and may fail to appreciate the logistics of implementation. It will also mean that key agencies do not feel that they have ownership of the recommendations.

The impact of HIA

Health impact assessment has now been carried out on a number of major policies, programmes, and projects and has had significant influence on policy-making and planning. Examples include the Greater London Assembly's HIA programme[17], the Finningley airport study[23] conducted by Doncaster Health Authority (which for the first time in the UK incorporated the establishment of an independent airport health impact group into the regulatory framework for an airport), and the St Helens and Knowsley PFI study[16] which was instrumental in attracting significant additional financial investment in the scheme at reduced interest rates from the European Investment Bank.

Some conceptual and methodological issues

Science or art?
Health impact assessment is a decision support process which draws on a scientific knowledge base. Each HIA is specific to a location in time, space, and local conditions—though its evidence base can be evaluated, and the rigor with which procedures and methods are implemented can (and should) be assessed.

Uncertainty
Uncertainties encountered during the undertaking of HIAs frequently dictate the need to make assumptions: these are often acceptable but should be declared explicitly.

Timing
Health impact assessment should take place early enough in the development of a project to permit constructive modifications to be carried out prior to its implementation, but late enough for a clear idea to have been formed as to its nature and content.

Depth
The financial and opportunity costs of undertaking HIA dictate the need both to screen candidate projects and also to have available a range of methods according to the depth of analysis required.

Politics
Although HIA is itself part of the political process, external political imperatives may sometimes inappropriately determine the outcome of the decision being assessed. Disagreements or power inequalities between different stakeholder factions may be similarly important. Health impact assessments will often be taken out of context to justify pre-set political positions. None of this 'policy-based evidence making' should deter us from continuing to use this innovative approach to promote healthy public policy.

References
1 WHO European Centre for Health Policy (1999). *Health impact assessment: main concepts and suggested approach*, Gothenburg consensus paper. ECHP, Brussels.
2 Birley MH (1995). *The health impact assessment of development projects*. HMSO, London.
3 Will S, Ardern K, Spencely M, Watkins S (1994). *A prospective health impact assessment of the proposed development of a second runway at Manchester International Airport*. Written submission to the public inquiry. Manchester and Stockport Health Commissions.

4 Scott-Samuel A (1996). Health impact assessment—an idea whose time has come. *BMJ*, **313**, 183–4.

5 Abrahams D, den Broeder L, Doyle C et al. (2004). *EPHIA—European policy health impact assessment: a guide*. IMPACT, University of Liverpool. Available at: http://www.ihia.org.uk/document/ephia.pdf (accessed 15 June 2005).

6 Commission of the European Communities (2002). *Communication from the Commission on impact assessment*, COM(2002)276 final. CEC, Brussels.

7 Milner S, Bailey C, Deans J, Pettigrew D (2003). *Integrated impact assessment: UK mapping project report*. Northumbria University, Newcastle. Accessed at: http://www.publichealth.nice.org.uk/page.aspx?o=525318 (accessed 15 January 2006).

8 Krieger N, Northridge M, Gruskin S et al. (2003). Assessing health impact assessment: multidisciplinary and international perspectives. *J Epidemiol Commun Health*, **57**, 659–62.

9 Public Health Advisory Committee (2004). *A guide to health impact assessment: a policy tool for New Zealand*. Public Health Advisory Committee, National Advisory Committee on Health and Disability, Wellington. Available at: http://www.nhc.govt.nz/PHAC/publications/GuideToHIA. pdf (accessed 15 June 2005).

10 Mahoney M, Simpson S, Harris E, Aldrich R, Stewart Williams J (2004). *Equity focused health impact assessment framework*. Australasian Collaboration for Health Equity Impact Assessment, Newcastle, NSW. Available at: http://chetre.med.unsw.edu.au/files/EFHIA_Framework.pdf (accessed 15 June 2005).

11 World Health Organization (2003). Special issue on HIA. *Bulletin of the World Health Organization*, **81**(6). Available at: http://www.who.int/bulletin/volumes/81/6/en/ (accessed 16 June 2005).

12 O'Keefe E, Scott-Samuel A (2002). Human rights and wrongs: could health impact assessment help? *J Law Med Ethics*, **30**, 734–8.

13 O'Keefe E, Scott-Samuel A (2006). Health impact assessment: towards globalization as if people mattered. In: Kawachi I, Wamala S. (eds) *Globalization and health*. Oxford University Press, New York.

14 Ison E (2002). *Rapid appraisal tool for health impact assessment. A task-based approach*. Available at: http://www.publichealth.nice.org.uk/page. aspx?o=525147 (accessed 15 January 2006).

15 Milner SJ, Bailey C, Deans J (2003). 'Fit for purpose' health impact assessment: a realistic way forward. *Public Health*, **117**, 295–300.

16 Ardern K (2003). *Rapid health impact assessment of the private finance initiative proposal: a whole system approach in St Helens and Knowsley*. South Liverpool Primary Care Trust, Liverpool. Available at: http://www.phel.nice.org.uk/hiadocs/Rapid_HIA_of_PFI_Proposal.pdf (accessed 15 June 2005).

17 Taylor L, Gowman N, Quigley R (2003). *Evaluating health impact assessment*. Health Development Agency, London. Available at: http://www.publichealth.nice.org/page.aspx?o=502589 (accessed 15 January 2006).

18 Kemm J, Ballard S, Harmer M (2001). *Health impact assessment of the new home energy efficiency scheme*. National Assembly for Wales, Cardiff.

19 Patterson J (2004). *Health impact assessment of the North Huyton New Deal for Communities programme*. North Huyton NDC and Knowsley Primary Care Trust, Huyton.

20 Barnes R (2004). HIA and urban regeneration: the Ferrier Estate, England. In: Kemm J, Parry J, Palmer S (eds) *Health impact assessment. Concepts, theory, techniques and applications*, pp. 299–307. Oxford University Press, Oxford.

21 Petts J, Wheeley S, Homan J, Niemeyer S (2003). *Risk literacy and the public MMR, air pollution and mobile phones*. Department of Health, London. Available at: http://www.dh.gov.uk/assetRoot/04/07/40/99/04074099.pdf (accessed 15 January 2006).

22 Abrahams D (2002). *Foresight Vehicle Initiative comprehensive health impact assessment. Executive summary*. IMPACT—International Health Impact Assessment Consortium, University of Liverpool. Available at: www.ihia.org.uk/document/impacthiareports/FVI.pdf (accessed 15 June 2005).

23 Abdel Aziz MI, Radford J, McCabe J (2000). *Health impact assessment, Finningley Airport*. Doncaster Health Authority. Available at: http://www.publichealth.nice.org.uk/media/hiadocs/79_finningley_airport_hiareport.pdf (accessed 15 January 2006).

1.6 Being explicit about values in public health

Nick Steel

Introduction

The practice of public health is a discipline rich in values. Ireland and California can ban public smoking because smoking is no longer valued by most people who live there. In contrast, attempts to reduce the death toll from road traffic collisions by restricting car use will not be successful so long as we continue to love our cars. Successful public health interventions work through the organized efforts of society. Their success both shapes and reflects social values. Social values influence the behaviour of individuals and communities, and so are important determinants of health. Be explicit about the values in your public health approaches and initiatives; it will serve you well. At least you will know whether you have to push the project uphill or just let it roll down, gathering support as it goes. Values are hard to measure, but that does not mean they are not important. J. K. Galbraith, the tallest Canadian economist, claimed that the denigration of value judgement is one of the devices by which the scientific establishment maintains its misconceptions.

Objectives

Reading this chapter will:
- give you techniques for making explicit the social values held by different groups and reflected in public health issues
- use explicit value judgement to challenge assumptions and influence the success (or otherwise) of public health interventions
- help to explain different approaches to measuring the value of health outcomes.

Values as a cross-cutting theme

Values in public health should not be considered as an isolated area of the discipline. They cut across nearly every area. It will be a rare meeting, policy statement, or plan of action that is not influenced by the values held dear by those responsible.

The importance of the social values held by different population groups is also mentioned in the following chapters: ethics in public health (Chapter 1.7), communicating risk (see Chapter 7.5), influencing governments via media advocacy (Chapter 4.7), and involving 'consumers' (Chapter 8.4).

Why is it important to be explicit about values in public health?

The development of a more open and evidence-based approach to decision-making in health care has shown how much personal values influence professional behaviour. Science is far from being value-free; science and values are inseparable. The challenge is neither to ignore them nor eliminate them, but to clarify those values and combine them with the science in a way that allows us to make the best decision, explicitly.

Two complementary approaches to being explicit about values in public health

The first approach is to make every effort to *measure* values, in the sense of utility or the desirability of a particular outcome, in order to make quantitative comparisons between alternatives. Examples are decision-analysis (Box 1.6.1) and quality-adjusted life years (QALYs) and disability-adjusted life years (DALYs) (Box 1.6.2). The second approach is more holistic, treating values as moral principles or standards; what we hold dear about the way we live. The broad effects of public health decisions are considered more qualitatively.

Box 1.6.1 Decision analysis

Decision analysis quantifies the effects of the different options in a decision.[1] It combines scientific information with valuations of the benefits and burdens of the options. The analysis is usually expressed as a decision tree. For each decision in the tree, the probability of each outcome is weighted by the value of the outcome. The probability should be based on the best research available. Values are expressed as a number between 0 and 1. For example, if a person would tolerate a 20% chance of dying to *avoid* a particular outcome, then that outcome has a value of 0.8 (80%) attached to it. A variety of methods have been developed to measure values (see below). Values will change over time and according to how people are asked about them. They will be different for people with a health problem than for a sample of the general population who might consider an illness more theoretically.

Box 1.6.2 QALYs and DALYs

QALYs are years of healthy life lived. Scientific information on life expectancy is weighted with the utility of different health states. They are used as an outcome measure in cost-utility analysis (see Box 1.6.3 and Chapter 1.4).

DALYs are years of healthy life lost. They use disability (rather than utility) weights, and are a measure of the burden of disease on a defined population[2] (see Chapter 2.9). The key choices are about:

- the potential years of life lost as a result of a death at a given age
- the relative value of a year of healthy life lived at different ages
- the discount rate, to allow for the greater value of human life and health in the present than the future
- the disability weights used to convert life lived with a disability to a common measure with premature death.

Measuring values

Values can be quantified by measuring preferences for health outcomes with techniques such as the standard gamble, the time trade-off, and visual analogue scales.[3] Because this is time-consuming and complex, it can be simpler to use a pre-scored multiattribute health status classification system. Three such systems are Quality of Well-Being, Health Utilities Index, and EuroQol.[3] These include aspects of health such as pain, disability, mood, self-care, social activities, and work.

Decision analysis can be used to provide guidelines for managing similar groups of patients. The analysis is run using a selection of probabilities and values within a reasonable range for:

- the estimated probability of each outcome used in the analysis
- the estimated incidence of side-effects
- the values used
- any financial cost estimates.

Treatment can then be tailored when required by matching the guidelines to the characteristics of the patient or population.[4]

The strength of decision analysis is that the values on which the decisions are based are explicit, and can be varied. The weakness lies in trying to replace the uncertainties, mysteries, and doubts that are human values by a number between 0 and 1. Using decision analysis to make decisions about groups of people may create ethical dilemmas if inequalities are increased as a result. For example, those with poor health may have low expectations, and put a low value on an intervention to improve their health. In contrast, a healthier group may have higher expectations and put a high value on an intervention to give them a relatively small health gain. A decision that incorporated these expressed values would risk increasing inequalities between the two groups.

The use of QALYs is limited by concerns over the validity of single indices of quality of life and over the effect on equity when QALYs are used to prioritize services.[3] The use of DALYs is limited by the assumption that the lives of disabled people have less value than those of people without disabilities.

Developing a holistic approach

Before applying the results of a decision analysis or cost–utility study, or any scientific evidence, the wider implications of such techniques should be considered. The perspectives of different groups in society need to be understood. Whose values are being considered? Most people can be considered to belong to one of three main groups:

- professional or technocrat (often termed 'technical')
- public (often termed 'user')
- politician (often termed 'funder').

Any one person can move quickly between these groups depending on their particular circumstances. Different perspectives lead different people (and even the same person at different times) to draw different conclusions from the same evidence. No evidence is truly objective: all evidence is value-laden. Hence it is rarely possible to change someone's behaviour by defeating them with logic. Exploring assumptions will improve the quality of decisions and their acceptability to diverse groups.

This broader approach can be fostered by reading widely. George Eliot's *Middlemarch* is an example of a well-known novel that explores the impact of values on scientific progress.[5] Robert Pirsig's *Zen and the Art of Motorcycle Maintenance* is an entertaining search for the indefinable quality that comes before the division of the world into science and values.[6] The New York University School of Medicine Database of Literature and Medicine is one source of suitable texts.[7]

Accepting that uncertainty and variation are inevitable will foster a broader approach to decisions. Stephen Jay Gould wrote about the inevitability of uncertainty after he was diagnosed with mesothelioma and discovered the low median survival time from the disease: 'variation is the hard reality, not a set of imperfect measures for a central tendency. Means and medians are the abstractions'.[8]

Techniques to help you be explicit about values in public health

- Be explicit about the nature of the problem, the choices available and the relevant outcomes (especially the outcomes as valued by different sorts of people).
- Collaborate with all those involved with the issue within your organization and outside it to incorporate as wide a range of perspectives as possible.
- Appraise the validity and relevance of the scientific evidence.
- Identify whose perspective is used to tell the story and present the evidence.
- Ask what has been left out.
- Think laterally to generate new ideas and challenge assumptions.[9]
- Think about the language and images used and the effect they have on the meaning.
- Identify which events are under human control and which are governed by chance.

- Distinguish the probabilities of outcomes from the values and be as precise as possible about each.
- Be explicit about assumptions and uncertainties.
- Consider a sensitivity analysis to explore how varying the values and probabilities changes the decision.
- Ascertain who appraised the value of outcomes, and how they did it. (The UK National Institute for Health and Clinical Excellence's (NICE) April 2005 draft guidance for consultation is a good example of organizational clarity about social value judgement (Box 1.6.3).

Box 1.6.3 National Institute for Health and Clinical Excellence (NICE) social value judgements consultation—key extracts[10]

Background

'Social value judgements relate to society rather than basic or clinical science: they take account of the ethical principles, preferences, culture and aspirations that should underpin the nature and extent of the care provided by the NHS.'

Moral principles

'Widely accepted moral principles that are expected to underpin clinical and public health practice: respect for autonomy, non-maleficence, beneficence, distributive justice.'

Economic evaluation

'The QALY embodies the important social value judgement that to count only gains in life expectancy, without considering the quality of the additional life years, omits important dimensions of human welfare. Value judgements embodied in QALYs are that health-related quality of life can be reasonably captured in terms of: physical mobility, ability to self-care, ability to carry out activities of daily living, absence of pain and discomfort, and absence of anxiety and depression.

There are also value judgements embodied in the ways in which these elements are combined and the scoring given to the various combinations of levels of functioning.'

Engaging other people

One way to engage other people is to give examples of work that failed due to values not being made explicit, or succeeded where the contribution of both science and values was clear. The success or failure of evidence and guideline implementation are often suitable examples (see Chapters 6.7 and 6.8).

Potential pitfalls

Decisions about treatment options are particularly sensitive to values when:

- the possible outcomes are either greatly different (e.g. death or disability) or very similar
- treatments have greatly different probabilities and types of complications
- choices are made between short-term and long-term outcomes
- an individual or group involved is particularly risk-averse
- an individual or group considers some possible outcomes particularly important.[11]

Overconfidence in either science or values is another potential pitfall. It can lead to 'group-think'—a group making a decision that looks at too few alternatives and becomes very selective in the sort of facts it sees and asks for.

Unpicking dogma

Combining values with science has been criticized for devaluing objective knowledge. In fact, it merely recognizes that all knowledge is subjective, and the important skill is to understand whose perspective is being used and how it affects the results. How people act is determined by an interaction between what they value and what they construe as reality. With the same information and alternatives, different people make different choices. Better choices are made when different values are explored and acknowledged as a central part of the public health task.

Conclusion

Health measures should always take account of relevant values where possible. An appreciation and acknowledgement of both the scientific base *and* value base will contribute to better, more sustainable decisions concerning the health of a population. It may be difficult to measure the success of combining science and values, but the benefits will be clear to all involved, both in terms of process and outcome.

References

1 Weinstein MC, Fineberg HV, Elstein AS *et al.* (1980). *Clinical decision analysis*. WB Saunders, Philadelphia, PA.
2 The World Bank (1993). *World development report 1993*. Oxford University Press, New York.
3 Drummond MF, O'Brien B, Stoddart GL, Torrance GW (1997). *Methods for the economic evaluation of health care programmes*. Oxford University Press, Oxford.
4 Lilford RJ, Pauker SG, Braunholtz DA, Chard J (1998). Decision analysis and the implementation of research findings. *BMJ*, **317**, 405–9.
5 Eliot G (1999). *Middlemarch*. Oxford University Press, Oxford.

6 Pirsig RM (1991). *Zen and the art of motorcycle maintenance*. Vintage Press, New York.

7 New York University School of Medicine (2005). *Literature, arts and medicine database*. Available at: http://endeavour.med.nyu.edu/lit-med/lit-med-db/index.html (accessed 8 September 2005).

8 Gould SJ (1998). The median isn't the message. In: Greenhalgh T, Hurwitz B (eds) *Narrative based medicine*, pp. 29–33. BMJ Books, London.

9 De Bono E (1990). *Lateral thinking*. Penguin Books, London.

10 National Institute for Health and Clinical Excellence (2005). *Social value judgements: guidelines for the Institute and its advisory bodies. Draft for consultation*. National Institute for Health and Clinical Excellence, London.

11 Kassirer JP (1994). Incorporating patients' preferences into medical decisions. *N Engl J Med*, **330**, 1895–6.

1.7 Understanding ethics in public health

Angus Dawson

Objectives

As a result of reading this chapter you will be:
- better informed about the role of ethics in public health
- better able to identify ethical problems in public health
- have some argumentative resources to help discuss ethics in public health (see Chapter 1.6).

Box 1.7.1 Definition

Public health ethics is concerned with the ethical issues that arise from all aspects of public health theory and practice.

Why is ethics important to public health?

A large literature has evolved over the last 30 years discussing ethical issues in medical ethics. However, the focus of this work has overwhelmingly been on clinical practice rather than public health. Public health interventions are different in two fundamental ways from clinical medicine, both of which have consequences for the ethical issues that inevitably arise:
- public health practice focuses on the health of populations and not just individuals
- public health action usually requires the actions of groups, populations, or governments, not just individuals, to bring about the proposed benefit.

These characteristics of the discipline raise important ethical issues. For example, the focus on the health of populations might mean that public health practitioners are in danger of:
- focusing on reducing harm or the risk of harm, even though the general public are not aware of, or don't care about, such harm
- sacrificing individual freedoms for the sake of improvement in the population's health despite the fact that the majority of the population might prefer the preservation of the former to the creation of the latter.

In addition, many public health interventions are controversial because they involve a commitment to the idea of creating and maintaining public goods and population health ('the improved health of the population is in everyone's interest …'). This is a reason why government action is often thought to be a necessary part of public health.

Public goods are goods that:
- cannot be constructed by the individual alone
- cannot be broken up into and enjoyed as individual private goods
- once created, any benefits are shared by all in that population.

For example, the existence of herd protection against a disease in a population might count as a public good. It involves a collective effort, no individual can take away their contribution to it, and those that have not contributed to it still benefit if they live in that society.[1]

Public health must involve ethics, because public health interventions impact upon not only individuals, their lives, environment, but critically upon their choices and behaviours. Ethical public health involves:
- being sensitive to all aspects/consequences of action and inactions
- taking ethical issues into account before a decision is made about an action or inaction.

There are many different arguments that might be constructed in relation to public health. Some of these will be illustrated in this chapter through a focus on just one topical issue, that of smoking. The same or similar arguments can be used in relation to many different public health interventions.

Is public health practice paternalistic?

It is a common accusation that public health activity is paternalistic, with the clear implication that this is held to be morally wrong. What does such a claim mean? Is it true?
- *Paternalism* can be defined as acting (or not acting) with the intention of reducing harm or bringing about greater good for the subject(s) of the action.

On this definition it is left open whether a paternalistic action is morally justifiable: this is held to be a separate judgement. Some believe (i.e. many liberals) that we can use a distinction between strong or weak paternalism to settle the issue of justifiability.[2]
- *Strong paternalism* is where an action will overrule the action or decision of a competent individual. (On this view this is usually held be unjustifiable.)
- *Weak paternalism* is where an action is performed on behalf of an incompetent individual, e.g. a young child, an adult with serious learning difficulties, an adult with dementia, etc. (On this view this is usually held to be justifiable.)

Let's assume for the purposes of argument that it is beyond doubt that both smoking and passive smoking cause harm.[3,4] If this is the case then harm can be caused not just to the smoker themselves but also to third parties (via passive smoking). We can now consider two cases

Box 1.7.1 Case A: I could act to stop you smoking
for your own good

This is paternalism—but is it justified? Many hold it is not, as it is wrong to interfere with someone's liberty of action. On this view, in such a situation we should not intervene except for providing information to the smoker about the risk of harm to themselves. Of course, such a view presupposes that the smoker freely chooses to smoke, and this might be doubted if the individual is addicted.

Box 1.7.2 Case B: I could act to stop you smoking
for the good of others

This is not paternalism. This is because it is harm to others that motivates the action, not the good of the individual smoker. The so-called 'harm to others principle' is recognized by liberals such as Feinberg. This means that if you act to stop smoking on the grounds of preventing harm to the population from passive smoking your actions are not paternalistic.

(Boxes 1.7.1 and 1.7.2) to see how the accusation of paternalism might work in relation to smoking.

Others think that whilst these classifications offer a useful rough guide to the issue of justifiability, such distinctions will not be the only relevant consideration. For example, in some cases we might think that a proposed intervention is (strongly) paternalistic, but still think we should perform it, as it is justified for other reasons (e.g. it will have a well-evidenced positive impact upon the public's health). This might be particularly important if you think that you have a responsibility for other people's health.

Does the state have a duty to protect its citizens?

The discussion so far has been concerned about the actions of individuals. However, once we begin to talk about some of the possible ways to prevent harm to others we necessarily begin to talk about actual or possible actions of government. Does the state have a duty to protect its citizens? Most will answer 'yes', in at least some cases (e.g. defence from foreign powers etc.). Here the justification may be in terms of harm to others. Such a justification can also be given for government action in relation to public health.

Box 1.7.3 **Case study: a ban on smoking in public places**

One form of protection from a known harm is to have a ban on smoking in public places (e.g. bars and restaurants). This has been very successful in a number of jurisdictions where it has been tried.[5-7] Note that there may be three different motivations for a government in proposing such a ban and only two of them will be paternalistic (although they might still be justifiable):

1. *Harm to others:* where the ban is motivated by health and safety concerns for bar staff and other (non-smoking) visitors to bars. Here the issue is harm to others and is not paternalistic.

2. *Protect smokers from (self-inflicted) harm:* where the ban is motivated by a wish to discourage smoking in general as a means of protecting smokers' own health by making it harder for them to smoke. This will be (strongly) paternalistic, although it may be justifiable.

3. *Culture and environment:* where the ban is a contribution to improving the population's health through a series of measures to make smoking less visible and acceptable. The aim is to try and ensure that new smokers are less likely to be recruited and to help existing smokers give up. This is likely to be both strongly and weakly paternalistic, although both may be justifiable.

Clearly the state will have some obligations to prevent harm to others where it can. This alone might be used to justify a ban on smoking in public (at least in some environments). However, what about state paternalism? Is paternalism justified in the smoking case?

What are the possible grounds for justified state paternalism?

There are a number of different possible justifications for state paternalism. The first is the fact that government action in such cases is focused on preventing known harms. There are many different ethical theories that might use this idea to justify public health action.[8] One possible justification might be supplied by the 'four principles' approach.[9] The four principles are as follows:

- beneficence (doing or bringing about good)
- non-maleficence (doing no harm)
- respect for autonomy
- justice.

The four principles might be used to justify paternalism in such cases by appeal to the principles of non-maleficence and/or beneficence and the idea that these prima facie principles out-weigh that of respecting autonomy (at least on this occasion). On this view, whilst not all individuals are asked for their consent they do benefit, even if their liberty is reduced or circumscribed in some way. Where the harm is serious enough a restriction on autonomous action may be justifiable.

Another potential source of justification is to look to the moral theory called consequentialism. Consequentialism is the idea that we should look to the result of actions and evaluate possible actions in terms of the sum of the potential harms and benefits resulting from those decisions. One early form of this view was known as utilitarianism (and was influential in bringing about much nineteenth-century legislation to improve the public's health). However, one reason why consequentialism is controversial is because it often focuses on the good for populations, rather than that of individuals. On this view, it may be that the state is obligated to bring about the best possible levels of welfare for its citizens. For example, a consequentialist justification for a ban on smoking could appeal to the benefit to be derived from all of the three reasons given in the case study above.

Thirdly, it might be possible to appeal to the idea of public goods as a justification for paternalism. The idea here is that the promotion and maintenance of such goods can only be performed by the state, and therefore this is a responsibility of the state. Perhaps a society that does everything it can to discourage smoking creates an important public good. If it is accepted that the promotion and maintenance of such public goods is important then public health action to improve the population's health (through a ban on smoking in public places) might be a form of justifiable paternalism even if it interfered with smokers' liberty to smoke. (This argument can be used in addition to any harm to others argument.)

Each of these three possible justifications for state paternalism might justify a ban on smoking in public through an attempt to focus on the health of the whole population. On this approach, it is better for the population if there are fewer smokers, and so action should be taken to try and ensure that there are the fewest possible number. This might be an argument for blurring the distinction between the original two cases (A and B as outlined above). If I prevent you from smoking, I am contributing to making smoking less acceptable and thereby likely to discourage others from smoking. If I let you indulge, society may be seen to be supporting your action as a reasonable and legitimate action. This might encourage others to smoke.

This idea can also be seen in the fact that a whole host of public health interventions do not focus upon individuals and their actions but upon the social or environmental conditions that might influence people to begin or continue smoking. Such interventions may be at least partly paternalistic. Examples might include:

- above-inflation tax increases on cigarettes
- increasingly visible and strong health warnings
- restricting tobacco advertising
- restricting access to cigarettes (e.g. age restrictions on purchasing cigarettes and ensuring that vending machines are not accessible to children).

Such activities are deliberate attempts to make smoking less easy and acceptable. The aim here is not just to reduce smoking, and thereby reduce smoking-related deaths, but also to improve the population's health. The purpose of such interventions is to manipulate the environment, reduce the triggers or opportunities for smoking, and so change the preferences of the members of the population for their own and the public's good. A ban on smoking in public will also contribute to this end.

However, at least some liberals might object to all these interventions, and argue that they are examples of what is wrong with public health. The argument might be that each one is paternalistic and also unjustifiable. This is because they all interfere with individual liberty (even when there are no harm-to-others concerns) and this is morally wrong. There is no easy way to respond where such deep disagreement exists.

Should the public be involved in the formation and delivery of public health policy?

Many public health activities seek to reduce harm to the whole population. Such interventions often involve action by the government on behalf of that population through legislation. At least some such actions are legitimate, because individuals cannot always create the relevant conditions to reduce harms to their health on their own. Arguably, this is the case in relation to smoking. Given the fact that such actions will be likely to restrict the actions of at least some individuals, is it appropriate to involve the public in formation of public health policy? If so, what is the best way to do so? Clearly care needs to be taken here. For example, disagreement is likely to exist in society on most policy issues, and the majority view is not necessarily the right view. Public health policy should take the public's views into account, but the 'public's view' cannot simply be applied as policy.[10]

In fact, there is not much evidence about people's attitudes to public health issues. What does exist suggests that people are willing to accept restrictions on their actions for the benefit of increased public health (although this differs depending upon the case to be considered). Interestingly, there is strong support for a ban on smoking in public places (from 68% of those surveyed).[5] Despite this both the recent UK Department of Health white paper on public health and the Wanless Report[11,12] rejected such a ban (at least for the moment). Presumably, this is because they are nervous about the implications of restricting individual liberty in this case. However, whilst a ban on smoking in public may be controversial, it is not obvious that it need be paternalistic, or even if it is, it might still be justifiable.

Conclusions

Public health is an area fraught with ethical issues because a common focus of public health activity is upon seeking to prevent harm and to change the behaviour of individuals or the environment. It will always help to bear this in mind and ask of any proposed action what the ethical issues are and how they should be addressed before the action is taken. However, in general, public health is concerned with the promotion of the health of populations. Whilst it must always be borne in mind that this might cause harm, it is also the source of much good.

Further resources

Anand S, Fabienne P, Sen A (2005) *Public health, ethics, and equity.* Oxford University Press, Oxford.

Beauchamp DE, Steinbock B (1999). *New ethics for the public's health.* Oxford University Press, Oxford.

Callahan D, Jennings B (2002). Ethics and public health: forging a strong relationship. *Am J Public Health,* **92**(2), 169–76.

Childress JF, Faden RR, Gaare RD *et al.* (2002). Public health ethics: mapping the terrain. *J Law Med Ethics,* **30**, 170–8.

Public Health Ethics Curriculum (linked to the Association of American Schools of Public Health). Available at: http://www.asph.org/document. cfm?page=723 (accessed 31 March 2005).

Verweij M (2000). *Preventive medicine: between obligation and aspiration.* Kluwer, Dordrecht.

References

1 Dawson A (2004). Vaccination and the prevention problem. *Bioethics,* **18**(6), 515–30.

2 Feinberg J (1973). *Social philosophy.* Prentice-Hall, Englewood Cliffs, NJ.

3 Department of Health (1998). *Smoking kills: a White Paper on tobacco.* The Stationary Office, London.

4 International Agency for Research on Cancer (2004). *Tobacco smoking and involuntary smoking,* IARC Monographs on the Evaluation of Carcinogenic Risks to Humans Vol. 83. IARC, Lyon.

5 King's Fund (2004). *Public attitudes to public health policy.* Kings Fund Publications, London.

6 BBC News (31 May 2004). *Ireland smoking ban a success.* Available at: http://news.bbc.co.uk/1/hi/business/3763471.stm (accessed 22 June 2005).

7 American Heart Association (22 October 2003). *New York city restaurant survey supports smoking ban.* Available at: www.americanheart. org/presenter.jhtml?identifier=3016321 (accessed: 22 June 2005).

8 Dawson A, Verweij M (eds). (2006) *Ethics, prevention and public health.* Oxford University Press, Oxford.

9 Beauchamp T, Childress J (2001). *Principles of biomedical ethics,* 5th edn. Oxford University Press, Oxford.

10 Dawson A (2005). Risk perceptions and ethical public health policy: MMR in the UK. *Poiesis and Praxis,* **3**(4), 229–41.

11 Department of Health (2004). *Choosing health: making healthy choices easier.* The Stationary Office, London.

12 Wanless D (2004). *Securing good health for the whole population.* HM Treasury, London.

1.8 Innovative ways to solve public health problems

J. A. Muir Gray

More of the same is not always the answer. More data, more staff, more analyses, more reports—these activities will not necessarily solve the problems faced by the public health professional. Different approaches to problem solving have been developed in other disciplines and can be used by public health professionals.

Resolving disputes using linguistic techniques

The public health professional is often entangled in endless debate where different individuals and organizations are arguing about what should be done about a particular problem such as health inequalities. Each party has their own argument, which they pursue with commitment and passion but make little progress. In this situation the public health professional can unlock problems and make progress by ensuring agreement on the terms being used and the propositions for change being put forward.

Agreeing to the meaning of terms

Much of the effort involved in solving problems, and sometimes all of the reasons for failing to do so, is due to the failure to define the terms being used. Words such as 'plan' and 'strategy', or 'consulting' and 'engaging', to take commonly used verbs, as well as nouns such as 'inequality' and 'inequity', can be a source of confusion, impair problem solving, and may become a problem in their own right unless steps are taken to reach a common understanding of the way in which the term will be used in this particular public health context. This is best done not by consulting the *Shorter Oxford English Dictionary*, although this, and Last's *Dictionary of Epidemiology*[1], can help, but by asking all the key stakeholders to work together to develop the meaning that will be used, for example by:

- assembling key stakeholders
- asking them to work in pairs for 3 minutes to agree the words that they associate with the term being discussed; the term 'quality', for example, could elicit the words 'standards', 'goodness', 'efficiency', and 'safety'
- writing these on a board or flip chart

- asking the stakeholders to group the words into sets. 'Standards' and 'goodness' emerge as being central to the meaning of quality—at this stage a definition such as that developed by Avedis Donabedian 'the quality of a service is the degree to which it conforms to preset standards of goodness'[2]—can be introduced. 'Efficiency' and 'safety' can then be pointed out as being aspects of a service, each of which can have its quality appraised
- writing down the meaning developed and agreed by the group.

Sometimes it is necessary to take steps to discontinue the use of a term which is consistently and frequently the cause of confusion and as such prevents understanding and progress. This is less frequently necessary in management than in clinical practice because management decision-making involves many terms which are created and enter widespread use until they themselves become displaced by later fashions. 'Benchmarking' and 'modernizing' are examples of such terms, and the same fate may, heaven forefend, befall 'evidence-based decision-making', but if it does cause more confusion than clarity then it should be dropped from decision-making discourse. Even in clinical practice, however, terms can cause confusion and may need to be deleted from debate.

In his highly praised biography, Ray Monk[3] describes how Ludwig Wittgenstein, when a technician in a research laboratory in Guy's Hospital in 1941, joined a Medical Research Council team whose leader had observed that 'there is in practice a wide variation in the application of the diagnosis of "shock" without an agreed meaning of the term' which was harmful to patients and 'renders it impossible to assess the efficacy of the various methods of treatment adopted'. He argued that 'there is good ground, therefore' for the view that it is better to avoid the diagnosis of 'shock' and to replace it by an accurate and complete record of a patient's state and progress, together with the treatment given.

Clarifying the meaning of propositions

It is not only single terms that cause confusion; sometimes the problem is created by failure to agree the meaning of propositions, for example, 'community engagement will increase the sense of empowerment of those whose health is worst'. Resolution of this type of problem is best done not by analysis of the individual words but by using the techniques developed by the logical positivists and most clearly articulated by A. J. Ayer:[4]

> The criteria which we use to test the genuineness of apparent statements of fact is the criterion of verifiability. We say that a sentence is factually significant to any given person, if, and only if, he knows how to verify the propositions which it purports to express – that is, if he knows what observations would lead him, under certain conditions, to accept the proposition as being true, or reject it as being false. And with regard to questions the procedure is the same. We enquire in every case what observations would lead us to answer the question, one way or the other; and, if none can be discovered, we must conclude that the sentence under consideration does not, as far as we are concerned, express a genuine question, however strongly its grammatical appearance may suggest that it does.

The logical positivists believe that no term should be examined in isolation—a study of the term 'efficiency' would be pointless—but investigated in the context of propositions, such as 'this hospital is more efficient than that hospital'. To define the meaning of this proposition, a logical positivist would not have recourse to a dictionary but instead seek to agree on the data that would need to be collected to confirm or refute it. Thus, for this particular proposition, the debate immediately becomes: 'How would you measure efficiency?'

The meaning of propositions can be elucidated by:

- asking stakeholders to work in pairs for 3 minutes
- recording the criteria suggested on a flip chart or board
- asking the group to assess the validity and feasibility of each criterion to agree how the impact, if any, of the proposed change could be measured.

This approach can irritate those whose basic training is in the social sciences because they may see this as a positivist, reductionist, or medical approach. It is therefore sensible, and correct, to adapt this approach not only for vaguer statements but also for propositions that appear to be self-evident, such as, 'our objective is to reduce the prevalence of smoking'.

Resolving linguistic differences can solve many public health problems, but significant obstacles can remain because the different disciplines that have to combine to solve a public health problem can have different views of reality.

Resolving multiple realities

Reality is a social construct.[5] What a person takes as reality is constructed by their upbringing and their professional training and created by the language they use. The view of reality held by the professionals and the public involved in tackling the problem is determined by their world view: to the anthropologist the problem is one of cultures and beliefs; to the sociologist the problem is one of social class or gender; to the politician the problem is one of values and beliefs; and to the community worker the problem is one of empowerment and disadvantage.

The public health professional needs to reconcile these views, and one method is to use the metaphor of the lens. Each professional can be asked to describe how the problem looks through their lens. This metaphor is better than using the metaphor of 'the model'. The model, for example, 'the public health model', implies that the reality must fit the model; the lens implies that there is a focus on part of a whole, just as the lens in an optician's spectacle frame may be placed in front of other lenses, each focusing on a part of the whole.

A second technique is to use John Rawl's 'veil of ignorance',[6] that is, to ask each professional to look through the veil of ignorance to imagine they do not know who they will be in the next life, imagining if possible that they are powerless and poor, rather than seeing the problem through their confident view of reality. For this approach to be successful requires each professional to accept not only that they have a biased view of a problem but also that the reality of the problem that they see is itself constructed by their concepts and described by their esoteric language.

For some professionals, however, such admissions prove very difficult to accept and they may need help to leave their secure certainty that they understand the reality of the situation. Storytelling can help.

Narrative-based public health

A story can help an individual or group leave a fixed position.

Age brings some consolation for the public health professional because the number of personal stories of successes (and, even more useful, failures) accumulates. If there is not an apposite personal story then the stories of others can be used, and two excellent sources are the collections of anthropologic essays on public health failures: *Health, Culture and Community* by Benjamin Paul[7] and *Anthropology in Public Health* by Robert A. Hahn[8].

The content of the story is important but so too is the manner of its telling. Even more so than when giving a talk or lecture, the objective must be to induce a state of trance in the audience. Trance induction can be brought about by the tone of voice and by the choice of words, and should start with the opening sentence. In a shared state the individual professionals can safely leave their bunkers and mingle in a common understanding of a problem and are more likely to find the means of mitigation, if not solving the problem. The use of theatre could also be useful and might play a part in helping a whole community come to terms with a problem and its solution, but such an approach requires a major commitment of resources. Mild trance induction, on the other hand, is relatively easy to achieve with practice, although the public health professional must have sufficient insight to be able to distinguish between trance induction and sleep induction.

References

1 Last JM (2001). *A dictionary of epidemiology*. 4th edn. Oxford University Press, New York.
2 Donabedian A (1980). The definition of quality: a conceptual exploration. In: *Explorations in quality assessment and monitoring. Volume I: The definition of quality and approaches to its assessment*. Health Administration Press, Ann Arbor, MI.
3 Monk R (1991). *Ludwig Wittgenstein: the duty of genius*. Vintage, London.
4 Ayer AJ (1936). *Language, truth and logic*. Penguin, London.
5 Berger PL, Luckman T (1967). *The social construction of reality*. Anchor Books, New York.
6 Rawls J (1971). *A theory of justice*. Harvard University Press, Boston, MA.
7 Paul B (1955). *Health, culture and community*. The Sage Foundation, New York.
8 Hahn RA (1999). *Anthropology in public health*. Oxford University Press, Oxford.

Introduction

If public health is the science and art of improving the health of populations, then measuring health status and assessing the health needs of populations are the universal starting points for most of its activities.

This part assumes a basic knowledge of epidemiological principles, and aims to link these to the challenges faced in public health practice. (Chapter 2.3 provides a refresher or an introduction to epidemiological principles for public health practitioners.)

In Chapter 2.1 we explore public health information, especially quantitative information—essentially involving counts, either of people at risk, of health events, of people with a disease, or of outcomes. This is complemented by a chapter outlining the principles, practice, and value of qualitative research (Chapter 2.2). Both forms of information are essential to most public health efforts, and in practice combining these approaches is almost always desirable.

Public health work would be much easier if the qualities and quantities it dealt with were clear-cut, binary states. In practice, risks, diseases, and outcomes are complex and dimensional. Clinicians are used to categorizing people as either having or not having conditions, but in practice the boundaries of almost all diseases are unclear, and a full range of severity exists from the hardly perceptible to the catastrophic. Establishing what will be counted as a 'case' and what will be excluded is an essential step, yet the precise boundaries can have enormous impacts on the numbers included. The somewhat arbitrary nature of the definitions of the boundaries of health states results in much of the variability in routinely collected data: without meticulous definition and attention, classification errors and biases abound.

Many health issues are fairly stable over time and can be satisfactorily dealt with through special studies or routinely collected data. However, some health challenges require specific data collection systems linked to mechanisms for taking early public health action. Chapters 2.4–2.6 cover three important areas of public health information: basic surveillance of risk factors and disease, the general skills in investigating unexpected changes in occurrence, and the specific issue if managing an apparent cluster.

Chapter 2.7 explores the world of registries, specifically cancer registries, forcing us to ask ourselves fundamental questions about their rationale, core function, the specific ways in which they help, and some myths about registries.

Assessing the health status of a population (Chapter 2.8) and summarizing population health (Chapter 2.9) are two important core activities. Summarizing health is increasingly important, as even now the general population appreciates the importance of quality, not just quantity, of life.

The final three chapters of this part deal with some of the most challenging quantitative issues facing public health practitioners in the twenty-first century. Although average health has improved in many countries around the world, this increase in average health is not matched by a decrease in the health inequalities. In fact a typical picture is for health to improve and health inequalities widen. The first step in addressing this is to develop valid and consistent methods for measuring and monitoring inequalities and inequities (Chapter 2.10). The penultimate chapter deals with some of the technical issues that need to be developed in order to find and appraise research evidence. The last chapter addresses the important issue of how we deliver and contextualize data, information, and evidence for the practitioner and policy maker, crucially in ways that suit the end user.

Throughout this part of the handbook, both the technical issues and the managerial or procedural issues are discussed. Sound information and concern for data quality and accurate analysis are part of the core scientific skills of public health practice. However, public health goes beyond analysis, and seeks to make a difference in the real world—from analysis to action. As a result, political, managerial, and procedural issues are central to the public health endeavour. Involving all stakeholders, especially patients and the public, helps to build an informed and active constituency to drive change. Nothing is more frustrating than completing a technically fine analysis of a public health problem only to find it ignored by those in a position to act. However logical the analysis, however technically correct the proposed action, nothing will happen without the support of the decision-makers and their public—winning emotional involvement in public health analysis is vital. Throughout this part, advice and checklists are offered to maximize the chances of achieving change.

DP

2.1 Understanding data, information, and knowledge

Barry Tennison

Objectives

The aim of this chapter is to help the public health practitioner to:
- appreciate the subtleties of the varied forms of information about the health of a population and related matters
- develop a toolkit for thinking about the complexity of information and its uses
- orientate themselves positively towards the decisions and actions needed, applying wisely and with good Judgement the information and knowledge available.

The classification (taxonomy) of types of information given in this chapter should help the public health practitioner to:
- assess the relevance, timeliness, accuracy, and completeness of available information
- decide which types of information are most appropriate for a particular public health task
- make optimal use of information which is not ideal, and assess the effects of its departure from perfection.

The use of the words 'data' and 'information'

Some people are purists. They will use the word 'data' (singular or plural) for raw numbers or other measures, reserving the word 'information' for what emerges when data are processed, analyzed, interpreted, and presented. This has the virtue of making clear the sequence of steps that are involved in turning observations about the world into a form that is useful to those who wish to draw conclusions, and to act. This always involves the use of Judgement in assessing the information as a source of evidence (alongside other evidence), and combining this judiciously with accepted best practice to arrive at usable knowledge. This process is summarized in Figure 2.1.1.

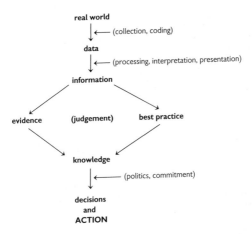

Figure 2.1.1 From reality to action

In practice, many people use 'data' and 'information' more or less interchangeably, perhaps on the grounds of the greyness of some of these distinctions and steps. However, in assessing the value of what emerges as information from these steps, the practitioner must bear in mind the fundamental issues which affect the quality of the data:

- *Validity*: are the data capturing the concept or quantity the practitioner intends? Are the definitions and methods of data collection explicit and clear?
- *Selection bias*: where the data mislead because they are not representative of the population or problem being considered, for example because of poor sampling.
- *Classification bias*: where there is a non-random effect on putting data into groupings, for example in non-blind assessments of health outcome.
- *Statistical significance*: where, although differences seem apparent, analysis shows that they are reasonably likely to have occurred by chance (see, for example, Marshall and Spiegelhalter[1]).

What kinds of data sources are there?

In most countries, there are many different sources of information on the health of the population.[2] Different types of information vary in their 'CART': Completeness, Accuracy, Relevance (and/or Representativeness), Timeliness.

Data sources also vary in the ease with which a 'base population' can be identified, for use in the denominator, or for calculating rates. Typical data sources for local areas are summarized in Table 2.1.1.

Table 2.1.1 Data sources

Source	Strengths	Weaknesses
1. Routine data sources		
Population estimates. Census or population registers	Usually reasonably accurate, especially if complemented by local authority (UK) or other government data	May be problems with small area estimates, especially between censuses
Birth/abortion notifications	Reasonably accurate—often several possible data sources	No complete data on spontaneous abortions. Sometimes non-standard coding used
Mortality records	Most reliable health data as death tends to be unequivocal. Total mortality reliable	Insensitive measure of health. Physician's cause of death specification often inaccurate/incomplete. Non-fatal disease not reflected in mortality figures
Morbidity measures: infectious disease notifications (see Chapter 2.4)	Certain diseases notifiable (mandatory). Generally adequate for monitoring trends	Often incomplete, sometimes inconsistently incomplete
Morbidity measures: disease registers (see Chapter 2.7)	Key group identified. Often don't cover whole country	May miss people due to no contact or non identification
Impairment, disability and handicap	Functional status often more relevant than disease status	Usually available from surveys only
Health services data: access and supply, utilization, activity, costs	May be potentially relevant especially if condition almost always results in health-care use, e.g. fractured femur	Likely to be incomplete. Data tend to identify health service activity and settings rather than receipt of (effective) interventions. Data quality may be poor
Data from other agencies—social care, housing, environmental risks, etc	May be relevant	May be poor quality. May be incomplete. Categories and definitions may be incompatible with other data
2. Surveys (see Chapter 2.8)		
National surveys, or surveys from other countries	Available. May be authoritative and highly relevant	Require 'modelling' to local population characteristic. May not be generalizable to local population. Quality variable
Previous local surveys	Relevant and usually appeal to a local audience	Quality variable
Local surveys to be commissioned	Can be tailor-made	Often expensive
3. Qualitative data		
Local descriptive accounts of environmental or social factors	May give a good understanding or stimulate research	The scale of health impact of identified problems may be difficult to assess
People's perceptions of how health problems affect them	May give a good understanding of what really affects people	Qualitative data can need careful handling, as details of context, background, and question wording can result in unstable responses

A 'population health information' system can help in assembling data sources on a population. Such systems often involve a partnership between different agencies involved with a population, and can allow coordination of health information activities. A comprehensive population health information system would ideally record both:

- personal health *events*—health-related occurrences or states pertaining to an identified person (examples are myocardial infarction or smoking status) and
- population health *factors*—health-related features or occurrences that apply to a population defined by some combination of person, time, and place (examples are exposure of a defined population to a health risk like a toxic spill or prevalence of smoking in teenage girls in a specified locality, derived from a survey)

Such a system would also allow both routine and *ad hoc* analyses in such a way that both events and factors are linked.

What does the information describe?

Information about the health of a population can cover:

1. *Demography*: the basic characteristics of the population, such as age, sex, geographic distribution, and mobility.
2. *Health-related characteristics or risk factors*, such as measures of deprivation, living conditions, employment, housing, or more medical factors or physiologic measurements (e.g. blood glucose levels).
3. *Health need data*, such as the distribution of the indications for an intervention such as hip replacement[3] or the distribution of different thresholds for intervention.
4. *Mortality*: the death experience of the population, including causes of death and variation according to the dimensions of person, place, and time.
5. *Morbidity*: the health or illness experience of the population, including prevalence and incidence of diseases.
6. *Health service use data*, such as diagnoses, interventions and procedures, and health outcomes of interventions; it may be useful to distinguish patient interactions with *agents* such as nurses or doctors from their use of *settings* such as hospital, day hospital, health centre, or home in using the health service.
7. *Health economic data*, often concerning the costs of interventions, and the distribution of activity and costs at marginal or average levels.

Clarity and judgement are needed about when one of these types of data is being used as a *proxy* for another. For example, where mortality data are firm and morbidity data poor in quality, with care, mortality may be seen as a good proxy for morbidity—this might work well for certain kinds of heart disease or cancer but very poorly for most mental health problems. Similarly, care is needed in moving from burden of disease (mortality, morbidity, or even more carefully, health service use) to health *need*.

In terms of how it is collected, assembled, and made available, information can be either:

- *Routine*: collected, assembled, and made available repeatedly, according to well-defined protocols and standards; such data are usually part of a

system of data collection by which information is:
- made available at regular intervals
- intended to allow tracking over time
- codified according to national or international standards (for example, using the International Classification of Diseases (ICD[4])).

- *Specially collected*: for a particular purpose, without the intention of regular repetition or adherence to standards (other than those needed for the specific study or task); such data are usually:
  - aimed at a specific, time-limited study or task
  - codified according to the task in hand and the wishes of the investigators (sometimes in ignorance of the availability of suitable standard codes and methods)
  - difficult to compare (between times, places, and people) with routine data and other specially collected data.

Most of the data published in medical journals fall in the category 'specially collected'.

Table 2.1.2 gives important examples of information according to these dimensions. Note that these are only *examples*, but the table may help to see where an existing, new, or proposed data source sits, and the corresponding opportunities and drawbacks.

Table 2.1.2 Information collected according to the dimensions 'routine' and 'specially collected'

	Routine data	**Specially collected data**
Demography	Census counts, birth registration	Survey of homeless, roofless, and rough sleepers
Risk factors	Census details, such as housing conditions	Survey of ethnicity and coronary risk factors. Local survey of tobacco use
Mortality	Death registration, coroner's records, medical examiner's records	Some cohort studies which capture deaths search for deaths probably due to suicide, using multiple sources
Morbidity	National health surveys (such as the Health Survey for England[12] or the National Health Interview Survey in the USA[13]). Disease notifications and registers	Case finding for an outbreak. Survey to establish prevalence of a specific disease. Most cohort studies
Health need	(mainly proxies)	Survey of prevalence of indications for specific intervention, such as hip replacement
Service use	Use of in-patient beds. Attendances at out-patient department, emergency room, or physician's office	Observational study of use of a hospital department. Follow-up study of outcomes of hip replacement
Economic	Accounts of health service organizations. Cost and price tables[14,15]	Costing of an existing or proposed service

Classification of intrinsic types of data

It is sometimes useful to categorize data as hard or soft (Table 2.1.3). In fact, there is a spectrum from 'hard' to 'soft' data: data are never completely hard or soft.

Table 2.1.3 Examples of data considered to be harder or softer

	Harder	Softer
Demography	Ethnic breakdown of a population according to a given ethnic classification. Proportion of houses with a specific amenity (e.g. a bath)	Narrative account of nature and composition of a neighborhood
Risk factors	Blood pressure. Proportion of smokers, non-smokers, and ex-smokers (according to precise definitions)	Patient experience of symptoms. Smoking 'careers' of teenagers
Mortality	Numbers dying of a specific disease. Survival data after specific interventions	Impact of deaths on the survivors
Morbidity	Prevalence of disease in a population at a moment in time. Numbers of admissions to a particular hospital	Reasons why a family doctor refers patients to hospital. Reported quality of treatment given by a particular hospital

Harder data tend to be:
- precise (or intended to be precise)
- often numerical; if not, then coded according to a firm protocol
- reproducible, and likely to be similar even if the data collectors or individuals studied are varied.

Softer data tend to be:
- qualitative, attempting to capture some of the subtlety of human experience
- often narrative or textual in form, at least as they are collected
- imbued with some subjectivity, due to the complexity of the personalities of the data collectors and the individuals studied.

(Note that some people will use the term 'soft' when they wish to imply that the data have inherent tendencies to imprecision, even if they are 'hard' in the sense of being numeric or strongly coded.)

Neither hard nor soft data are intrinsically better than the other. The utility of the information (in terms of better decision-making) often comes from combining the two:
- harder data usually allow more precise analysis and comparisons, but may fail to capture subtleties of human experience and preferences
- softer data usually capture more of the 'truth' about the world, but often at the expense of emphasizing the uniqueness of circumstances, rather than aiding comparisons and conclusions.

The important thing to assess is *fitness for purpose*: are the existing or proposed data fit for the purpose for which they are intended, the conclusion to be drawn, the decision to be made, or the action to be taken? For example, for deciding the allocation of resources, one requires relatively hard data to obtain a degree of precision and transparency, so that the Judgements involved are explicit. On the other hand, soft data may be useful in deciding on a change in the pattern of services provided, for example when a client population (such as teenagers) seems to make poor use of current services: a well-designed qualitative survey may reveal some of the reasons, and a potential service configuration response. Softer data are also essential when capturing patient preference[5] or professional experiences[6,7].

Absolute and comparative information

Often data about one location, one time, or one population are difficult to interpret in isolation; or worse, seem to beg obvious conclusions when, in fact, *comparison* with similar data elsewhere, previously, or in another population suggests a different conclusion or decision.

Comparative data are available on a local, regional, national,[8] or international[9] level. The WHO publishes comparative data between countries, for example on comparative performance of health systems.[10]

Assessing the appropriateness and usefulness of particular information

Experience shows the truth of the adage that the information you think you want is seldom the information you actually need; and the information you have seldom matches either need or want [often attributed to Finagle: in full, Finagle's law is often quoted thus 'The information you have is not what you want; the information you want is not what you need; the information you need is not what you can get; the information you can get costs more than you want to pay' (or a variation thereof)]. The pragmatic public health practitioner must learn to cope with what is possible, not to set impossible standards, and to make the appropriate allowances, professionally, for shortcomings of the available information. Above all, public health practitioners must not allow themselves or others to despair and to declare tasks impossible without the necessary information (which is in fact unavailable or infeasible).

Below is a checklist of issues to consider when assessing data or a data source for fitness for purpose. None of these issues is absolute, and the balance of advantage and disadvantage must be assessed using judgement.

Checklist for assessing appropriateness and usefulness of data and data sources

Technical issues:
- Are the definitions sufficiently clear and appropriate?
- Are the target and study populations sufficiently clear?
- Are the data collection methods sufficiently clear and sound?
- How complete, accurate, relevant, and timely are the data? How much does this matter?
- Do any differences that appear reach statistical significance, and what are the confidence limits or intervals? (consider the use of a Bayesian approach[11]).

Issues relating to the conclusion or decision involved:
- Is the study population sufficiently representative of the target population for the purpose of the decision or proposed action?
- Do we need absolute or relative estimates to make the best decision?
- What precision is needed for the decision (taking into account confounding factors, random variation, and the influence of external factors such as resource availability, professional opinion, and politics)?
- Would a simpler or existing data source suffice, for example by using comparative data; by extrapolating or interpolating, with care; or by transferring data from a similar or analogous situation?
- Would qualitative information suffice (or be best), when habit automatically suggests quantitative data?

Conclusion

All too often, when faced with a decision, there is a call for more information (or worse, a new information system). Frequently, either the available data are in fact, with care and interpretation, fit for the purpose for the decision needed; or the costs (including money, skills, burden of effort, and delay) of the new information or system is not commensurable with the problem faced. The above checklist, and this chapter, should help the practitioner to find a pragmatic but wise balance between what is needed and what is feasible and adequate.

Further resources

Health Canada Online. http://www.hc-sc.gc.ca/english/ (accessed 29 March 2005).

Rigby M (ed.) (2004). *Vision and value in health information*. Radcliffe Medical Press, Oxford.

UK National Electronic Library for Health. http://www.nelh.nhs.uk/ (accessed 29 March 2005).

US Department of Health & Human Services. http://www.os.dhhs.gov/reference/index.shtml (accessed 29 March 2005).

References

1 Marshall EC, Spiegelhalter DJ (1998). Reliability of league tables of in vitro fertilisation clinics: retrospective analysis of live birth rates. *BMJ*, **316**, 1701–5.

2 Detels R, McEwen J, Beaglehole R, Tanaka H (eds) (2002). *Oxford textbook of public health*. Oxford University Press, New York.

3 Frankel S, Eachus J, Pearson N *et al.* (1999). Population requirement for primary hip-replacement surgery: a cross-sectional study. *Lancet*, **353**(9161), 1304–9.

4 World Health Organization. *The WHO family of international classifications*. Available at: http://www.who.int/classifications/en/ (accessed 20 March 2005).

5 Silvestri G, Pritchard R, Welch HG (1998). Preferences for chemotherapy in patients with advanced non-small cell lung cancer: descriptive study based on scripted interviews. *BMJ*, **317**, 771–5.

6 Jain A, Ogden J (1999). General practitioners' experiences of patients' complaints: qualitative study. *BMJ*, **318**, 1596–9.

7 Dowie R (1983). *General practitioners and consultants: a study of outpatient referrals*. King Edward's Hospital Fund for London, London.

8 National Statisitics, Official UK statistics. Available at: http://www.statistics.gov.uk (accessed 20 March 2005); Statistics Canada, Canadian statistics. Available at: http://www40.statcan.ca/z01/cs0002_e.htm (accessed 8 September 2005); National Centre for Health Statistics, US statistics. Available at: http://www.cdc.gov/nchs/ (accessed 21 March 2005).

9 World Health Organization. *WHO Statistical Information System (WHOSIS)*. Available at: http://www.who.int/whosis/ (accessed 21 March 2005).

10 World Health Organization. *Health systems performance*. Available at: http://www. who.int/health-systems-performance/ (accessed 21 March 2005).

11 Spiegelhalter DJ, Myles JP, Jones DR, Abrams KR (1999). Methods in health service research: an introduction to Bayesian methods in health technology assessment. *BMJ*, **319**, 508–12.

12 Department of Health. *Health Survey for England*. Available at: http://www.dh.gov.uk/PublicationsAndStatistics/PublishedSurvey/HealthSurveyForEngland/fs/en (accessed 20 March 2005).

13 National Centre for Health Statistics. *National Health Interview Survey (NHIS)*. Available at: www.cdc.gov/nchs/nhis.htm (accessed 20 March 2005).

14 Department of Health. *Reference costs*. Available at: http://www.dh.gov.uk/PolicyAndGuidance/OrganisationPolicy/FinanceAndPlanning/NHSReferenceCosts/ (accessed 21 January 2006).

15 Centre s for Medicare & Medicaid Services. *Cost reports*. Available at: http://www.cms.hhs.gov/CostReports/ (accessed 21 January 2006).

2.2 Using qualitative methods

Tom Ling

Objective of this chapter

The purpose of this chapter is to identify the main techniques of qualitative analysis, to identify when to use them, and to indicate how to take these skills further.

What is qualitative research?

Qualitative research explores experiences, attitudes, values, emotions, and practices and locates these within their social context. It recognizes that human beings in their daily lives make sense of the world and it seeks to understand the meanings they create. Implicitly, if not explicitly, it is assumed that the way that people make sense of the world matters because it helps to explain their behaviour, choices, relationships, and so on. It can therefore tell us about situations as varied as policy-making, prescribing, use of new technology in health care, or decisions about exercise. It gives us rich and complex accounts of human agency in its social context. Typically, it aims to provide 'in depth' insights rather than 'broadly' based analysis of parts of, or whole, populations.

Quantitative and qualitative research

Qualitative research is sometimes defined in opposition to quantitative methods (e.g. see p.60 of Blaxter's book[1]). This is unfortunate for two reasons. First, it is not very helpful to define something by what it isn't. The practical consequence of this is that researchers might tend to see qualitative research as a second best only to be used when the numbers are not available. Secondly, and more importantly, quantitative and qualitative research are not opposing disciplines but are part of a continuum of research methodologies and are very often used in conjunction with each other. For example, there is an area of quantitative research which is also concerned with attitudes, beliefs, and so on. This includes attitudinal surveys, 'tick box' questionnaires, and Delphi methods which are usually described as quantitative approaches because they try to use quantitative measures to identify strengths of feeling, or preferences, or percentages who agree with a certain statement. They are, however, often trying to get at similar sorts of questions (although trying to understand general characteristics of whole populations). In practice, policy-makers and practitioners increasingly feel more comfortable when offered both quantitative and qualitative evidence on such matters. Qualitative research can sometimes also have an emotional impact that quantitative research lacks (a tradition of research that goes back at least to Engels' *Conditions of the Working Class in England*).

Combining quantitative and qualitative data

Despite the often complementary practices of qualitative and quantitative research, it is worth noting that there can be different ontologic and epistemologic claims underlying these approaches. This suggests that care should be taken before simply adding together quantitative and qualitative data and analyses. Briefly, qualitative approaches often emphasize a constructivist ontology, seeing evidence about social life as being 'constructed' through the meanings that individuals create as they engage in dialog with others.[2] For the qualitative researcher it is therefore often important to see the social act in its 'natural' setting rather than conduct an experiment or complete a survey. Epistemologically, 'truth' about the world is discovered by interpreting the meanings of these dialogues and, at least to some degree, requires the researcher to make sense of the way that others interpret the world. This contrasts with a tendency for quantitative approaches to claim that they are identifying evidence about a population that is 'objective', and that knowledge can be created by building theories based upon this 'independent' evidence.[3]

How does qualitative research help public health practice?

As John Gabbay has put it 'The academic base for public health is necessarily eclectic and broad-ranging'.[4] Methods and skills need to be developed that are fit for the diverse needs of the public health practitioner. This has given the public health tradition both its eclecticism (or even 'disarray') and its dynamism.

It is important to use qualitative methods only to address qualitative questions. For example, implementing a healthy eating or smoking cessation campaign requires an understanding of how people want information to be made available, how to influence behaviour, and why previous campaigns have or have not worked. It would be appropriate, therefore, to discover how the target audiences makes sense of the world, how they shop, how they make choices and prioritize, and why they might change their behaviour. Quantitative approaches, for example using a survey or a questionnaire, would be very helpful in getting an understanding of certain dimensions of this problem; typically questions which begin with 'how often', 'how many', 'what proportion', and so on. Quantitative data would, for example, help us to understand how large the potential population is and to divide this population into relevant groups in order to target messages more effectively. However, knowing how many people belong to a group might not tell us enough about the motivations and values of that group. For example, it might not explain why some people react positively to a campaign and others do not.

In looking at how children make choices about diet, it is helpful to spend time in a school playground or dining room observing when and how food is eaten. Observations might be supplemented by asking children to keep a diary or running in-depth interviews (individually or in groups) with children based upon the initial findings to see how they reflect upon their own behaviour and views and those of others around them. Hopefully this would provide a better understanding of the complex context within which children actually make decisions about what to eat. A strong case can be made for combining this sort of qualitative data with quantitative research.

What tools are available to the qualitative researcher?

The domains of qualitative research each examine meaningful social behaviour in its social setting. Practically, this usually involves examining one or more of the following:

- what people say and do in their 'natural' settings
- what people say when researchers ask them questions about their world views and behaviour
- what people write about their world in reports, plans, diaries, historic documents, newspapers, and so on.

Each of these domains has associated research tools.

What do people say and do in their 'natural' settings?

The main techniques used to find out what people actually do are *ethnography* and *participant observation*. To a greater or lesser extent, this involves researchers in immersing themselves in the social context of the things being researched (see p.137 of Devine[5]). The technique has its origins in anthropology and the study of pre-industrial society (Malinowski's study of the Trobriand Islands is a classic example) and it was then applied to contemporary industrialized settings, especially in the United States, by researchers such as Herbert Bloomer, Howard Becker, and Erving Goffman.

Covert and overt research

Before starting this sort of work key choices must be made. First, the researcher must choose between *covert* and overt work. In covert research, those being researched do not know that research is being conducted. This brings some advantages but significant disadvantages (see p.296 of Bryman[6]). On the one hand, it removes the need to negotiate access and it ensures a 'natural' response from those being observed. On the other hand, there are practical problems of how to take notes, the danger of being uncovered, and ethical problems based on the invasion of privacy and failing to ensure that human subjects in research give informed consent. Using a practice from marketing, some researchers into public services have advocated the use of 'mystery shoppers' as a way of covertly observing how services are functioning (although the level of cultural understanding required in this technique is often limited). Ethical concerns do not necessarily 'trump' all other worries but in practice it is often decisive in pushing researchers towards overt research, and even 'mystery shopping' raises significant concerns over privacy (and damage to the reputation) of those being researched.

Overt observation/ethnography requires access to be secured. This might be formal (a letter to the chief executive of the organization, for example) or informal (a group of young people who are being researched have to accept the researcher). The next problem is how involved or detached to be. According to Gold's famous classification[7] the researcher must choose where to sit on a continuum from complete participation to complete observation. To a degree, this will be determined by questions of legality and propriety (for example, researchers cannot participate as surgeons if they are not trained to do so), but there are many examples of successful research being conducted at each point along this continuum and it may be worth noting that the complete observer is less obtrusive than might be imagined—people soon learn to ignore the researcher in the corner scribbling his or her field notes. There is a further potential problem which arises when the research is into illegal activities (recreational drug use, for example) which can involve the researcher in illegal acts. As with all such ethical issues there is a need to balance the potential benefit of the research with the concerns for the researcher and those being researched.

Sampling

The next task is to identify *an appropriate sample* or case. In practice this is often begun by intuitively identifying a group to 'hang out with' with and then being introduced to others by a process known as 'snowballing' where the researcher is introduced to friends and acquaintances (see p.16 of Taylor[8] for a good example of this). This approach is widely regarded as a perfectly legitimate approach, but in public health there may be concerns about the apparently random nature of the contacts made. Another approach is to collect data systematically and inductively derive a theory. Then, when sufficient data have been collected, the original theoretic assumptions may be reassessed, new theoretic claims be developed, and more data collected. This is therefore an iterative process, known as 'grounded theory' because the theory is 'grounded' in the data. The search for data is not random but nor does it claim to be based on statistical sampling. Instead it is referred to as theoretic sampling (which can refer to people, events, or processes):

> Theoretical sampling is done in order to discover categories and their properties and to suggest the interrelationships into a theory. Statistical sampling is done to obtain evidence on distributions of people among categories to be used in descriptions and verifications.
>
> Glaser and Strauss[9] p.62

For more on theoretic sampling and grounded theory start with Chapter 14 of Bryman[6] and go on to Strauss and Corbin[10] and Charmaz.[11] However, even theoretic sampling is open to the criticism that the data are atypical and both approaches use non-probabilistic sampling when selecting case studies.

This leaves a crucial question hanging: how do we know when sufficient data have been collected so that we can assess and adapt our theoretic claims? The answer builds on the intuition that if the researcher is repeatedly told the same thing by a wide range of participants then eventually it is assumed that this carries enough weight to make it part of the researcher's working assumptions (at least until proved differently). More formally, a category is said to be saturated with data when the continuing fieldwork produces no new data, when the (theoretically) relevant properties of the object of study have been fully explored, and when the interrelationships between the category and other relevant categories have been identified and validated (see p.212 of Strauss and Corbin[10]). For example, imagine a study examining the impact on patient compliance examining a nurse prescriber communicating in a novel way about patients' prescriptions. The key categories might be the communication of information, the recollection and attitude of patients, and the evidence that the patient has complied. The theory might be that providing the information in at least three different ways (say oral, written, and backed up by telephone) supports higher levels of compliance. The fieldwork would explore both the context and practice. Consistent confirming evidence would not prove (in a positivist sense) the theory but it would build up strong supporting evidence and theoretic saturation would be reached when no new evidence was forthcoming.

Field notes
Once access has been secured the next problem is to collect data. It is accepted that observers cannot collect 'purely' objective facts but it is expected that they should reflect on their own assumptions and attitudes and be clear about these to themselves and to those reading the research. For example, researchers should reflect on the dangers of 'going native' (see Lee-Treweek[12]). The data collection takes the form of field notes. This typically involves taking as many notes as possible (and acceptable) at the time they take place and then at least once a day writing these up as completely as possible. Notes can also be made to a dictaphone and then transcribed. Photographs may also be very helpful. Typically field notes both describe what the ethnographer took to be happening (an expression often used in field notes is 'I took this to mean . . . ') and may also include an effort to explain how the ethnographer felt about these events in an effort to indicate how the subjective views of the researcher will (inevitably) shape the field notes. The effort is not to achieve pure 'objectivity' but, rather, to achieve some disengagement and reflexivity. (For more on taking field notes in a medical setting, see Atkinson[13]).

Conversation analysis
Researchers are interested in what people say in a context where people are in a conversation (such as phoning NHS Direct). The latter case can

be used to produce transcripts and analysed like other qualitative data (see below) or can be analysed through conversation analysis (CA).

Conversation analysis is a detailed description and analysis of a conversation, including not only what was said but also noting pauses, breaths, and emphases. It therefore provides us with fine-grained accounts of conversations. In public health this might, for example, help us to analyse what happens when someone contacts the health-care system, a clinician gives advice, or information is provided. However, CA practitioners insist that meaning is embedded in the conversation and they are reluctant to make wider claims. However, a more relaxed approach might use it to reveal how interruptions, embarrassment, confusion, or anxieties manifest themselves in conversations in ways which inhibit effective communication. (For more on how this might be applied in a health setting, see Silverman[14].)

What do people say when researchers ask them questions?

Qualitative researchers spend a lot of time asking questions to individuals or groups. While more quantitative approaches often ask respondents to tick boxes, to rank, or to scale, more qualitative interviews and groupwork are more open ended. They are rarely completely unstructured, however, and will typically be 'guided', 'facilitated', or 'moderated'. The most frequently used techniques are the face-to-face interview and the focus group.

The interview

Interviewees should be selected because they have something useful to say about the thing being investigated. This might be because they have some privileged access to information and understanding, and we often refer to these as key informant interviews. Usually this is because of their role. For example, we might interview the directors of medical research units to understand how they think that research is best translated into improvements in medical practice. But it might also be because they have had an important experience of an event or process. Also key informants might be key academics who have studied the issue at length (although increasingly the preference is for a systematic literature review rather than one academic's view). In addition to key informants, we might want to interview people who in some sense are typical users or providers of a service. However, being 'typical' here means that they have had some experience which is likely to be widely shared rather than being 'typical' in the sense used in statistical sampling.

The researcher must then devise an interview schedule. This will allow room for interviewees to explain their feelings and understandings and to identify what they believe to be relevant. Too much 'closing down' of the issue may mean that the interview reflects too closely the understanding of the interviewer rather than the interviewee (which rather defeats the point of the interview). At the least structured end, interviews might involve a small number of prompts from the interviewer and then be very conversational. A more structured approach involves the interviewer identifying in advance a sequence of topics to be covered. The questions should be ones which the interviewer is equipped to answer so, for example, a patient might be asked 'how did you feel when you first came onto the ward?' rather than 'does this ward represent good value for money for the NHS?'. They should also be sensitive to the ethical context and asked in a clear, non-patronizing way, with sufficient acceptance of pauses and digressions to allow the interviewee to explain their understanding. Finally, the questions should demonstrate that the interviewer has adequately prepared by understanding the context of the interview. It is often the case that qualitative interviews involve one interviewer and another taking notes and observing (and possibly ensuring that the whole topic had been covered). (See Kvale[15] for more on what makes a good interviewer and Chapter 15 of Bryman[6] for a clear introduction to the issues around qualitative interviewing.)

Audio recordings are good practice if the purpose is to identify how the interviewee feels about and understands an issue because many nuances of meaning can be lost when committed to paper. This is less important if the purpose is a more exploratory interview concerned with identifying key issues or capturing expert opinion, for example. Notes, carefully written up after the interview, might be sufficient for this purpose (and a great deal cheaper and easier than producing transcripts). A practical alternative is to use notes for most of the interview but to transcribe key sections.

Finally, almost every experienced qualitative researcher would agree that wherever possible it is advisable to conduct pilot interviews to test the interview schedule and to make sure that the questions and guidance offered by the researcher make sense to those being interviewed. Failure to do so can result in useless data collection.

Group work

An alternative to the interview is group work. The focus group, in particular, has emerged as a key tool in qualitative research (it has also become a much misused term). Focus group work has two key dimensions: first it is on a clearly focused theme which the participants have shared experience of (so there should be some homogeneity in the group at least in terms of their experience); secondly, it involves listening to how members of a group discuss and interact when considering this theme (because this allows issues to come to the surface that might not appear in one-to-one interviews). It helps us understand how wider members of the selected group might react to and assess the theme under discussion. In terms of group dynamics, most practitioners believe that groups of between six and twelve people work best. These might be stratified by class, age, gender, or some other category in order to ensure some homogeneity of experience.

Focus groups should be recorded and notes taken. Often the recording can be used to enrich the note taking afterwards but sometimes whole transcripts are produced from the recordings. Recording group work is, however, practically very difficult and it is often not clear who is speaking at any one time. If transcripts are to be produced sufficient time should be allocated for this and for analyzing the outputs which are generally more rich and complex than interview transcripts. The analysis should (but often does not) take account of the interactions within the group. (For more on conducting focus groups see Mannheim and Rich.[16])

What people write

People and organizations write all sorts of things ranging from personal 'to do lists' through to annual reports. These may be found in archives (and increasingly on the internet) or may need to be discovered through other means. It is also possible for researchers to ask others to produce written documents in the form of diaries or statements, for example. In all cases researchers will want to ask the key questions of who, why, where, how, and when.

However, the researcher will then be required to take a view on what the document means. Discourse analysis is a term used to cover a range of approaches to 'uncovering' meaning (although this can be applied to both text and spoken words, unlike CA which is used only for spoken conversations). Discourse analysis looks at how meaning is constructed through the use of words, but it is especially interested in how the power of language lies in its ability to construct meanings which depend upon underlying discourses. These may even become part of 'common sense'. Mental illness would be a famous example of how a condition has been constructed differently during the past 200 years and how treatments and social responses have been shaped by these underlying discourses. In this very important sense, language is a 'practice in its own right' (Gill[17] p.176) because it has real effects. However, there are conflicting discourses at any one time and White Papers, newspaper articles, or annual reports can all construct their world in different ways. Discourse analysis seeks to uncover these constructions. And most typically this is done by a careful, sceptical reading (see Gill[17] and Potter[18]).

Analyzing qualitative data

There is no end to the availability of qualitative data on most research questions; no moment when the researcher can say with certainty 'I have enough'. Consequently researchers may often become overwhelmed by the quantity and complexity of the data they collect. In public health research this can be frustrating. The golden rule, therefore, is not to wait until 'all' the data have been collected before starting to think about how they can be analyzed. At a common sense level this involves developing some very provisional hypotheses about the issue being analyzed; collecting some early findings; revising the assumptions; collect more data; and continue this cycle of induction until the data and the explanation come into line. A commonly applied technique within this approach is that of grounded theory which we outlined above. In this approach the data collection and the data analysis phases of research are closely linked.

We have already introduced the idea of grounded theory above. A crucial stage in making this work involves 'coding'. This involves examining the transcripts of interviews, focus groups, diaries or whatever and first of all coding these at a general level. This means developing concepts, for example in a series of interviews on communicating with clinicians we might begin to categorize statements into 'respect', 'confusion', 'source of information', or 'family friend'. Gradually these might come together around a core category which becomes the 'storyline' (see Strauss and Corbin[19]). Inevitably much richness will be lost through this process. Equally inevitably, the choice of codes can be criticized as being subjective. However, this may be the cost of trying to organize large amounts of complex data and to make sense of this in a way that allows us to make some generalizable claims. This process of coding is now most typically carried out using a software package such as QSR Nvivo[20] and NUD*IST.[21]

Conclusions

We therefore have a picture of qualitative research as an iterative process. Robust conclusions can be arrived at through testing clear hypotheses using theoretic sampling, well-conducted interviews and group work, and inductive reasoning. But it is perhaps more likely than in quantitative research that these processes will need to be done in parallel, and for this reason findings are likely to be emergent. Whilst it can be argued that well-conducted qualitative research is therefore the equal of quantitative research it is worth stressing that they are most commonly, and often most beneficially, best conducted as a partnership.

Further resources

ESDS Qualidata. http://www.essex.ac.uk/qualidata/ (accessed 23 June 2005).

FQS. Ethnography and Health Care: Focus on Nursing. Available at: http://www.qualitative-research.net/fqs-texte/1–00/1–00hodgson-e.htm (accessed 23 June 2005).

Online Gateway for Qualitative Research. http://www.qualitative-research.net/ (accessed 23 June 2005).

Social Science Information Gateway. http://www.sosig.ac.uk/research_tools/ (accessed 23 June 2005).

The Qualitative Report. Available at: http://www.nova.edu/ssss/QR/qualres.html (accessed 23 June 2005).

W. K. Kellogg Foundation Evaluation Handbook. Available at: http://www.wkkf.org/Pubs/Tools/Evaluation/Pub770.pdf (accessed 23 June 2005).

References

1 Blaxter L, Hughes C, Tight M (1996). *How to research*. Open University Press, Buckingham.

2 Benton T (1977). *Philosophical foundations of the three sociologies*. Routledge Kegan Paul, London.

3 Bryman A (1998). Quantitative and qualitative research strategies in knowing the social world. In: May T, Williams M (eds) *Knowing the social world*. Open University Press, Buckingham.

4 Gabbay J (1999). The socially constructed dilemmas of academic public health. In: Griffiths S, Hunter DJ (eds) *Perspectives in public health*. Radcliffe Medical Press, Oxford.

5 Devine F (1995). Qualitative analysis. In: Marsh D, Stoker G (eds) *Theory and methods in political science*. Macmillan, London.

6 Bryman A (2004). *Social research methods*, 2nd edn. Oxford University Press, Oxford.

7 Gold RL (1958). Roles in sociological fieldwork. *Social Forces*, **36**, 217–23.

8 Taylor A (1993). *Women drug users: an ethnography of an injecting community*. Clarendon Press, Oxford.

9 Glaser BG, Strauss AL (1967). *The discovery of grounded theory: strategies for qualitative research*. Aldine, Chicago, IL.

10 Strauss AL, Corbin JM (1998). *Basics of qualitative research: techniques and procedures for developing grounded theory*. Sage, Thousand Oaks, CA.

11 Charmaz K (2004). Grounded theory. In: Bryman A, Liao TF (eds) *The Sage encyclopedia of social science methods*, Vols 1–3. Sage, Thousand Oaks, CA.

12 Lee-Treweek G (2000). The insight of emotional danger: research experiences in a home for the elderly. In: Lee-Treweek G, Linkogle S (eds) *Danger in the field: risk and ethics in social research*. Routledge, London.

13 Atkinson P (1981). *The clinical experience*. Gower, Farnborough.

14 Silverman D (1994). Analysing naturally occurring data on AIDS Counselling: some methodological and practical issues. In: Boulton M (ed) *Challenge and innovation: methodological advances in social research on HIV/AIDS*. Taylor and Francis, London.

15 Kvale S (1996). *Interviews: an introduction to qualitative research interviewing*. Sage, Thousand Oaks, CA.

16 Mannheim JB, Rich RC (1995). *Empirical political analysis: research methods in political science*, 4th edn. Longman, New York.

17 Gill R (2000). Discourse analysis. In: Bauer MW, Gaskell G (eds) *Qualitative researching with text, image and sound*. Sage, London.

18 Potter J (2004). Discourse analysis. In: Hardy M, Bryman A (eds) *Handbook of data analysis*. Sage, London.

19 Strauss A, Corbin JM (1990). *Basics of qualitative research: grounded theory procedures and techniques*. Sage, Newbury Park, CA.

20 Richards L (1999). Data alive! The thinking behind NVivo. *Qual Health Res*, **9**(3), 412–28. Available at: http://www.qualitative-research.net/fqs-texte/2–02/2–02welsh-e.pdf (accessed 24 June 2005).

21 Crowley C, Harré R, Tagg C (2002). Qualitative research and computing: methodological issues and practices in using QSR NVivo and NUD*IST. *Int J Soc Res Methodol*, **5**(3), 193–7.

2.3 Epidemiological understanding: an overview of basic concepts and study designs

Anjum Memon

Objectives

The aim of this chapter is to help the public health practitioner to:
- appreciate the various uses of epidemiology
- define and distinguish between key measures of disease frequency
- understand the main features of epidemiological study designs
- organize disease frequency data into a two-by-two table, and calculate and interpret measures of impact and association
- define and distinguish between bias, confounding, and random error and appreciate their role in epidemiology
- understand the epidemiological approach to associations and causation.

What is epidemiology?

Epidemiology is the basic science of public health. It describes, quantifies, and postulates causal mechanisms for disease in populations, and provides evidence to guide public health policy and action and clinical practice to protect, restore, and promote health.

The applications of epidemiology in public health can be summarized as follows:
- To describe the spectrum and extent of disease in the population— what is the burden of obesity in the population?
- To identify factors that increase or decrease the risk of disease—what factors increase the risk of, or protect against, transmission of HIV infection?
- To study the natural history and prognosis of disease—does early diagnosis of prostate cancer through screening for prostate-specific antigen improve survival in patients?
- To monitor and predict disease trends in the population—what impact will the increasing prevalence of obesity have on future disease trends and health-care needs?

- To provide evidence for developing public health policy and making regulatory decisions—will a smoking ban in bars reduce the incidence of smoking-related disease in workers?
- To evaluate the efficacy of preventive and therapeutic interventions—do combinations of statins, aspirin, and beta blockers improve survival in patients with coronary heart disease?
- To evaluate public health programmes—is the smoking cessation programme helping people to quit smoking?
- To evaluate the effectiveness of health services—are known contacts of persons with STDs followed up and treated?

Measuring disease frequency

Epidemiology is a quantitative science. The ability to measure carefully and accurately the frequency of disease forms the foundation of descriptive epidemiology.

Incidence

Incidence (or *incident cases*) is a count of *new cases* of disease in the population during a specified time period. The *incidence rate* is the number of *new cases* of a disease in a defined population within a specified time period, divided by the number of persons at risk (or person-time) of developing the disease during that time period.

- Incidence rate measures the rapidity (or 'speed') at which new cases of disease are occurring in the population within a time period. It has three essential elements: a numerator (the number of new cases), a denominator (the number of persons at risk or person-time), and time dimension (the beginning and end of the period during which the cases accrue). It is normally expressed in a particular convention (e.g. cancer incidence in adults is typically expressed as per 100,000 population).
- Increase in incidence of a disease in the population can be due to: in-migration of susceptible persons, a change in diagnostic criteria, improved case ascertainment, introduction of a new diagnostic/screening test, introduction of new, or changes in exposure to existing, etiologic agent(s).
- Incidence rate is calculated from data collected by disease registers (e.g. cancer registry), cohort studies, and clinical, field, and community trials. It is used for predicting the risk of disease; research on causes and treatment of disease; to describe trends of disease over time; and for evaluating the effectiveness of prevention programmes.

Prevalence

Prevalence is the number of *existing cases* of a disease in a defined population at a notional point in time (*point prevalence*—do you have migraine now?) or at any time during a certain period (*period prevalence*—have you had migraine in the last 12 months?), divided by the number of persons in the population at that time.

- Prevalence is a measure of the extent of health problem or burden of disease in the population, and is normally expressed as a proportion (e.g. 4.3% of men in England had diabetes in 2003). It is most useful for describing diseases with a gradual onset and long duration (e.g. hypertension, osteoarthritis).
- Prevalence clearly depends on the incidence and the duration of disease.
- Increase in prevalence of a disease in the population can be due to: in-migration of cases, increase in incidence, and/or longer duration of disease (e.g. due to better treatment).
- Prevalence is calculated from data collected by cross-sectional studies and surveys.
- Prevalence data are used for planning health services, resource allocation, and organization of prevention programmes.

Some other commonly used measures of disease frequency and impact that you should know include: cumulative incidence; crude-, age-, and cause-specific mortality rates; age-standardized (or adjusted) rate; standardized mortality ratio; proportional mortality ratio; livebirth rate; infant mortality rate; maternal mortality rate; attack rate; case fatality rate; years of potential life lost; survival rate.

Epidemiological study designs

All studies examine associations between exposure and disease—ecologic and cross-sectional studies are good for generating hypotheses, and case–control, cohort, and experimental studies are best for testing them and establishing causality (cause and effect relationship). In all but ecologic studies, the unit of observation and analysis is the individual. The selection of study design depends on the research question, validity, feasibility, efficiency, and ethical concerns.

Box 2.3.1 Types of epidemiological studies

Observational
- Ecological (correlation studies)
- Cross-sectional (surveys, prevalence studies)
- Case–control
- Cohort (incidence, longitudinal, follow-up studies)

Experimental (intervention studies)
- Clinical trials
- Field trials
- Community trials (cluster randomized trial)

Ecologic studies

The objective of ecologic studies is to examine the association between exposure and occurrence of disease with population-level data (i.e. the units of analysis are populations rather than individuals). Their key features are:

- Ecologic studies compare aggregate exposure and disease across different populations over the same time period or within the same population over time.
- They are excellent for generating hypotheses (particularly when the disease is of unknown etiology) but they cannot establish causality.
- They are generally inexpensive and quick to conduct if routine data on exposure (e.g. per capita income, mean ambient temperature, air/water quality, weather conditions, smoking prevalence, per capita intake/annual sale of food items/alcohol) and disease (e.g. incidence/mortality rates, prevalence) are available.
- They are useful for examining the effect of short-term variations in exposure within the same population (e.g. effect of temperature on mortality in the elderly) and evaluating the impact of public health interventions by comparing aggregate-level information before and after the intervention (e.g. fluoridation of drinking water, seat belt law).

Ecologic studies have a number of *limitations*:

- they are subject to confounding as information on potential confounder(s) is generally not available
- associations at the population level do not necessarily represent associations at the individual level (*ecologic fallacy* or ecologic bias).

The outcome measure of an ecological study is the *correlation coefficient*. Examples of the type of questions addressed include: Is per capita daily meat consumption associated with colon cancer in different countries? Is per capita wine consumption associated with death rates from coronary heart disease (CHD) in different countries?

Cross-sectional studies

The objective of cross-sectional studies is to determine the prevalence of an exposure and/or disease in a defined population at one particular time. Their key features are:

- Cross-sectional studies take a 'snapshot' of the sample of individuals in the population at one particular time. They are conducted to determine the burden of exposure and/or disease in the population, assess knowledge, attitude, and practice in relation to health-related issues (KAP studies), public health monitoring, and planning interventions and health services, and to generate hypotheses and examine association between exposure and disease.
- Unlike case–control and cohort studies, the study population is commonly selected without regard to exposure or disease status, and you can examine multiple exposures (e.g. smoking, high cholesterol, family history) and outcomes (CHD, asthma, diabetes) simultaneously in each individual.
- They can be conducted in a relatively short time; and when based on a representative sample, their findings can be generalized to the whole population.

- Sequential health surveys (e.g. the Health Survey for England) are the best method for monitoring trends in behavioural/lifestyle risk factors over time.

Cross-sectional studies have the limitation that it is generally not possible to establish a temporal sequence between exposure and disease onset.

Examples of questions addressed by a cross-sectional study include: What proportion of adults served by a primary health centre over the last year have hypertension? What are the views of school pupils on sexual violence and on the risk of HIV infection?

(Note that a census—which not only enumerates the population but also assesses the prevalence of various characteristics—and opinion and political polls are basically cross-sectional studies).

Case–control studies

The objective of case–control studies is to study associations of a disease with an exposure(s) or factor(s): subjects are defined as cases (persons with disease) and controls (persons without disease), and past exposure and/or biologic markers are compared. The key features of case–control studies are:

- Case–control studies are conducted to generate and test etiologic hypotheses, evaluation of screening and prevention programmes, vaccine and treatment efficacy, and outbreak investigation.
- It is possible to study associations of a disease with several exposures and characteristics, and measure potential confounding factors.
- They are relatively inexpensive and conducted in a short time, and are efficient for rare diseases and those with long induction/latent period.

The outcome measure of a case–control study is a ratio of ratios (exposed and unexposed cases and controls) and hence expressed as an odds ratio (OR).

Case–control studies have some limitations:

- they are subject to problems with control selection and matching between cases and controls
- recall bias
- sometimes it is difficult to establish a clear temporal sequence between exposure and disease
- they are inefficient for rare exposures.

Examples of case–control studies include: Is vaginal cancer in daughters associated with maternal exposure to diethylstilbestrol during pregnancy? Is cervical cancer associated with smoking? Does reduced exposure to common infections in infancy increases the risk of childhood leukemia?

Cohort studies

The objective of cohort studies is to study associations of an exposure(s) with a disease and/or several health outcomes; participants are grouped according to exposure (exposed/unexposed) and followed over time to compare the incidence of health outcomes. For a *prospective cohort* past or current exposure is determined at the beginning of study (baseline) and participants are followed into the future to observe the outcome. For a *historic* (or *retrospective*) *cohort* participants are grouped on the basis of historic exposure data at a defined time in the past (baseline) and the outcome up to the present time is observed (i.e. both the exposures and outcomes have already occurred in the past, and the investigator reconstructs the outcomes between the defined time of exposure in the past and the present).

Key features of cohort studies are:

- Cohort studies are conducted to test etiologic hypotheses, understand physiology, pathogenesis, prognosis, and natural history of disease, and evaluation of screening and prevention programmes and vaccine and treatment efficacy.
- The study design is the most robust in observational epidemiology. It is possible to establish temporal sequence as the exposure is assessed at baseline and incidence (or mortality) rates of disease among the exposed and unexposed groups are determined.
- In prospective studies, the length of the follow-up period can range from a few days/weeks for infectious disease to several years/decades for diseases such as cancer or cardiovascular disease.
- It is possible to study associations of an exposure with several outcomes, and also to study multiple exposure (when a general population cohort is selected irrespective of any particular exposure, e.g. the Framingham and European prospective investigation into cancer and nutrition (EPIC) studies).
- Prospective studies are less vulnerable to bias because the outcomes have not occurred when the cohort is assembled and the exposure is assessed at the beginning of the study.
- Historic studies take less time and money to conduct, and are commonly used for studying outcomes of occupational and clinical exposures.

The outcome measures of a cohort study are the incidence (and/or mortality) rates in the exposed and unexposed groups. From these measures, one can calculate relative risk, attributable risk, and population attributable risk.

Cohort studies have a number of limitations:

- Prospective studies are relatively expensive to conduct, take a long time to yield results, and are usually inefficient when studying rare outcomes. Subjects lost to follow-up (generally >10%) may undermine the validity of the study.
- In historic studies the available data on exposure, outcome, and other key variables may be inadequate.

Examples of cohort studies include:

- prospective studies: the British doctors' smoking study; the Framingham heart study; the EPIC study
- historic studies: risk of bladder cancer in chemical industry workers; risk of childhood leukemia in individuals who received blood transfusions in infancy.

Experimental studies

Experimental studies are designated experiments where the investigator assigns individuals (or communities) to two or more groups that either receive or do not receive a preventive or therapeutic treatment.

The active manipulation of the exposure by the investigator is the hallmark of these studies. Like a prospective cohort study, the groups are then followed into the future to observe the outcome(s). There are three main types of experimental study:

- *Clinical trials* are conducted to evaluate the treatment, complications, and prognosis of disease, and measures for secondary prevention of disease. In most trials, treatments are assigned by randomization, using random number assignment. Randomization has two main objectives: it ensures that the treatment assignment (i.e. exposure) is unbiased and it produces comparability between the groups with respect to factors (i.e. baseline characteristics) that might affect the rate of outcome (i.e. controls for known and unknown confounding factors). When it is ethically feasible to conduct them, randomized clinical trails provide the best evidence to establish a causal association.
- *Field trials* are conducted to study primary prevention of disease (e.g. Salk (polio) vaccine trial of 1954; hepatitis B vaccine trial).
- *Community trials* (cluster randomized trial) are also conducted to study the primary prevention of disease, but the exposure is assigned to clusters of people (or communities) rather than individuals (e.g. drinking water fluoridation trials in the 1940s; improving health-education and medical services for treating sexually transmitted diseases to reduce the incidence of HIV infection).

Figure 2.3.1 summarizes the variuos study designs used in observational epidemiology.

Comparison is fundamental to epidemiology. You can compare the incidence or mortality rates in the exposed/unexposed groups in two ways. They can be subtracted from one another (*absolute comparisons*—risk or rate difference, attributable risk) or divided by one another (*relative comparisons*—risk or rate ratio, relative risk, odds ratio). *Absolute* measures describe the public health impact of an exposure (e.g. population attributable risk) and potential for prevention, and *relative* measures describe the strength of the association between an exposure and outcome.

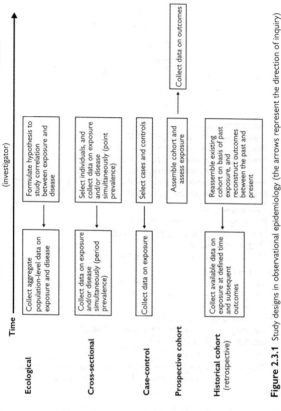

Figure 2.3.1 Study designs in observational epidemiology (the arrows represent the direction of inquiry)

Box 2.3.2 The 2 × 2 table in epidemiology

		Disease:		Total
		Yes	No	
Exposure:	Yes	A	B	A + B
	No	C	D	C + D
		A + C	B + D	N

Cross-sectional study
- Prevalence (exposure) = $(A + B)/N$
- Prevalence (disease) = $(A + C)/N$
- Prevalence of disease in exposed = $A/(A + B)$
- Prevalence of disease in unexposed = $C/(C + D)$
- Prevalence of exposure in diseased = $A/(A + C)$
- Prevalence of exposure in non-diseased = $B/(B + D)$

Case–control study
- Proprtion of cases exposed = $A/(A + C)$
- Proportion of controls exposed = $B/(B + D)$
- Odds ratio = AD/BC
- Odds ratio (matched pairs) = B/C (ratio of discordant pairs)

Cohort study
- Incidence rate in exposed = $A/(A + B)$ (absolute risk)
- Incidence rate in unexposed = $C/(C + D)$ *(absolute risk)*
- Attributable risk = incidence rate in exposed — incidence rate in unexposed (risk difference)
- Relative risk = incidence rate in exposed/incidence rate in unexposed (risk ratio)

Other related study designs and concepts you should know about include numbers needed to harm and numbers needed to treat.

Issues in deriving causal inferences from epidemiological studies

To be able to judge and draw causal inferences from epidemiological findings you need to understand the concepts of bias, confounding, and random error (Box 2.3.3), as well as the guidelines for judging epidemiological research and associations.

Box 2.3.3 Bias, confounding, and random error

Bias is a systematic error (committed by the investigator) either in the design, data collection procedures, analyses, or reporting of a study.
Confounding reflects the fact that observational epidemiological research is conducted among free-living humans with unevenly distributed characteristics.
Random error is the probability that the observed association is due to 'chance'.

Bias (systematic error)

Bias is any trend either in the study design, data collection procedures, analyses, reporting, or a combination of these factors that can lead to conclusions that are systematically different from the truth.

The main types of bias are:

- *Selection bias* occurs when there are systematic differences in the characteristics (i.e. those which are related to exposure and/or outcome) of persons who take part in a study and characteristics of those who do not (e.g. low participation by heavy smokers in studies of smoking and disease; high participation by health-conscious individuals—or those with family history of cancer—in voluntary cancer screening).
- *Information bias* occurs when there are systematic differences in the way information on exposure and/or outcome is collected. This leads to a different quality (accuracy) of information between the comparison groups (e.g. using different methods and/or instruments to measure blood pressure to classify hypertension).

Confounding

The word 'confounding' derives from the Latin *confundere*, to mix together. Confounding is a distortion or mixing of effects between an exposure, an outcome, and a third extraneous variable known as a confounder (see Figure 2.3.2).

A confounding factor has three requirements, it must: (i) be associated with the disease (i.e. either as a cause or a proxy for a cause, but not as an effect of the disease), (ii) be associated with the exposure (e.g. among controls in a case-control study or among the source population of a cohort study), and (iii) not be an effect of the exposure (i.e. should not be an intermediate step in the causal pathway from exposure to disease).

In observational studies, increasing study size will not make any difference to the amount of confounding. The study size does matter in randomized clinical trials as any confounders (known and unknown) are more likely to be balanced across the study groups and it is less likely that there will be any confounding.

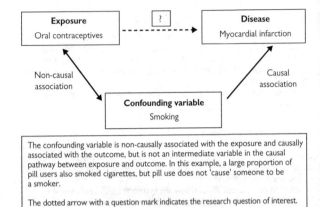

The confounding variable is non-causally associated with the exposure and causally associated with the outcome, but is not an intermediate variable in the causal pathway between exposure and outcome. In this example, a large proportion of pill users also smoked cigarettes, but pill use does not 'cause' someone to be a smoker.

The dotted arrow with a question mark indicates the research question of interest.

Figure 2.3.2 The nature of the association between the confounding variable, exposure, and disease (smoking, oral contraceptives, and myocarial infarction)

Random error (chance)

Random error is the portion of variation in a measurement that has no apparent connection to any other measurement or variable, generally regarded as due to 'chance' (an uncontrollable force that seems to have no assignable cause).

- Random error leads to a false association between the exposure and disease that arises due to chance.
- In epidemiological studies, random error originates from three sources: individual biologic variation, sampling variability, and measurement errors (errors in assessing the exposure and disease).
- It can never be completely eliminated since you can study only a sample of the population; individual variation always occurs and no measurement is perfectly accurate. It can be greatly reduced by careful measurement of exposure and disease and adequate study size (i.e. increasing the number of subjects and/or the length of follow-up time).
- There are two methods for quantifying random error: the P value (with a threshold of 0.05), and confidence interval (CI) estimation (calculated around a point estimate, which is either a measure of disease frequency (incidence rate, prevalence) or association (relative risk, odds ratio). The width of the CI is determined by random error stemming from sampling variability and measurement error, and by an arbitrary certainty factor, which is usually set at 95%. Measures of association should always be presented with CIs.

Box 2.3.4 Association or causation? Guidelines for judging epidemiological research and associations

- *Temporal sequence*—did exposure to the risk factor(s) precede outcome?
- *Strength of association*—how strong is the effect (relative risk or odds ratio)? It is important to understand that statistical associations do not necessarily imply causal associations. Some epidemiologists suggest that RR > 3.0 in cohort studies, or OR > 4.0 in case–control studies, provide strong support for causal association.
- *Dose–response relationship*—is increasing exposure (i.e. amount and/or duration of exposure) associated with an increasing disease risk?
- *Replication of the findings*—has a similar effect been seen in different persons, in different places, with different study designs, circumstances, and times?
- *Biologic plausibility*—does the association make sense in the light of current biological knowledge?
- *Consideration of alternate explanations*—is the association due to bias, confounding, or random error (have the investigators considered other possible explanations, and to what extent they have ruled out such explanations?).
- *Cessation of exposure*—does the risk of disease decline when exposure is reduced or eliminated?
- *Coherence with other knowledge*—does the cause-and-effect interpretation seriously conflict with what is known about the natural history and biology of the disease?
- *Specificity*—is the exposure associated with only one disease? This is the weakest of all guidelines, as only a few exposures (e.g. the rabies virus) lead to only one outcome.

Further resources

Aschengrau A, Seage GR III (2003). *Essential epidemiology in public health*. Jones and Bartlett, Sudbury, MA.

Epidemiology On-Line: http://www.sph.unc.edu/courses/eric/index.html (accessed 9 September 2005).

Friis RH, Sellers TA (2004). *Epidemiology for public health practice*, 3rd edn. Jones and Bartlett, Sudbury, MA.

Gordis L (2004). *Epidemiology*, 3rd edn. WB Saunders, Philadelphia, PA.

Last JM (2001). *A dictionary of epidemiology*, 4th edn. Oxford University Press, Oxford.

Rothman KJ (2002). *Epidemiology: an introduction*. Oxford University Press, Oxford.

The WWW Virtual Library: Medicine and Health: Epidemiology. http://www.epibiostat.ucsf.edu/epidem/epidem.html (accessed 9 September 2005).

Webb P, Bain C, Pirozzo S (2005). *Essential epidemiology: an introduction for students and health professionals*. Cambridge University Press, Cambridge.

2.4 Monitoring disease and risk factors: surveillance

Daniel M. Sosin and
Richard S. Hopkins

What is surveillance?

Public health surveillance is 'the ongoing, systematic collection, analysis, interpretation, and dissemination of data about a health-related event for use in public health action to reduce morbidity and mortality and to improve health'.[1] Thus public health surveillance is a continual process of monitoring health and health indicators and is important for a wide range of acute and chronic conditions. Examples of health-related events include episodes of illness or injury, diagnosis of chronic conditions, risk behaviours for adverse health outcomes (e.g. tobacco use or non-use of seatbelts), or completion of a health-care procedure (e.g. Pap smear or measles immunization). The principles of public health surveillance are the same for communicable and non-communicable diseases; however, the experience has been more plentiful with communicable diseases.

Historically, infectious disease surveillance has depended upon legally mandated disease reporting by health-care providers, laboratories, and health-care systems. Increasingly, surveillance for both infectious and non-communicable disease events relies on surveys and data collected for other purposes where public health benefits secondarily (e.g. administrative data, electronic medical records, vital registration). Electronic management and submission of data to public health agencies afford the possibility of instantaneous reporting and review of disease, injury and health indicator data, including laboratory results, at the time they are recorded by the provider.

Syndromic surveillance is an investigational approach where health department staff, assisted by automated data acquisition and generation of statistical signals, monitor disease indicators continually to detect outbreaks of disease earlier and more completely than might otherwise be possible with traditional methods for reporting disease.[2] Signals detected by these methods then need further investigation to determine what they represent.

Surveillance should be conducted in a standardized and consistent manner and should be designed to support public health action (e.g. treatment, guidance, policies, or programmes).

Why conduct surveillance?

Public health surveillance is used to support interventions in individual cases and communities; understand the natural history of a disease or injury; estimate the magnitude of disease and risk factors in a target population; identify patterns and changes in agents, conditions, and practices; conduct exploratory research; and identify research gaps. Purposes of surveillance systems can be classified into three main categories: case management, outbreak detection and management, and programme management. Individual cases of diseases of public health interest (e.g. tuberculosis) are routinely reported to public health authorities to ensure proper disease management for both the individual and the community (e.g. investigation to locate and treat exposed contacts to an infectious disease or toxin). Public health authorities use surveillance data to detect, track the course and extent of, and manage outbreaks (e.g. severe bloody diarrhea and secondary hemolytic uremic syndrome due to ground beef contaminated with *Escherichia coli* O157:H7, or birth defects due to introduction of a new medication, or cancers due to a new occupational hazard). They also use surveillance data for the planning and continuous evaluation necessary to ensure that programmes to prevent and control disease at the community level are effective (e.g. immunizations to prevent childhood diseases, or 'back to sleep' campaigns to prevent sudden infant death syndrome, or interventions to improve quality of clinical care).

Designing a surveillance system

The first step in designing a surveillance system is to state its purpose clearly. The relative importance of many system attributes depends on the purpose (Table 2.4.1). For example:

- A system that is sufficiently *timely* to support programme planning with a several-year time horizon may not be sufficiently timely for outbreak recognition or immediate control measures.
- When resources are scarce, an automated alarm system for outbreak detection may need to be set with low *sensitivity* and high *positive predictive value* (PPV). For case management and programme management, PPV reflects the probability that a case in the database is one being sought by the system and *negative predictive value* (NPV) reflects the probability that persons not in the database do not have the condition under surveillance. For outbreak management, PPV reflects the probability that a system signal identifies an outbreak of the type being sought, and NPV reflects the probability that no signal from the system means that no outbreak is occurring.
- If reassurance that an outbreak is not occurring when there is no signal is an important desired feature of the system, a high NPV for outbreaks is important.
- *Data quality* needs to be particularly high when medical treatment decisions will be made on the basis of data in the system. When surveillance is used as a screening tool to detect events requiring further investigation, lower data quality may be tolerated. Costly investments in prevention programmes also demand high-quality data for planning and evaluation purposes.

Table 2.4.1 Relative importance (five-point scale) of surveillance system performance attributes that vary by purpose of surveillance

Attribute	Purpose of surveillance		
	Case management	Outbreak detection	Programme planning and evaluation
Timeliness	****	*****	*
Sensitivity	****	****	***
Positive predictive value	****	***	****
Negative predictive value	**	*****	***
Data quality	*****	***	****
Representativeness	**	**	****
Flexibility	***	****	*
Stability	****	*****	***

- *Flexibility* reflects the ability of a system to change as needs change. Outbreak detection systems particularly require flexibility to adapt to changing threats and levels of risk over time.
- *Stability*, reflected by the resilience of the system to external changes and consistency in operation over long periods of time, is more important in systems for outbreak detection.

System characteristics also vary with the primary purpose of the system (Table 2.4.2):

- *Data sources* are most diverse for programme management and least diverse for case management where individual treatment decisions require a follow-up with personal identifiers. Outbreak detection can often be done with data that do not contain *personal identifiers*, yet timely investigation of cases that may be part of an outbreak may require that identifiers be accessible. Cultural norms and rules of use and protection of personal data for public health purposes can vary by jurisdiction. At any time when personally identified data are collected for public health purposes, utmost care must be taken to meet ethical and legal standards and ensure privacy and confidentiality of the data. Data that are not needed should not be collected.
- *Data collection* may be manual or electronic. The point in a distributed collection system at which switching from manual records to auto-mated ones makes sense will depend on the level of technology and trained staff realistically available as well as the volume of reports and the timeliness needed. In most settings, surveillance data are collected at the most local level in the system and gradually aggregated as they are passed up the chain to surveillance units responsible for larger areas (e.g. county, district, province, or country). More recently, technologic advances have permitted a reversal of this flow. When the data

Table 2.4.2 Surveillance system design characteristics by purpose of surveillance

System design characteristic	Case management	Outbreak detection	Programme planning and evaluation
Data sources	Case reports from clinicians, health-care facilities, schools, or laboratories	Case reports; electronic health records; administrative health-care data; highly specific lab data (e.g. PulseNet and other molecular methods); news reports; environmental and workplace monitoring for hazards and exposures; poison centre records; sales of over-the-counter or prescription drugs; calls to nurse hotlines	All previous plus: repeated population-based surveys (e.g. Behavioural Risk Factor Surveillance System in the US); vital registration; census data; social services data; public safety data; registries; periodic evaluation data collections from programme delivery sites
Collection method	Reports by mail, phone, fax, E-mail, web site, electronic lab reporting (ELR); infection control practitioners and health-care organizations	Direct electronic acquisition of records coded by ICD9-CM, chief complaint, or other early diagnostic information; case reports; ELR	All; personal report; observation (e.g. seat belt use)
Collection frequency	Reported on a set interval after a case is identified at a reporting source (e.g. 24 h or 1 week)	Case reports as they occur, or batch reporting on a frequent (e.g. daily) or continuous (real-time) basis	Extended periodic interval (e.g. annually)
Data processing	Limited (tabulation and sorting for case investigation and follow-up)	Automated steps for organizing and detecting aberrations	Extensive cleaning and updating of data
Statistical and epidemiological analysis	Standard and simple measures of central tendency and time plots; direct action case by case; line lists and histograms	Complex analytic routines for pattern recognition; stratified analysis for risk groups; combination of data from multiple sources	Routine tables and more advanced modelling/projections (e.g. time series, complex stratified and cluster models)
Reporting and dissemination	Case managers (public health); clinicians; case reporters	Public health practitioners at local, state, federal levels; emergency responders; news media; public	Programme managers; policy-makers; news media; public

source for surveillance is inherently centralized, data may be collected in a central office and be made available promptly to local public health units.

- *Analysis* of surveillance data should be appropriate to the task at hand. Localized acute disease surveillance may need no more than line lists of cases, cases plotted over time (i.e. epidemic curves), and simple mapping. Systems with many streams of data, especially case-based data with demographic detail (e.g. age, race, sex, ethnicity, occupation, and location of residence) may benefit from automated aberration detection and from more complex displays. Increased availability of highly detailed molecular subtyping of organisms causing disease (e.g. PulseNet) also creates a need for software to identify similar isolates and identify apparent clustering among a multitude of cases.
- *Descriptive and analytic epidemiology* (e.g. calculations of rates by sub-groups and time intervals, mapping of cases and rates, age adjustment, and calculation of relative risks) is useful in all surveillance activity but especially in support of programme planning and evaluation.
- Surveillance data, summaries, analyses, and recommendations should be *disseminated* regularly to suppliers of data, those with a need to know for clinical and public health purposes, and the general public.

Public health informatics

Public health informatics has been defined as 'the systematic application of information and computer science and technology to public health practice, research, and learning'.[3] Modern surveillance systems increasingly acquire electronic data and rely on information and computer science to optimize the collection, storage, and use of these data. As more clinical records are computerized by using standardized messaging (e.g. HL-7) and vocabulary standards (e.g. LOINC and SnoMED) and emerging national and international standards for electronic health records, rapid and complete transfer of such data into surveillance systems is becoming more feasible. Informatics expertise should be engaged early in the design of surveillance systems.

Evaluating a surveillance system

Surveillance systems should be evaluated regularly and modified promptly as needed. Evaluations of all types of surveillance systems can be guided by the 'Updated guidelines for evaluating public health surveillance systems'.[1] Systems designed for outbreak detection have some specific characteristics that need attention during evaluation, as indicated in the 'Framework for evaluating public health surveillance systems for early detection of outbreaks'.[2] Evaluations should be undertaken in consultation with system stakeholders, to whom results should also be disseminated.

Table 2.4.1 shows performance attributes assessed in surveillance system evaluation that are likely to vary by purpose. Additional attributes that are common to all surveillance systems are also important. Acceptability—the willingness and authority of participants to contribute to data collection, analysis, and use—is important in all systems that depend on timely and high-quality data. Cost is always important, but thresholds for acceptable costs will differ based on the condition and on the purpose/use of the data. Ultimately, the performance of a surveillance system depends on its usefulness for accomplishing its stated purpose. To the extent possible, usefulness should be expressed by the prevention and control actions taken as a result of analysis and interpretation of data from the system.

General principles for effective surveillance systems

The key contributions of public health professionals to establishing, running, and quality assurance of surveillance systems are to understand the strengths and limitations of the data for the intended purpose of the system and to analyze the data frequently so that utility and quality can be assured. The following principles should be diligently applied:

- Have clear objectives and design the system to meet those objectives.
- Collect only the data needed to meet the explicit objectives.
- Collect direct measures of the condition of interest (e.g. office visits for respiratory disease) before indirect markers (e.g. absenteeism, over-the-counter drug purchases).
- Value and build personal relationships, as well as laws, rules, and technology.
- Demonstrate the public health uses of the data to reporters (e.g. clinicians and laboratories).
- Provide authoritative consultation to reporters, as this will lead to reporting.
- Identify and remove barriers to rapid reporting of cases.
- Build redundancies to minimize the impact of reporting gaps.
- Analyze and interpret data by time, place, and person routinely and frequently.
- Integrate the analysis and interpretation of data across all the systems your organization manages.
- Convey confidence about the value of surveillance, epidemiology, and public health practice.

Further resources

Teutsch SM, Churchill RE (eds) (2000). *Principles and practice of public health surveillance.* Oxford University Press, New York.

References

1 Centres for Disease Control and Prevention (2001). Updated guidelines for evaluating public health surveillance systems: recommendations from the guidelines working group. *Morbidity and Mortality Weekly Report,* **50**(RR-13), 1–35. Available at: http://www.cdc.gov/mmwr/preview/mmwrhtml/rr5013a1.htm (accessed 21 January 2006).

2 Centres for Disease Control and Prevention (2004). Framework for evaluating public health surveillance systems for early detection of outbreaks; recommendations from the CDC Working Group. *Morbidity and Mortality Weekly Report,* **53**(RR-5), 1–13. Available at: http://www.cdc.gov/mmwr/preview/mmwrhtml/rr5305a1.htm (accessed 21 January 2006).

3 O'Carroll PW, Yasnoff WA, Ward ME, Ripp LH, Martin EL (eds) (2003). *Public health informatics and information systems.* Springer-Verlag, New York.

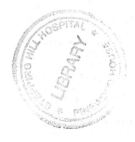

2.5 Investigating changes in occurrence

Ibrahim Abubakar

The detection of changes in disease incidence or prevalence is frequently encountered in public health practice. Organizations or individuals investigating a potential problem should be systematic but also flexible in their method of analysis and subsequent use of statistical tests.

Objectives

This chapter presents a systematic approach to investigating and monitoring changes in disease occurrence. It is focused on detecting an artefact to avoid unnecessary detailed investigation. A generic method applicable to various scenarios/diseases is provided, as well as a guide to further sources of epidemiological and statistical material and advice. It does not cover the detail required for the investigation of a putative cluster (see Chapter 2.6), preventing epidemics of communicable disease (see Chapter 3.1), or etiologic research.

Importance for public health

The usual observation that interests the public health practitioner is a higher occurrence of a disease. However, low occurrence of a disease may prompt an investigation.[1] In most cases the observation of an apparently high incidence of a disease is not a significant event and a thorough investigation is unnecessary. Doing nothing or a brief review may be adequate. Key steps to enable the identification of observations not requiring a detailed review are discussed in this chapter. The main concern for most service practitioners is the anxiety over potentially missing an important finding and ensuring that a real problem is promptly identified and dealt with. There may also be associated media and public interest.

Four key steps when investigating changes in incidence/prevalence

The four steps (Box 2.5.1) for investigating changes in incidence/ prevalence are:
- the identification of a potential problem
- excluding an artefact

- excluding chance
- further investigation of the problem.

The stages of investigation are not fixed. Local judgement and discretion are always required. For instance, prior local knowledge of the practice of a particular clinician may explain the observed differences.

Box 2.5.1 Key stages when investigating a high incidence/prevalence

1. A potential problem identified
2. Excluding an artefact—is the observation real?

Numerator errors—are there differences in:
- disease recognition?
- coding rules and procedures?
- classification codes?
- accuracy of coding age at death?

Denominator errors—check for:
- changes in age distribution of population
- errors in enumeration of population at risk.

3. Exclude chance by considering the following:
- confidence intervals
- comparing observed and expected numbers—Poisson
- statistical process control.

Real differences in prevalence can arise from changes in:
- fatality
- survival
- incidence of disease
- incubation/latent period.

4. Further investigation of the problem
- do nothing
- investigate: genetic differences; environmental differences.

The identification of a potential problem

Changes in disease occurrence usually come to light following routine surveillance or monitoring of routinely collected data (see Chapter 2.1). Other ways include reporting by concerned individuals and partner agencies, and occasionally the media. The collection of information and the recording of details of the reported number of cases and rates are important at this stage. A case definition should be agreed, i.e. what constitutes the disease of interest.

Excluding an artefact

The three possible explanations for an apparent increase in the rate of disease are chance occurrence, an artefact, or a real increase. The first step should be to ascertain that one is not dealing with an artefact. An artefact is defined in this context as a misleading observed difference arising from an artificial character in the way the data are defined, collected, or presented due usually to an extraneous (human) factor.[2]

(An artefact is a type of bias. The word bias is not used in this chapter to avoid confusing the term 'artefact' with 'bias' in the broader sense defined as 'deviation of results or inferences from the truth, or processes leading to such deviation' in Last's *Dictionary of Epidemiology*.) Put more simply, is the observation real?

It is better to use rates rather than crude numbers

The measure of disease occurrence presented may be an increase in a number, a rate, or a proportion. A comparison of the crude number of cases between areas or over time may show variation due to differences in the size of the population from which the cases arose. It is therefore essential that rates are calculated before any meaningful comparison can be attempted. An example of this type of error involves an attempt to draw conclusions based on hypothetical data on all patients with diabetic ketoacidosis (DKA) in a diabetology unit during a 10-yr period. Table 2.5.1 presents the age distribution of DKA patients by town.

Table 2.5.1 Age distribution of DKA patients in town A and town B

Age (yr)	Town A (%)	Town B (%)
0–24	5	4
25–34	8	14
35–70	33 (72)	16 (47)
Total	46	34

Looking at these data about 72% of DKA in town A occurred in those aged 35 to 70 yr of age, while 47% of DKA occurred in patients of that age in town B. It would be tempting to suggest that DKA is more likely among adults in town A compared with B. However, one cannot draw this conclusion from these data. The denominator may easily show that the reason for the difference is that the residents of town A are older than those in town B.

An artefactual difference in observed rates can be either due to numerator and/or denominator errors.[3]

Numerator errors

Numerator errors can arise from any stage of the measurement process that generates the data. Differences can arise from three broad dimensions of measurement:

- conceptualization—how the variables upon which the data are based are defined
- operational factors—what procedures or rules are used to quantify the variables
- accuracy—how valid and reliable the measured values are.

Potential sources of error include differences in disease recognition and ascertainment and coding problems.

Differences in disease recognition and ascertainment can be due to:

- changes in the case definition, e.g. changing the definition of diabetes mellitus can suddenly mean individuals previously classified as having impaired glucose tolerance are reclassified as having diabetes
- changes in awareness of the condition including differences in clinical recognition due to the presence of an expert or specialist in the area
- enhanced case finding in an area or hospital
- differences or changes in the accuracy/type of diagnostic tests used or due to laboratory errors.

Changes in International Classification of Disease (ICD) codes should be taken into account when comparing changes in rates over time. Comparability between ICD revisions is hampered by contradictory demands, including meeting the needs of an ever widening number of users, incorporation of advances in the understanding of the biology of disease, and preservation of the continuity of time series which form the basis of the revisions.[4] An example of change in clinical definition can result from the introduction of guidelines for the diagnosis and management of the condition. Figure 2.5.1 shows the trend in prostate cancer in the east of England. The fall in incidence in 1996 coincided with the introduction of guidelines.

Discussion with local clinicians can reveal differences due to the presence of a specialist or enhanced case ascertainment in a particular centre. A comparison of data from different sources, for instance clinician reports versus laboratory evidence of the disease, may reveal the source of the problem.

Coding problems include:

- differences in coding rules and procedures
- differences in classification of codes
- accuracy of coding of disease and errors in the recording of cases.

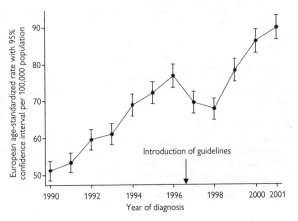

Figure 2.5.1 Incidence of prostate cancer, 1990–2001, east of England

Box 2.5.2 An example of the importance of coding differences

A common condition where variation in coding practice can lead to misleading differences in mortality rates is hip fractures. Differences were observed in hip fracture mortality rates between local authority areas in Cambridgeshire, UK using routine data. A local audit investigating the variation revealed significant differences in coding practice between areas accounting for most of the difference. Death certificates in patients who have had a hip fracture in the local authorities with the lowest death rates did not include hip fracture as a cause or contributing cause.

In order to check if coding problems are an issue:
- check the data source and ensure that the same clinical codes have been used
- obtain information from the data source about the quality of the data in terms of how valid they are, how the data are entered, and how accurate they are likely to be
- compare the rate of various diseases that have different etiologies
- a validation study may be undertaken to compare information in a small number of 'case notes' or other crude data source with reported death or hospital episodes data.

Denominator errors

Denominator errors can arise from errors in the enumeration of the population at risk or characteristics of the population. Several numeric fallacies in public health have to do with a failure to identify an appropriate denominator or population figure. The main sources of error are:
- use of the wrong denominator
- calculation of a rate at country level and extrapolation to a local level
- failure to account for confounding.

The population used to calculate the rates of disease should be checked to ensure that the relevant denominator was used. This check should include:
- a check on the source of the data. Is it census data or some other statistic such as total hospital admissions? Use new census data rather than projected estimates if available.
- ascertaining that the population is not under-enumerated in a census
- ensuring that the right age group, gender or socio-economic group are used.

Box 2.5.3 Example of denominator error

A situation where rates are misrepresented due to problems with denominators will arise when a section of the population is under-enumerated in a census. Rates of disease in the group will be artificially increased. For instance, this occurs in the US where 'Black American' men as a racial group are under-enumerated in the census. This implies that some of the observed higher rates of disease based on an incorrect small denominator among Black American men compared with White American men may in part be a result of this artefact.

If an artefact is found that explains the observed difference, no further investigation is necessary. However, if a real change is still suspected after excluding an artefact, then, standardized rates should be calculated controlling for confounding. Adjust for factors such as age, race, sex, and socio-economic deprivation and hospital case mix where appropriate, using indirectly standardized mortality or morbidity ratios (SMR), or alternatively using directly standardized mortality/morbidity rates. Remember to check whether you are comparing like with like. For instance the rate of disease may be higher than the national average but when compared with other areas within the country with similar risk factors it may not appear so high.

Excluding chance

Any identified difference between rates should be checked for statistical significance to exclude chance. Commonly used statistical approaches include:

- Chi-squared tests of observed versus expected frequencies (based on the Poisson distribution for low-frequency data).
- Comparison of standardized rates and calculation of confidence intervals around the standardized rate and comparator. Poisson regression may be used to control for confounding. The formulae in Boxes 2.5.4 are unstable with a small number of events and would suggest the use of appropriate statistical software if the number of events O is less than 25. For further discussion on this subject refer to texts such as INphoRM issue 5.[5]

Box 2.5.4 Confidence intervals around rates

Upper 95% confidence limit $= \text{rate}(\lambda) \times \exp(1.96\sqrt{1/O})$

Lower 95% confidence limit $= \dfrac{\text{rate}(\lambda)}{\exp(1.96\sqrt{1/O})}$

where O = number of events in Y person—years of observation.

Box 2.5.5 Confidence intervals around standardized mortality or morbidity ratios

$\text{SMR} = \dfrac{\text{observed}}{\text{expected}} \times 100$

Standard error $= \dfrac{\text{SMR}}{\sqrt{O}}$

95% confidence intervals for SMR:

$$\left(\dfrac{O}{E} \times 100\right) \pm \left(\dfrac{\sqrt{O}}{E} \times 100\right)$$

where O = number observed and E = number expected.

- Statistical process control. This is an alternative approach to detect outliers. It indicates whether the process is stable and detects when significant or special cause variation has occurred. (For details of these methods consult publications by the Eastern Region Public Health Observatory[6,7] or Wheeler[8].)
- Time series analysis is an alternative approach that accounts for the fact that data points taken over time may have an internal structure (such as autocorrelation, trend, or seasonal variation) that should be accounted for. The method is not used to exclude chance but to obtain an understanding of the underlying forces and structure that produced the observed data. A process called 'smoothing' minimizes or cancels out random variation. Fitted models are useful for monitoring and forecasting. Most statistical software can be used for time series analysis.

If the number of cases is too small to give meaningful rates, pooling across geographic areas (if a sensible larger area exists) or time may be possible. A commonly used method for reducing minor variation is to plot a moving average of the rates. The smaller the number of cases and the greater the standard error of the rate the more attention needs to be paid to questions of possible artefact. One should either avoid multiple testing or include a Bonferroni correction if the variables under consideration are independent.

Use of geographic information systems (GIS)
Mapping the data may be helpful. Powerful GIS are available for the investigation of an observed high rate of disease. Maps may be used to test hypotheses but it is sensible to contact organizations with expertise in using the software for advice before undertaking further GIS analysis.

Interpreting data
Should the data for a given time period appear out of line with what might be expected, check the data source in question to see whether the trend could be explained on the basis of local circumstances, custom, or practice. A review of the evidence for an apparent change over time, drawing on the experience of epidemiologists, laboratory specialists, information analysts, the hospital coding department, and clinicians may be required.

Remember that a statistically significant difference is not necessarily an important difference that should always be acted upon. Other factors should be taken into account, including the size of the difference, the importance of the disease(s) under consideration, and whether specific public health action can make a difference.

When considering prevalence specifically, possible reasons for a real difference include changes in fatality, survival, incubation/latency period, and incidence.

An increase in the incidence/prevalence of disease can be due to genetic or environmental/lifestyle factors. Once any of these is ascertained to be the cause of a high rate of disease, public health action should be taken to manage the cause of higher incidence, poor survival, or increased fatality. If the reasons for a higher rate are not obvious a local study may be necessary.

Box 2.5.6 Interpreting data: example

Changes in the incidence of prostate cancer provides an example of a real change in occurrence. Large increases in the incidence of prostate cancer have occurred throughout the world, partly due to increasing diagnosis. Mortality has remained stable. An increase in the number of children born after 1945 who will be in their mid-50s in the early part of the 21st century coupled with the trends in increasing life expectancy, will result in an increase in absolute terms in the number of cases of prostate cancer diagnosed. In the absence of improvements in treatment and with prospects for prevention by modification of lifestyle remote within current knowledge, there will also be an increase in the number of deaths from prostate cancer worldwide. The situation would be further augmented by the presence of a temporal trend in risk that is widely reported from many countries and unlikely to be entirely artefactual.[9]

Caveat for infections

Possible explanations for differences in the occurrence of infections include short-term fluctuations of incidence in time masquerading as differences or errors arising from an artefact. Real differences are usually due to changes in:[10]

- host susceptibility
- agent virulence
- environment
- incubation/latency period.

Pseudo outbreaks can occur due to artefacts.[11] Cases of infectious disease are usually linked, and to ascertain that an outbreak has occurred one has to demonstrate that the number of cases have exceeded the number expected for the given place and time. Table 2.5.2 provides a guide based on Poisson distribution that can be used to initiate an investigation.[12] Reaching an alert level for two consecutive weeks should call for an outbreak control meeting. This should always be within the context of knowledge of local incidence and known transmission between cases.

Table 2.5.2 Suggested thresholds for investigation of infectious disease within a district

Usual weekly rate[a]	Observed number of cases in one week	
	Check[b]	Alert[b]
1	3	4
2	5	6
3	6	8

[a] Allowing for seasonal variation.
[b] Check 1 in 20 probability and alert 1 in 100 probability of chance occurrence.
(Source: Bouchier report[10])

Further investigation of the problem

If, having taken into account the role of chance and artefact, you conclude that a real increase has occurred there are a number of options to consider. These include:

• Log the incident. You can be more confident that no further investigation is warranted at this stage when the consequence of no action is negligible.

• Undertake a local study. The decision to investigate the reasons for a higher incidence within the area will depend on the importance of the disease in terms of severity, economic impact, infectiousness, and media and political pressures.

The local public health service may not be the appropriate body to conduct a detailed investigation as the financial and academic resources required may not be available. Collaboration with a local university public health department, hospital clinicians, or national bodies may be the appropriate channel to investigate the risk factors and possible solutions to the increase. Remember that qualitative information/studies can aid understanding and may help to explore possible solutions.

Other steps may include:

• action at a national or regional level, e.g. lobbying
• other organizations—work in partnership
• remember the media may be interested.

The steps required for a more detailed study are outside the scope of this chapter but will include identifying a clear hypothesis, study protocol and design, ethical approval, funding, statistics, and the publication of findings.

Potential difficulties

Various difficulties may be encountered when investigating an observed increase or decrease in disease occurrence, including:

• poor quality of data sources
• small numbers
• unhelpful and distracting public/media interest
• cost.

Further resources

England and Wales Association of Public Health Observatories (PHOs). http://www.apho.org.uk (accessed 23 June 2005).

Hamilton JD (1994). *Time series analysis*. Princeton University Press, Princeton, NJ.

International Association of Cancer Registries. http://www.iacr.com.fr/iacr.htm (accessed 23 June 2005).

National Statistics. Home of official UK statistics. http://www.statistics.gov.uk (accessed 23 June 2005).

Small Area Statistics Health Unit, Imperial College, London. http://www.sahsu.org/ (accessed 23 June 2005).

Wheeler DJ (1995). *Advanced topics in statistical process control. The power of Shewhart's charts*. SPC Press. Knoxville, TN.

References

1 Allardyce J, Morrison G, Van Os J, Kelly J, Murray RM, McCreadie RG (2000). Schizophrenia is not disappearing in south-west Scotland. *Br J Psychiat*, **177**, 38–41.

2 *Oxford English Dictionary* (2000). *OED Online*, 2nd edn. Oxford University Press, Oxford.

3 Lilienfeld AM, Lilienfeld DE (1980). *Foundations of epidemiology*. Oxford University Press, New York.

4 Muir CS, Fraumeni JF Jr, Doll R (1994). The interpretation of time trends. *Cancer Surv*, **19–20**, 5–21.

5 Abubakar I (2005). *INphoRM 5: Investigating outliers*. ERPHO, Cambridge. Available at: http://www.erpho.org.uk/viewResource.aspx?id=11454 (accessed 21 January 2006).

6 Battersby J, Flowers J (2004). *INphoRM 4: Presenting performance indicators: alternative approaches*. ERPHO, Cambridge. Available at http://www.erpho.org.uk/viewResource.aspx?id=7518 (accessed 21 January 2006).

7 Flowers J (2004). *Statistical process control*. ERPHO, Cambridge. Available at: http://www.erpho.org.uk/viewResource.aspx?id=10305 (accessed 21 January 2006).

8 Wheeler DJ, Chambers DS (1992). *Understanding statistical process control*, 2nd edn. SPC Press, Knoxville, TN.

9 Boyle P, Maisonneuve P, Napalkov P (1995). Geographical and temporal patterns of incidence and mortality from prostate cancer. *Urology*, **46**(3, Suppl. A), 47–55.

10 Bhopal RS (1991). A framework for investigating geographical variation in diseases, based on a study of Legionnaires' disease. *J Public Health Med*, **13**(4), 281–9.

11 Casemore DP (1992). A pseudo-outbreak of cryptosporidiosis. *Commun Dis Rep CDR Rev* **2**(6), R66–R67.

12 Bouchier I (1998). *The third report of the expert group on cryptosporidium in water supplies*. DEFRA and Department of Health, London.

2.6 Investigating alleged clusters

Patrick Saunders, Andrew Kibble, and Amanda Burls

Introduction

Community anxieties about the effects of environmental contamination on public health have increased in recent years. This chapter details the methods used to investigate alleged clusters of disease. In order to make it as practical and as real as possible we have chosen to base it on the methods used to investigate alleged clusters of diseases with potential association with exposure to environmental chemicals. While community exposure to low levels of chemicals is unlikely to have a dramatic effect on public health, the potential for exposure is real as is the toxicity of many chemicals and the genuine nature of the concerns of local populations. Chemical releases receive considerable publicity and press attention, and surveillance systems indicate an upward trend in the number of chemical releases.[1]

Community suspicions about unusual diseases or levels of disease can be easily raised. A person with a disease may be looking for a cause and focus on a local environmental issue. This understandable reaction can readily lead to a campaign raising awareness and recruiting further cases which, of course, may be entirely unrelated. These campaigns can be extremely difficult to respond to effectively. Community concerns must be taken seriously and treated professionally. Not only could the campaign be right but the fact that people are so animated to take action at least implies some degree of ill-health if using a broad definition of health.

Such studies are notoriously prone to error, and while professional knowledge and expertise have steadily improved, public expectation has outstripped this progress. Clusters of cases may occur purely by chance, and with few exceptions there is actually little scientific or public health purpose to investigating in detail every individual disease cluster.[2] However, to concerned lay people these clusters can be remarkable and confirm their suspicions of a major health scare. Allaying these concerns without seeming to avoid the issue is a major challenge. Deciding whether to investigate is the first important step in a successful response. Unless this is done rationally, investigations may be carried out unnecessarily or be refused inappropriately. Doing nothing is not an option. It is important that public health practitioners have the confidence to employ the correct method at the right time and the confidence and justification, when appropriate, not to conduct a study.

Given the importance of these responsibilities, a number of countries *require* these studies to be conducted. In the UK, for example, health service guidelines require the surveillance of both sources of environmental contamination and potentially environmentally related diseases.[3,4]

A number of agencies have produced guidance addressing some of these issues but none specifically deals with all.[5-10] All these guidelines share some common themes, including the importance of treating complaints about unusual disease distribution with care and caution and generally endorsing an incremental approach, i.e. begin with relatively simple but robust methods and only proceed to more sophisticated analyses if positive results are obtained that justify further study.

Before the investigation

Intelligence on potential sources of environmental contamination

There has been a significant shift in the approach of environmental law from one of response to an incident to one of prior control and approval. In many countries data on existing and historic sources of potential environmental contamination can be accessed through prior authorization of industries, local air quality review and assessment, chemical incident surveillance systems, inventories of contaminated land, and site emergency plans etc. Such information can provide useful background information to any site-specific investigations (e.g. identifying potential environmental confounders) and can provide an indication of the sort of hazards existing and the appropriate resources necessary to respond to them.

Point of contact/responsible individual

There should ideally be a nominated individual acting as a first point of contact. This person must have appropriate training in dealing with the public and be supported by a system that ensures the recording and release of appropriate details. This can be achieved through the use of standardized pro forma which should be retained for audit purposes. The first contact should also be used to make an initial assessment of the level and direction of concern.

Review committee

A review committee should be developed to act as an expert forum for investigations. Access to an expert group to offer advice in difficult cases (perhaps even arbitration in disputes) is essential. Placing this responsibility outside the remit of any one particular agency will also lend validity to the decision and will incorporate some degree of both validation (important scientifically) and independence (important in dealing with the media and public) to the investigation.

Initial response (stage 1)

Reported health problem

When the agency is alerted to a community concern by individual member(s) of the public, it is important that as much relevant information as possible is obtained on first contact. This will enable an early assessment and ensure that the response is treated professionally.

The symptoms reported must be clearly and consistently documented, e.g. are people reporting the same type of symptoms, are conditions self-reported or clinically confirmed? Allegations from individuals do not necessarily mean that the whole community is worried about potential health effects of contamination. Self-appointed pressure groups do not necessarily represent the views of the community. Unfounded concern can lead to property blight and the wider community may actually want an agency to reassure others that there is no public health concern.

Plausibility

This stage requires assessing whether the reported relationship makes sense given what is known about biology and the mechanisms of health and disease, and the temporal and spatial relationships between the disease and the putative source. Is there any evidence that the alleged exposure will result in the effect reported? There is little point initiating a study if the pollutant under investigation cannot cause the effect reported. However, for most diseases, environmental risk factors are poorly understood and in many cases the concerns will be about disease(s) in general rather than specific disease/exposure linkages.

For many diseases, there is a latency period between the point of first exposure and the development of clinical disease. For some cancers this could be decades. Therefore, the address on diagnosis is not necessarily the address at the time of exposure and the agency must decide whether the effect reported is plausible in terms of the likely period and extent of exposure.

Some basic assessment of the geographic relationship between cases and alleged source can also be made at this stage of the investigative process.

Exposure verification

There is a range of information sources (see stage 2) which can be assessed for any evidence of a real or potential exposure. A preliminary investigation of the putative source can reveal whether it has been the subject of previous complaints or could be the source of relevant environmental pollution. However, such a judgement can be extremely difficult to make, e.g. reported symptoms will often be generalized and may not provide any meaningful information on the plausibility of chemical exposure. It is important to establish the number, characteristics, distribution, and timing of complainants. Further assessment of the source is not warranted at this stage.

Environmental hazard

The existence of viable source–pathway–receptor relationships should be considered. Each component needs to be identified and evaluated in order to assess risk. A toxic substance has to be present and there has to be a viable exposure pathway(s) to a target or receptor. If no pathway exists, the contamination may well be a hazard (i.e. there could be an intrinsic toxicity), but it will not present a risk (i.e. the chemical cannot come into contact with a vulnerable target). This is particularly important where specific chemical/disease relationships are being alleged. Again the issue of biologic and temporal plausibility will need to be considered when examining any viable source–pathway–receptor relationships.

Apparent excess of cases

If the plausibility criteria are met it may be possible at this stage to ascertain whether the number of cases reported is excessive. For example, region-wide rates of various diseases can be used as an initial screening tool.

Scoping review

At this early stage an initial scoping literature search will provide useful background information on the nature of the process, toxicologic mechanisms, biologic plausibility, and the volume and quality of the literature and help refine the potential research question.

The decision to continue

By now it should be possible to make some initial Judgements. If the referral is clearly unfounded or even malicious in nature then it would be appropriate to stop any further investigation and document the concern for future reference. If a health-based or environmental standard has been exceeded at the site of interest, the appropriate industry regulator should take action. In the case of no apparent disease excess and no environmental standard being exceeded, the investigation should stop. If there is an apparent excess of cases (as reported by the complainant) and a plausible link with an environmental hazard then it would be appropriate to move to stage 2. However, in many cases there will be few, if any, environmental data available. In these cases, if the type of site means that contamination was, or is, feasible then the investigation should proceed to stage 2 particularly if there are concerns that the alleged exposures occurred some time ago. If there is no possibility of prior exposure and data indicate that there is no relevant environmental contamination, the investigation can stop. For example, there would be little need to continue if the only possible source/hazard is a landfill site known to contain inert materials. In this case, the investigator should stop and report back to the community. In the event of no plausible exposure but a potential excess of disease, the issue should be considered by the agency and, if necessary, referred to the review committee.

Verification of cases and potential excess (stage 2)

Introduction

The aim of this stage is to determine whether a detailed environmental and epidemiological assessment is justified. Appropriate spatial and temporal boundaries should be developed. This will require consideration of factors including meteorologic conditions, operational conditions, emissions, land use change, possible period of exposure, and latency period. Detailed environmental monitoring or modelling is not required at this stage but the investigator should obtain sufficient information to decide whether the source of the contamination is biologically, spatially, and temporally plausible given the health problems reported. Wherever possible, multisite studies should be considered.

Verification of cases

Case details including any evidence of exposure should be obtained and diagnoses confirmed. The latter may need the input of GPs, hospital departments, and routine data sources such as cancer registration systems. This is particularly important when dealing with investigations carried out by pressure groups or concerned individuals that purport to show an excess of disease. An active surveillance system for potentially environmentally related diseases would provide valuable *a priori* intelligence.

Literature review refined

The literature search should now be refined and papers obtained at this stage. This should be carried out in a systematic way focusing on the peer-reviewed literature (see Chapter 2.11) but should also include good quality grey literature if possible. The review committee should be able to provide support.

Test for excess cases

An observed/expected (O/E) analysis using a suitable reference population is appropriate at this stage. The simplest method of analysis is to choose a study area and compare the observed number of cases in that area with the number of cases that would be expected if the area had the same incidence rate as a larger reference area or population. This analysis, while relatively simple, still requires good-quality data and there are methodological issues that need to be considered when interpreting the results. Two methods are commonly used—indirect and direct standardization—although indirect has become the standard methodology.

An O/E comparison might show differences. However, if the prevalence of the condition is related to age or deprivation, an increase in disease levels could be due to large numbers of elderly or poor people in that population. Analysis should take account of such factors as age and gender, and where necessary other factors which may (but not always) need controlling, for example deprivation. It is important to recognize the risk of over-adjustment for social class (any association with environmental factors may be 'adjusted away', since deprived people also are typically much more exposed to environmental hazards).

A clear explanation of the computation of the expected number is given in a number of reference works.[11]

Problems and limitations

People living in areas in the vicinity of a source of pollution (e.g. a factory) can identify themselves as being under risk and it may often be tempting to initiate studies in order to clarify the cause of these apparent risks. By their very nature, these studies are *post hoc* since they were prompted by complaints of apparent 'clusters' of ill-health. *Post hoc* hypotheses may lead to bias by focusing on narrow time bands and specific areas where an excess risk has been observed. Other potential weaknesses with this type of analysis include small numbers, multiple testing, inadequate control for confounders, and, almost invariably, absence of exposure *measures*.[2,12,13] Advice on methodological issues is available from a number of sources.[5,6,9,13–15]

If an association is suggested, the investigation can move to stage 3, otherwise stop, document, and report back to the community.

Environmental and exposure assessment (stage 3)

Monitoring and analysis

It is important to appreciate that measurement of exposure may be extremely difficult but it is a key requirement for drawing conclusions of causality from epidemiological investigations of health outcome. Studies of disease clusters typically involve poor or missing exposure measures. Most use a surrogate or some other indirect measure of exposure with little or no regard to the impact of meteorologic conditions or process characteristics (e.g. stack height, efflux velocity, and plume temperature). Exposure zones are often several kilometres beyond the site or point of release, introducing considerable exposure misclassification and possibilities for confounding co-exposures from other industries. The inclusion of people who may not be exposed may dilute any effect that may be estimated and might result in a true greater effect downwind of the point source being missed. Individuals will also move within and outside these zones (to work, school, etc.) and many people will not reside within the zone for most of the day.

Accurate assessment of exposure is a basic requirement for estimation of its effect. Advances in environmental modelling, particularly air dispersion modelling, can help improve exposure estimates. This requires the input of specialist environmental expertise.

It is possible that routine environmental monitoring data may be available. In the UK, ambient air measurements at ground level are automatically collected across selected monitoring sites, which can be classified according to their location, e.g. city centre, urban background, industrial, and rural. Where such automated monitoring sites are located near to point sources, they can provide valuable data on likely levels of exposure, but in many cases monitoring sites may not be advantageously located or are unable to measure specific pollutants of concern. Therefore, it may be appropriate to commission environmental monitoring.

If the concentrations of chemicals are below a recognized standard, the nature of the investigation should be reconsidered. This does not necessarily mean it should be stopped, as many standards are relatively old, some may be under review, and there are very few chemicals which have actually been evaluated for their health risk. A toxicologic input will be particularly important in the interpretation of the environmental data.

Any monitoring or modelling must focus on compounds that could produce the effects under investigation. It should not be undertaken unless the potential problem is clearly understood or defined (i.e. there must be some plausibility). Inadequate monitoring/modelling is likely to do more harm than good.[8]

Site details will also need confirmation, and should include a site visit with appropriate experts to confirm the plausibility of an exposure pathway.

The decision to continue

If there is evidence of a potentially significant chemical exposure (chemical, level, pathway, spatial and temporal plausibility) and the health effect is plausible, proceed to stage 4. Otherwise consider referral to the review committee or stop and document.

Epidemiological assessment (stage 4)

Boundaries

It is useful to engage the concerned community in confirming the most appropriate spatial and temporal boundaries. This can help engender a real sense of being involved in the design of the study. It can also provide the researchers with pre-defined boundaries. The areas of concern may not necessarily reflect the realities of exposure assessment. The investigators should consider how meteorologic, operational, and technical factors may affect exposure and whether additional environmental sampling and modelling may be necessary to refine the area of exposure. The area of interest may also be manipulated to assess whether there is a risk with proximity, e.g. examining areas at different distances from a putative source.

Identifying all cases within the spatial and temporal boundaries

Appropriate case finding techniques should be employed. If the study is relying on routine data sets, the investigators must assure themselves of the data quality and be aware of the limitations of each data source used. This may have significance in determining the spatial boundaries of the study, e.g. cancer registration may only be available for a specific period.

Agree an appropriate method

If there are no resources available, such as academic units, to assist in developing an appropriate method the review committee should provide advice. At its simplest this may be a refinement of the O/E analysis performed in stage 2 and/or the use of a dispersal model to identify exposed populations more accurately. It may be more appropriate to use a more sophisticated analysis[5] such as Bayesian mapping or link the study to a larger multisite study. If this stage still shows an apparent excess of disease the issue should be referred to the review committee to assess the quality of the study and to determine the need and method for more sophisticated epidemiological or other research studies.

Biomarkers of exposure may also be considered appropriate in some circumstances.

Communication strategy

The statutory agencies should seek the involvement of the affected or concerned communities. It is not enough to simply make information available for use by the public. When conducting investigations, involving the community must be an integral part of the process and should be planned for. Worry and concern can lead to stress or anxiety which can exacerbate existing conditions or result in an increase in the reporting of symptoms including those which do not have a toxicologic basis. Openness with the community can help alleviate community and individual concerns and help generate a more positive working relationship with the community. If the result of the study shows no significant excess of disease, this information needs to be communicated effectively. Guidance is available from a number of sources including the Department of Health[16] and the ATSDR.[17]

References
1 Kibble A, Dyer J, Wheeldon C, Saunders PJ (2003). Public health surveillance for chemical incidents. *Lancet*, **357**(9265), 1365.
2 Rothman KJ (1990). A sobering start for the cluster busters' conference. *Am J Epidemiol*, **132**(1, Suppl.), S6–S13.
3 NHS Management Executive (1993). *Health Service Guidelines HSG(93)38: arrangements to deal with health aspects of chemical contamination incidents*. Department of Health, Health Aspects of the Environment and Food Division, London.
4 NHS Management Executive (1993). *Health Service Guidelines HSG(93)56: public health responsiblities of the NHS and the roles of others*. Department of Health, Health Aspects of the Environment and Food Division, London.
5 Alexander FE, Cuzick J (1996). Methods for the assessment of disease clusters. In: Eliott P, Cuzick J, English D, Stern R (eds) *Geographical and environmental epidemiology methods for small-area studies*, pp. 238–50. Oxford University Press, Oxford.

6 Alexander FE, Boyle P (1996). *Methods for investigating localised clustering of disease*, IARC Scientific Publication No. 135. International Agency for Research on Cancer, Lyon.

7 Centres for Disease Control (1990). Guidelines for investigating clusters of health events. *Morbidity and Mortality Weekly Report*, **39**(RR-11), 1–23.

8 Department of Health (2000). *Good practice guidelines for investigating the health impact of local industrial emissions*. Department of Health, London.

9 Leukaemia Research Fund (1997). *Handbook and guide to the investigation of clusters of disease*. Leukaemia Research Fund Centre for Clinical Epidemiology, University of Leeds, Leeds.

10 Rothenberg RB, Thacker SB (1996). Guidelines for the investigation of clusters of adverse health events. In: Eliott P, Cuzick J, English D, Stern R (eds) *Geographical and environmental epidemiology methods for small-area studies*, pp. 264–77. Oxford University Press, Oxford.

11 Kirkwood BR (1997). *Measures of mortality and morbidity. Essentials of medical statistics*, pp. 106–17 Blackwell Scientific Publications, Oxford.

12 Neutra R, Swan S, Mack T (1992). Clusters galore: insights about environmental clusters from probability theory. *Sci Total Environ*, **127**(1–2), 187–200.

13 Urquhart J (1996). Studies of disease clustering: problems of interpretation. In: Eliott P, Cuzick J, English D, Stern R (eds) *Geographical and environmental epidemiology methods for small-area studies*, pp. 278–85. Oxford University Press, Oxford.

14 Elliott P, Wakefield JC, Best NG, Briggs BJ (2000). *Spatial epidemiology—methods and applications*. Oxford University Press, Oxford.

15 Hills M (1996). Some comments on methods for investigating disease risk around a point source. In: Eliott P, Cuzick J, English D, Stern R (eds) *Geographical and environmental epidemiology methods for small-area studies*, pp. 231–7. Oxford University Press, Oxford.

16 Department of Health (1997). *Communicating about risks to public health pointers to good practice*. EOR Division, Department of Health, London.

17 Agency for Toxic Substances and Disease Registry. *A primer on health risk communication principles and practices* Available at: http://www.atsdr.cdc.gov/HEC/primer.html (accessed 21 January 2006).

2.7 Assessing longer-term health trends: registers

Jem Rashbass and John Newton

Objectives

The objectives of this chapter are to enable you to
- understand disease registers in general
- understand cancer registries in particular
- use them efficiently
- be aware of the traps for the unwary
- appreciate the future of disease registers.

Introduction

A disease register is a file of data on all cases of a particular disease or health condition, limited to a defined population. There is a wide range of registries each focused on specific health issues. One recent count in England identified around 250 specific disease registers.[1]

This chapter aims to provide
- a brief overview of registers and how to get best use of them
- a more detailed account of one of the most comprehensive: the cancer registries.

Registries (the organizations that support registers) arrange systems to collect, collate, and quality assure data on new cases of the condition of interest; they may also collect follow-up (longitudinal) data on identified cases. The resulting records are intended to be permanent, and the data are periodically analysed, tabulated, and reported.

Epidemiological registers can be based on:
- disease, e.g. cancer, psychiatric illness, coronary heart disease, and diabetes
- risk factors, e.g. specific exposures (for example radiation industry workers or genetic factors, including twin status)
- interventions or treatments, for example cochlear implants or renal transplants.

Registers can also be oriented toward service provision rather than epidemiology, but can nevertheless be useful for public health purposes. For example, 'at risk' registers for children might be used to ensure adequate protection for such children, and registers of disabled people run by local authorities have a similar purpose. Communicable disease notification provides an analogous function. However, registers of patients seen or treated in a particular hospital or clinical setting, that are not population based, can be difficult to use for general epidemiological purposes. They may be used as a source of cases for case–control studies[2]—although selection biases are common. In general, clinical data-bases that are not population-based are more useful for technology assessment and quality improvement than for epidemiological purposes.

The data collected by registries vary widely, but often include personal identifiers, socio-demographic information, disease status (possibly including stage and severity), details of treatments and other interventions, and eventual outcomes.

A registry must establish systems to:

- maintain a reliable notification or identification of cases within the studied population
- ensure comparability of inclusion criteria onto the register: for a diagnosis, strict rules are needed to identify the studied condition, within an agreed classification
- minimize under-coverage—cases not being included when they should be
- ensure that duplication of cases within the register does not occur
- keep the register updated—removing those who have recovered, died, or moved out of the area.

Most registers require patient consent to collect and hold the data. However, in the UK, legislation has allowed cancer registries (and some others) to collect identifiable patient information without prior informed consent (Section 60, Health and Social Care Act 2001)—this important caveat is currently subject to annual review by the Patient Information Advisory Group (PIAG[1]) in England and Wales. Any research use of the registry data can only occur with the appropriate ethical approval, especially if identifiable data are held or shared with outside researchers.

Maintaining a register is time and labor intensive and can be expensive. Maintaining motivation and interest is essential and often depends on the person organizing the register. Registers tend to get out of date quickly, and a rigorous process of quality assurance must be in place if the data are to be of high quality.

Many registries are likely to change significantly as health records become electronic and patients can be identified with minimal ambiguity with a unique identifier (for example the UK National Health Service (NHS) number). Electronic records improve data accessibility and timeliness, while the unique identifier facilitates linkage to other data sets. Electronic data are not necessarily more accurate than paper records, and may conceal other errors, but they are easier to collect. It pays to remain skeptical of data quality and look for evidence of validity. In the future a national electronic health record system covering the whole UK population could greatly reduce the need for discrete disease registers, and could deliver near real-time disease monitoring and surveillance.

How can registers help?

If case ascertainment is high, prevalence and incidence rates can be computed. Analysis of risks and etiology can be explored, using individual as well as area characteristics. With follow-up data, outcomes can be measured, e.g. survival rates for cancer. If registers are maintained over time they can produce evidence of change in, for example, epidemics or in the effectiveness of interventions.

Registers can be used to assist in the management of chronic disease in clinical settings, triggering follow-up care for people with, for example, diabetes or asthma within a primary care practice. Registers can also form the basis for clinical audit and quality improvement efforts.

An example of a disease register: a cancer registry

The cancer registration system is a unique world-wide resource, there being regional cancer registries covering between 1 and 15 million people in most countries in the world. Each registry is essentially a detailed list of all the cancers that have occurred since each registry was established (e.g. in the UK this was usually around 1970).

Cancer registries in Europe work together through the European Network of Cancer Registries. World-wide, the International Association of Cancer Registries coordinates registry activities. The entire population is covered in the UK and Republic of Ireland, Scandinavia, The Netherlands and Germany (from 1999), Canada and nearly so in the USA. Registries in other countries have complete coverage for subpopulations. Others are hospital based. International details can be found in *Cancer Incidence in Five Continents.*[3]

Important features

Three important features of cancer registries should be remembered:

- cancer registries contain details of *diagnosed* cancers—they cannot tell you about cancers which we take to our grave without diagnosis
- the record starts at diagnosis and collects details of the patient and the tumor (stage and grade) at that time—and there is increasingly information on treatment in the first 6 months
- most are population based, providing a denominator for numbers of tumors in relation to the population of which the patients were members.

What is on the register?

Registries differ very slightly, but the minimum content is nationally defined. In the UK, for example, the registry includes details of:

- the patient—name, address, postcode, date of birth, sex, their doctors, NHS number
- the tumor—site, histological type, and possibly grade and stage at diagnosis (how advanced the tumor is)
- date of diagnosis
- treatment during the first 6 months after date of diagnosis and cause of death.

Many registries will keep extra data on each patient and tumor, and there will be links between multiple tumors in the same patient. The NHS number allows linkage to other datasets where a patient is identified by their NHS number.

In the UK the Office for National Statistics compiles mortality statistics which refer to date of death and residence at death. Survival data refer to place and date of diagnosis.

What the data can be used for?

For each type of tumor and type of patient, it is possible to analyze:

- *Incidence* of cancer, and trends in incidence. These can be used to make projections in demand and to help judge the effectiveness of preventive strategies. Given the knowledge of the population size, migration, and all cause mortality, projections of incidence are fairly reliable for up to 10 years.
- *Survival* of people with cancer, and trends in survival. Trends in survival can be used to make projections and to help judge the effectiveness of treatment.
- *Linkage analysis*—since all cancer registry data now contain a unique patient identifier, the NHS number, records can be linked to any other data set that uses this identifier. For example, hospital episode statistics (HES data) from the UK Department of Health can be used to track in-patient events for patients diagnosed with cancer. In the future, it will be possible to link to any data held within the complete health record (for example medication, co-morbidities, lifestyle).

Using cancer registry data

All registries produce routine reports, usually on incidence and survival, so if your enquiry is simple just take the report off the shelf. If the enquiry is more complex, or if you are not quite sure what you need, the registry will advise you. However, there are some questions you will always be asked, so you must know:

- which cancers you are interested in—cancers are classified by site (lung, brain, rectum, etc.) and type (adenocarcinoma, teratoma, etc.)
- which people you are interested in—by age, or date of birth, year or age band, e.g. 35–40, or born between 1920 and 1930, sex, area of residence (in the UK usually health district, but any combination of postcodes can be used, but must be in the region covered by the registry)
- the year of diagnosis.

Most registries are willing to provide data from which individuals cannot be identified although there are issues around even anonymous data which may be 'disclosive' if the population is small or the tumor relatively rare in the age group. If individuals need to be identified or the data are potentially disclosive then release will depend on other factors, mainly related to ethical and confidentiality issues. These are spelt out in the UK Association of Cancer Registries Policy Document[4] whose procedures are similar to those established by the International Association of Cancer Registries. To summarize, you can have named data if you are the patient or the patient's doctor, or you want the data for the benefit of the patient or the direct benefit of others or for audit. For genetic counselling you need the consent of living relations, and for research you need research ethics committee permission.

Analyzing the data

Before you obtain the data, you must have a reasonably detailed idea of what you intend to do with them. Essentially, as with any investigation of this kind, the analytical skills you need are epidemiological and statistical, but it pays to be quite clear which problems you are trying to solve, and whether the questions you ask will do it. All registries employ statisticians or epidemiologists, and part of their job is to advise on the use and the limitations of the data.

The limitations of the data

Cancer registries are the main source of epidemiological information on cancer, although there are limits to the information they can provide. They will *not* tell you:

- About cancer more than 30 years ago (at least for the whole of the UK)—before that, you have to rely on mortality information; other countries are similar though many have been started more recently
- About hospital activity; they will tell you about patients resident in that region, but patients from outside the registry region will be entered on their home registry, and patients from outside the UK probably will fall through the net
- About patients diagnosed within the last year—registries cannot provide survival data for a period longer than the time since diagnosis, e.g. 5-year survival in patients diagnosed the previous year. Actually, approximations and projections can be made but they are not particularly accurate
- What has happened between 6 months after diagnosis and death. Unless there is active follow-up, some deaths may be missed—this also applies to local recurrence and prolonged treatment.

Myths and shortcomings

Data collection takes time, especially when it is manual, and therefore registers are unlikely to have a complete up-to-date collection of data. Cancer registries usually have complete data that are about 1 year old, while the UK Office of National Statistics publish the data after 18 months. With the increase in electronic data feeds to registries data are being collected more rapidly and statistics are being released on-line more quickly. The data are never entirely complete because occasional data may appear many years after diagnosis.

A register is only as good as the data that are available to it. Remember, electronic data are no more accurate than paper data—but they may be easier to obtain and simpler to import into the register and therefore avoid some of the human errors that occur during data entry. If the diagnosis or the death certificate is wrong then even a complete data set will be flawed. Be skeptical and question all your data sources—even registers!

Further resources

International Association on Research on Cancer. *Epidemiology database* http://www-dep.iarc.fr/ (accessed 25 June 2005).

Cancer Research UK. *Statistics. Cancer facts and figures.* Available at: http: www.cruk.org. uk/aboutcancer/statistics/ (accessed 25 June 2005).

National Statistics, UK. *Cancer.* Available at: http:www.statistics.gov.uk/ CCI/nscl.asp?id=6279 (accessed 25 June 2005).

National Cancer Institute (USA). *SEER (surveillance, epidemiology and end results).* http://seer.cancer.gov (accessed 25 June 2005).

References

1 Newton J, Garner S (2002). *Disease registers in England. Report for the Department of Health policy research programme.* Available at: www.erpho.org.uk/viewResource.aspx?id=12531 (accessed 21 January 2006).

2 Black N, Barker M, Payne M (2004). Cross sectional survey of multi-centre clinical database in the United Kingdom. *BMJ*, **328**, 1478–81.

3 Parkin DM, Whelan SL, Ferlay J, Teppo L, Thomas DB (2003). *Cancer incidence in five continents*, Vol. VIII. IARC, Lyon.

4 UK Association of Cancer Registries. *Guidelines on the release of confidential data.* Avilable at: http://www.ukacr.org/confidentiality/ (accessed 25 June 2005).

2.8 Assessing health status

Peter Gentle, David Pencheon, and
Julian Flowers

Objectives

Assessing the health of a population is a fundamental part of many public
health activities. Doing assessments well is challenging—there are usually
problems in obtaining the necessary data and in balancing alternative
approaches. Assessing of health status is an essential part of:
- a needs assessment
- an equity audit
- a policy/planning review
- target setting
- resource allocation
- evaluation/research of current/potential services/interventions.

The objective of this chapter is to identify the principles of assessing the
health of a defined population and to provide some practical advice.

Assessing population health status

There are many types of population health assessment, but the usual
steps in performing an assessment are:
- define the purpose of the assessment
- define the population concerned (and any comparator populations)
- define the aspects of health to be considered
- identify and review existing data sources: are good local data available?
  are routine local or national statistics available? are relevant published
  surveys available?
- select the most appropriate existing data
- make good use of the data, analyze appropriately (e.g. adjusting for
  population composition, deriving suitable measures and perhaps
  modelling future trends)
- consider if specific issues require specially collected data: should a
  special survey be undertaken?
- consider the use of comparators
- address issues of confidentiality and disclosure
- interpret and communicate the results of the assessment
- evaluate your efforts.

Be clear about the purpose

The starting point, defining the purpose, is especially important. A tendency to have an extensive unfocused list of objectives must be resisted, as well as the temptation to examine interesting but irrelevant issues.

The most important reasons for assessing the health status of a defined population are to:

- support *needs assessment*, establishing whether particular health problems exist in a given population, characterizing the problems, and identifying the potential for avoidable mortality and morbidity (see Chapter 1.3)
- support a *health equity audit*; establishing quantitatively the mismatch between need and supply for a defined population/service, doing something about it, and reviewing the effectiveness of such action (see Chapters 2.10 and 5.5)
- support *policy making* through informing the public, professional groups, and decision-makers about the nature and distribution of health challenges, and the definition of the problem; this includes a health impact assessment (see Chapter 1.5)
- support *planning and implementation*, improving resource allocation, target setting, and helping targeting of health and other services (see Chapters 4.5 and 4.6), and inform *health impact assessment* (see Chapter 1.5)
- support *evaluation* of interventions, programmes, or policies (see Part 6)
- prioritize the most important areas where *research* is needed.

Define the aspects of health to be considered

Health can have a variety of meanings; for example the World Health Organization takes a very broad view. Health is seen as having physical, emotional, and social dimensions. In practice, although you may want to (or be well advised to) use a more restrictive definition, you should always be aware of broad aspects of health (Box 2.8.1).

Box 2.8.1 The World Health Organization's view of health

Health is the extent to which an individual or group is able:
- to satisfy needs
- to realize aspirations
- to change or cope with their environment.

Health is a resource for everyday life, not the objective for living: it is a positive concept emphasizing social and personal resources as well as physical capabilities.[1]

Profiles of the health status of populations can present data on both
• the determinants of health status
• the measures of the status itself
These should relate eventually to measurable outcomes. Assessments may relate to health overall or just cover one or more aspects.

The determinants of health may be endogenous and exogenous. They include (adapted from Ruwaard et al.[2]):

• susceptibilities: markers, genetic factors (e.g. prevalence of sickle cell trait, apoE4 gene), or endogenous susceptibilities
• physical, emotional, social, economic, and environmental influences
• health attitudes and health-related behaviours
• health protection, collective prevention, health promotion
• health and social care, both somatic and mental.

The measures of health status includes:

• self-assessed health status (including the experience of having the health problem)
• symptom incidence and prevalence
• disease incidence and prevalence
• impairment, disability, or handicap
• mortality.

Who defines health for a particular study may be crucial. It may be the individual with a health problem, or a professional expert, or society as represented by government policy (see Chapters 1.3 to 1.7).

Define the population

Defining the population of interest is critical. Population size, structure, and the period of observation covered can have powerful effects on the numbers of cases of disease or disability: data are therefore usually expressed as proportions (e.g. the number of people with diabetes per thousand population at a particular point in time) or rates (the number of new cases per thousand population per year). For certain purposes such rates may need adjustment for potential confounding variables (e.g. age, sex, socio-economic status, or ethnicity) to allow valid comparison with other populations.

Often geographic identifiers are used to frame the population studied, for example postcodes. Problems can arise with population estimates for small areas, especially those projected from a census that is relatively distant in time. If small areas are being studied, errors in estimates of population numbers and composition can result in dramatic but erroneous findings.

Review the available data

Comprehensive population health assessments are based on a wide range of data of different types. In order to maintain some framework to all the data items being used, consider the simple dimensions of data as used by Stevens and Gillam:[3]

* local versus national data
* routine versus *ad hoc* data
* quantitative versus qualitative.

The inter-relationship of these dimensions can be represented as a cube (Figure 2.8.1).

While *local data* are required for assessing the health of the local population, they may not be available, and so *national (or indeed international) data* may be used if the local population is felt to be typical of the nation as a whole. Data from similar localities (e.g. in terms of levels of deprivation) or national data may of course be used for comparative purposes.

Many data are collected *routinely* by census offices, health service providers, local and central government, and others. In addition, some of the many *ad hoc* studies that have been carried out locally or elsewhere may be relevant to a particular issue. Weaknesses of routine data collection systems include non-standard or inconsistent approaches to coding and data collection, and limited availability due to cost and privacy policies.

Quantitative data are usually necessary to answer questions such as 'How many people have a particular condition?'. *Qualitative approaches* are well suited for exploring such issues as what it is like to be disabled, or perceptions about the effects and tolerability of risks from industrial pollutants.

Qualitative data can be very valuable and tend to be insufficiently used.

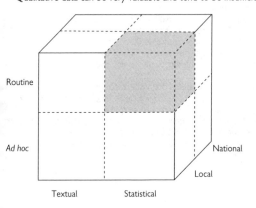

Figure 2.8.1 The data cube, showing three important dimensions of data used for health assessment (adapted from Stevens and Gillam[3])

Many useful data are recorded as part of clinical care or collected by health-care providers. However, very great care is needed in using such data: not all people with a health condition receive treatment (or they may be treated by other providers). Clinicians usually record information just for clinical purposes rather than for analytic purposes. The absence of a positive record (e.g. of smoking) may mean a true negative or that the information was not sought. The definition of a condition (and whether to treat it) may vary substantially from clinician to clinician, causing large differences between areas. Issues of confidentiality must be addressed.

Select data carefully

At first sight there seem to be so many data available that assessing health should not be much of a challenge. However, Finagle's law is usually proved correct in public health work.

Box 2.8.2 Finagle's law of information

In full, Finagle's law is often quoted thus: 'The information you have is not what you want; the information you want is not what you need; the information you need is not what you can get; the information you can get costs more than you want to pay' (or a variation thereof).

There are detailed descriptions of sources and approaches to using health-related data elsewhere in this handbook (see Chapter 2.1). Relevant, detailed, and accurate data are seldom available directly, and so data collected for other purposes have to be used appropriately to give an indirect assessment.

In considering the use of any data, think about how they have been obtained. People often assume that the quality and relevance of the data is satisfactory for the intended purpose. But those recording the data may well not use consistent terms or criteria and this can have a major impact. Remember that it is usually better to use good data from elsewhere than poor local data.

Remember that organizations that collect data often publish only some of them and may make other data available. They will often advise on data quality and relevance for particular purposes.

The use of international data needs great care as different countries may use different definitions and data collection processes.

When the source has been identified a number of questions should be asked (Table 2.8.1).

Table 2.8.1 Questions to be asked of data

Validity of data for your purpose	
Relevance	Are the data relevant to the issue?
Definition	Have the data items been defined usefully for your purpose?
Conceptual bias	Are there conceptual biases in the data source (e.g. has data collection been structured to benefit the organization that has produced the data?)
Timeliness	Are the data still relevant?
Generalizability	Are the data relevant to your population?
Technical quality of data	
Recording	Have the data been entered properly according to the definitions?
Completeness	Have all been included—or a random sample used?
Bias	Are there classification or selection biases?
Appropriate aggregation	If the data are already aggregated, has this been done properly?
Quality of the analytic methods	
Appropriate adjustment or modelling	Can adjustment be made for your population structure, e.g. age/sex standardization, weighting for social group or ethnic composition? Is modelling necessary?
Summary measures used	Are the summary measures useful? (e.g. do you require a measure of absolute risk while only relative risk is reported?)
Statistical significance	Are the numbers big enough to allow an adequately precise estimate?
Practical questions	
	Will confidentiality policies allow the relevant use of the data?
	What is the cost likely to be?
	Are the data available in machine analyzable form?

Make good use of the data

Those assessing the health of populations should always be suspicious of any data, but they should not be paralyzed by the above list of potential problems with data sources. Don't let perfection be the enemy of the useful. The essential issue is: are the data you are using fit for purpose? If the purpose remains clear, direct or indirect measures of the studied risks or health problems can usually be derived, sometimes by assembling fragments of evidence from a number of different sources.

In progressing from data to information, the five forms of health information identified by Ruwaard et al.[4] form a useful framework:

- recording the situation at one moment in time for individual variables
- recording trends over time for individual variables
- simultaneously recording a series of different variables
- describing relationships between different indicators
- making forecasts with the help of modelling.

The purpose of the assessment will determine the nature of the analyses chosen. Common purposes include:

- comparing findings for the population with other similar populations or larger populations, or comparing health status observed with that expected for the type of population
- describing the relative health of parts of the population (areas or social groups), identifying inequalities
- comparing health trends over time
- estimating the extent of potentially preventable health problems
- describing the likely health impact of environmental and social factors
- describing the impact of health problems in terms of people's experience of health problems.

Some general approaches that may help include:

- using data from larger populations or special studies, if thought to be comparable
- adjusting data statistically for confounders, e.g. allowing for population age, sex, and social differences
- using evidence-based proxy measures (e.g. estimating all deaths due to smoking from those due to lung cancer)[5]
- combining data from several years, to reduce statistical uncertainty
- giving broad estimates or ranges if uncertainties exist (observed differences may be very large)
- making logical deductions from patterns of data
- seeing whether different analyses give similar results.

A number of technical analyses on the available data might be helpful, for example:

- elementary measures such as prevalence (point or period), incidence, etc.
- calculating relative rates or ratios of standardized mortality or morbidity, e.g. standardized mortality ratio (SMR)
- calculating years of life lost before a given age (e.g. before age 70) in the studied population, perhaps by risk factor or condition
- calculating and comparing life tables and life expectancy.

One challenge is analysing data on both mortality and morbidity patterns together. Chronic conditions such as arthritis and depression cause a great deal of disability, but relatively few deaths. A number of methods of measuring and comparing the burden of disease by suitably combining disability and death data have been developed, including:

- disability-free life expectancy[6]
- disability-adjusted life years (DALYs)[7,8] (see Figure 2.8.2).

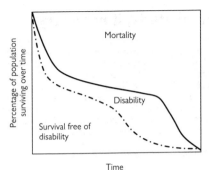

Figure 2.8.2 Disability-adjusted life years over time (adapted from Murray et al.[9])

(For more details of summary measures of health which combine measures of mortality and morbidity see Chapter 2.9.) On occasions, data from different systems can be linked if a unique or probabilistic identifier is available.

Assessing health status using spatially referred data requires particular thought. Geographic information systems[10] can be used to map and analyse differences in any of the risk or health status measures. Be aware of the strengths and weakness of assessing and disseminating health status information in geographic format (Table 2.8.2).

Table 2.8.2 Strengths and weakness of assessing health using spatial data and maps

Strengths	Visually arresting
	Most readers immediately identify with the areas
	Use of colours can be used to show gradients without the use of numbers
	Can suggest patterns not visible in tables of numbers
Weaknesses	Analysis by geography may mask more important patterns by subpopulations ('most poor people don't live in poor areas')
	Thematic maps using averages will inevitably mask many individuals with attributes of interest (risk doesn't suddenly change at county boundaries to a different uniform pan-county risk)
	There may be considerable uncertainty about data shown for areas with small populations. If these areas are coloured then seriously false impressions may be given.

Carry out a local study, if necessary

Health issues can be sufficiently pressing and the available data so limited that a case exists for conducting a specific study with fresh data collection. At national or state level, this situation arises relatively frequently. At local level, a survey or longitudinal study should only be carried out if time is available and the value of the data to be provided justifies the cost. Again, it is essential to be clear about the purpose. There is always a tendency to ask too many interesting questions or record too many findings. As well as being unnecessarily expensive, this may reduce the response rate, for example if a questionnaire appears too complex. Key features of a successful survey are:

- a clear aim
- well designed, with enough statistical power to address the studied issue
- good instrument selection, ensuring measures are valid, reliable, and repeatable
- good planning and management of the study logistics and resources, including interviewer training and data recording
- adequate arrangements for timely data entry, analysis, and reporting.

Consider the use of comparators

Assessing the health of a population may be undertaken to answer two rather different questions, firstly what is the actual extent of a health problem and secondly how does it compare with previous years, other areas and other social groupings. For example in examining the need for initiatives to reduce smoking, all that may be required is the number of deaths and extent of ill health associated with smoking locally. Information that locally this data is 10% lower or higher than the national average may well be redundant and indeed may divert attention from the principal data. However on other occasions comparative data will be required to highlight problems that are becoming more important with the passage of time or are particularly acute locally and need to be addressed in ways that are different from those required for most other areas.

Comparisons are of particular relevance when considering inequalities and inequities (see Chapter 2.10). Remember that an inequality measure is a description of a difference, a variation, a distribution (and ultimately, in the case of an inequity, an unfair, unjustifiable difference where need and supply are inappropriately matched, the extreme case being described classically by Julian Tudor Hart as the 'inverse case law'[11])

Address issues of confidentiality and disclosure

Assessing health status, especially at a small area level, increases the risk of inappropriate and unnecessary disclosure of person-level data. This is a highly complex and evolving area, as there are both technical issues and societal issues, notably around balancing the benefits to society with the risks to individuals (a common theme in the practice of public health).

For the purposes of this handbook, there are some important principles to remember (see box 2.8.3).

Box 2.8.3 Disclosure, confidentiality in population health information

1. Public health practice relies on the secondary use of health information in aggregated and record level form for surveillance, health monitoring, epidemiological, and research purposes. Most information used in public health practice is derived from data collected on individuals, often for other primary reasons.[12]

2. Public health practitioners rarely need to be able to identify the actual names of individuals, but do need person identifiers to be able to *discriminate* between individuals, or to confirm that two records belong to the same individual for *linkage* purposes. Data that are de-identified through anonymization or pseudonymization may prevent adequate discrimination or linkage.

3. There is a range of legal protection,[13,14] codes of practice,[15] and protocols applied to data (and statistics derived from data) which are largely designed to protect individual privacy (i.e. disclosure of information over and above that which is already publicly available without consent).

4. Some of the safeguards designed to protect confidentiality have made it increasingly difficult to access or share data for legitimate purposes. It is becoming increasingly apparent that the balance between individual risk and population benefit appears heavily weighted to the former.[16,17]

5. Within the UK National Health Service the HORUS principles define good practice in data use—data should be Held securely and confidentially, Obtained fairly and efficiently, Recorded accurately and reliably, Used effectively and ethically, and Shared appropriately and lawfully. Applying such principles can enable the more effective sharing and use of data in order to protect and improve health, and improve health care.

6. Although health statistics and aggregated data are in effect anonymized, there maybe inadvertent disclosure on occasion.[18] Increasingly, statistical outputs and the raw data that are used to generate them are subject to statistical disclosure control procedures in order to reduce the risk that inadvertent disclosures occur. These procedures (which include data suppression, controlled rounding,[15,19,20] and aggregation of data in tables) are applied when data tables are shared which contain cells with small numbers of events.[21]

7. Although these techniques are applied by national statistical bodies, they are difficult to apply by local practitioners in generating or sharing local data, and may severely damage the usefulness of local data. There is inconsistency between datasets about many of the rules (e.g. what constitutes small numbers, populations at risk, whether zeros in a data table are disclosive and so on[15,20,22]).

8. As a result there is increasing confusion amongst practitioners about what can be shared with whom and how.

9. Practitioners and organizations may become so risk averse (due to uncertainty and confusion) that legitimate data sharing will not take place, with the consequence that information and analysis that will benefit the public is not understood.
10. It is crucial that a framework for data sharing, access, and use which balances both individual privacy and the need to use the aggregated or record level data from individuals for legitimate non-clinical health purposes is developed.

Communicate results effectively

Occasionally a large set of data is to be produced for reference purposes, for subsequent expert analysis. But usually the information is used to inform the process of identifying opportunities to improve health, and while experts may be involved the information usually needs to be communicated to a general audience. The communication methods required need careful consideration and coordination. This becomes most apparent when communicating with the press (see Chapters 4.7 and 7.4).

When communicating results, a full description of the analytic methods used together with their limitations and assumptions may well be inappropriate. If so the assessor must take great care to provide a fair assessment and ensure that the typical audience will gain the right impression (for example by resisting the temptation to use a false origin for a bar chart, even if it spoils the impact). The assessor must, however, be prepared and able to justify the methods in detail if requested.

Key points about health status analyses to consider in a written or oral communication are:
- think through its purpose
- don't leave it to the reader to deduce relevant points from a mass of data—quote specific data to make a point
- ensure confidentiality for participants in surveys, and ensure this is made clear to everyone
- don't be too sophisticated—many people in the target audience will not have much background knowledge of the issue.

Evaluate your health status assessment

Those of us engaged in public health emphasize the importance of assessment to others. This should begin at home. It is important that our work is assessed using tools such as audit—perhaps using the headings of this chapter.

Further resources

Last JM (1998). *Public health and human ecology*. Appleton and Lange, Stamford, CT.

McDowell I, Newell C (1996). *Measuring health. A guide to rating scales and questionnaires*. Oxford University Press, New York.

Murray SA, Graham LJC (1995). Practice based health needs assessment. *BMJ*, **310**, 1443–8.

Stevens A, Raftery J (eds) (1997). *Health care needs assessment*, 2nd series. Radcliffe Medical Press, Oxford.

Streiner DL, Norman GR (1995). *Health measurement scales: a practical guide to their development and use*, 2nd edn. Oxford University Press, Oxford.

UK Academy of Medical Sciences (2006). *Personal data for public good: using health information in medical research*. Available at: http://www. acmedsci.ac.uk/images/project/Personal.pdf (accessed 21 January 2006).

UK Council for Science and Technology (2005). *Better use of personal information: opportunities and risks*. Available at: http://www2.cst.gov.uk/ cst/reports/files/personal-information/report.pdf (accessed 21 January 2006).

Wright J (ed.) (1998). *Health needs assessment in practice*. BMJ Books, London.

References

1 World Health Organization (1946). *WHO constitution*. Available at: http://www. who.int/trade/glossary/story046/en/ (accessed 25 June 2005).

2 Ruwaard D, Kramers PGN, van den Berg Jeths A, Achterberg PW (1994). *Public health status and forecasts: the health status of the Dutch population over the period 1950–2010*, pp. 30–3. National Institute of Public Health and Environmental Protection, Bilthoven, The Netherlands. Sdu Uitgeverij, The Hague.

3 Stevens A, Gillam S (1998). Needs assessment: from theory to practice. *BMJ*, **316**, 1448–52.

4 Ruwaard D, Kramers PGN, van den Berg Jeths A, Achterberg PW (1994). *Public health status and forecasts: the health status of the Dutch population over the period 1950–2010*, pp. 159–61. National Institute of Public Health and Environmental Protection, Bilthoven, The Netherlands. Sdu Uitgeverij, The Hague.

5 Peto R, Lopez AD, Boreham J, Thun M, Heath C Jr (1992). Mortality from tobacco in developed countries: indirect estimation from national vital statistics. *Lancet*, **339**(8804), 1268–78.

6 Robine JM, Romieu I, Cambois E (1999). Health expectancy indicators. *Bull World Health Org*, **77**(2), 181–5.

7 Morrow RH, Hyder AA, Murray CJ, Lopez AD (1998). Measuring the burden of disease. *Lancet*, **352**(9143), 1859–60.

8 Murray CJ, Lopez AD (1997). Global mortality, disability, and the contribution of risk factors: Global Burden of Disease Study. *Lancet*, **349**(9063), 1436–42.

9 Murray CJL, Salomon JA, Mathers C (1999). *A critical examination of summary measures of population health*. World Health Organization, Geneva (GPE discussion paper No. 12, quoted in *WHO World Health Report 2000*).

10 de Lepper MJC, Scholetn HJ, Stern RM (eds) (1995). *The added value of geographical information systems in public and environmental health*. Kluwer, Dordrecht (on behalf of the World Health Organization for Europe).

11 Tudor Hart J (1971). The inverse care law. *Lancet*, **1**, 405–12.

12 Verity C, Nicoll A (2002). Consent, confidentiality, and the threat to public health surveillance. *BMJ*, **324**(7347), 1210–13.

13 Boyd P (2003). The requirements of the Data Protection Act 1998 for the processing of medical data. *J Med Ethics*, **29**(1), 34–5.

14 Higgins J (2003). The Patient Information Advisory Group and the use of patient identifiable data. *J Health Serv Res Policy*, **8**(Suppl 1), S1–11.

15 Office of National Statistics (2003). *National Statistics code of practice. Protocol on data access and confidentiality.* Office for National Statistics, London.

16 Lowrance WW (2002). *Learning from experience. Privacy and the secondary use of data in health research.* The Nuffield Trust, London.

17 Coleman MP, Evans BG, Barrett G (2003). Confidentiality and the public interest in medical research–will we ever get it right? *Clin Med*, **3**(3), 219–28.

18 Police examine 'cleft palate' abortion. BBC News. 28 Oct 2002. Available at: http://news.bbc.co.uk/1/hi/england/2367917.htm (accessed 21 January 2006).

19 Office of National Statistics (2003). *National Statistics code of practice. Protocol on data matching.* Office for National Statistics, London.

20 SD2HES (2003). *The HES protocol. Instructions for handling the data.* Department of Health, London.

21 Goldblatt P, Willmer R (2003). *Copyright arid disclosure for Compendium 2002* (letter to the NHS). Department of Health, Office of National Statistics, London. Available at: http://tinyurl.com/byfmq (accessed 21 January 2006).

22 UK Association of Cancer registries. *cancer registration, confidentiality and consent.* Available at: http://www.vkacr.org.uk/UKACR_statements.htm (accessed 21 January 2006).

2.9 Summarizing health status

Jean-Marie Robine

Objectives

This chapter introduces you to the main current summary measures of population health and their principal characteristics.

Definition

Summary measures of population health, known today as health expectancies, are defined as measures that combine mortality and morbidity data to represent overall population health on a single metric.

Why summarize population health status?

Summary measures of population health allow us to answer the question of whether overall life expectancy is increasing faster or slower than life expectancy spent in good health (for instance without chronic disease or functional limitation). This question led to the development of a new family of indicators, health expectancies. The general model of health transition proposed by the World Health Organization (WHO) in 1984 distinguished overall life expectancy, disability-free life expectancy, and morbidity-free life expectancy.[1] Its strength lies in its ability to assess the likelihood of different health scenarios expressed as interrelationships between these three measures: a pandemic of chronic diseases and disabilities,[2,3] a compression of morbidity,[4] or contradictory evolutions including the scenario of dynamic equilibrium (Figure 2.9.1).[5]

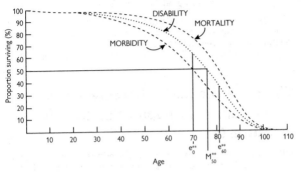

Figure 2.9.1 The general model of health transition.[1] e_0^{**} and e_{60}^{**} are the number of years of autonomous life expected at birth and at age 60, respectively. M_{50}^{**} is the age to which 50% of females could expect to survive without loss of autonomy. (Figure used by kind permission of the World Health Organization.)

Background

Research on such measures, combining mortality and morbidity data at the population level, dates back to the 1960s. The first method of calculation was proposed by Sullivan in 1971.[6] Soon research took two directions, one, following the work of Sullivan, gave priority to availability of data and simplicity of calculation, whilst the other, following the work of Bush and his collaborators,[7,8] focused on several methodological refinements, including the multistate approach[9,10] and weighting combinations.[11] Methodological papers compare the various approaches.[12–14]

Health expectancies have been increasingly used in industrialized countries to assess the evolution of a population's health status, *in particular that of older people*.[15] Being independent of the size of populations and of their age structure, health expectancies allow direct comparison of the different groups that make up populations: e.g. sexes, socio-professional categories, regions.

Since 1989, an international research network, REVES (Réseau Espérance de Vie en Santé/Network on Health Expectancy), has coordinated research on summary measures.

A number of international agencies (the OECD[16], WHO[1]) have underlined the need for such measures. In the final communiqué of its 1997 summit in Denver, the G8 encouraged collaborative biomedical and behavioural research to improve active life expectancy and reduce disability.

The health expectancy approach has now been extended to incorporate the modern concepts of the disablement process: chronic morbidity, functional limitation, activity restriction, and physical dependency, and progressively more attention has been devoted to mental health expectancy.[17]

What are the main characteristics of the summary population health measures?

Table 2.9.1 summarizes the principal characteristics of health expectancies. For more information on data requirements and the methods of calculation see Further resources, p.166.

Table 2.9.1 Principal characteristics of the health expectancies

Method of calculation	Decomposition of the years lived by the population of a life table between two ages into the years lived in good health and the years lived in poor health
Prevalence life table (Sullivan)	Use of the observed cross-sectional prevalence to estimate the period prevalence of health problems introduced in the summary indicator
Multistate life table	Use of observed transitions between health states and death to compute the period prevalence of health problem introduced in the summary indicator
Combination of items and dimensions	
No combination	Decomposition of the years lived in simple complementary states, such as in two states (with and without disability) or three states (with severe disability, with moderate disability, and without disability)
Boolean combination	Decomposition of the years lived in complex complementary states, such as 'without disability and in good perceived health' versus 'other'
Weighted combination	Combination of the years lived in several health states through health weights, leading to a single number of health adjusted years

Basic operations: good and poor health as sums and as proportions

- The sum of complementary health expectancies is always equal to life expectancy (LE)—for example, disability-free life expectancy (DFLE), plus life expectancy with disability (LEWD) is equal to total life expectancy (DFLE + LEWD = LE).
- Health expectancies can also be divided. For instance, the ratio disability-free life expectancy to total life expectancy indicates the proportion of life expectancy lived without disability (generally expressed as a percentage).

The WHO summary measure: health-adjusted life expectancy (HALE)

Since 2000, the WHO has used a summary measure of population health to assess overall population health and judge how well the objective of good health is being achieved by different countries. WHO chose, at first, to use a measure termed 'disability-adjusted life expectancy' (DALE). DALE is estimated from three kinds of information:

- the fraction of population surviving to each age, calculated from birth and death rates
- the prevalence of each type of disability at each age
- the weight assigned to each type of disability (which may or may not vary with age).

Survival at each age is adjusted downwards by the sum of all the disability effects, each of which is the product of a weight and the complement of a prevalence (the share of the population not suffering that disability). These adjusted survival shares are then divided by the initial population, before any mortality occurred, to give the average number of equivalent healthy life years that a newborn member of a population could expect to live.[19]

In 2001, WHO renamed this summary indicator health-adjusted life expectancy (HALE) and more simply called it 'healthy life expectancy'.[20] HALE is based on life expectancy at birth but includes an adjustment for time spent in poor health. It is most easily understood as the equivalent number of years in full health that a newborn can expect to live based on current rates of ill-health and mortality.[21,22]

For the 2000 report, a great deal of data were simulated, but year after year more empiric data were collected through population surveys such as the WHO Multi-country Household Survey Study[17] and the World Health Survey.[18] Therefore, estimates of healthy life expectancy published for nearly 200 countries by WHO are not directly comparable from year to year because of changes in methodology. WHO has not published new estimates since the 2002 estimates published in the report for 2003.

The US Healthy People summary measure: years of healthy life (YHL)

In the US, the two overarching national health goals identified for Healthy People 2010 are to
- increase the quality and years of healthy life
- eliminate health disparities.

As an initial effort in the development of summary measures of health, the National Centre for Health Statistics (NCHS) sponsored a workshop which underlined that:

> No single measure can adequately incorporate all aspects of health and mortality. A set of summary measures including both mortality and various aspects of morbidity or health that can be calculated from existing or collectable data should be proposed for Healthy People 2010.

Thus the set of summary measures recommended for monitoring progress toward the first goal of Healthy People 2010, include the following:
- years of healthy life defined as life without disability
- years of healthy life (YHL) (as used for Healthy People 2000)
- years of healthy life without functioning problems
- years of healthy life without specific diseases
- years of healthy life in excellent or very good health
- years of healthy life lived with good health behaviour.

All of the proposed summary measures can be constructed with available data and should be available for major subgroups of the population.[23,24] The methods used for calculating these various health expectancies are explained in a statistical note.[25] Trends in life expectancy free of limitation of activity by sex and race have been available since 1985 as well as several estimations using different definitions of health for the year 1995.[22]

The EU structural indicator: healthy life years (HLY)

In 2005, the Commission of the European Union, selected healthy life years (HLY), defined as disability-free life expectancy, as one of the structural indicators to be examined every year, during the European Spring Council.

According to the Commission, the demographic measure of life expectancy, which has often been used as a measure of a nation's health, has limited utility because it does not provide an estimate of how healthy people are during their lifespan. The European population is ageing, and as the post-war generation reaches retirement the pace of that ageing will increase dramatically, with profound social effects. One major difficulty in planning for future health and long-term care needs, however, is the lack of agreed estimates of future numbers and needs:

- HLY could provide some of these estimations. The Commission is aware that the health status of a population is inherently difficult to measure because it is often defined differently among individuals, populations, cultures, and even across time periods.
- Many of the studies of health expectancy focus on measures such as physical impairment or disability in functional tasks or the presence of a specific chronic disease. However, self-assessed health, being much more global and subjective in nature, can incorporate a variety of aspects of health including cognitive and emotional as well as physical status. It can therefore provide insights into the needs of an ageing society. Hence, self-assessed health measures such as HLY may be a particularly important indicator of the potential demand for health services and long-term care needs.
- The two components of the calculation of the HLY are mortality tables and self-perceived disability (as assessed by health surveys). From 1995 to 2001, data from the Eurostat European Community Household Panel (ECHP) survey have been used for the EU-15 Member States. Its successor, the Eurostat EU-Statistics on Income and Living Conditions Survey (EU-SILC) will be used from 2004 or 2005 onwards for the present EU-25 Member States. Trend in disability-free life expectancy for the EU-15 are available since 1995.[26]

The HLY is completed by a set of summary measures computed by the European Health Expectancy Monitoring Unit (EHEMU), including an activity limitation-free life expectancy, a chronic condition-free life expectancy, a self-perceived health expectancy, and a life expectancy in good health combining the three previous indicators (no activity limitations, chronic condition, and very good or good perceived health). The data come from the EU-SILC survey.

Some European countries such as the United Kingdom[27,28] and Denmark[29] have their own national series of summary indicators.

Future harmonization

The two indicators, the 'years of healthy life defined as life without disability' used in the United States for Healthy People 2010 and the 'healthy life years' (defined as disability-free life expectancy) used in the European Union as a structural indicator, are very similar in their method of computation (the Sullivan method) and data used (observed cross-sectional prevalence) but not identical. Similar indicators are also used in other OECD countries (Australia, Canada, or Japan).

As for life expectancy at birth, the main (potential) interest of a summary measure of population health is to be comparable between various countries. Therefore, the next step will be to harmonize the health data from cross-sectional health surveys.

Box 2.9.2 **Main websites on summary measure of population health**

European Union: public health. http://europa.eu.int/comm/health/ (accessed 25 June 2005)

National Statistics. Home of UK national statistics. http://www.statistics.gov.uk/ (keyword health expectancy) (accessed 25 June 2005)

Réseau Espérance de Vie en Santé (REVES). http://www.reves.net (accessed 25 June 2005)

US Healthy People 2010. http://www.healthypeople.gov/ (accessed 25 June 2005)

World Health Organization. http://www.who.int/en/ (accessed 25 June 2005)

Further resources

Bone MR, Bebbington AC, Jagger C, Morgan K, Nicolaas G (1995). *Health expectancy and its uses.* Department of Health, London.

Jagger C (1999). Health expectancy calculation by the Sullivan method: a practical guide. In: *European concerted action on the harmonization of health expectancy calculations in Europe,* NRPS publication no 68, pp. 1–36. Nihon University Population Research Institute, Tokyo.

Jagger C, Reyes-Frausto S (2003). *Monitoring health by healthy active life expectancy.* Trent Public Health Observatory, Leicester.

Robine J-M, Jagger C, Egidi V (eds) (2000). *Selection of a coherent set of health indicators: a first step towards a user's guide to health expectancies for the European Union: final report of the Euro-REVES II project supported by the European Commission.* Euro-REVES, Montpellier.

Robine J-M, Jagger C, Mathers CD, Crimmins EM, Suzman R (eds) (2003). *Determining health expectancies.* John Wiley, Chichester.

References

1 World Health Organization (1984). The uses of epidemiology in the study of the elderly: report of a WHO scientific group on the epidemiology of aging. *World Health Org Tech Rep Ser,* **706,** 1–84.

2 Kramer M (1980). The rising pandemic of mental disorders and associated chronic diseases and disabilities. *Acta Psychiatr Scand,* **62**(Suppl. 285), 382–97.

3 Gruenberg EM (1977). The failures of success. *Milbank Memorial Fund Q,* **55**(1), 3–24.

4 Fries JF (1980). Aging, natural death, and the compression of morbidity. *N Engl J Med,* **303**(3), 130–5.

5 Manton KG (1982). Changing concepts of morbidity and mortality in the elderly population. *Milbank Memorial Fund Q,* **60,** 183–244.

6 Sullivan DF (1971). A single index of mortality and morbidity. *Health Services Mental Health Administration Health Reports* **86,** 347–54.

7 Fanshel S, Bush JW (1970). A health-status index and its application to health-services outcomes. *Operations Res,* **18**(6), 1021–66.

8 Bush JW, Chen MM, Zaremba J (1971). Estimating health programme outcomes using a Markov equilibrium analysis of disease development. *Am J Public Health*, **61**(12), 2362–75.

9 Land KL, Guralnik JM, Blazer DG (1994). Estimating increment-decrement life tables with multiple covariates from panel data: the case of active life expectancy. *Demography*, **31**(2), 297–319.

10 Laditka SB, Wolf DA (1998). New methods for analysing active life expectancy. *J. Aging Health*, **10**(2), 214–41.

11 Murray CJL, Salomon JA, Mathers CD, Lopez AD (eds) (2002). *Summary measures of population health.* World Health Organization, Geneva.

12 Crimmins EM, Saito Y, Hayward MD (1993). Sullivan and multi-state methods of estimating active life expectancy: two methods, two answers. In: Robine J-M, Mathers CD, Bone MR, Romieu I (eds) *Calculation of health expectancies: harmonization, consensus achieved and future perspectives/Calcul des espérances de vie en santé : harmonisation, acquis et perspectives*, pp. 155–60. John Libbey Eurotext, Montrouge.

13 Mathers CD, Robine J-M (1997). How good is Sullivan's method for monitoring changes in population health expectancies. *J Epidemiol Commun Health*, **51**, 80–6.

14 Cambois E, Robine J-M, Brouard N (1999). Life expectancies applied to specific statuses: a history of the indicators and the methods of calculation. *Population: an English Selection*, **11**, 7–34.

15 Robine J-M, Romieu I, Cambois E (1999). Health expectancy indicators. *Bull WHO*, **77**(2), 181–5.

16 McWhinnie JR (1981). Disability assessment in population surveys: results of the OECD common development effort. *Rev Epidémiol Santé Publique*, **29**, 413–19.

17 Robine J-M, Jagger C, Romieu I (eds) (2002). *Selection of a coherent set of health indicators for the European Union. Phase II: final report* [of the Euro-REVES II project supported by the European Commission]. Euro-REVES, Montpellier.

18 Denver Summit of the Eight. Final communique. 1997. Available at: http://www.g8.utoronto.ca/summit/1997denver/g8final.htm (accessed 21 January 2006).

19 World Health Organization (2000). *The world health report 2000: health systems: improving performance.* World Health Organization, Geneva.

20 World Health Organization (2001). *The world health report 2001: mental health: new understanding, new hope.* World Health Organization, Geneva.

21 World Health Organization (2002). *The world health report 2002: reducing risk: promoting healthy life.* World Health Organization, Geneva.

22 World Health Organization (2003). *The world health report 2003: shaping the future.* World Health Organization, Geneva.

23 Wagener DK, Molla MT, Crimmins EM, Pamuk ER, Madans JH (2001). *Summary measures of population health: addressing the first goal of healthy people 2010, improving health expectancy.* Statistical notes no.22, pp.1–13. National Centre for Health Statistics, Hyattsville, MD.

24 Molla MT, Madans JH, Wagener DK, Crimmins EM (2003). *Summary measures of population health: report of findings on methodological and data issues*: Publication No. 2004–1258. US DHHS, Hyattsville, MD.

25 Molla MT, Wagener DK, Madans JH (2001). *Summary measures of population health: Methods for calculating healthy life expectancy*. Healthy People Statistical notes, no. 21. National Centre for Health Statistics, Hyattsville, MD.

26 European Commission: Public Health (2005). *Healthy life years in the core of the Lisbon strategy*. Available at: http://www.europa.eu.int/comm/health/ph_information/indicators/lifeyears_en.htm (accessed 25 June 2005).

27 Office of National Statistics (2004). Healthy life expectancy in Great Britain. *Health Statist Q*, **22**, 2.

28 Bajekal M (2005). Healthy life expectancy by area deprivation: magnitude and trends in England, 1994–1999. *Health Statist Q*, **25**, 18–27.

29 Bronnum-Hansen H (2005). Health expectancy in Denmark, 1987–2000. *Eur J Public Health*, **15**(1), 20–5.

2.10 Measuring and monitoring health inequalities and auditing inequity

Julian Flowers

Introduction

Reducing inequalities and inequities in health and health care is now a key objective of health systems nationally[1] and internationally.[2] In England, the process of 'health equity audit' has been formalized to encourage a consistent, quantified, and performance-managed approach to tackle inequalities and inequities.[3]

As with all policy initiatives, measurement and monitoring is essential. For health inequalities this has added complexity: we need to be able to assess and monitor not just *overall* health, but the *distribution* of health within the populations we serve. As health inequality now forms an important part of the performance framework for public health, robust and defensible measurement is imperative.

Objectives

This chapter is intended to provide practitioners (who have responsibility for a population in a geographic area) with:
- a framework for understanding measures of health inequality
- an understanding of the strengths and weaknesses of different measures of health inequality, how these measures can be used in assessing health inequality locally, and the need to use more than one measure to monitor health inequality
- a brief overview of the process of equity audit.

What are health inequality and equity?

Health inequality

Health inequality refers not simply to differences in health status or outcome but to differences that are unacceptable and avoidable. However, there is less agreement about how to *quantify* inequality. The Black Report measured *socio-economic inequality in health*; it demonstrated both absolute and relative *differences* in health determinants, status, and outcomes between social class groupings in the population (based on the UK Registrar General's occupational groupings of social class).[4-6] The World Health Organization, however, discusses *total* inequality—the sum total of differences in health between individuals, for which there is an effort to produce a summary measure.[7] National policy in England focuses more on group differences, or on *dimensions* of inequality by virtue of who someone is (gender, ethnicity, or social class) or where they live.[1]

In practice, people often use the idea of *health gaps* to describe local inequality, generally meaning the difference in health between those with the best and worst health, or between the wealthiest and the poorest groups.

These differences in perspective and interpretation influence how inequality is measured and can lead to confusion and uncertainty about *what* inequalities exist and whether or not they are improving. When trying to demonstrate the presence of health inequality five questions may help (Box 2.10.1).

Box 2.10.1 Five questions to ask about measures of health inequality

1. *Inequality, poor health, or deprivation?* Often inequality is confused with poor health or deprivation—all may coexist within an area or any of them could exist on their own: (a) socio-economic variation in health is often used synonymously with health inequality—this will only be true if health and deprivation are correlated; (b) poor health *of* an area does not equate with inequality *within* an area.

2. *Inequality of what?* For what aspect of health, e.g. mortality, life expectancy, low birth weight, is inequality being measured? Some advocate a single summary measure to encapsulate inequality such as child mortality while others use multiple health measures that refer to the particular groups.

3. *What dimensions of inequality?* Which groups we are comparing, e.g. gender, ethnic group, socio-economic status, geographic area? All are potentially subject to the ecologic fallacy. In addition, area-based inequality is non-scalable (see later).

4. *Using what metric or index of inequality?* What summary measure is being used to quantify inequality, e.g. absolute range, interquartile range, Gini coefficient? Does it include a socio-economic dimension?

5. *Relative or absolute inequality?*

What is health equity?

Health equity usually refers to the extent to which health care (or more health-related services/opportunities) meets the needs of the population.[8] The classic example of inequity in healthcare is the 'inverse care law',[9] which has been found to exist for a range of services.[10-15] Health economists often talk of horizontal equity (equal care for equal need) and vertical equity (unequal care for unequal need). Inequality and equity may legitimately coexist but equality and inequity should not. For example, the English national target to achieve a revascularization rate of 750 per million population would create *equality* but not equity because needs vary. Figure 2.10.1 shows the relationship between inequality and inequity. Redressing inequity in an effort to reduce inequality has been supported in England by a process of health equity audit[7,8,16] (see later in this chapter).

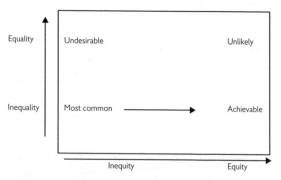

Figure 2.10.1 Schematic diagram showing the relationship between inequality and inequity. The most desirable scenario is to move an unequal *and* inequitable service to one that is unequal but equitable

Commonly used summary measures of inequality

There have been several reviews of measures of health inequality.[17–24] Measures of inequality applied to the evaluation of *health* inequality have been developed by economists,[18,19] information scientists,[25] epidemiologists,[17,24] and by social statisticians;[20] some of the more frequently used are summarised in Table 2.10.1. There is no agreed measure of inequality—all have strengths and weakness as the following example illustrates.

Table 2.10.1 Inequality measures/metrics/indices which could be used for assessing inequalities within an area

Index	Definition/interpretation	Advantages	Data requirements	Socio-economic inequality dimension	Absolute/relative
Range (of extremes)	Difference between highest and lowest rates	Easy to interpret and calculate but there will always be a highest and lowest	Small area rates	No	Absolute
Ratio (of extremes)	Ratio of highest and lowest rates	Easy to interpret and calculate	Small area rates	No	Relative
Average:worst fifth *difference* (e.g. England national inequality measure)	Difference between lowest quintile and population average rate	See Range	Area rates	No	Absolute
Average:worst fifth *ratio*	Ratio of lowest quintile and population average rate	See Range	Small area rates	No	Relative
Coefficient of variation	Ratio of standard deviation to mean	Widely understood statistic	Small area rates	No	Relative
Gini coefficient	Mean difference between rates in all areas. It measures extent to which poor health is concentrated in areas with worst health. Takes values between 0 and 1, where 0 implies equal rates in all areas, and 1 that all deaths occur in one area only	Can compare inequality over time or between health outcomes	Small area rates ranked from lowest to highest rate	No	Relative
Odds ratio	Odds of poor health in low social group relative to upper group	Easily understood by epidemiologists	Individual-level data	Yes	Relative

Table 2.10.1 (Contd.)

Index	Definition/ interpretation	Advantages	Data requirements	Socio-economic inequality dimension	Absolute/ relative
Health concentration index (HCI)	Summary of the extent to which inequalities in health systematically associated with socio-economic status. If all deaths are in the most deprived area, HCI will be −1, if all rates are equal, it will be 0	See Gini	Small area rates ranked in order of decreasing socio-economic status	Yes	Relative
Slope index of inequality (SII)	Slope of the regression line associating mean health status in socio-economic groups and relative rank in the socio-economic distribution. Can be interpreted as the excess poor health rate per unit increase in deprivation. Slope of 0 = no socio-economic gradient. The SII can be thought of as the average change in the health status rates moving from the lowest socio-economic class to the highest.	See Gini	Small area rates, populations, socio-economic status	Yes	Absolute
Relative index of inequality (RII)	[Slope index of inequality (SII)] divided by [average health of the population]	See Gini	Small area rates, populations, socio-economic status	Yes	Relative

Example of measures of inequality

Table 2.10.2 Hypothetical data illustrating change in health inequality over time

Area	Deprivation	Population	Time 1 No of deaths	Death rate per 1000	Time 2 No of deaths	Death rate per 1000	Proportion of the population	Relative rank*	Cumulative % population	Time 1 Cumulative % deaths	Time 2 Cumulative % deaths
A	Least	1000	4	4	4	4	0.2	0.1	20	7	7
B	2nd least	1000	8	8	6	6	0.2	0.3	40	20	19
C	Middle	1000	12	12	10	10	0.2	0.5	60	40	37
D	2nd most	1000	16	16	14	14	0.2	0.7	80	67	64
E	Most	1000	20	20	20	20	0.2	0.9	100	100	100
Total or Average		5000	60	12	54	10.8	1.0				

*needed to calculate the slope index of inequality and relative index of inequality.

Table 2.10.3 Summary measures of inequality and their change over time

Summary measure	Time 1	Time 2	Change over time
Range of extremes	16 deaths/1000	16 deaths/1000	None
Ratio of extremes	5	5	None
Average worst-fifth difference	8 deaths/1000	10 deaths/1000	Increase
Average worst-fifth ratio	1.67	1.9	Increase
Coefficient of variation	0.53	0.59	Increase
Gini coefficient	0.33*	0.37	Increase
Health concentration index	−0.2*	−0.3	Increase
Slope index of inequality	−6.8 deaths/1000	−7.2 deaths/1000*	Increase
Relative slope index of inequality	−57%	−68%*	Increase

*$P < 0.001$.

Imagine a population spread throughout five localities (A–E) with the populations and death rates for two time periods as shown in Table 2.10.2. There is *health improvement*—the overall death rate decreases from 12 to 10.8 per 1000 with a reduction in mortality of 2 per 1000 population in each of the areas apart from the least and most deprived. There is a socio-economic gradient in poor health with a correlation between deprivation and mortality.

What happens to the *inequality* in death rates between time 1 and time 2?

We can calculate the values of a range of inequality measures (Table 2.10.3) (details of the calculations can be obtained from the author on request).

How can these figures be interpreted?

- The Gini coefficient is significantly different from 0 indicating that there is health inequality. The health concentration index and slope index of inequality both show that there is a *socio-economic gradient* in ill-health which increases over time (a more negative value indicates a worsening gradient).
- The slope index of inequality indicates the excess deaths due to inequality.
- In this example the comparison of extremes shows no change but inequality increases because of changes *within* the distribution.

Using more than one measure (including absolute and relative measures) can help to determine *if* inequalities exist, the *scale* or burden of inequality, *where* inequality exists (e.g. which group or area), and, if repeated, *how it changes over time*.

Visualizing inequality

We often communicate the presence of health inequality graphically using bar charts or thematic maps but these are not effective tools for demonstrating change over time.

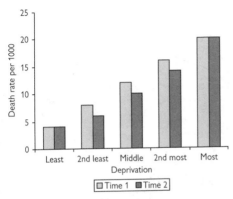

Figure 2.10.2 Death rates by locality at time 1 and time 2. (See data in Table 2.10.2.) In this figure we are comparing the distribution of mortality rates over the 5 areas (A–E) at Time 1, with a different distribution of mortality over the 5 areas in Time 2. See Table 2.10.3. for the many different ways of describing this change in distribution using quantitative summary measures.

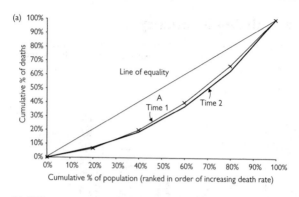

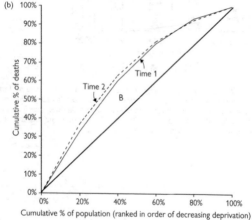

Figure 2.10.3 (a) Lorenz curves for time 1 and time 2. We have plotted the cumulative proportion of deaths against the cumulative proportion of the population for each of our localities, ranked in order of decreasing health (increasing death rate). The gradient of the curves at each point is the death rate, the area A is used to calculate the Gini coefficient, and the diagonal line is the line of equality where equal population shares have equal health shares. The Lorenz curve for time 2 lies further from the line of equality than that for time 1, indicating the increase in inequality over time. (b) Health concentration curves for time 1 and time 2. We have plotted the cumulative proportion of deaths against the cumulative proportion of the population for each of our localities, ranked in order of decreasing deprivation. The gradient of the curves at each point is the death rate, the area B is used to calculate the health concentration index, and the diagonal line is the line of equality where equal population shares have equal health shares. The health concentration curve for time 2 lies further from the line of equality than that for time 1, indicating the increasing concentration of poor health in the most deprived areas

Using the data in Table 2.10.2 we can construct a bar chart (Figure 2.10.2), where we can see the socio-economic gradient and the improvement in health, but it is hard to judge change in health inequality.

An alternative way of charting the variation in death rates is the Lorenz curve, where the cumulative proportion of deaths in each area, ranked by increasing death rate, is plotted against cumulative proportion of the population (these can also be plotted for age-standardized rates by using an adjusted population). If, instead, areas are ranked by decreasing deprivation, this produces the health concentration curve.[19] Figures 2.10.3a and b show these curves for the data in Table 2.10.2. The further the curve is from the diagonal the greater the inequality: we can see clearly the increase over time.

Some pitfalls for the unwary in monitoring health inequality

There are several methodological problems associated with the measurement of inequality[23] and here we highlight some of those related to monitoring and target setting.

Sensitivity to change

Some of the measures used to summarize inequality are not appropriately sensitive to changes over time within the distribution of health. For example, if we 'transferred' health from the second worst off in the population to the second best off, the gap between worst and best off might stay the same, but most would agree that we have probably *increased* the inequality. Measures like the range or health gap measures violate a fundamental attribute of inequality known as the *transferability principle*—if we transfer a resource from the better off to the worse off, our metric of inequality should reflect that change and decrease accordingly.

Non-scalability of geographic health inequality targets

Targets for reducing inequality between areas are not directly translatable to within-area inequality—that is, health inequality targets are not geographically scalable. If there were, for example, a national area-based target to reduce inequality *between* areas by X%, but instead, every area reduced the inequality *within* their areas by the same X%, the inequality *between* areas, as measured nationally, would not necessarily change. Lesson: distinguish "between area inequality" and "within area inequality". (This phenomenon does not apply to inequality when analysed through groups of people rather than geographical areas; reducing inequalities locally within children *will* influence the national inequalities within children.) Therefore, we must be explicit about the geographic scale at which inequality is being assessed and inequality targets need to be differentially applied at different geographic scales. An example of this can be seen with the development of 'spearhead' local authorities in England where, in an effort to reduce national inequality, additional resources have been focused on the quintile of areas within England with the poorest health.

The direction paradox

This arises when we assess inequality using an indicator that relates to a metric we wish to see increase (such as life expectancy) and related indicators that we wish to see decrease (such as cancer or circulatory disease mortality) *and* when we are using an absolute range measure as our inequality metric. One would except that the as the inequality in important causes of mortality (circulatory and cancer) reduce, one would expect the inequalities in life expectancy to likewise reduce. This is *not* necessarily the case. When this occurs, it is purely a mathematical phenomenon, and is purely a consequence of the values of the health indicators moving in different directions.

Absolute–relative paradoxes

A related paradox which further emphasizes the complexities of monitoring health inequality (and which again is a mathematical phenomenon), is that it is possible for relative inequality to increase as absolute inequality is falling, and vice versa. This paradox is illustrated in Figure 2.10.4.

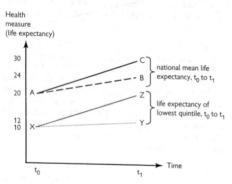

Figure 2.10.4 Let ABC represent potential changes in the *national mean* life expectancy and XYZ changes in the *lowest quintile* of life expectancy. If A = 20 and X = 10 then at time t_0, inequality can be described either as an *absolute* difference (gap) A−X = 10 or *relative* difference (ratio) A/X = 2.

If the absolute *gap* remains constant over time, A will increase to C (30) at time t_1, and B will increase to Z (20) at time t_1. The gap C–Z will still be 10 but the ratio will have fallen from 2 to 1.5.

If however the *ratio* remains constant over time at 2, A will increase to B (24) and X to Y (12), then B–Y will = 12; i.e. the gap has increased.

It can be seen therefore that if the trajectory of national mean improvement lies between AB and AC and that of the lowest quintile lies between XY and XZ, the ratio will decrease at the same time as the absolute gap increases.

If we use a measure which decreases over time falls e.g. circulatory mortality rates, the opposite will be true

Equity audit

We often demonstrate the existence of inequity by showing the lack of, or even an inverted relationship between, some aspect of *need* and associated health-care provision or utilization. Dixon *et al.*[26] provide a good summary of the existence and extent of inequity within the UK National Health Service. We can use some of the methods outlined above to both quantify and visualize *inequity* to make it easier to compare potential areas for equity audit and detect change over time. For example, a modified form of the Lorenz curve can be drawn where we rank areas by increasing need rather than health—this could be summarized in a single figure with an index like the health concentration index to give an equity index to allow us track change over time.

The equity audit cycle

Identifying potential inequities and having the tools to quantify and monitor them are only steps in an iterative cyclical process designed to help to reduce inequity through action. There are parallels with clinical audit as we identify deficiencies in service provision to meet need, identify barriers to meeting need, and seek to change practice, attitudes, or resource allocation to try and redress some of the imbalances (see Figure 2.10.5). In England, equity audit is now mandatory for Primary Care Trusts and action and progress is assessed as part of the routine performance monitoring process.

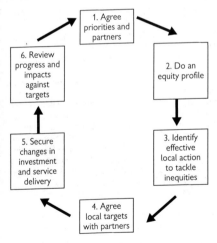

Figure 2.10.5 The equity audit cycle

Equity audit is still, however, in its infancy but some examples of the topics and key issues are shown in Box 2.10.2.[27]

- *Topics*—provision of tertiary cardiac services compared to need, equity of smoking cessation services compared to burden of smoking illness (e.g. measured by smoking attributable mortality), lung cancer surgery, health visitor distribution, gender prescribing of aspirin for coronary heart disease.
- *Level of comparison?*—Often small areas within Primary Care Trusts.
- *What dimensions of inequality?*—Spatial, socio-economic, deprivation, age, gender.
- *Issues?*—Data requirements, advice on good practice, methodological support.

Conclusions

Robust measurement of health inequalities is essential to support policy, target setting, and monitoring performance. An understanding of the range of potential measures and their strengths and weaknesses, the potential pitfalls in monitoring, and clarity of description can greatly help in focusing appropriate action to reduce heath inequality. Equity audit provides an important tool for practical action.

References

1 Department of Health (2003). *Tackling health inequalities. A programme for action.* Department of Health, London.
2 Brundtland GH, Frenk J, Murray CJ (2003). WHO assessment of health systems performance. *Lancet*, **361**(9375), 2155.
3 Department of Health (2003). *Health equity audit: a guide for the NHS.* Department of Health, London.
4 Black D, Morris JN, Smith C, Townsend P (1992). *Inequalities in health: the Black report.* Pelican, Harmondsworth.
5 Sociologies of Health and Illness ELearning Databank (SHIELD). *The Black Report and inequalities in health.* Available at: http://www.ucel.ac.uk/shield/ black_report/ (accessed 25 June 2005).
6 Socialist Health Association. *The Black Report* 1980. Available at: http://www.sochealth.co.uk/history/black.htm (accessed 25 June 2005).
7 Gakidou E, King G (2002). Measuring total health inequality: adding individual variation to group-level differences. *Int J Equity Health*, **1**(1), 3.
8 Hamer L, Jacobson B, Flowers J, Johnstone F (2003). *Equity audit made simple: a briefing for Primary Care Trusts.* Department of Health. London.
9 Tudor-Hart J (1971). The inverse care law. *Lancet*, **1**(7696), 405–12.
10 Langham S, Basnett I, McCartney P et al. (2003). Addressing the inverse care law in cardiac services. *J Public Health Med*, **25**(3), 202–7.
11 O'Dea JF, Kilham RJ (2002). The inverse care law is alive and well in general practice. *Med J Aust* **177**(2), 78–9.
12 Webb E (1998). Children and the inverse care law. *BMJ*, **316**(7144), 1588–91.

13 Brown S, Lumley J (1993). Antenatal care: a case of the inverse care law? *Aust J Public Health*, **17**(2), 95–103.

14 Smith CJ (1986). Equity in the distribution of health and welfare services: can we rely on the state to reverse the 'inverse care law?'. *Soc Sci Med*, **23**(10), 1067–78.

15 Hart JT (1971). The inverse care law. *Lancet*, **1**(7696), 405–12.

16 Flowers J, Pencheon D (2002). *Introduction to health equity audit*. Eastern Region Public Health Observatory, Cambridge. Available at: http://www.erpho.org.uk/viewResource.aspx?id=6282 (accessed 22 January 2006).

17 Manor O, Matthews S, Power C (1997). Comparing measures of health inequality. *Soc Sci Med*, **45**(5), 761–71.

18 Wagstaff A, van Doorslaer E (2004). Overall versus socioeconomic health inequality: a measurement framework and two empirical illustrations. *Health Econ*, **13**(3), 297–301.

19 Wagstaff A, Paci P, van Doorslaer E (1991). On the measurement of inequalities in health. *Soc Sci Med*, **33**(5), 545–57.

20 Carr-Hill R, Chalmers-Dixon P (2003). *A review of methods for monitoring and measuring social inequality, deprivation and health inequality*. South East Public Health Observatory, Oxford.

21 Regidor E (2004). Measures of health inequalities: part 2. *J Epidemiol Commun Health*, **58**(11), 900–3.

22 Regidor E (2004). Measures of health inequalities: part 1. *J Epidemiol Commun Health*, **58**(10), 858–61.

23 Kunst AE, Groenhof F, Borgan JK et al. Socio-economic inequalities in mortality. Methodological problems illustrated with three examples from Europe. *Rev Epidemiol Sante Publique*, **46**(6), 467–79.

24 Mackenbach JP, Kunst AE (1997). Measuring the magnitude of socio-economic inequalities in health: an overview of available measures illustrated with two examples from Europe. *Soc Sci Med*, **44**(6), 757–71.

25 Conceição P, Ferreira P (2000). *The young person's guide to the Theil index: suggesting intuitive interpretations and exploring analytical applications*. Massachusetts Institute of Technology/UTIP. Available at: http://papers.ssrn.com/sol3/papers.cfm?abstractid=228703 (accessed 22 January 2006).

26 Dixon A, Le Grand J, Henderson J, Murray R, Poteliakhoff E (2003). Is the NHS equitable? A review of the evidence. *LSE Health and Social Care Discussion Paper 11*. London School of Economics, London.

27 Aspinall PJ, Jacobson B (2005). *Health equity audit: a baseline survey of Primary Care Trusts in England*. London Health Observatory, London. Available at: http://www.publichealth.nice.org.uk/page.aspx?o=50332 (accessed 21 May 2006)

2.11 Finding and appraising evidence

Anne Brice, Amanda Burls, and Alison Hill

Objectives

Making good public health decisions requires integrating good *information* (much of it routine; see Chapters 2.1 and 2.8) with good *research evidence*. However, there is a vast quantity of research evidence available, much of it of poor quality. This chapter aims to help you find and appraise research evidence efficiently, so the best, most relevant research evidence is used to improve health.

Finding research evidence

What sort of evidence do you need?

Before searching for evidence, you need to know what sort of evidence to look for. To do this you need to:
- have a clearly formulated question
- know what study design would best answer the question you have (see below).

To formulate your question you need to specify, for the context of your decision, the
- Population (to whom is the decision being applied)
- Exposure (e.g. an intervention if the question is about effectiveness, or a risk factor if the question is about harm)
- Comparator
- Outcome(s)
- Time (period or time horizon you are interested in).

For clinical questions you will often find that the acronym PICO is used (Population or participant, Intervention or indicator, Comparator or control, Outcome).

Table 2.11.1 Best primary research design for different questions

Type of question	Study design	Comment
Effectiveness	Randomized controlled trial	
Etiology	Case–control	Cohort studies also provide information on etiology
Harm	Cohort	
Prognosis	Inception cohort	
Diagnosis	Diagnostic test study	
Patient experience (e.g. of illness, treatment or service)	Qualitative studies	Within this there are many designs including: questionnaires, focus groups, interviews
Value for money	Economic evaluation (e.g. cost-effectiveness study or cost–benefit study)	

Table 2.11.1 shows the best primary research design for different questions. If an appropriate study design has not been used then the study is unlikely to provide information of value to your decision. If available, a good quality up-to-date systematic review of studies of the appropriate design will give the best overview.

The question you have formulated, and the best study design to answer the question, will help to shape your search for evidence, and we explain the process in the section below.

Finding the evidence

It can be difficult to find the best research evidence, and to know when you have found it. Developments in technology, particularly electronic databases via the Internet, mean that you can access a huge range of resources. However, you need a systematic and reproducible approach to avoid wasting time, missing relevant literature, or having to wade through large quantities of irrelevant citations. Searching techniques need to be *sensitive* (to get as much of the information you *do* need as possible) and *specific* (to minimize the amount of retrieved information that you *do not* need).

Box 2.11.1

Searching for evidence is a research methodology like any other. As such, in communicating how it was done, the techniques (e.g. search strategy) should be made explicit to demonstrate reproducibility.

Searching for literature is not a linear process. Search strategies may need to be refined in the light of citations retrieved in order to improve the identification of relevant papers—often called 'iterative searching'.

Sources of information

Evidence can be found in a wide range of sources. There are between 20,000 and 30,000 biomedical journals and about 17,000 new biomedical books are published every year. Therefore you need a clearly defined question and knowledge of which source to search.

Sources include guidelines, the Cochrane Library, Medline/PubMed, primary and secondary journals, grey literature, and textbooks. These resources can be accessed in a number of ways, for example via specific databases or via national/international portals [e.g. the National Library for Health (www.library.nhs.uk) in the UK].

A detailed description of sources and their advantages and disadvantages can be found on the CASP website.[1]

Selecting sources

Deciding which sources to search and the nature of your strategy will depend on many factors, including the purpose of your search and the time available. Using a protocol can help you plan your approach and ensure that the search is reproducible. A sample protocol is included in Figure 2.11.1. Another useful protocol can be found on the website of the School of Health and Related Research in Sheffield, UK.[2]

Doing the search

When creating a search strategy it is essential to go back to your carefully formulated question. This will help you identify relevant terms on which to base your search, and to build the blocks of your search strategy. Start with a broad, or sensitive, search. This will find a lot of material, much of which may not be relevant. It is important not to limit or narrow the search too quickly as this may exclude vital evidence from your search results. For example, in order to search as broadly as possible in Medline we need to know how to:

• perform a MeSH search
• perform a text word, or free-text search.

For each concept within the search identify the relevant MeSH terms, and also keywords and synonyms to search as free text. Using techniques such as

• exploding the thesaurus terms
• applying all subheadings
• using truncation and wild cards

will help ensure that useful evidence is not excluded. The search can always be refined later if the results are not as expected. As indexing quality is variable, it is important to build a search strategy using a combination of both MeSH terms and text words, and combine the results using Boolean logic 'operators' such as 'AND' and 'OR' and 'NOT'.

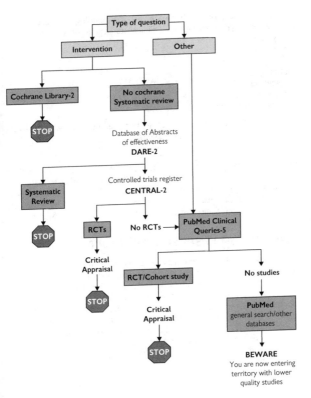

Figure 2.11.1 Protocol for a search strategy. (Reproduced with the kind permission of Paul Glasziou and Carl Heneghan)

Searching for quality
To narrow a search, and increase its specificity, requires systematically excluding the least useful articles. The most useful criterion on which to search for quality papers is to look at the methods being used. A few randomized controlled trials are likely to give much more useful evidence than 10 times as many anecdotal case studies, if evidence of effect is being sought.

Using search filters
Search filters are tried and tested literature search strategies that provide a more effective way of refining your search to find high-quality evidence appropriate to your type of question. They can be used to identify systematic review and randomized controlled trial literature on Medline,

and in other databases. There are also methodological search filters which will help you retrieve sound clinical studies that deal with:

- diagnosis
- prognosis
- therapy
- etiology
- guidelines
- treatment outcomes
- evidence-based health-care methods.

You can find out more about these filters at http://www.phru.nhs.uk/casp/filters.htm (accessed 26 June 2005).

Summary of search strategies

Search strategies should be explicit and reproducible. Start with a broad search, and then narrow by quality filters. Remember to match the search strategy to the question, and that searching is an iterative process. For more help in searching for evidence go to http://nhs.netg.co.uk/websvm/login.asp (requires registration: accessed 26 June 2005).

Appraising research evidence

Critical appraisal is the systematic assessment of research evidence. No research is perfect. The purpose of appraising a study is not to find fault because it is less than ideal, but rather to identify what, if anything, is of value that could help inform your decision. You mind find it helpful to think of the word critical as meaning to find value (i.e. critique), rather than just considering a more common interpretation of the word (to find fault/criticize).

When critically appraising any study you need to be able to tell:

- what question the researchers set out to answer
- whether they used an appropriate study design
- what they did
- what they found
- the implications of the findings in your context

... or even more simply:

- why did they start? (concise, answerable question in full)
- what did they do? (methods—the right methods? done correctly?)
- what did they find? (results—in numbers and words)
- what does it mean? (relevance—so what?).

Screening questions for any study

Given the vast number of potential studies available, you need to triage papers for their potential usefulness. Thus, the first question to ask is 'Is a clear question being addressed?'. You need to ensure here that you can identify all the components of the question (PECOT) that we described at the start of this chapter. If the answer is no, or you cannot tell, then the paper is unlikely to be useful (in fact, it is likely to be positively unhelpful—it might support your prior belief and thus you ascribe it too much value, and find it difficult to forget).

The next question is 'Did the researchers use an appropriate study design for the question they were asking?'. Remember it is usually only worth proceeding to appraise a study in more depth if it has a clear question and appropriate study design.

Appraising the validity of studies of different designs

We use studies to try and predict the probable consequences of our decisions. Thus we need to know to what extent a study's findings are likely to reflect the 'truth'. For example, if a study finds the death rate in those treated with a new treatment is half that in patients given the standard treatment, we would like to be convinced that this is because the new treatment actually halves the death rate and was not simply due to the way study was done. Systematic deviation of results from the truth because of the way a study is conducted is known as *bias*.

An important element of critical appraisal is to check that potential biases were both identified and minimized. Since different study designs are prone to different biases, there are specific questions you need to focus on to check their validity. We provide the following checklists as an *aide-mémoire* for the important biases you need to check for when appraising studies of different designs.

This chapter cannot teach you critical appraisal skills, which requires practice and experience, therefore resources for further learning are provided at the end of the chapter.

Box 2.11.2 Randomized controlled trials (RCTs)

- Was the allocation of patients to treatments randomized?
- Was this allocation concealed?
- Were the groups similar at the start of the trial, in terms of factors that might effect the outcome such as age, sex, and social class?
- Were patients, health workers, and study personnel 'blind' to treatment?
- Apart from the experimental intervention, were the groups treated equally?
- Were all of the patients who entered the trial properly accounted for at its conclusion?
- Were patients analyzed in the groups to which they were randomized?

Box 2.11.3 Systematic reviews

To be valid a review should systematically identify and evaluate all appropriately designed studies that address the question being considered and, where appropriate, combine their results. If this is not done properly there is the potential for bias and the results will not be trustworthy even when the included papers were well conducted.

- Did the reviewers try to identify all relevant studies?
- Did the reviewers assess the quality of the included studies?
- If the results of the studies have been combined, was it reasonable to do so?

Box 2.11.4 Cohort studies

- Was the cohort recruited in an acceptable way?
- Was the exposure accurately measured to minimize bias?
- Was the outcome accurately measured to minimize bias?
- Have the authors identified all important confounding factors?
- Have they taken account of the confounding factors in the design and/or analysis?
- Was the follow up of subjects complete enough?
- Was the follow up of subjects long enough?

Box 2.11.5 Economic evaluations

- Was a comprehensive description of the competing alternatives given (i.e. can you tell who did what to whom, where, and how often)?
- Was there evidence that the programme's effectiveness had been established?
- Were all important and relevant consequences and costs for each alternative identified?
- Were consequences and costs measured accurately in appropriate units (e.g. hours of nursing time, number of physician visits, years of life gained) prior to valuation?
- Were consequences and costs valued credibly?
- Were consequences and costs adjusted for differential timings (discounting)?
- Was an incremental analysis of the consequences and costs of alternatives performed?
- Was a sensitivity analysis performed?

Box 2.11.6 Diagnostic tests

- Did all patients get the diagnostic test and the reference standard?
- Could the results of the test of interest have been influenced by the results of the reference standard?
- Is the disease status of the tested population clearly established?
- Were the methods for performing the test described in sufficient detail?

Box 2.11.7 Qualitative studies

- Was the recruitment strategy appropriate to the aims of the research?
- Were the data collected in a way that addresses the research issue?
- Has the relationship between researchers and participants been adequately considered?
- Have ethical issues been taken into consideration?
- Was the data analysis sufficiently rigorous?

Making sense of results

One should not waste time looking at the 'results' of a study where the methods lack sufficient validity. However, even if the study methods are trustworthy, it is important to consider the results critically. Also consider the way the results are expressed as this might influence the reader's interpretation and subsequent decision-making.

What are the results?

- How were the outcomes expressed [e.g. odds ratios, risk ratios, risk differences, numbers needed to treat (NNTs), or, in a diagnostic test study, likelihood ratios]?
- What was the bottom-line or estimate for each outcome?
- What is the uncertainty surrounding this estimate? (i.e. the precision of the result) Ideally these will be reported as confidence intervals.

What do they mean?

- How likely is it that this result occurred simply by chance? (The p value estimates how frequently such a result would be seen by chance.)
- How important is this result for the patient or policy decisions? It is important to consider other ways of expressing the results as the way in which results are expressed can influence how important they appear. For example, try to calculate the NNT if results are reported as relative risks or, in diagnostic test studies, the likelihood ratios where results are expressed as sensitivity and specificity.
- Were all important outcomes considered? (e.g. did the study explicitly considered adverse events?).

Box 2.11.8 Example of communicating the same evidence with different emphasis . . .

Consider the following results. If nicotine replacement therapy increases the 6-month quit rate from 10% to 17%, there are at least two ways of communicating these results. On the one hand it nearly doubles the quit rate, and on the other hand, because the NNT is about 14 [i.e. 1/(0.17–0.1)], then for every 14 people who take nicotine replacement therapy, 13 of them gain no additional benefit (approximately 2 out of the 14 quitted, although about one would have quit anyway . . .).

Can the results be applied to the local population?

You need to consider whether there are any important differences between the local population or setting and the study population or setting that would mean that the results would be likely to be different locally.

Are the benefits worth the harms and costs?

This is usually not explicitly considered in individual studies. However, the bottom-line is that the probable benefits of a decision need to outweigh the probable harms and costs. To make this judgement public health practitioners will usually need to draw on their wider experience and background knowledge. Bear in mind that, when making policy decisions this usually requires a consideration of the opportunity cost as well.

Further resources

If you want to see the checklists in more detail, with hints, they are available on the CASP website http://www.phru.nhs.uk/casp/casp.htm (accessed 26 June).

The Evidence Based Medicine Working Group, a group of clinicians at McMaster University, Hamilton, Canada, and colleagues across North America, have created a set of guides, published in the Journal of the American Medical Association.[3] References for these are available at the School of Health and Related Research (SCHARR) netting the evidence website in the UK (www.shef.ac.uk/~scharr/ir/userg.html) (accessed 26 June 2005).

For more help on searching techniques contact your local health librarian, or look at a demonstration of some basic techniques, using some of the learning materials held at http://nhs.netg.co.uk/websvm/login.asp (free registration required: accessed 26 June 2005).

See also the following publications and websites:

CASP (2005). *CASP: Evidence-based Health Care Workbook and CD-ROM.* Update software. Oxford.

EBM Teaching Tips online. *Evidence-based practice tips.* Available at: http://www.ebmtips.net/ci001.asp (accessed 22 January 2006).

Gray JAM (2001). *Evidence-based healthcare, how to make health policy and management decisions*, 2nd edn. Churchill Livingstone, London.

Greenhalgh T (2000). *How to read a paper: the basics of evidence based medicine*, 2nd edn. BMJ Books, London.

Oxford Centre for Evidence Based Medicine. Available at: http://www.cebm.net/ (accessed 26 June 2005).

Sackett DL, Richardson WS, Rosenberg W, Haynes RB (2000). *Evidence-based medicine: how to practice and teach EBM*, 2nd edn. Churchill Livingstone, London.

References

1 CASPfew. *Sources of evidence.* Available at: http://www.phru.nhs.uk/casp/sources_of_evidence.htm (accessed 22 January 2006).

2 School of Health and Related Research in Sheffield, UK (SCHARR). *Seeking the evidence: a protocol.* Available at: www.shef.ac.uk/uni/academic/R-Z/scharr/ir/proto.html (accessed 26 June 2005).

3 Oxman AD, Sackett DL, Guyatt G (1993). Users' guides to the medical literature. I. How to get started. The Evidence-Based Medicine Working Group. *J Am Med Assoc*, **270**, 2093–5.

2.12 Providing data and evidence for practitioners and policy makers

Julius Weinberg and David Pencheon

Objective

This chapter outlines some of the more important issues concerned with delivering knowledge to practitioners.

Introduction

Although epidemiology is essentially a methodological discipline, public health is a discipline which is essentially about outcomes—the methods are secondary—and it is highly pragmatic. The most common and important *content* that these disciplines both generate and use are data and evidence. The terms data and evidence are widely used and have multiple meanings.

By data, we usually mean numerical information that is collected routinely and that is used to monitor health of the populations (surveillance data) or the activity of health-related services. Data (plural) tends to refer to numerical information—usually counts 'how many' and 'how much'. It is worth remembering that counts *per se* are rarely useful unless there is a meaningful comparator. 'Compared with what' is (or should be) one of the most frequent responses to isolated data. Many data issues in public health involve taking one number, dividing it by another, and comparing the result with a third. Such data can monitor trends, reorder priorities, assess need, and, if done well, often enough, and with the right statistical processes, may even provide early warning of issues that need addressing urgently. Data (especially routine data) provide mainly a descriptive overview of a population's health. Information can be considered to be the product of processing and evaluating (raw) data. The degree of processing required to turn data into information may depend on the level of expertise of the recipient (see Chapter 2.1).

Evidence is usually the word given to knowledge generated from research. This can be etiological research (to what extent does A cause B?), interventional research (does intervention C reduce/prevent/ameliorate the risk factor/outcome D?). Evidence tends to be a richer mixture of words and numbers (when compared with simple data)—literally something that helps you understand the world around you more clearly, and, one hopes, in a less biased way. After all, experience, however valuable

in most areas of life, can be one of the most important causes of ignorance. In the legal world the word evidence is used to describe the material which shows that something has occurred 'beyond a reasonable
doubt'; this could be a mixture of accounts from witnesses, the police,
expert opinion, and forensic science. Evidence comes from many sources,
is of variable quality, and requires interpretation. This is also the case
when considering empirical evidence, arising from observation or
experiment.

In order to be effective, you will normally use three types of knowledge:

- Knowledge derived from research—evidence.
- Knowledge derived from routinely collected or audit data—statistics.
- Knowledge derived from the experience (experience from patients,
  fellow professionals, partner organisations . . .).

Important steps in providing data and evidence for practitioners and policy makers

There has always been a mismatch between the generation of evidence
and data and their communication to the right people in the right way at
the right time. Some of the reasons for this can be overcome with careful
organization and preparation.

There are often a wealth of descriptive data about a population (often
from routine data, supplemented by local surveys), although rarely are
they made available in a way that makes it easy for practitioners to take
effective action.

The main problems in providing data and evidence for practitioners
and policy makers are:

- There are many types of knowledge—data, evidence, and best practice
  often get confused.
- They are not available in real time.
- There is a lack of consistency in information definitions.
- There is lack of meaningful comparators (aggregation, drill down ...).
- Knowledge is made available in a solution-focused way not a problem-
  focused way.
- There is a lack of a common language to describe domains.
- We communicate evidence in unhelpful ways.
- There are too many people doing this badly.
- We do not always balance harm, benefit' and cost explicitly.
- We are often too ready to broadcast evidence without listening to
  the users.
- Policy makers often don't want evidence.

There are many types of knowledge—data, evidence, and best practice often get confused

One of the most important roles of a public health practitioner is to help develop an organized approach to considering problems and solutions—combining 'content' and 'process'. As such, try to be clear to people with whom you are trying to work that there are different sorts of knowledge, all of which can help but in different ways, and, critically, only when they are assembled and articulated in a clear balanced way. For instance, anecdotes are powerful ways of exemplifying what the more generalizable, systematic data and evidence suggest. They are powerful ways to raise issues (to be validated by data and evidence), but they are *not* valid, on their own, to direct expensive and significant policy and action that might influence many people's lives.

They are not always up to date

We all dream of a population-based information system that can tell us the prevalence, incidence, activity, risks, outcomes, etc. at the touch of a button. Sadly, with the exception of some communicable disease data, precious little information is available in near real time. Do not, however, let others use this as an excuse for lack of analysis, debate, and action. The reason why data are not always timely is that they are expensive to collect, and often do not change quickly. There are far bigger challenges, and benefits to be gained, in using and adapting the current systems and knowledge we already have more effectively.

Lack of consistency in information definitions

There are times to let a thousand flowers bloom, and times to be centralist. Definitions of data to be used in local, national, and international analysis (which must involve meaningful comparisons) must be consistent. National and international health bodies have an important responsibility to move towards consistency in data definitions.

Lack of meaningful comparators (aggregation, drill down . . .)

A particularly powerful way of helping practitioners is to offer data in ways that can be queried if necessary. Comparators can be everything in analysis. Too often we offer data in a way that does not help practitioners ask the obvious questions:

- Should I be worried about this?
- How does this compare with other places?
- Has this been changing over time in a way and at a rate that is acceptable?
- Are these differences (inequalities) justifiable or are they inequitable (unfair)?
- What is the quality of this evidence?
- Is it applicable to situations like mine?—can I drill down and see the methods used?

Made available in a solution-focused way not a problem-focused way

Most systems to help practitioners are deigned with answers. Realistically, most practitioners start with problems. The best systems to help practitioners and policy makers work by starting with the most common problems and help people work through them. Good information sources supplement their products in terms of questions not answers (frequently asked questions: FAQs) (see the UK National Electronic Library of Infection (NeLI) antimicrobial resistance website for an example[1]).

Lack of a common language to describe domains

Most people have a different ways of organizing the public health world. A little more consistency can greatly help communication. One person in a meeting might be thinking of diseases, another will be thinking of risk factors, a third will be thinking of geographic settings, a fourth of populations at risk, whilst the finance officer will be thinking resources. There has yet to be an international classification for public health in the same way as we have the International Classification for Disease (ICD), although there are national bodies working on it in Australia[2] and the UK.[3]

We communicate evidence in unhelpful ways

Rather than say 'an absolute risk reduction of 7%' consider saying 'that out of 100 people who take this new treatment, on average the number people who will die after 5 years will fall from about 17 to about 10'. It is important to be highly fluent in the use of absolute and relative risks, and the importance of using natural frequencies to communicate risk and uncertainty.[4]

An inappropriate dose of evidence can be as damaging to a desired policy outcome as the wrong dose of a drug to a patient. The full panoply of evidence (statistics, charts, meta-analyses, etc.) does not always need to be marshalled. A key committee or individual may only have time to see a carefully crafted synopsis as long as the supporting material which underpins the synopsis is available somewhere accessible. Overkill (in terms of quantity, and especially in terms of timeliness) may kill the decision-making process. Evidence that is 'good enough' before a key decision is taken is clearly of more value than the perfect evidence after the event. Never let the perfect be the enemy of the sufficient.

The committee, the researcher, and the busy on-call clinician, all need the evidence packaged differently. However, they need to be able to find, or make Judgements on, the quality of the evidence, its relevance to the questions they are asking, and whether it is up to date.

There are too many people doing this badly

How often should the evidence be disseminated, paraded, or sought? Over-use of the evidence can cause unforeseen reactions; in some cases with perverse outcomes. Continued exposure to the antismoking or antidrug abuse messages may cause some subsections of society to rebel and perpetuate (or worst still, adopt) the behaviours which one is trying to avoid.

As economic considerations become increasingly important[5] the cost of actually accruing evidence must be set against the efficiencies to be made using it. The frequency of establishing evidence is particularly relevant in two areas:

- it is better to have a few experts doing it regularly, rather than everyone doing it sporadically (and poorly)
- the cost of repeating it (e.g. updating Cochrane reviews,) must be set against the expected benefits that might accrue.

We do not always balance harm, benefit, and cost explicitly

What is the likelihood that implementing the evidence causes more good than harm? How broadly are the effects known? Considerations of this sort are particularly important when health policies are being developed. There is evidence that introducing user charges may reduce inappropriate attendance, but it might lead to an adverse impact on the most disadvantaged. At an individual level, suppressing ventricular ectopics, more common after myocardial infarction, and done in the best faith to reduce post-infarct death rates, in fact increased the risk of sudden death rather than decreasing it,[6] something that was established only after careful research.

We broadcast evidence too often and listen too seldom

Seek to understand first, and then be understood. Knowing the most important facts (descriptive data, etiological or interventional evidence…) about an area and/or specific population allows you to talk/write with much more authority than a person or organization who believes, thinks, or claims certain issues to be true, important, etc. The key issue with data is to choose the right data (with the right comparators) that will change the particular minds (and hearts) of the people in front of you. It is almost always a good investment of time and effort to seek to understand the perspective, anxieties, and motivations of the people you are working with. This can greatly increase the impact of what you are saying, especially if you can combine population data (with which people can often not identify) with more personalized data, or even powerful anecdotes, as long as anecdotes are not your (or their) *only* source of evidence or justification.

Policy makers often don't want evidence

Lastly, it is useful to remember that policy makers, especially politicians, do not always welcome evidence. In many ways, good-quality evidence, well generated and explicitly disseminated, can make an issue less political as there may be less debate. If you have evidence that the dearly held beliefs of your minister are simply wrong, think carefully about how you help them see the light. Do not fall into the trap of producing spurious or biased evidence merely to satisfy a policy position (policy-based evidence making).

Summary

Evidence and data are provided for a reason—usually (but not exclusively) to change and improve the quality of decision-making (a public health professional armed with good data and evidence in a well-organized fashion, and who has the skill and confidence to raise and debate issues opportunistically, without the need berate, harangue, or sermonize, can be very effective). There is a paucity of good evidence on how the evidence base can best be used to effect change. This has always been, and still is, one of the major challenges in public health.

The essential database of evidence can only be determined by a dialog between those who are using it and those generating it. There is not a one-way flow of evidence from generators to users. The best people to understand the profound evidence gaps we have are the users. They need to be a meaningful part of any strategic planning of research and knowledge management. This needs to be an iterative process whereby the lack of data and evidence in key areas can be identified and fed into the relevant research and surveillance agenda.

Similarly, there is always a need to ensure that the learning from everyday interactions with patients, practices, procedures, and policies people can be captured, made systematic and disseminated (or made available) such that as many 'daily activities of working' can generate useful information to improve the quality of practice. The personal knowledge and evidence of each practitioner should ideally be validated and made available systematically.

Further resources

Karolinska Gapminder. Making sense of the world by having fun with statistics! Available at: http://www.gapminder.org/ (accessed 29 June 2005).

Smith AFM (1996). Mad cows and ecstasy: chance and choice in an evidence-based society. *J R Statist Soc*, **159**(3), 367–83.

References

1 The National electronic Library of Infection (NeLI). *Bugs & drugs on the web*, *NeLI antimicrobial resistance website*. Available at: http://www.antibioticresistance. org.uk/ (accessed 14 September 2005).

2 Public Health Classifications Project, National Public Health Partnership of Australia. Available at: http://www.nphp.gov.au/workprog/phi/ (accessed 22 January 2006).

3 Public Health Information Tagging Standard and National Public Health Language. Available at: http://www.phits.org/ (accessed 22 January 2006).

4 Gigerenzer G (2003). *Reckoning with risk: learning to live with uncertainty*. Penguin, London.

5 Wanless D (2004). *Securing good health for the whole population. Final report*. UK Department of Health, London. Available at: http://www.dh.gov. uk/assetRoot/04/07/61/34/04076134.pdf (accessed 29 June 2005).

6 Ruberman W, Weinblatt E, Goldberg J et al. (1977). Ventricular premature beats and mortality after myocardial infarction. *N Engl J Med*, **297**, 750–7. (Cited in Sackett DL, Richardson WS, Rosenberg WMC, Haynes RB (1997). *Evidence-based medicine: how to practice and teach EBM*. Churchill Livingstone, New York.)

Direct action

Introduction

All too often public health is seen as an abstract subject with well-meaning practitioners wrestling with fearsome but nebulous giants such as poverty social deprivation, inequality, and the global tobacco industry. This, it is true, is part of the agenda of public health, and the contribution of the practitioner can only be indirect, exerted by the influence they have on national or global policy makers. This is certainly a very important function of public health, but legislation is only one means by which public health acts to improve the health of populations. Practitioners are also directly responsible for a wide range of services and know just as sharply as any clinician the enjoyment that a successful intervention produces, as well as the fear and apprehension which is felt when something goes wrong with controlling an outbreak or managing a screening programme.

Public health, unlike clinical practice, however, is at best a zero-gratitude job, Practitioners do not receive Christmas cards or bottles of whisky from grateful members of the public. When things are working well in public health no-one says thank you, but as soon as they start to go wrong the press can turn on public health with energy and hostility.

The indirect influence of the public health practitioner plays a part in policy-making. However, the practitioner who is directly responsible for services has both to make and to take decisions, often with imperfect information on which to base a decision.

Having taken a decision to deliver a pubic health service in a particular way, the same practitioner is usually responsible for putting that decision into action. On some occasions it is possible for the practitioner to do this by mobilizing resources for which they are directly accountable; often, however, one's own resources are inadequate and persuasion and push are required to bring others on board.

Taking decisions and taking action

The practitioner who is directly responsible for services has firstly to make decisions, often with imperfect information. Having taken a decision to deliver a public health service in a particular way, the same practitioner is usually responsible for implementing it. On some occasions it is possible for the practitioner to do this by mobilizing resources for which they are directly accountable. If so, they should be asking the perennial 10 questions (the 10 things to consider when you are asked to take action about a specific problem):

- Is this issue really a problem?
- If so, does the proposed action really address this problem?
- If so, are *you* the best person to address it?
- If so, is *now* the best time to do it?
- If so, who else will be involved and how?

- What are the resources available?
- What are the likely costs involved?
- What are the opportunities?
- What are the barriers?
- How will you know if you are being (or have been) successful?

Life is rarely simple—even if answers are available to these questions, very few issues can be addressed meaningfully without the involvement of others; persuasion and advocacy are required to bring the resources and power of others to bear.

Where the buck stops

If a policy goes wrong it is possible to blame many factors other than public health practitioners. However, when a service fails, for example when a second youngster dies of meningitis, the public health practitioner and the team need to account for the actions taken or not taken. This may sound alarming, but many people become public health practitioners not to escape clinical decision-making but to take equally difficult decisions, and to take action to make a difference, on a bigger canvas.

Such actions have made a significant contribution to the public's health. It is claimed that, of the 30 extra years of life expectancy gained in the 20th century, 25 of these years can be attributed to advances in public health.[1]

Of all the achievements made, the 10 great public health achievements of the 20th century in the United States are claimed to be:[2]

- vaccination
- improved motor-vehicle safety
- safer workplaces
- control of infectious diseases
- decline in deaths from coronary heart disease and stroke
- safer and healthier foods
- healthier mothers and babies
- family planning
- fluoridation of drinking water
- recognition of tobacco as a health hazard.

In this part of the handbook ways in which public health practitioners and organizations take direct action to improve the health of populations are described; for each of them the public health practitioner will be held accountable. Important ways of taking direct action range from reaching and empowering communities, through to societal efforts to protect and sustain the environment in general and the workplace in particular. Specific public health tasks such as screening, outbreak management, and handling disasters are broken down into specific tasks and competencies. This section includes chapters on working with many diverse groups of people, from community development workers to 'hard to reach' populations. Finally there are two chapters on how public health skills and approaches can be used in other settings, such as in poorer countries or in primary care.

Public health and civil engineering

The public health professional needs to work academically but needs to be a civil engineer. If public health is health improvement and protection through the organized efforts of society, the organization of society is a task as big, as difficult, and sometimes as dangerous as driving a tunnel through a mountain or building a dam. It is civil engineering on a grand scale. The public health professional needs good enough evidence but will have to make a judgement because the best evidence is rarely available.

The context of civil engineering changes; different projects are required in different times. Since the first edition of this book was published in 2001 the emphasis on health protection within public health has increased in scope and importance, and this edition of the book recognizes that.

Being sure of your resignation point

In management terms public health professionals are accountable to somebody, usually at the top of the organization, and that person is not a public health professional. It is essential for a public health professional to know the type of issue on which they would resign; if you do not know your resignation issues, you do not have a clear enough view of the application of ethics to professional practice.

References

1. Bunker JP, Frazier HS, Mostellar F (1994). Improving health: measuring effects of medical care. *Milbank Q*, **72**, 225–58.
2. Centres for Disease Control and Prevention (1999). Ten great public health achievements—United States, 1900–1999. *Morbidity and Mortality Weekly Report*, **48**(12), 241–3. Available at: www.cdc.gov/mmwr/preview/mmwrhtml/00056796.htm (accessed 14 September 2005).

JAMG

3.1 Preventing epidemics of communicable disease

Sarah O'Brien

In human/microbe interactions new diseases, like severe acute respiratory syndrome (SARS), emerge and old diseases, like tuberculosis, re-emerge. Far from being defeated, communicable diseases are always a threat either naturally or, potentially, as a result of bioterrorist action.

Objectives

After reading this chapter you will be able to:
- define the terms 'epidemic' and 'outbreak'
- explain the principles of preventing communicable disease
- explain the key features of different types of outbreaks or epidemics
- outline the key steps in investigating an outbreak or epidemic.

Definitions

Probably the most commonly used definition is that of Abram Benenson, who defined an epidemic as 'the occurrence in a community or region of cases of illness (or an outbreak) with a frequency clearly in excess of normal expectancy'. The meaning of the term 'epidemic' is broad, in particular:
- both communicable diseases, e.g. meningitis, and non-communicable diseases, e.g. obesity, are included—in this chapter, however, we will concentrate on communicable diseases
- numbers of cases, geographic extent, and the time period are all unspecified.

There are several meanings of the term 'outbreak':
- two or more related (i.e. epidemiologically linked) cases of a similar disease—an acute event like food poisoning after a wedding breakfast may present in this way
- an increase in the observed incidence of cases over the expected number within a given time period—this way of detecting outbreaks, through routine surveillance, implies a less acute onset but, paradoxically, may be more serious than the first example. This is because the problem was detected later, there is no immediate indication as to source and many more cases may be pending

• a single case of a serious disease—a single case of botulism or smallpox constitutes a public health emergency and would trigger a very detailed investigation.

Why does preventing epidemics matter?

In 2001 the World Health Organization (WHO) estimated that communicable diseases led to 14.7 million deaths, or 26% of global mortality (Table 3.1.1) whilst the International Agency for Research on Cancer (IARC) assessed that 26% of cancers in the developing world and 8% of cancers in the industrialized world are attributable to an infectious agent (Table 3.1.2). Reducing mortality and morbidity therefore means tackling these preventable infections.

Table 3.1.1 WHO estimates of global mortality from infectious diseases, 2001 (adapted from Kindshauer[1])

Infectious disease	Deaths (millions)
Respiratory infections	3.9
Acquired immunodeficiency syndrome	2.9
Diarrhoeal disease	1.9
Malaria	1.1

Table 3.1.2 Infections and cancers, 2000 (IARC estimates) (adapted from Kindshauer[1])

Infectious agent	Cancer site	Proportion of cancers due to infection
Human papilloma virus	Cervix	100
Helicobacter pylori	Stomach	50
Hepatitis B virus	Liver	55

What are the approaches to the prevention of epidemics?

Classically, prevention activities are threefold: primary, secondary, and tertiary.

Primary prevention—aiming to prevent disease onset

In the context of communicable diseases various options include:

- Eliminating the organism:
  - controlling organisms in their natural reservoir, e.g. maintaining *Brucella*-free cattle herds to prevent human brucellosis.
- Environmental protection:
  - ensuring a safe drinking water supply, with proper separation of sewage from drinking water (taken for granted in high and middle income countries!)
  - safeguarding the food supply.

These two approaches are both discussed further in the next chapter.

- Interrupting the chain of transmission:
  - controlling the insect vector for arthropod-borne diseases like West Nile Virus, an emerging cause of encephalitis in North America
  - controlling the rodent vector for diseases like leptospirosis and salmonellosis
  - modifying behaviour, such as practicing safe sex or avoiding injecting drug use, to prevent the spread of sexually transmitted diseases and blood-borne viruses like hepatitis B, hepatitis C, and human immunodeficiency virus
  - personal hygiene—a simple yet effective means for controlling communicable diseases.
- Reducing susceptibility in the host:
  - reversing malnutrition and micronutrient deficiency to boost individuals' immunity in low-income countries helps to prevent the spread of, for example, tuberculosis
  - vaccination—perhaps the most successful example of primary prevention, on one hand leading to the global eradication of small-pox and on the other to a sustained reduction in the incidence and consequences of childhood diseases. Childhood vaccination schedules vary by country, but an up-to-date list is posted on the WHO website at http://www.who.int/vaccines/GlobalSummary/Immunization/ScheduleSelect.cfm (accessed 14 September 2005). This is a very useful website to consult when assessing whether children moving into the community from overseas are likely to have completed their courses of vaccinations or not.
- Health education and community participation:
  - promoting vector control programmes, in particular the use of personal protection like insect repellents and mosquito nets
  - supporting personal hygiene and food hygiene measures in preventing gastroenteritis
  - endorsing vaccination campaigns.

The options here include:
- screening: where there is an asymptomatic or pre-symptomatic period
  in the infection process screening programmes are useful
- outbreak/epidemic investigation.

The main aims of epidemic/outbreak investigation are:
- to identify the causative agent, route of transmission, and risk factors
  for the outbreak
- to develop and implement control and prevention strategies and provide advice to prevent a similar event in the future.

Tertiary prevention—limiting the consequences of
established disease

One example of this is providing artificial limbs for a child who has
needed amputations following severe meningococcal septicaemia.

What are the key elements of
epidemic or outbreak investigation
and management?

Epidemic/outbreak investigation needs to be systematic and rapid.
Conventionally the investigation and management of outbreaks/epidemics
is divided into stages, though in practice these often run in parallel. The
technical stages are as follows.

Establish that an outbreak has truly occurred

Examination of surveillance data and local knowledge are invaluable in
determining whether or not an epidemic/outbreak is occurring. However,
consider artefactual reasons why an epidemic/outbreak might appear to
have occurred. These include:
- changes in reporting practice
- introduction of new microbiological methods
- increasing awareness of an infection in the community leading to
  increased reports
- a laboratory contamination incident.

Confirm the diagnosis

Arrange for appropriate specimens to be obtained and examined. The
types of specimens needed depend upon the precise circumstances so
seek the advice of an expert in microbiology. If nothing else, being
warned of an impending influx of specimens allows the laboratory staff to
organize their work, prioritizing outbreak samples. Agree with laboratory
staff how to identify outbreak-related samples. Since laboratory diagnosis
takes time and must not delay investigations, look for a degree of com-
monality of symptoms to form a case definition.

Create a case definition

The case definition comprises clinical criteria, which should be simple and
objective, with limitations on time, place, and person. Sometimes various

levels of case definition will be needed: possible (patients with similar symptoms) and confirmed (where a laboratory diagnosis is added to the definition for a probable case).

Count cases (case finding)

Where an outbreak is centred on an event or discrete location (e.g. a hotel or hall of residence) contacting everyone who might have been exposed and finding out if they have symptoms is relatively easy. Where the extent of the outbreak is less well defined trawl through laboratory returns or approach general practitioners to find additional cases. Whatever method is adopted, it is important that the case definition is applied without bias. Typically information from cases is recorded in a questionnaire.

- Personal demographic data: name, address, date of birth, gender, and occupation.
- Clinical details: date of onset of illness, a listing of symptoms from which the case can select those affecting them, duration of illness, days off work and need for admission to hospital, outcome of illness.
- Data items determined by the nature of the outbreak: for example travel history, immunisation history, exposure to possible causal sources such as food, water, recreational, environmental, places visited, shopping habits, contacts with ill persons or animals all depending on circumstances.

Draw an epidemic curve

Simply plot the number of cases over time on a graph. By convention cases are represented as square boxes. The shape of the epidemic curve provides evidence of the nature of the outbreak. A point-source epidemic curve, where exposure has been limited in time, usually shows a sharp upswing and a fairly rapid tail-off (Figure 3.1.1). A propagated, or continuing source, epidemic curve tends to be flatter in shape and continues over a much longer time (Figure 3.1.2). In an outbreak transmitted from person to person epidemic waves can be seen. The epidemic curve should be updated on a daily basis. In an outbreak of legionnaires' disease, plotting cases on a map can also yield helpful clues to potential sources of contamination.

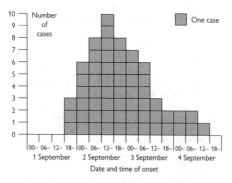

Figure 3.1.1 An example of a point source epidemic curve

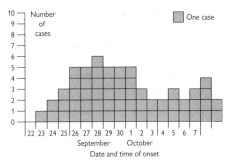

Figure 3.1.2 An example of a propagated source epidemic curve

Determine who is at risk

In certain situations this is obvious, e.g. a food poisoning outbreak at a wedding breakfast where those at risk are the guests. But also consider other parties who might have dined at the same establishment but not been part of the wedding party.

Generate and test hypotheses for exposure

Collate information about symptoms, circumstances, and diagnosis to form a hypothesis about the cause of an outbreak. The hypotheses may be tested using analytical epidemiology, but do not use cases who were interviewed to form the hypothesis. Decide on the appropriate study design. If the event is so well delineated that all those at risk, both ill and well, can be identified, then a cohort study is appropriate. If all those at risk cannot be delineated, e.g. where a general excess of disease is apparent in the community but its origin is not, a case–control study is appropriate:

- Data capture from the cohort, or cases and controls is usually using a standard structured questionnaire. If possible, develop questionnaires on the Web to avoid the need for separate data entry, but make sure that data are secure. E-mailing questionnaires also achieves rapid responses.
- Control selection (case–control study): controls must have had the opportunity of exposure to the hypothesized source, and in a community outbreak select the controls from that community. Consider the need for matching (e.g. within 10% for age) and avoid over-matching. Matching on too many variables leaves you nothing to test for, because, by definition, cases and controls are identical with respect to matched variables. Controls can be nominated by cases or recruited at random (e.g. random digit dialing). The pros and cons are outlined in Table 3.1.3.
- Data analysis: in a cohort study, where denominators are known, compare the attack rates in those who consumed a given food with the attack rate in those who did not to generate relative risks (Table 3.1.4). In a case–control study the odds of becoming ill are generated (Table 3.1.5). In each instance calculate 95% confidence intervals (CIs) and use an appropriate statistical test (seek advice from a statistician). If more than one exposure is significantly associated with illness, look at strategies for dealing with confounding, e.g. stratified analysis or logistic regression modelling.

Alternative methods for analysis include case–case studies[2] and case–cross-over studies.[3]

Table 3.1.3 Pros and cons of control selection in epidemic/outbreak investigations

Control type	Advantages	Disadvantages
Hospital or laboratory	Easy to access. Cases and controls comparable in terms of medical care	Patients may have other conditions that are associated with the disease of interest
Case-nominated	Easy to access. Useful for rare conditions. Participation rate usually good	Risk of over-matching—friends, relatives, or neighbours may share exposures with the cases
Community	Avoids bias inherent in using case-nominated controls	Method of recruitment may introduce new biases. Participation rate likely to be lower than with case-nominated controls

Table 3.1.4 An example of how to present results from a single risk variable analysis in a retrospective cohort study

Variable	Category definitions	Ill	Not ill	Attack rate	Relative risk	95% CI for the relative risk	P value
Coleslaw	Yes	21	23	48	1.13	(0.62, 2.09)	0.89
	No	8	11	42			
	Missing	1	3				
Pasta salad	Yes	26	24	52	2.43	(0.86, 6.85)	0.08
	No	3	11	21			
	Missing	1	2				
Italian ciabatta and butter	Yes	16	14	53	1.39	(0.81, 2.40)	0.34
	No	13	21	38			
	Missing	1	2				
Lemon cheese-cake	Yes	9	11	45	0.92	(0.52, 1.64)	1.00
	No	20	21	49			
	Missing	1					
Strawberry gateau	Yes	13	17	43	0.92	(0.54, 1.58)	0.96
	No	16	18	47			
	Missing	1	2				
Orange juice	Yes	28	22	56	3.92	(1.06, 14.48)	0.01
	No	2	12	14			
	Missing	0	3				

Table 3.1.5 An example of how to present results from a single risk variable analysis in a case–control study (in this instance the analysis was matched)

Variable	Exposed (%)		MOR*	95% CI		P Value
	Cases	Controls		Lower	Upper	
Cold food from takeaway cafes	46 (58)	34 (26)	3.46	1.84	6.50	<0.001
Eat any eggs	56 (71)	67 (51)	2.41	1.26	4.61	0.006
Egg prepared away from home	35 (60)	14 (18)	25.74	3.24	204.55	<0.001
Any cold cows milk drunk	56 (71)	107 (81)	0.48	0.24	0.99	0.04
Sandwiches, rolls etc. bought in plastic packs	47 (59)	26 (20)	4.34	2.33	8.07	<0.001
Ham sandwiches etc.	10 (13)	5 (4)	3.68	1.12	12.07	0.02
Prawn/other seafood sandwiches etc.	6 (8)	3 (2)	4.52	1.05	19.46	0.03
Egg mayonnaise sandwiches etc.	13 (16)	1 (1)	18.11	2.33	140.51	0.0001

Note: the percentage of cases and controls exposed ignoring matching.
*Matched odds ratio.

Consider what additional evidence is needed

Do you need additional laboratory tests, e.g. food, water, or environmental samples? What have investigations by your professional colleagues shown? For example in a food poisoning outbreak environmental health officers will collect important details such as food preparation and storage practices and carry out an inspection of the implicated premises. In an outbreak of legionnaires' disease a specialist inspection by an environmental engineer may be needed. Combining information from the epidemiologic, environmental, and microbiological investigations allows the investigating team to develop a picture of what went wrong and why, and helps them formulate both immediate control measures and measures to prevent a recurrence in the longer term.

Implement control measures

These can be initiated at any stage of the investigation, as soon as there is sufficient evidence to act upon. Seek specialist advice if necessary. The aims are to prevent new primary cases and secondary spread.

Write up your findings

Keep contemporaneous notes as you go along—this saves heartache in court later! At the end of the outbreak write up your findings in an outbreak control team report. As well as serving as a record of what you did and what was found, lessons learned should be highlighted so that others may learn from what happened.

Box 3.1.1 Key elements of outbreak/epidemic investigation and management

- Establish that an outbreak has truly occurred
- Confirm the diagnosis
- Create a case definition
- Find and count cases
- Draw an epidemic curve
- Determine who is at risk
- Generate and test hypotheses for exposure
- Consider what additional evidence is needed
- Implement control measures
- Write up your findings

What are the skills and competencies needed to achieve these tasks?

Public health professionals investigating outbreaks need expertise in the following areas:
- surveillance
- epidemiologic study design
- statistics
- leadership
- management of programmes
- evaluation
- communication.

A sense of humor also helps! Skills such as microbiology and environmental health are vested in other team members.

What is actually involved in getting something done?

Have a plan beforehand, exercise it regularly, and update it annually. It helps to know your colleagues before you come together in a crisis. Make sure that you can mobilize people to help 24 hours a day, set up an incident room, and access specialist advice.

Who are the other people that might need to be involved?

This depends to a certain extent on the nature of the outbreak/epidemic. For example, in an outbreak of foodborne disease the core team often comprises a public health practitioner with specialized training, an environmental health officer or sanitarian, a microbiologist, and a statistician. It might be appropriate to include a specialist food microbiologist, a clinician, and a veterinarian, depending on the exact circumstances. Assistance from a press officer usually proves invaluable.

Potential pitfalls in outbreak/epidemic investigation

Probably the biggest potential pitfall is attempting to run an investigation single-handed. Outbreak/epidemic investigation is genuinely a team effort. Do not rely on being able to conduct an investigation solely during office hours. By the time an outbreak comes to light many of the cases may have recovered. This means that they are back at work during the day-time, just like you are! The best times to conduct interviews tend to be during the evening, up to 9.00 p.m., and at weekends, although make sure that you are aware of the major sporting fixtures—ringing people during a major cup final is not likely to increase the response rate!

Do not have more than one person speaking to the press. Agree at the outset who will do it, and stick to it.

Use your common sense—a good descriptive study can provide better evidence than a poor analytic one!

Dogma, myths, and fallacies

It is sometimes said that there is no point in investigating point-source outbreaks because they are, by definition, over. The answer to that is that you cannot know an outbreak is over unless you have at least conducted a preliminary investigation.

Requests for standard questionnaires are often made. Whilst it is true that certain elements, e.g. demographic and clinical details, rarely change, in reality there is no such thing as a standard outbreak. The danger is of being blinded by biologic plausibility and, if taken to its logical conclusion, outbreaks of salmonellosis associated with contaminated lettuce or melons would never have been identified and controlled. Similarly we would still be chasing contaminated hamburgers as the cause of outbreaks of *Escherichia coli* O157, ignoring transmission from the environment and animals. Standard questionnaires are not a substitute for thinking.

What are the key determinants of success?

Skill, speed including the ability to mobilize sufficient resources at very short notice, a pre-determined plan, flexibility, and political clout.

How will you know when/if you have been successful?

Continued monitoring of the epidemic curve and routine surveillance data should show no new cases or a reduction in incidence.

Further resources

Giesecke J (2002). *Modern infectious diseases epidemiology*, 2nd edn. Arnold, London.

Gregg MB (ed.) (1996). *Field epidemiology*. Oxford University Press, Oxford.

Connolly MA (ed.) (2005). *Communicable disease control in emergencies. A field manual*. World Health Organization, Geneva.

Palmer SR (1995). Outbreak investigation: the need for 'quick and clean' epidemiology. *Int J Epidemiol*, **24**(Suppl. 1): S34–S38.

References

1 Kindshauer MK (ed.) (2003). *Communicable diseases 2002—global defence against the infectious disease threat*, WHO/CDS/2003.15. World Health Organization, Geneva. Available at: http://www.who.int/infectious-disease-news/cds2002/intro.pdf (accessed 23 January 2006).

2 McCarthy N, Giesecke J (1999). Case-case comparisons to study causation of common infectious diseases. *Int J Epidemiol*, **28**(4), 764–8.

3 Haegebaert S, Duche L, Desenclos JC (2003). The use of the case-crossover design in a continuous common source food-borne outbreak. *Epidemiol Infect*, **131**(2), 809–13.

3.2 Protecting health, sustaining the environment

Roscoe Taylor and Charles Guest

Threats to public health from environmental hazards are continually emerging, with impacts ranging from small-scale or local, to widespread exposures affecting whole populations.

Public health has its developmental roots in the identification and control of environmental health threats. Poor sanitation, contamination of the food or water supply leading to outbreaks of infectious disease, or air pollution episodes causing increased respiratory morbidity and mortality were triggers for major advances in health protection.

It remains a primary function of environmental health practitioners to identify environmental hazards and understand, predict, prevent, monitor, and respond to the threats that they present. While enforcement of statutory provisions was the mainstay of practice in the past, the emphasis now is more on prevention—calling into play a broad range of strategies including advocacy, intersectoral collaboration, and community development models in addition to development of policy, standards, and guidelines.

Objectives

This chapter should help you to understand:
- environmental health in the rapidly changing context of health protection
- the interrelationship between health and the environment
- the process of identifying, evaluating, and planning a response to an environmental health threat, and
- ecologic sustainability as a legitimate consideration in public health practice.

Why is this an important public health issue?

Environmental health practice at the grassroots level—such as the work carried out by local governments to ensure the safety of food and water—continues to form part of the bedrock of public health protection.

But it is also abundantly clear that ecosystem degradation threatens health at the global level, on a massive scale, and in ways that are likely to affect disadvantaged people and developing nations most severely.[1,2] The attention of nations to such fundamental long-term problems as climate change, deforestation, loss of biodiversity, fisheries depletion, and other consequences of environmental degradation, is being diverted, at our peril, by global conflict and the 'war on terror'.

Social and economic factors are powerful determinants not only of the health of the population but also the environment. Ultimately the two are inextricably related. Public health practice now usually assumes that healthy environments, including healthy social and economic conditions, are needed to improve the health of the population. However, differing beliefs about what constitute 'healthy economic conditions' continue to hamper community understanding of the difference between 'sustainable development' and 'unlimited growth'.

Although environmental health and sustainability are, ultimately, the same thing, the practice often fails this rhetoric. While the reasons for this may seem beyond the control of individual practitioners, the importance of community mobilization should not be underestimated.

Definitions

Environmental health is defined broadly as 'the segment of public health that is concerned with assessing, understanding, and controlling the impacts of people on their environment and the impacts of the environment on them'.[3] The discipline involves the theory and practice of assessing, correcting, controlling, and preventing those factors in the environment that can potentially affect adversely the health of present and future generations. Environmental health practitioners may operate at local (municipal), regional, or national and international levels, and be involved in a wide range of issues across many sectors. The occupational environment is generally excluded from consideration, but practitioners in both domains often share similar approaches.

Health protection is the avoidance or reduction of potential harm from exposures through organized efforts, including direct action with individuals or communities, regulation, legislation, or other measures. In recent years, health protection has been a major consideration in public health governance; many health departments have reorganized their functions according to health protection, health promotion, and quality of care assurance. Health protection may include environmental health services, food and water safety, communicable disease control, tobacco control, injury prevention, and other activities that aim to minimize preventable health risks.

Hazard is the intrinsic capacity of an agent, a condition, or a situation to produce an adverse health or environmental effect. Whilst information about a source of emissions and environmental concentrations of contaminants—the hazard—is essential to environmental health protection, it does not indicate how much toxin actually reaches the individual.

An agent may be hazardous but not necessarily result in a risk until exposure occurs and a dose is delivered to target organs.

Exposure refers to actual contact with an agent, usually chemical, physical, or biologic.

Exposure assessment is the estimation of the magnitude, frequency, duration, and pathway of contact of an agent encountered by humans in the course of their activities. Exposure pathways include inhalation, ingestion, or dermal contact. In contrast to dose, exposure does not necessarily indicate absorption, metabolism, storage, or excretion of a toxin.

Dose is the stated quantity of a substance to which an organism is exposed. The *applied dose* is the amount of the substance in contact with the primary absorption sites (e.g. skin, lungs, gut) and available for absorption. The *absorbed dose* is the amount crossing a specific absorption site. The *delivered dose* is the amount actually available for interaction with any particular organ or cell which may be particularly difficult or impossible to measure.

Dose–response assessment is the determination of the relationship between the magnitude of a dose or level of exposure to hazard, and the incidence or severity of the associated effect.

Risk assessment is the process of estimating the potential impact of a chemical, physical, microbiologic, or psychosocial hazard on a specified human population or ecologic system under a specific set of conditions and for a certain timeframe. Where information on good dose–response relationship, exposure, and other factors is available, risks may be quantifiable. However, risk assessments must also take into account qualitative information influencing the nature of health effects in the context of particular communities.

Risk management is the process of evaluating alternative actions, selecting options, and implementing them in response to risk assessments. The decision-making process draws on scientific, technological, social, economic, and political information and requires value judgements. The more transparent these value judgements the better it is for communication of health risk. The influences of risk perception and community outrage must also be acknowledged.

Health impact assessment utilizes risk assessment techniques in relation to development proposals that may have consequences for environmental health (see Chapter 1.5). Increasingly, consideration of equity is being introduced into health impact assessment (see Chapter 2.10).

Systematic approaches to managing an environmental health threat

In order to assess and then protect against a potential environmental health threat, it is useful to adopt a consistent framework for assessing health risk. The steps involved are:[4]

- identification of the hazard
- determining the relationship between the hazard and the effect (dose–response assessment)

- exposure assessment
- risk characterization
- risk management.

In practice, this process is often iterative rather than linear. Risk management strategies must sometimes be developed before all the information is available.

The recent international trend towards adoption of risk management frameworks in guidelines for drinking water quality, incorporating a multiple-barriers approach to hazards from catchment to tap, provides an excellent example of a systems approach to a profoundly important environmental health issue.[5,6]

Hazard identification

Before embarking on a formal risk assessment the specific issues should be identified with key stakeholders. Specific concerns and their context should be identified. It is most important to establish if the issue is actually amenable to risk assessment. Successful management requires transparency and a strong involvement of the affected communities as far as possible in every aspect of the process. Hazard identification generally relies on prior knowledge and published literature, including animal toxicology and epidemiological studies.

Dose–response assessment

Dose–response information is also derived from prior knowledge and the literature. However, there are often gaps in such data. This is partly due to difficulties in measuring exposure and dose in human studies (which tend to be opportunistic and retrospective), but methodological weaknesses are also common. Even when human data are available, it may be difficult to extrapolate dose–response relationships from high-exposure studies to situations involving low exposures.

Exposure assessment

Commonly, environmental exposures (e.g. via soil, water, or ambient air) present lower dose rates and total doses than those experienced through personal ('lifestyle') behaviours or occupational sources. Such exposures may incur relatively small increases in risk. However, because they are perceived as being outside the control of individuals, there is often a large 'outrage' factor. It is important to understand and accept that such issues may require attention that seems out of proportion to their physical health impact if they are involuntary (see Chapter 7.5).

Risk characterization

Environmental factors with only a small, perhaps unmeasureable, additional risk at the individual level can still have a major impact on populations if many people are exposed, for example low-level childhood lead exposure, or particulate pollution of airsheds and cardiovascular disease. Rose's 'prevention paradox' is very relevant to environmental health and can be used to illustrate how small reductions of exposure across a population may reap significant health benefits overall, whilst offering little to the individual.[7]

Risk management

Some environmental hazards are amenable to control more readily than lifestyle exposure factors and therefore present opportunities for efficient and effective public health interventions. This is analogous to 'engineered' injury prevention measures that separate the person from the hazard.

In establishing priorities when there are multiple environmental health problems, consider:
- the urgency of the threat (see Chapter 3.5)
- the number of people affected, and their experience of the impacts;
- whether the exposure is increasing
- the consequences of 'doing nothing'
- the vulnerability and identifiability of population subgroups
- the amenability of issues to investigation
- the availability of interventions or remedies.

Periodic, systematic review is important to ensure that priorities are not only reactive. For example, there is an urgent need to address long-term environmental issues (including the abatement of greenhouse gas emissions) by considering the health perspective, as well as the health impacts of immediate problems related to the environment. Our preoccupations include food, water, fuel, and waste disposal (particularly in developing countries), together with unemployment, violence, drugs, and debt (everywhere). Ecosystem disruption is occurring, but in terms of societal change remains a largely neglected threat whilst these more immediate issues demand attention.

Maintaining a healthy environment and mitigating risk

Maintenance of a healthy environment requires a systematic approach that may include a range of strategies such as:
- legislation and other regulation, with enforcement
- healthy public policy
- appropriate guidelines and standards
- economic incentives
- demonstration projects
- interventions to bring about attitudinal change
- community involvement
- accurate information
- intersectoral action.

Although legislative controls and regulatory mechanisms may be available to deal with an environmental health threat (and are sometimes essential as a back-up measure), this is not usually the first course of action. It is preferable to establish collaborative approaches and to work with stakeholders, including affected communities, from an early stage in developing risk management strategies.

A capacity for monitoring and surveillance is necessary for verifying that control measures are working.

There is increasing reflection on the influence of globalization on public health, and it is important to use every opportunity to recognize and support inclusion of the environment as a 'global public good for health'.[8]

Options for risk management

In formulating a response it may be helpful to broadly categorize the spectrum of potential strategies that may be available to control or prevent risks, for example:

Reducing the hazard at its source
- Alteration of systems and human behaviours that underlie the production of a hazard, e.g. transport systems, peaceful means of conflict resolution, water catchment contamination.
- Enforced shutdown of activity.
- Cleaner processing systems.
- Improved emission controls.

Reducing community exposure to ongoing hazards
- Removal of contaminant from a medium (e.g. drinking water treatment).
- Physical separation from the source: relocation of activity; buffer zones between the sources of emissions and the community; barriers, e.g. noise barriers, clean topsoil cover, creation of shade.
- Altering behaviours to reduce exposure: dietary consumption, e.g. reducing intake of mercury-contaminated fish; avoidance, e.g. preventing recreational water contact during blue-green algal blooms; regulation of environmental tobacco smoke.

Protection at the individual level
- Wearing personal protective equipment.
- Biological measures, e.g. hepatitis A vaccination to reduce the risk of the disease from an unsafe food or water supply.

Note that options in 'Reducing the hazard at its source' are in general preferable as, unlike the later options, they address the root causes and tend to be more equitable and sustainable.

Ecologically sustainable development

Neglect of root causes world-wide reflects the difficulties we face in promoting ecologically sustainable development (ESD). We need to increase the efficiency and use of renewable resources and to decrease the production of waste and hazardous materials; to protect ecosystems and the diversity of species; and to develop analytic tools for long-term economic, environmental, and socially responsible decision-making (Box 3.2.1).

Box 3.2.1 Ecologically sustainable development (ESD) and human health

Principles for ecologically sustainable development:
- live off 'interest' (renewable resources) rather than (non-renewable) 'capital'
- aim for diversity and variety
- 'closed cycle' system designs (e.g. waste water recycling)
- population levels should be in balance with available resources
- work with rather than against natural topography and biologic systems.

It is essential that ecologically sustainable development is linked to investment. Programmes in public health and other sectors should aim to:
- focus on what is possible
- solve small problems to influence larger ones
- involve people's creativity and energy
- foster the responsibility of those who pollute or degrade.

Some programmes that have aimed to promote sustainability and health have had low participation rates. New projects and programmes that bring the questions of sustainability in the indefinite future into focus in the present are required. These may be developed by:
- identifying the critical quality-of-life issues in a region
- establishing how these issues relate to longer-term sustainability issues
- identifying simultaneous solutions for sustainability and quality-of-life issues
- obtaining resources to make solutions happen.

Sustainable health programmes should simultaneously promote:
- economic efficiency
- social equity
- environmental responsibility
- human livability.

Many institutions are now committing to ESD, at least in principle.[9] For example, the notion of 'triple bottom line' reporting of social, economic, and environmental consequences has gained currency to assist in determining sustainability. Public health practitioners should use these or other structures—such as 'state of the environment' reports by governments, or municipal planning processes—as opportunities to advocate for inclusion of environmental health concerns as components of comprehensive approaches to planning and policy-making that protect and promote health (see Box 3.2.2).

Box 3.2.2 Using an organized community structure for environmental and health benefit

Tasmania Together: a 20-year social, environmental, and economic plan

Tasmania *Together* is a pioneering project that allows the people of Tasmania (an island state of Australia) to have a say in their long-term social, economic, and environmental future, in the form of a long-term plan for the state's development for a period of 20 years. It provides a framework for planning, budgeting, and policy priorities for the government and non-government sectors.

As a system of community goal setting and decision-making, it is enshrined in law (and not tied to the fortunes of any particular government). It is used to guide decision-making at the highest levels of the state public service.

Tasmania *Together* includes 24 goals and 212 benchmarks that were of most concern to the people during more than 2½ years of community consultation. These benchmarks are helping to shape government policy, service delivery, and budgets into the future, and are linked to local government, industry, and communities.

Progress is monitored by an independent statutory authority, the Tasmania *Together* Progress Board, to report directly to parliament and ensure that recommendations are implemented.

Tasmania *Together*. http://www.tasmaniatogether.tas.gov.au/
(accessed 14 March 2005).

Wood smoke and premature mortality

Some Tasmanian cities and towns have significant levels of particulate air pollution during winter, when inversion layers trap smoke from wood heaters (wood has been a relatively cheap source of fuel for many years). Combined with educational programmes on correct operation of wood burners to minimize pollution, a 'buy back' scheme was initiated by government to encourage cleaner forms of heating. This led to reductions in annual breaches of ambient air standards, but available funding was becoming exhausted and the project threatened whilst further substantial progress was still required.

An opportunity arose for government agencies collectively to use a portion of gambling levy money to help address a range of health-related Tasmania *Together* benchmarks. Given the evidence showing links between particulate pollution and premature mortality—particularly in relation to cardiovascular mortality—the benchmark of reducing premature years of life lost (PYLL) by 10% over 5 years was used as the basis for inclusion of funding for extension of the community education programme, as one of a range of projects and programmes. This is an (unfortunately too rare) example of health sector interests directly supporting the work of the environment sector.

Uncertainty and the precautionary principle

Whilst an evidence-based approach should underpin environmental health action there are many instances where adequate information is lacking. In such circumstances, a precautionary approach should apply, recognizing the existence of uncertainty and ignorance and accepting that lack of full scientific certainty should not be used as a reason to postpone preventative measures (see Box 3.2.3).

Box 3.2.3 The precautionary principle

One of the outcomes of the United Nations Conference on Environment and Development (also known as the Earth Summit) held in Rio de Janeiro, Brazil, in June 1992 was the adoption of the Rio Declaration on Environment and Development, which contains 27 principles to underpin sustainable development.

One of these principles is Principle 15, which states:

'In order to protect the environment, the precautionary approach shall be widely applied by States according to their capabilities. Where there are threats of serious or irreversible damage, lack of full scientific certainty shall not be used as a reason for postponing cost-effective measures to prevent environmental degradation.'

The 'cost-effective' component of this principle can be neglected by protagonists, leading to conflict between stakeholders about the appropriate response to an issue. Nevertheless, proponents of environmental modification need to be able to demonstrate that, to a very high degree of probability, a project will not cause significant harm, either to the environment or to health.

In the development of standards and guidelines, it is common for government policy to be defined not in terms of the precautionary principle but on a science-based conservative approach which underpins risk assessment and risk management regimes.

Health risk assessments need to be explicit about uncertainties. Looking for bias and identifying what further information could reduce the uncertainty also assists in setting priorities in research and monitoring.

What are the competencies needed to achieve these tasks?

The domain of environmental health practice is very broad, potentially requiring knowledge of principles underlying food, water, air and soil quality, waste disposal, drugs and poisons, vector control, communicable diseases, health promotion, healthy cities and municipal health planning, disaster planning, preparedness and response, and, increasingly, ecosystem health.

Necessary competencies may include communication and 'people skills', advocacy, policy, and planning together with an understanding of epidemiology, toxicology, microbiology, and a range of other biologic, physical and social sciences—and an ability to recognize when additional specialist input is needed.

Who are the other people that might need to be involved?

In conjunction with the breadth of inputs mentioned above, efforts to protect public health from environmental threats typically require engagement with many government and non-government sectors outside health, and issue-specific community groups. Development of a shared understanding with such partners is a key strategy, for example in prevention of injury by altering the physical environment through town planning measures, or in minimizing exposure to air pollutants from vehicle emissions.

Potential pitfalls

Epidemiological studies of adverse health outcomes from environmental exposures can provide critical evidence. But health studies also have limitations and can be a weak link in health risk assessments. Inadequate measurement of exposure is a particularly common failing when attempting to assess whether current health outcomes are attributable to past environmental exposures. Other problems may include lag times between exposures and potential health effects, health effects may be poorly defined, and low-level effects may be very difficult to distinguish from 'background' incidences of common health problems. There may be groups within a population that are more susceptible to certain hazards, or more highly exposed, or both (e.g. children), and to whom standard risk assessment assumptions do not apply. Compounding of risk by other exposures or possible synergism between co-pollutants may also lead to underestimates of risk, or alternatively the significance of such risks may be over-played.

Communities often call for a 'study' of their own health status when concerned about impacts from an existing exposure. However, epidemiological investigations in relation to environmental exposures should not be undertaken lightly and many factors need to be considered in examining their feasibility.[10] Such studies are often inconclusive (particularly in small populations) and may sometimes actually delay implementation of reasonable precautionary measures to reduce exposure.

It is often more appropriate and efficient to carry out thorough exposure assessment and rely on pre-existing information (e.g. dose–response data of a known toxicant, or application of environmental standards or guidelines) to help interpret the exposure data.

Lessons from success and failure

Successful environmental health practice is usually invisible, while failures often attract attention.

Successes

Locally there are many examples of benefit from activities under the auspices of the World Health Organization's Healthy Cities programme and Local Agenda 21. Consider the local action to create shade protection against UV light exposure (Box 3.2.4).

Disasters such as earthquakes and tsunamis powerfully illustrate the essential nature of local environmental health measures in reducing morbidity and mortality during recovery phases.

Major reductions in population exposure to lead have been achieved through systems changes across a wide range of activities and settings.

Environmental health action is leading to reduced harm from exposure to environmental tobacco smoke and to indoor air emissions from unflued gas heaters.

The global success of the Montreal Protocol in reducing the output of ozone-damaging emissions may allow recovery of the ozone layer. Ratification of the Kyoto Protocol has been a step towards combating global warming but the protocol itself cannot yet be claimed a 'success'.

Failures

Construction of dams to increase certainty of water supply for irrigation-based agriculture has been a widespread practice resulting in short-term economic gain but sometimes adverse long-term social and ecologic consequences.[11]

The fatal water-borne disease outbreak in the community of Walkerton in Canada was a model example of systems failure, and the experience is now being used constructively to help water authorities understand the need for a more active approach to risk management.[12]

Failure to consider the principles of ESD remains common in the health-care system. The Australian Hospital Association and Environment Protection Agency, for example, developed a green health care project but were unable to achieve satisfactory levels of participation.[13] The rising costs of waste disposal and energy bills have probably been more important than the actions of pressure groups in alerting managers to the need to consider the challenges of sustainability more actively. Nevertheless, the aim of environmentally responsible health care could become a valuable focus for a public health perspective on sustainability.[14]

Box 3.2.4 Creating shade: a case study

A high mortality rate from skin cancer (particularly malignant melanoma), arising from excessive exposure to sunlight and UV radiation, is a major public health issue in Australia. Extensive promotional efforts have led to high public awareness but have not been sufficiently effective in encouraging people to adopt 'sunsmart' behaviours.

More sustainable approaches combine individual and community responsibility through interventions such as the creation of shade—however, there is no legislative mandate regarding provision of shade.

Local governments are very well placed to implement shade creation policies, but at this stage only some have adopted such policies. Research into barriers and facilitative factors combined with shade audits in local government areas demonstrated the following 'critical success' factors:

- support from elected council members
- quarantined funding for provision of natural and manufactured shade
- appointment of an officer to facilitate actions emanating from the shade creation policy whilst maintaining links with staff in all local government departments (including planning, engineering, parks and gardens, finance, executive officers, and environmental health)
- transferring responsibility for shade creation to other parties, for example by including shade provision as a condition of approval of development applications for facilities to be used by the public
- active inclusion of community members and groups in development, adoption, and implementation phases of the policy.

Adapted from The National Environmental Health Strategy,
enHealth Council of Australia (1999)

http://www.health.gov.au/pubhlth/publicat/document/
metadata/envstrat.htm (accessed 14 March 2005).

Key determinants of success

In acute situations where environmental exposures clearly threaten health, adequate legislation and emergency powers to support public health interventions may be essential to ensure that exposures are abated as soon as possible.

Risk assessment and management practices need to be sound and accountable. Knowing where and when to seek advice on technically complex matters is vital: cultivate contacts who can rapidly steer you in the right direction if they do not know themselves.

Empowerment and support of local authorities and communities to integrate environment, health, and sustainable development in local strategies is fundamental to the creation of healthy environments.[15]

How will you know if you have been successful?

- Reduced exposure to a hazard (usually easier to measure than health outcomes).
- 'Process' measures such as improvements in policy or community satisfaction with the process of risk assessment and management.
- Reduced morbidity or mortality associated with the exposure, when health surveillance/epidemiological methods allow.
- Programme outcomes include explicit sustainability criteria.

Further resources

Harr J (1996). *A civil action*. Vintage Press, New York. (A courtroom drama that shows the difficulties of establishing environmental causation of disease—and of obtaining justice.)

Grossman LA, Vaughan RG (1999). *A documentary companion to A Civil Action*. Foundation Press, New York.

Grossman LA, Vaughan RG (2000). *A documentary companion to A Civil Action—teacher's manual*. Foundation Press, New York.

World Health Organization (1993). *Health, environment and development: approaches to drafting country-level strategies for human well-being under Agenda 21*. World Health Organization, Geneva.

Health impact assessment websites:

Health Canada. http://www.hc-sc.gc.ca/ewh-semt/pubs/eval/index_e.html (accessed 24 January 2006).

London Health Commission (2000). *A short guide to health impact assessment—informing health decisions*. http://www.londonshealth.gov.uk/pdf/hiaguide.pdf (accessed 20 April 2005).

World Health Organization. *Health impact assessment*. http://www.who.int/hia/en

World Health Organization Regional Office for Europe. *Health impact assessment methods and strategies*. http://www.who.dk/healthimpact

References

1 McMichael AJ (1993). *Planetary overload: global environmental change and the health of the human species*. Cambridge University Press, Cambridge.

2 McMichael AJ, Campbell-Lendrum DH, Corvalán CF *et al.* (2003). *Climate change and human health—risks and responses*. World Health Organization, Geneva.

3 Moeller DW (2005). *Environmental health*, 3rd edn. Harvard University Press, Cambridge, MA.

4 Commonwealth Department of Health and Ageing (for enHealth Council) (2002). *Environmental health risk assessment: guidelines for assessing human health risks from environmental hazards: June 2002*. Available at: http://www.health.gov.au/internet/wcms/Publishing.nsf/Content/health-pubhlth-publicat-document-metadata-env_hra.htm (accessed 14 March 2005).

5 Australian Government NHMRC/NRMMC (2004). *Australian drinking water guidelines*. National Health and Medical Research Council, Natural Resource Management Ministerial Council 2004. Available at: http://www.nhmrc.gov.au/publications/synopses/eh19syn.htm (accessed 13 March 2005).

6 World Health Organization (2004). *Guidelines for drinking water quality*, 3rd edn, Vol. 1 Recommendations. World Health Organization, Geneva. Available at: http://www.who.int/water_sanitation_health/dwq/gdwq3/en/ (accessed 13 March 2005).

7 Rose G (1992). *The strategy of preventive medicine*. Oxford University Press, Oxford.

8 Smith R, Beaglehole R, Woodward D, Drager N (eds) (2003). *Global public goods for health—health economic and public health perspectives*. Oxford University Press, Oxford.

9 Harvard University Gazette (2004). *Six new sustainability principles adopted*. Available at: http://www.news.harvard.edu/gazette/2004/10.14/09-sustain.html (accessed 24 January 2006).

10 Agency for Toxic Substances and Disease Registry (1996). *Guidance for ATSDR health studies*. US Department of Health and Human Services, Washington, DC. Available at: http://www.atsdr.cdc.gov/HS/gd1.html (accessed 14 March 2005).

11 Brewster D (1999). Environmental management for vector control. Is it worth a dam if it worsens malaria? *BMJ*, **319**, 651–2.

12 Hrudey SE, Hrudey EJ (2004). *Safe drinking water—lessons from recent outbreaks in affluent nations*. IWA Publishing, London.

13 Australian Hospital Association (1996). *Green health care. Environmental assessment manual*. Australian Hospital Association, Canberra.

14 Pierce J, Jameton A (2004). *The ethics of environmentally responsible health care*. Oxford University Press, New York.

15 World Health Organization Regional Office for Europe (2005). *Healthy cities and urban governance*. Available at: http://www.euro.who.int/healthy-cities (accessed 14 March 2005).

3.3 Protecting and promoting health in the workplace

Tar-Ching Aw, Stuart Whitaker, and Malcolm Harrington

For many people lack of work, unemployment, is a cause of ill-health but the workplace itself poses many preventable health hazards.

Objectives

After reading this chapter you will be able to understand:
* the nature and scope of occupational health practice and
* how efforts to protect and promote health in the workplace will contribute to general public health.

Definition

Occupational health deals with the two-way interaction between health and work. It encompasses:
* prevention of occupationally related illness or injury resulting from exposure to workplace hazards
* ensuring that workers with pre-existing illnesses or disability are able to continue working without undue risk to their health or those of third parties
* promoting general health and safe working practices in the workplace.

Why is this an important public health issue?

Individuals at work constitute a significant proportion of the general population. Maintenance of their state of health is key to ensuring the well-being of their co-workers, their families, the employer, and the nation.

Approaches to occupational health

Preventing occupationally-related illness or injury

- Identifying hazards in the work setting.
- Determining the population exposed to such hazards.
- Assessing the risks from exposure to the hazards (risk assessment).
- Taking appropriate preventive action by one or more of the following actions to reduce those risks: elimination, substitution, or containment of the hazards; limiting the numbers of workers exposed; reducing the time each person is required to spend at specific work areas where hazards are not easily eliminated; and providing personal protective equipment, as a last resort.
- Auditing and reassessing the efficacy of the preventive measures.
- Considering the need for a suitable health surveillance programme or periodic monitoring system for the workforce.

Workers with pre-existing illnesses or disability

- Identifying relevant risk factors, e.g. atopy, previous asthma, or previous history of several episodes of low back pain, so that suitable advice, job placement, and work modification can be considered.
- Assessment of job duties.
- Pre-placement assessment and advice.
- Health surveillance, including periodic review of health status and sickness absence record.

For some occupational groups, e.g. health-care workers, specific tasks include checking the immune status and providing immunization as required. An example is determination of the hepatitis B immune status for health-care workers.

Promoting general health in the workplace

The main tasks involved in health promotion at the workplace are:

- *Specific*: Suitable and sufficient information, instruction, and training in working safely should be provided where there are recognized hazards in the workplace.
- *General*: The workplace can be used as a setting to address non-occupational, lifestyle factors that affect general public health. Examples are advice and information on alcohol intake, smoking, diet, exercise, safe driving, and precautions in the course of travelling or working abroad. The workplace, along with other venues such as the school, the home, and the local community, is an important setting for the delivery of health education and health promotion. Health promotion initiatives in the workplace can include measures such as changing the food provided in the works canteen, establishing a no-smoking policy. or providing subsidized membership to sports and exercise facilities.

The potential disadvantage of focusing on workplace health promotion is the diversion of attention and resources away from measures to assess and control the more serious occupational health and safety risks.

What are the tasks needed to achieve effective change?

- Proper assessment of risks by a competent person.
- Commitment at the highest level to rectify the problem.
- Clear strategy for implementing preventive measures.
- Good communication between preventive medicine professionals and management and the workforce. Publicity through in-house newsletters, seminars, and effective use of the media are crucial elements for creating effective change.
- Timely implementation of measures.
- Review and evaluation of success or failure.

It is essential that the workforce is not only informed but is actively engaged in the whole process of change where appropriate

Who are the other people that might need to be involved?

- Management at all levels, as they ultimately have the responsibility for managing occupational health issues and controlling the access to resources.
- The workforce and their representatives, as the measures proposed will affect them. Worker cooperation and participation is essential for the measures to succeed.
- Occupational health and safety and public health professionals:
  - occupational physicians and nurses, with clinical skill to assess health effects
  - occupational hygienists, who are experts in assessment of exposure to workplace hazards
  - occupational psychologists
  - safety practitioners
  - ergonomists
  - health promotion personnel
  - toxicologists
  - epidemiologists
  - other health practitioners and specialists.

In order to engage the workforce with the actions being taken to protect and promote their health, it is important to understand that genuine teamwork is crucial.

What are the potential pitfalls in occupational health?

- Misinterpretation of motives for action by either management or the workforce.
- Misguided and ill-informed media coverage.

- Inappropriate risk perception.
- Inappropriate or inaccurate health belief models.
- Lack of attention to social and cultural values.

Fallacies in occupational health

Fallacy 1: The data are abundant

For many occupational hazards there is often a lack of good data on the effects of exposure on human health. This is either because a good system for gathering information on health effects is non-existent, that compliance with current reporting requirements for occupational ill-health is poor, or that there are conflicting animal data, and human epidemiological data are limited.

Fallacy 2: If there are no data, exhortation will be sufficient

Until accurate data on the incidence and prevalence of work-related conditions become available, it may be difficult to impress upon the public, employers, and government the extent of any problem.

Fallacy 3: Most clinicians are well trained in occupational health

Training in occupational medicine and occupational health in medical and nursing schools is limited. Consequently, medical and nursing professionals often have only a very general understanding of what can be done to prevent ill-health and injury at the workplace.

Case studies—occupational health incidents

- *The Bhopal disaster:*[1] an explosion in the workplace led to acute and chronic health effects among the workforce and surrounding community. The chemical agent involved was methyl isocyanate.
- *The Chernobyl incident:*[2] effects from an out-of-control 'industrial process', partly related to operator fatigue, became a major public health problem (occupational and environmental). The agents involved were radioactive materials.
- The dibromochloropropane (DBCP) problem:[3] questions on male infertility and inability to start a family amongst a US workforce led to occupational and industry-wide epidemiological investigations that then identified DBCP as the cause. This resulted in cessation of manufacture of DBCP for use as a pesticide.
- Gynecomastia in a pharmaceutical company:[4] concerns regarding enlargement of male breasts in Puerto Rico led to investigations showing that for some potent biologically active workplace materials the level of containment to prevent health effects may need to be greatly increased. The agents involved were estrogenic compounds.

- Asbestos exposure:[5] pulmonary fibrosis, bronchogenic carcinoma, and pleural and peritoneal mesothelioma occurred in workers exposed to asbestos fibers. The risk of lung cancer for asbestos exposure was noted to be multiplied where there was concomitant cigarette smoking. Similar health effects occurred from secondary exposure of wives who had to clean the asbestos-contaminated overalls of these workers.
- Vinyl chloride monomer:[6] a cluster of four cases of a very rare malignancy—angiosarcoma of the liver—occurred amongst workers responsible for cleaning polymerization chambers for manufacture of polyvinyl chloride (PVC). Prompt preventive action led to rapid reduction in worker exposure to the chemical agent—vinyl chloride monomer. This is a gas that is polymerized to form the relatively inert and non-toxic PVC. Corroborative animal evidence of similar tumors in rodents came to light at about the same time.

Four important lessons

1. Prompt public health action may be needed even if not all of the desired information is available. Do not let the desire for perfection hinder the need for pragmatism.
2. Clusters of a rare disease (mesothelioma, angiosarcoma) are often easier to identify as resulting from an occupational exposure than more common pathology such as lung cancer or spontaneous abortions.
3. Effects on the workforce, the wider community, and the environment can result from workplace hazards.
4. Public health vigilance and clinical case reports can both lead to identification of health hazards in the workplace.

Predictors of success and failure

Success

- A good team of occupational and public health professionals can identify problems early in order to initiate effective preventive action.
- Sympathetic and supportive management and workforce aids this process.

Failure

- Health promotion in the workplace should not be done at the expense of control of workplace hazards.
- A multidisciplinary approach will not work if coordination of activities is poor and there is a lack of understanding of the roles of each team member.
- An over-reliance on the medical model may prove to be ineffective in addressing the problems encountered in the workplace. Identification of cases, correct diagnosis, treatment, and reporting procedures, important though those activities are, will do little to prevent further cases from occurring unless risks to health can be communicated effectively to the public, politicians, decision-makers, employers, and employees. All of these groups have a part to play in ensuring that effective action is taken to prevent exposure to hazardous working conditions.

How will you know if you have been successful?

Criteria for success:
- reduction in the incidence and prevalence of occupational ill-health
- and injury
- reduction of risk or frequency of hazardous exposures
- improved knowledge of risks and awareness by the working population
- positive changes in behaviour and attitudes towards occupational risks by the working population
- an absence of inappropriate adverse media publicity.

Further resources

Books

Adams P, Baxter PA, Aw TC, Cockcroft A, Harrington JM (ed.) (2000). *Hunter's diseases of occupations*, 9th edn. Edward Arnold, London.

Cox RAF, Edwards FC, Palmer K (ed.) (2000). *Fitness for work: the medical aspects*, 3rd edn. Oxford University Press, Oxford.

Harrington JM, Gill FS, Aw TC, Gardiner K (1998). *Pocket consultant: occupational health*, 4th edn. Blackwell Science, Oxford.

Sadhra SS, Rampal KG (ed.) (1999). *Occupational health: risk assessment and management*. Blackwell Science, Oxford.

Occupational health journals

Occupational and Environmental Medicine
Scandinavian Journal of Work, Environment and Health
American Journal of Industrial Medicine

Journal papers

Gochfeld M (2005). Chronologic history of occupational medicine. *J Occup Environ Med*, **47**(2), 96–114.

Greenberg M (2004). The British approach to asbestos standard setting: 1928–2000. *Am J Ind Med*, **46**, 534–41.

Databases

Available on CD-ROM: (contact info@mdx.com and http://www.ovid.com)
TOMES (Toxicology, Occupational Medicine and Environmental Series).
HSELINE (Health and Safety Executive, UK).
NIOSHTIC (National Institute for Occupational Safety and Health, USA).
CISDOC (International Labour Office, Geneva).

Websites

American Conference of Governmental Industrial Hygienists, Inc. http://www.acgih.org/home.htm
Faculty of Occupational Medicine, UK. http://www.facoccmed.ac.uk/
Finnish Institute of Occupational Health. http://www.ttl.fi/internet/english
Health and Safety Executive, UK. http://www.hse.gov.uk/

References

1 Cullinan P, Acquilla S, Ramana Dhara V (1997). Respiratory morbidity 10 years after the Union Carbide gas leak at Bhopal: a cross-sectional survey. *BMJ*, **314**, 338–42.

2 World Health Organization (1996). *Health consequences of the Chernobyl accident. Scientific report.* WHO, Geneva.

3 Whorton D, Krauss RM, Marshall S, Milby TH (1977). *Infertility in male pesticide workers. Lancet*, **2** (8051), 1259–61.

4 Harrington JM, Stein GF, Rivera RO, de Morales AV (1978). Occupational hazards of formulating oral contraceptives—a survey of plant employees. *Arch Environ Health*, **33**, 12–15.

5 Berry G, Newhouse ML (1982). Mortality of workers manufacturing friction materials using asbestos. *Br J Ind Med*, **39**, 344–8.

6 Baxter PJ, Anthony PP, MacSween RNM, Scheuer PJ (1997). Angiosarcoma of the liver in Great Britain 1963–73. *BMJ*, **2**, 919–21.

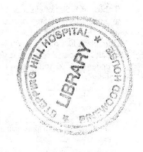

3.4 Facilitating community action

Anna Donald

Objectives

After reading this chapter you will understand the social determinants of health and ways to change them in the community.

Background

Social interventions at a community or population level are powerful ways of improving the health of individuals, because social factors are the most powerful determinants of health (Table 3.4.1). Being in a lower social class or having few years in formal education is more dangerous to one's health than having high cholesterol or exercising little.[1] In most rich countries, lifestyle factors such as smoking, excess drinking, and obesity combine to explain about one-third of differences in health outcomes. Most of the remaining difference is explained by different exposures to social factors, such as parental occupation, education, income, housing and transport, and political stability.[2]

Table 3.4.1 Size of effect on health following universal access to health and social services. Standardized mortality ratios for social classes, men aged 20–64 yrs, England and Wales, 1951. (Reproduced with permission from Blane D, Brunner E, Wilkinson R (1996). The evolution of public health policy: an Anglocentric view of the last fifty years. In: Blane D, Brunner E, Wilkinson R (eds) *Health and social organization*. Routledge, London.)

	Social class				
	I	II	III	IV	V
From the Decennial Supplement (1941–51)	98	98	101	94	118
As adjusted by Registrar General (1959)	86	92	101	104	118

How do social factors affect health?

Most social factors affect the degree to which people are able to control their actions in different spheres of life (work, home, leisure); how many physical hazards they are exposed to; and the degree of social support they enjoy.

At a biologic level social factors seem to affect the human body cumulatively through neuroendocrine, immunologic, and hemostatic mechanisms.[3] For example, people who are unemployed or who only have a few years of schooling are more likely to be depressed, and in turn are three to five times more likely to have a heart attack.[4] Those with poorly insulated houses are more likely to be cold, which in turn is a potent risk factor for cardiac events.[5] Secondly, a poor social environment adversely affects health by making it more likely that people will smoke, drink, eat to excess and be exposed to environmental hazards. For example, mortality rates in Russia have risen exponentially since the collapse of a stable legal and political system, at least in part mediated through excess drinking, as well as through exposure to cold and violence.[6] In Western countries, about half of childhood accidents are associated with poor design and maintenance of people's homes.[7] For policy purposes, it is more powerful to analyze social rather than biologic factors because social factors are generally more amenable to change and their improvement is likely to have greater and more lasting results. They can be analyzed using two frameworks: effects across the life course and cross-sectional analysis.

Effects across the life course

Longitudinal studies have found that individuals are particularly susceptible to the effects of different factors at different times in their lives. Although poverty and poor living standards exacerbate all of them, fetuses and babies are particularly susceptible to poor nutrition, children to parental depression, poor housing, and unsafe play areas, adolescents to social isolation, adults to unemployment and low-paid jobs, and elderly people to social isolation, cold, and pollution.[8]

Cross-sectional analysis

At all life stages, people are exposed to social factors which work at different levels (Figure 3.4.1).

General socio-economic, cultural and environmental conditions

↓

Living and working conditions
(education, employment, work environment, health care, housing)

↓

Social and community networks

↓

Lifestyle

↓

Person

Figure 3.4.1 Social factors influencing health (adapted from Drever and Whitehead[9])

Why is the social environment a public health issue?

The social environment is a public health issue because it has such a big impact on health and because public health workers can do so much to improve it. Unlike most health professionals, who are restricted to helping individuals on a case-by-case basis, public health workers can change institutions and laws that organize the social environment at a population level.

What can be done to improve the social environment at the community level?

Table 3.4.2 describes interventions that evidence has found improve social factors. Here are six steps which are common to any change management process:

1. Choose a model for change.
2. Prepare with data: identify the main problems; assess the size and scope of each problem; assess available resources and costs.
3. Prioritize options.
4. Plan each strategy: describe tasks and barriers.
5. Evaluate.
6. Build loyalty and trust.

Choose a model for change

In general, more collaborative approaches involving members of the community take longer, but achieve more lasting change, provided analytic and practical skills are 'cascaded' effectively. Communities may need different strategies at different times to match their confidence, experience, and available resources.

Prepare with data

Identify the main problems

It helps to structure each problem in terms of exposure, population affected, intervention(s) needed, level at which to act; outcomes to be achieved, and time period for intervention and follow-up period.

Assess the size and scope of each problem

It is important to know the likely contributing factors to the problem and the context in which it manifests.

Different data collection methods include direct observation, interviews with key stakeholders, rapid appraisal mechanisms, focus groups, 'town hall' meetings, formal needs assessment, routine data (statistics or qualitative surveys), and specialist surveys (see Chapters 2.1 and 2.8). Methods should be ethical and should optimize scientific reliability and feasibility.

Table 3.4.2 Examples of effective interventions to improve social risk factors (adapted from Acheson[10])

Exposure	Intervention	Examples of outcomes
Poverty	Redistributive mechanisms such as taxes and subsidies. Day care centres and pre-school programmes. Parental (especially maternal) education. Family planning programmes and access to contraception for adolescents and young adults. Media campaign to increase uptake of benefits. Local employment programmes	Improved all-cause mortality and morbidity
Psychosocial stress	Better job control. Crime-reduction policies, including community policing programmes and lighting of public walkways	Reduced cardiac events and all-cause mortality
Poor nutrition	Interactive health education. Surplus food schemes. Local food cooperatives. Business partnerships to make quality food available in low-income areas. Smoke reduction programmes	Reduced cardiac events in adulthood. Reduced cancer incidence
Parental depression	Mother–baby education units. Maternal education. Parental social support: home visits at critical periods	Reduced mental health disorders. Reduced child accidents. Reduced all-cause mortality
Poor housing	Smoke alarms. Insulation and heating subsidies. Planning to link housing with social networks and access to goods and services	Reduced death from fires. Reduced cardiac events. Reduced depression and all-cause mortality
Crime	Community policing programmes	Reduced stress. Reduced cardiac and all-cause mortality
Poor transport policies	Safe, maintained walking and cycling paths. Improved public transport. Child safety interventions (e.g. traffic calming devices). Subsidized public transport for deprived populations	Reduced obesity. Reduced respiratory disease from vehicle emissions. Reduced child accident rates. Reduced social isolation

You can compile information to develop a 'health profile' of the community. Health profiles commonly include: socio-economic data (age, sex, income/expenditure, area), health status (morbidity and mortality from different conditions), functional status, quality of life, specific health risks, distribution of health-care resources, and use of health care (see Chapters 2.1 and 2.8). Triangulation (data from several sources) can improve estimates from imperfect sources.

Assess costs and available resources

Resources may include money, skills and experience, time, organizational capacity, partners, and political influence. Costs may be assessed with cost–benefit analysis or simple budgeting. Assessment should include evaluation of the likely effectiveness of each intervention; opportunity costs of doing one thing rather than another; and non-monetary costs of interventions, including distress, dislocation, or reduced productivity resulting from changes to the social environment. (Such non-monetary costs are known as 'negative externalities' in economics.)

Prioritize options

It is rarely possible to address all issues at once. Problems can be prioritized in terms of how much disease and economic or social burden they place on society and how feasible they are to address. A problem may also be a priority for symbolic reasons rather than for immediate health gain. Depending on the nature of the problem, decision-tree analysis may help to separate options with uncertain outcomes.[11]

Plan each strategy: describe tasks and barriers

Describe systematically how to achieve different objectives as well as analyzing possible barriers. A simple grid of four overlapping realms—psychological, political, professional, and technical—can help to prompt and classify tasks and potential pitfalls (Table 3.4.3).

Table 3.4.3 Examples of tasks and barriers affecting most programmes for change

Realm	Examples of tasks involved	Examples of potential barriers
Psychological	Engage people in ways that matter to them. Identify and support people who are effective community change agents (sometimes called 'product champions'). Use language that empowers, not excludes	Resistance of all kinds arising from key stakeholders' fear of loss of role, power, identity, social networks
Political	Ensure key stakeholder support. Phrase policies in language of current discourse	Failure to engage popular change agents. Poor timing, given political agenda
Professional	Identify and plan to meet professional and legal requirements, if any, for proposed changes. Identify and secure resources. Set budgets	Regulations obstructing proposed changes
Technical	Secure equipment and map out process for data collection. Secure equipment and map out process for each change needed. Ensure requisite technical skills are available	Insufficient local skills or equipment to collect information

Evaluate

Programmes usually require evaluation to improve future cycles of the programme, to close down ineffective or harmful programmes, and to empower participants. Although demanding of programme leaders, openness about negative feedback usually inspires more confidence in the long run than no evaluation efforts. Like initial data collection, evaluation methods can be fairly informal and inexpensive, or highly structured. They include surveys of key stakeholders, routinely collected and specially collected data, or formal epidemiological trials (including randomized controlled trials), ecological trials, and before-and-after trials. Evaluation (including action research) should be planned from the beginning of the project and should include some kind of control group for comparison.

Build loyalty and trust

Efforts are usually wasted if agents of change do not obtain the loyalty and trust of community members. Different strategies and lots of time are usually needed to build loyalty and trust, or 'social capital';[12] staff levels and time-frames for projects need to be set accordingly.

Further resources

Benzeval M, Judge K, Whitehead M (ed.) (1995). *Tackling inequalities in health: an agenda for action*. King's Fund, London.

Durch JS, Bailey LA, Stoto MA (ed.) (1997). *Improving health in the community: a role for performance monitoring*. National Academy Press, Washington, DC.

Jacobson B, Smith A, Whitehead M (1988). *The nation's health: a strategy for the 1990s*. King's Fund, London.

Kuh D, Ben-Shlomo Y (1997). *A life course approach to chronic disease epidemiology*. Oxford University Press, Oxford.

Wilkinson R (1997). *Unhealthy societies: the afflictions of inequality*. Routledge, London.

Wilkinson R, Marmot M (ed.) (1998). *Social determinants of health: the solid facts*. World Health Organization, Geneva.

Wilkinson R, Marmot M (ed.) (1999). *Social determinants of health*. Oxford University Press, Oxford.

References

1 Rose G (1985). Sick individuals and sick populations. *Int J Epidemiol*, **14**, 32–8.

2 Marmot MG, Davey Smith G, Stansfeld S, Patel C, North F, Head J (1991). Health inequalities among British civil servants: the Whitehall II study. *Lancet*, **337**, 1387–93.

3 Stansfeld S, Marmot MG (ed.) (2000). *Stress and heart disease*. BMJ Publications, London.

4 Hemingway H, Marmot MG (1999). Evidence based cardiology: psychosocial factors in the aetiology and prognosis of coronary heart disease: systematic review of prospective cohort studies. *BMJ*, **318**, 1460–7.

5 Lloyd EL (1999). The role of cold in ischaemic heart disease: a review. *Public Health*, **105**, 205–15.

6 Walberg P, McKee M, Shkolnikov V, Chenet L, Leon DA (1998). Economic change, crime, and mortality crisis in Russia: regional analysis. *BMJ*, **317**, 312–18.

7 Department of Trade and Industry (1991). *Home and leisure accident research: twelfth annual report, 1988 data*. Department of Trade and Industry, Consumer Safety Unit, London.

8 Bartley M, Blane D, Montgomery S (1997). Education and debate. Socio-economic determinants of health: health and the life course: why safety nets matter. *BMJ*, **314**, 1194.

9 Drever F, Whitehead M (ed.) (1997). *Health Inequalities*, Decennial Supplement, series DS No. 15. HMSO, London.

10 Acheson D (1998). *Report on the inquiry into health inequalities*. The Stationery Office, London.

11 Lilford RJ, Pauker SG, Braunholtz DA, Chard J (1998). Getting research findings into practice: decision analysis and the implementation of research findings. *BMJ*, **317**, 405–9.

12 Pratt J, Plamping D, Gordon P (1999). *Working whole systems*. King's Fund, London.

3.5 Managing disasters and other public health crises

Paul Bolton

Objective

After reading this chapter you will be familiar with a basic public health approach to disasters and other crises.

Classification and definition

The term 'disaster' is used in many different ways. To get an overview of all the ways in which the word is used see Box 3.5.1.

Box 3.5.1 Natural and human disasters

Disasters of *natural* origin:
- sudden onset (earthquakes, landslides, floods, etc.)
- slower onset (drought, famine, etc.).

Disasters of *human* origin:
- industrial (e.g. Chernobyl)
- transportation (e.g. train crash)
- complex emergencies (e.g. wars, civil strife, and other disasters causing displaced persons and refugees).

Adapted from Noji[1]

This chapter focuses on the more complex disasters, with the understanding that any of the issues and approaches described apply equally to other types of disasters and lesser crises.

In a descriptive sense, a public health crisis is an event(s) that overwhelms the capacity of local systems to maintain a community's health. Therefore, outside resources are temporarily required. Crises can range from specific health issues—such as a disease outbreak in an otherwise unaffected community—to a full-scale disaster with property destruction and/or population displacement and multiple public health issues. The tsunami in December 2004 exemplified how big the challenge can be, but smaller disasters pose equally severe threats to public health.

Principles of response

The public health response to any disaster or crises is based on these principles:
1. Securing the basics that all humans require to maintain health.
2. Determining the current and likely health threats to the affected community, given the local environment and the community's resources, knowledge, and behaviour.
3. Finding and providing the resources required to address points 1 and 2.

The first action is a rapid assessment of points 1 and 2 in order to initiate step 3 as soon as possible. Too often assessment is delayed due to a misguided fear of delaying assistance. Instead organizations may rush to supply materials and personnel without checking what is actually needed. After a major disaster these supplies can choke the transport system with unneeded goods while needed goods cannot get through. Even in a limited crisis, time and money may be wasted sorting through, storing, and/or destroying useless donated supplies. The World Health Organization (WHO) have issued guidelines on drug and equipment donations during disasters that have helped improve this situation. These guidelines are available from WHO whose home page for disaster information is http://www.who.int/topics/disasters/en/ (accessed 30 January 2006).

Remember to quickly assess first, by the aphorism 'don't just do something, stand there (and assess)'. If conducting an assessment for a particular agency, then any assessments should include coordination with local government, community leaders, and other assisting and coordinating organizations, such as the UN or 'non-governmental organizations' (NGOs). This is necessary to determine their capacities and intentions and to avoid duplication of efforts.

This chapter concentrates on the initial rapid assessment as the basis for response. More detailed assessments and response should be done after the practitioner has been joined by persons skilled in the necessary techniques.

The initial rapid assessment

Assessment involves determining what is needed, and how much. What is needed is decided by considering the principles mentioned above.

Consider the basics required for health

Clean water and sanitation
Each person requires a minimum of 15 litres/day; three for drinking (more in hot weather or with exertion), two for food preparation, five for personal hygiene, and four for cleaning clothes and food utensils. Drinking water need not be pure, as long as it is reasonably clear, free of toxic substances and fecal contamination, and has acceptable taste. Simple kits for testing water quality are widely available. Where water is compromised, you should consult with a water and sanitation engineer to reconstruct damaged systems or set up temporary new ones.

Food

Food aid is most often required after disasters of human origin and when people have been displaced from their usual food sources. After natural disasters, crops usually remain intact and people usually do not leave the area, so that large supplies of food are not required. An exception to this can be in cases of flooding.

When outside supplies of food are required the major considerations are adequate calories, adequate micronutrients, acceptability to the local population, and ease of preparation. To survive, a population requires an average of at least 2100 kcal/person/day. If a population is already malnourished, or the emergency lasts months, they will require more. Acceptability to the population refers to supplying foods that people are familiar with and will eat. Ease of preparation is an important factor: if foods require cooking then supplies of fuel (such as piped gas or firewood) must be available. Alternatively, cooked meals may be provided directly in the short term.

When food must be supplied a nutritional survey conducted by nutritional experts should be done as soon as possible to determine the correct food needs. Securing and transporting adequate supplies of food will require the expertise of a food logistician.

Shelter and clothing

People are best housed in their own homes, except if a disaster has rendered these structures unsafe. They should never be moved from their homes just to ease provision of assistance. If shelter must be provided, people should be housed in small groups, such as families or groups of families, to reduce general crowding and exposure to disease. In cold weather, attention to insulation and heating is necessary.

Additional clothing is rarely required as people already have clothes appropriate to their environment and manage to retain sufficient supplies. Exceptions may occur where a population is displaced from a hot to a cold area. However, facilities for washing clothes are more frequently required. Estimating and supplying shelter and clothing material needs fall under general logistics.

Health services

Adequate health care provides treatment for illness, reassurance to the population who will feel unsafe without it, and forms the basis of the health information system (see below). 'Adequate' means reasonable access to drugs, equipment, and infrastructure necessary to treat likely problems, as well as trained staff skilled in treating those problems with those facilities. This is important to remember in considering what type, if any, of outside medical staff are required. For example, an internist accustomed to Western illnesses and advanced diagnostic facilities is not considered adequate staff for a crisis in a tropical area with limited resources; a skilled local nurse is more likely to be more useful. Good 'access' means that people know about the services, how they are eligible for them, and do not have to travel so far, wait so long, or pay so much as to make them disinclined to use them. Setting up these services requires clinical, pharmaceutical, and medical supply personnel with emergency experience.

Medical personnel will also need to assess the potential for epidemics, and assess the need for vaccination. Keep in mind that epidemics cannot occur unless the causative organism is present. For example, cholera cannot occur in a community, no matter how crowded or how poor the sanitation, without the presence of *Vibrio cholerae*. Therefore epidemic risk assessment includes finding out about the previous disease patterns of both the area of the disaster and the affected population. Among disaster-affected populations exposed to exhaustion, malnutrition, and crowding, measles vaccination assumes prime importance, due to increased susceptibility, morbidity, and mortality under these conditions. Measles vaccination is recommended for children aged 6 months to 12 years. This is particularly important among populations for which measles vaccine coverage prior to the disaster was low. Coverage of other routine child vaccinations should be maintained, although not as urgently as the provision of measles vaccination.

For large-scale emergencies WHO provides a recommended list of drugs and materials, including quantities, to serve 10,000 people for 3 months. These materials are available in kit forms.[2]

Information

This is often neglected but is nevertheless a fundamental requirement of the disaster response. In unaccustomed circumstances people require new information on how to maintain their health. They also require information on what is happening and what is likely to happen. In the absence of information rumor will take over, causing insecurity and mistrust of those handling the emergency. Rumors may even force inappropriate diversion of resources to minor or non-existent problems, to appease the population. Therefore, a system of good communication between those assessing the situation and in charge, and the affected population, is vital. Any accessible means of transmitting information is appropriate, as long as it communicates directly with the population and not through a third party, to avoid distortion. Collaboration with local persons in designing the messages is important to ensure a style and approach which is understandable to the population. Methods can include radio and TV, pamphlets, posters, advice by health workers in the clinics, and even megaphones.

Consider the current and likely health threats, given local conditions

Current health problems

Describing population health should include measurement of crude mortality rates, causes of mortality, and the nature of health problems—their current incidence and severity (including case fatality rates) and potential for change. Rates are important to determining disease trends in the face of varying population size. Measuring rates requires both numerators (the frequency of events, such as illness or death) and denominators (an estimate of population size).

For the initial assessment, numerator information can be gathered by visiting the available treatment centres, talking with staff, and reviewing daily records of diagnoses and treatment. These records form the basis of the HIS, which should be established as part of the initial assessment. In most cases setting up the HIS requires developing case definitions for the important health problems and establishing treatment protocols to ensure sufficient medical supplies for treatment and prevention. Case definitions are required because laboratory facilities are usually not adequate to test all suspected cases of illness. Rather, the (usually limited) testing facilities are used to confirm the presence of specific illnesses among the population (particularly those with epidemic potential such as meningitis) by testing the first suspect cases, and to develop case definitions for these diseases once confirmed. These case definitions are then used to diagnose subsequent suspected cases.

If the affected population is spread over a wide are and transport is poor, an effort should also be made to visit areas far from the treatment centres to ask people about the problems affecting them. In these situations, rates calculated on the basis of the HIS are likely to be underestimates, since many people will not attend the health centres. However, by visiting outlying areas you should still be able to form a general idea of the main problems and trends.

Denominators can be difficult to calculate (see below). Although much less useful, proportional mortality ratios can be used if the denominator cannot be determined with any confidence.

All efforts should be made to identify the leaders among the population, to meet them early on, get their impressions of the main problems, and enlist their support for your efforts.

Another important aspect of current health and disease threat is the health knowledge and behaviour of the population. Failure to take precautions, such as washing hands, can render populations more susceptible to illness. Such behaviours are relatively more important when one is dealing with overcrowding, or with a specific health crisis like a single transmissible disease. Local knowledge and behaviour can be assessed by direct observation, and by interviews in which local people are asked how they prevent particular illnesses of concern, such as diarrhoea. Gaps in knowledge and behaviour form part of the information needs discussed previously.

General condition of the population

Talk with health workers and walk through the community. Observe and talk with people. The aim is to form an overall impression of the state of nutrition and available supplies, including clean water and food, cooking supplies and fuel, shelter and clothing, particularly in a cold environment:

- assess whether people appear to be getting enough supplies
- observe how people get water, to estimate the risk and potential for contamination
- ask how people are disposing of their feces
- estimate the adequacy of access to medical treatment, given the distance, available transport, cost, and degree of crowding of the clinics.

Condition of the environment

Assess the need for shelter in terms of the weather. Get a weather report. Observe the water sources and whether the water from these sources looks clean or turbid. Observe where people are defecating, the adequacy of available latrines, water drainage, and the likelihood that the water supply and feces will come in contact. If there is a sewerage system, investigate whether the system has been damaged, whether it is being attended to, and whether water treatment supplies are adequate.

If the area is known to harbor transmissible disease, then monitor for those diseases as part of the disease surveillance system (see below). Supplies needed to address these illnesses must be investigated and prepared by the health team and logisticians. As previously noted, remember that transmissible agents can only occur if the agent is present in the environment. Information on disease endemicity is usually available from local authorities, and from regional health organizations like the Pan-American Health Organization (PAHO).

Injuries and diseases augmented by crowding—such as any respiratory or gastrointestinal infections—will be more likely where populations have left their homes and are crowded into an unfamiliar environment.

Security issues

These may be both health problems in their own right, such as violence, or threats which preclude access to resources and affect behaviour. For example, people may be unable to go to a clinic or collect supplies if this exposes them to danger. Similarly health personnel may be unwilling to work or unable to do their jobs. Even limited health emergencies may engender violence, often through ill-feeling and rumor due to lack of information. Security can be assessed by talking with local people about how secure they feel. Addressing these issues requires close cooperation with the police or even the military.

Having assessed what is needed, assess how much must be provided. This depends on how much is required less how much is available, which comes down to the size of the population and local capacity.

Size of the affected or vulnerable population

This is one of the most important pieces of information about the population. Without this 'denominator' the amounts of resources required cannot be assessed. Moreover, rates cannot be calculated, making it impossible, in public health terms, to determine the size of a problem or trends by prevalence or incidence.

Early in an emergency rough estimates are acceptable, and can be based on pre-existing information, estimates of knowledgeable persons, or even, in the case of a mass displacement of people to an open area, 'eyeballing' from a high piece of ground. Later more sophisticated sampling and survey methods should be used by a demographer or epidemiologist, or even a count if possible.

Demography of the affected population

Usually some groups are more vulnerable to problems than others. In a limited crisis, such as a disease outbreak, this may be because of disease susceptibility, for example children are more susceptible to measles. In a full-scale disaster with crowding and limited resources, some groups are at a disadvantage in securing their needs. This is particularly true in developing countries and can include women, particularly if pregnant or lactating, children, especially those without adult protectors, elderly people, and people with disabilities. The size and location of these groups should be determined and particular attention given to meeting their needs.

Assessing capacity

In meeting needs the emphasis should be on reconstructing or supporting the system that met those needs before the emergency, rather than on creating a parallel system. Determine what that system was or is and who is in charge. Work with that person to identify what they need to meet the current crisis, and try to provide it. This is particularly true after a disaster, yet this simple principle is often ignored. Where a system has been damaged rather than simply overwhelmed, this does not mean reconstituting it the way it was, but rather providing those elements required to meet demand. For example, during an emergency you may not rebuild a destroyed hospital but instead provide tents, supplies, etc.

Compared with the creation of a new system, reconstruction:
- requires fewer outside resources
- uses locally appropriate resources, and so will be sustainable
- builds local capacity to address this emergency, other problems, and future emergencies
- provides employment
- uses people who know the local population best
- restores a sense of self-reliance.

Assessing local systems in detail requires persons skilled in that field, for example a sanitation engineer to assess sewerage or a health information specialist or epidemiologist to assess a health information system. As always, suitable local people with these skills are preferable to outsiders because these will be the people who will maintain these systems in the long term.

Surveillance

After the initial assessment, a surveillance system must be created to monitor health trends and detect incipient epidemics. In any displaced and crowded population, surveillance should include measles and the common serious diseases known to occur among the population and in the geographic area. These may include important epidemic diseases like cholera and other diarrhoeal diseases, dysentery, malaria, dengue fever, meningitis, hepatitis, typhoid and paratyphoid, typhus, and viral encephalitis.

Surveillance information must be provided to all involved, including the affected population and those in charge politically. It will provide the information to determine whether the response to the crisis is effective. The surveillance system must be capable of rapidly investigating and either confirming or debunking rumors.

Setting up surveillance will require consultation with the other organizations providing health assistance to agree on standard case definitions and reporting formats. Access to a laboratory will be required to confirm diagnoses, particularly in the early phases of an epidemic. The system should be under the direction of an epidemiologist.

Logistics

For all external supplies, consider:
- where to get them in sufficient quality and quantity
- how to pay for them
- how quickly they are needed
- available transportation methods for these requirements
- how the situation is likely to change.

All these considerations will require cooperation between an experienced logistician and local people familiar with local suppliers and markets.

Skills and knowledge

After a disaster, the following skills and knowledge are required:
- rapid assessment and survey skills
- clinical
- water and sanitation
- food and nutrition
- logistics
- familiarity with local language, culture, environment, and the affected population
- relationships with important local persons whose assistance and support will be needed
- sensitivity in dealing with the affected population
- ability to communicate ideas and problems well, and to write coherent and clear reports
- ability to deal with the media.

Personnel

These skills and knowledge translate into the following personnel:
- project director
- epidemiologist
- logistician
- local people familiar with local culture and language
- water and sanitation expert
- nutritionist
- clinical staff familiar with likely problems and resources.

Fallacies

In his book *The public health consequences of disasters*,[1] Eric Noji describes some of the important myths and realities about disasters collected by the Pan-American Health Organization. Awareness of these myths is useful in approaching emergency response:

1. Foreign medical volunteers are always needed.
2. Any kind of international assistance is urgently required.
3. Epidemics are inevitable after disasters.
4. Disasters bring out the worst in people.
5. Affected populations are too shocked and helpless to help themselves.
6. Disasters kill randomly.
7. Locating disaster victims in temporary settlements is the best shelter solution.
8. Food aid is always required after natural disasters.
9. Clothing is always needed.
10. Conditions return to normal after a few weeks.

All of these myths, except 4 and 10, have been dealt with previously in this chapter. Most workers would agree that disasters overwhelmingly bring out the positive side of human nature, and that community spirit is usually enhanced. Far from resolving quickly, the effects of most disasters last for years, or even decades. This is true even in developed countries, where increased debt and interruption in economic activity can create long-term financial burdens.

Conclusion

As a public health professional or team there is much you can do to help in a disaster. Effective disaster and crisis response is predicated on rapid assessment of the situation prior to initiating a response, and on focusing on the public health principles outlined in this chapter.

Further resources

Heymann DL (ed.) (2005). *Control of communicable diseases manual*. American Public Health Association, Washington, DC.

Hanquet G (ed.) (1997) *Refugee health: an approach to emergency situations*. Macmillan/Medecins Sans Frontieres, London.

Office for Foreign Disaster Assistance. *Field operations guide*. Available at: http://www.usaid.gov/our_work/humanitarian_assistance/disaster _assistance/resources/pdf/fog_v4.pdf (accessed 30 January 2006).

Perrin P (1966). *War and public health*. International Committee of the Red Cross, Geneva.

References

1 Noji E (ed.) (1997). *The public health consequences of disasters*. Oxford University Press, New York.
2 World Health Organization (1998). *The new emergency health kit*, WHO document WHO/DAP/98.10. World Health Organization, Geneva.

3.6 Assuring screening programmes

Angela Raffle, Alex Barratt, and J.A. Muir Gray

All screening programmes do harm, some do good as well.

UK National Screening Committee

Objectives

After reading this chapter, you will:
- understand why screening needs a programme not just a test
- recognize the biases that limit the validity of observational evidence
- be clearer about the public health tasks in screening
- understand that values and beliefs shape screening policy as much as evidence.

What screening is and is not—definitions

Screening is the testing of people who do not suspect they have a problem. It is done:
- to reduce risk of future ill-health (e.g. screen for raised blood pressure, intervene with drugs, reduce risk of stroke)
- to give information (e.g. screen pregnant woman, identify if an unborn baby has Down's syndrome, couple keeps baby but is forewarned).

Tests or inquiries once disease is symptomatic are not screening. They are for prompt recognition or for clinical management.

Screening involves a system not just a test

There are two ways of looking at a screening system. You can consider everything that must be in place to deliver a service. This helps you ensure that high-quality programmes are delivered to your population. The elements include:
- a register (see Chapter 2.7) for issuing invitations and reminders
- a system for checking that follow-up steps happen
- screening tests
- investigations

- interventions
- information and support for participants
- staff training
- policy-making
- coordination locally and nationally
- setting standards and ensuring they are met
- commissioning research to improve screening.

You can also consider the basics steps that a participant goes through. This looks like a flow diagram; it helps with understanding what screening does.

What screening does

You need to know the range, and likelihood, of different consequences in order to make decisions about policy. Individuals need this information so they can decide whether to participate. Whether a consequence is judged 'good' or 'bad' varies from person to person. The flow diagram in Figure 3.6.1 can help you map the consequences.

A screening test is not a diagnostic test. It is only like a sieve. It sorts large numbers of low-risk people into a group at higher risk, who then go on to a diagnostic phase, and those at lower risk (but not no risk).

The main consequences, using breast screening as an example, are listed below. The individual may:

- be reassured at the time of screening and not get the disease, i.e. have a normal mammogram and not develop breast cancer
- be reassured but get the disease, i.e. have a normal mammogram but subsequently be diagnosed with breast cancer
- have a life-impacting disease averted, i.e. screen-detected breast cancer whose treatment prevents death from breast cancer
- have an intervention but develop life-impacting disease, i.e. screen-detected breast cancer but still die of breast cancer despite intervention
- have an intervention with a possibility of adverse effects, for a symptomless phenomenon, i.e. screen-detected ductal carcinoma *in situ* (DCIS) that would have caused no problem
- have an intervention but with no extra benefit, with an equally good prognosis if diagnosed symptomatically, i.e. screen-detected low-grade breast cancer that would have been curable on symptomatic presentation
- have an abnormality of uncertain significance detected, leading to follow-up, surveillance, possible intervention, and uncertain benefit, i.e. mammographic changes leading to annual repeat mammography.

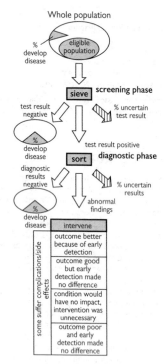

Figure 3.6.1 The screening process

Who is helped and who is harmed?

As a public health practitioner you will see that the people genuinely helped are those who, as a direct result of screen detection, avoid death or serious disease. The perception of most participants and clinicians can be very different. Almost everyone with a screen-detected abnormality feels thankful, and some clinicians believe they have cured all the people detected. This is the 'popularity paradox'. Over-detection is a major screening-related harm, yet it contributes to the popularity of screening through the illusion that large numbers of people are helped. A nurse in the UK cervical screening programme will see over 150 women with screen-detected abnormality for each one who has serious disease prevented.[1] For 10,000 men age 50, the number who would die of prostate cancer is 30, yet 4200 of them will have histologically confirmed prostate cancer if screened,[2] which leads to substantial harm from treatment-related deaths and side-effects such as incontinence and impotence.

Balancing harm, benefit, and affordability

There is always a trade-off between benefit, harm, and affordability. The numbers flowing into different parts of the system are influenced by:

- the acceptability and accessibility of screening, e.g. convenience, publicity, information
- the definition of the eligible group, e.g. changing the age range or frequency of testing
- changing the numbers of people defined positive or at high risk by the screening test, e.g. by more tests, by double or treble reading, or by changing the 'cut-offs' between low risk and high risk
- changing the number of positive or high-risk people diagnosed with the disease, e.g. multiple investigations or changing the cut-off value used to distinguish people with the disease from those who do not have it.

Measuring the impact of screening

Observational evidence can be highly misleading because of biases (see Chapter 2.3) that make outcome in screened people look good even if screening makes no difference.

Three key biases in screening

- *The healthy screenee effect.* People who come for screening tend to be healthier than those who do not.
- *Length time bias.* Screening is best at picking up long-lasting, slow-growing disease. This pulls good-prognosis cases into the observed group, whereas rapidly progressive, and therefore poor-prognosis, cases are detected less frequently by screening.
- *Lead time bias.* The survival time for people with screen-detected disease is longer simply because they are detected at an earlier point in the natural history of the disease.

Five sources of evidencce and information for evaluating screening in the population

Measures of test performance tell little about the impact on health of the whole programme so are not in this list.

- *Randomized controlled trials* (RCTs). People are recruited, then randomly assigned to receive screening or usual care. RCTs need to be large and last a long time but are less expensive than allowing unevaluated screening to develop. They are the only reliable source of evidence of benefit and harm.
- *Time trend studies.* These involve observation of trends in incidence and deaths once screening is in place. They are useful if properly conducted, and comparison with countries or regions without screening can help.
- *Case–control studies.* These compare past screening in people with the disease or who have died from the disease, and controls. Even with matching and validation of screening history they still consistently overestimate the effect of screening[3] because of confounding.
- *Modelling studies.* These make theoretical predictions about screening outcomes and examine the effect of varying frequency, age range, intervention threshold, etc. They are strongest if based on RCT evidence.

• *Pilot or demonstration projects.* These can solve practical issues. They are never reliable for assessing benefit and harm.

If more than one study of a particular method has been done, a systematic review of all the evidence should be prepared.

Presenting information about benefits and harms

Concern about rates of uptake has meant that benefits of screening have been emphasized more than harms. This slanted approach disregards the rights of autonomous adults to reach informed decisions and is no longer considered appropriate or ethical. Policy in the UK and elsewhere now requires that balanced information be available to people considering screening. Decision aids for presenting such information are starting to be developed.[4]

Practical tasks—implementing screening programmes

Starting a programme from scratch

It helps if you have:
• an agreed national policy and roll-out plan
• ring-fenced resources which can be spent only on screening
• training centres and demonstration sites
• consumer involvement
• reliable information technology.

Some of your challenges locally are:
• agreeing the boundary of the local programme—administrative and provider catchments seldom match
• getting cooperation from all organizations with a part to play
• communicating understanding of the programme to staff, participants, and the public.

Sorting out a mess

Haphazard testing often starts ahead of national policy. Converting this to a quality-assured equitable screening programme is difficult, but can be done. The major problems are:
• there is inconsistent training and practice but everyone thinks their way is right
• commercial, private practice, and research vested interests abound
• you meet resistance when you change from intense screening for a few to less intense for all.

Carrying on screening

Once a programme is up and running things will go wrong unless you keep an eye on it. Make sure there is:
• a nominated public health lead who knows the key players and understands the performance data
• a coordinating group meeting one to three times a year
• an annual report including a forward plan
• regular training/updating for all staff.

Quality assurance

Achieving quality depends on:
- system design and resources, e.g. staff training
- monitoring and readjustment, e.g. region-wide collation of annual performance data.

Quality is not solely about effectiveness. The seven components in Donabedian's definition of quality[5] include equity. Exclusive pursuit of effectiveness increases resource use irrespective of opportunity cost.

Here is an example of a quality assurance standard, taken from the programme to reduce risk of sight-threatening retinopathy in people with insulin-dependent diabetes:[6]
- *objective*—to take retinal photographs which must be of adequate quality
- *criteria*—the percentage of patients whose photographs are ungradeable for at least one eye, excluding eyes with cataracts
- *minimum standard* (all programmes must meet)—per cent ungradeable less than 10%
- *achievable standard* (current top quartile)—per cent ungradeable less than 5%.

Practical tasks—controlling unwanted screening

You need to be able to stop unwanted screening in order to protect the public from diversion of resources and direct harm. Unwanted screening arises because:
- new screening self-starts irrespective of evidence. Drivers include market forces, consumer pressure, clinician enthusiasm, and media pressure, usually with a complex and manipulative interrelationship between them;
- within existing programmes there is pressure to intensify irrespective of marginal cost–benefit . This is a response to inherent limitations (undetectable cases, cases outside the eligible group).

Key steps are to:
- understand why people want the screening—go and meet with and listen to clinicians, pressure groups, and campaigning journalists
- explicitly acknowledge the reasons why people want it—don't dismiss concerns or belittle their interpretation of evidence
- assemble and communicate evidence and information about the consequences the screening would really have, and about alternate ways of addressing the problem
- carefully introduce specific policy measures, such as refusing requests for tests.

Screening and the law

Out-of-court settlements are commonplace. In rare cases that are defended, the judgement may relate to standards you would expect from diagnosis, not screening. Judges are influenced by the fact that an expert witness finds abnormality in the test that the screener judged normal. This ignores:

- outcome bias—the witness knows the outcome for the subject, the screener does not
- context bias—the witness is an experienced doctor and has days to look at the sample, the screener is competent only at screening and had a few minutes.

Equipped with careful preparation and an expert lawyer who understands screening it is possible to successfully defend a service that meets recognized standards. We think it vital that health departments enable this to happen more often.

Making screening policy

Who makes policy decisions about screening?

Generally decisions are regional or national. They may relate to:

- state-funded provision of quality-assured national programmes (as in the UK)
- state reimbursement for approved screening, with provision by public and private providers (as in Australia)
- recommendations to consumers, who decide if they can afford a health policy that includes the screening (as in the USA).

What factors influence screening policy?

In theory you base your policy on evidence and resources. In practice values and beliefs have a profound influence. See the case study in Box 3.6.1.

Box 3.6.1 Case study

When the USA National Institutes of Health (NIH) recommended in January 1997 that evidence was insufficient to recommend screening mammography for all women in their forties the response was dramatic:

- At the news conference the panel was accused of condemning American women to death.
- The panel's chairman was summoned to a Senate subcommittee.
- The Senate voted 98 to 0 in favour of supporting mammography for this age group.
- The head of the NIH said he was shocked by the report and asked for the evidence to be looked at again

By March 1997 the panel had changed its recommendation and advised that women in their forties should get a screening mammogram every 1 to 2 years.

The *New England Journal of Medicine* published a review article[7] lamenting the lack of logic. But what the Senate was articulating were the values of American society. If mammography offers any potential for health gain how dare anyone recommend that the individual should not have it?

Many other societies take a collectivist approach and 'take it as read' that the rights of an individual to have any intervention that could be beneficial has to be balanced with the needs of others who require a share of the health-care resource.

The public health role is to present information for decision-making a clearly as we can, but the wise politician, who needs to survive the next election, may take a decision that matches public values and beliefs. In the UK, for example, we have an evidence-based national decision against introducing a prostate cancer screening programme, but the NHS provides prostate-specific antigen (PSA) testing for individual men. The strong belief in PSA testing among the public and politicians made it politically unacceptable to have an outright embargo.

The last word

Screening, like most other public health services, is at best a zero-gratitude business.

Further resources

Barratt A, Irwig I, Glasziou P et al. (1999). Users' guides to the medical literature XVII. How to use guidelines and recommendations about screening. *J Am Med Assoc*, **281**, 2029–34.

National Electronic Library for Health, Screening Specialist Library http://libraries.nelh.nhs.uk/ screening/ (accessed 20 September 2005).

Russell LB (1994). *Educated guesses, making policy decisions about screening tests*. University of California Press, Berkeley, CA.

References

1 Raffle AE, Alden B, Quinn M, Babb PJ, Brett MT (2003). Outcomes of screening to prevent cancer: analysis of cumulative incidence of cervical abnormality and modelling of cases and deaths prevented. *BMJ*, **326**, 901–4.

2 Frankel S, Davey Smith G, Donovan J, Neal D (2003). Screening for prostate cancer. *Lancet*, **361**, 1122–8.

3 Moss SM (1991). Case-control studies of screening. *Int J Epidemiol*, **20**, 1–6.

4 Barratt A, Trevena L, Davey HM, McCaffery K (2004). Use of decision aids to support informed choices about screening. *BMJ*, **329**, 507–10.

5 Donabedian A (2003). *An introduction to quality assurance in health care*. Oxford University Press, Oxford.

6 National screening programme for sight-threatening retinopathy. http://www.nscretinopathy.org.uk (accessed 30 January 2006).

7 Fletcher SW (1997). Whither scientific deliberation in health policy recommendation? Alice in the wonderland of breast-cancer screening. *New Engl J Med*, **336**, 1180–3.

3.7 The public health response to 'hard to reach' populations

Julia Carr, Don Matheson, and
David Tipene-Leach

Those who have most to gain from health improvement are often the
most difficult to reach.

Objectives

After reading this chapter you will:
- understand the relevance of historical, structural, and environmental
  influences creating so-called 'hard to reach' populations
- understand responses likely to be effective in improving the health of
  marginalized populations and which approaches are likely to
  perpetuate inequalities
- consider appropriate public health principles and frameworks when
  approaching an issue affecting marginalized populations.

Definition

When the health status of populations most affected by inequity and
alienation fails to improve despite the best efforts of conventional public
health approaches, these groups are deemed 'hard to reach'. The term is
generally applied to those marginalized by poverty, ethnicity, geography,
and different cultural or behavioural norms (e.g. intravenous drug use or
sexual orientation).

Why is this issue important?

By using terms such as 'hard to reach' dominant groups subtly reinforce a
political system that denies certain groups or individuals access to wealth,
opportunities, health care, and knowledge.[1] While the term 'hard to
reach' reflects historical reality (that many public health programmes have
had little impact on the populations with the lowest health status), it
implies that their poor health outcomes are somehow a problem of their
own making, a result of barriers erected between themselves and the

expertise that could 'deliver' better health. It is important to utilize language consistent with public health's commitment to social justice; language that speaks of reciprocity and interdependence to replace terms that reflect a 'deficit' model with terms that reflect health as a right.

The framework in which health is understood influences the actions taken. If we focus on the context of people's lives, on issues such as power, dominance, dispossession, paternalism, and racism and their implication for how diseases are created, distributed, and treated, this leads to a different approach from a framework that perceives health as a privilege or an individual responsibility.[2]

The belief that poor health is generally a result of 'unhealthy' choices leads to the 'educative' approaches seen so commonly. The belief behind the activity is that you can improve health by marketing a certain way of living. Extra attention and innovative methods to 'target' certain social groups focus on lifestyle 'choices'—diet, smoking and exercise.

Conceptualizing health as a right, and 'health for all' a collective re-sponsibility, leads to a different set of responses. The World Health Organization (WHO) model of health promotion of the early 1980s emerged from increasing recognition that health education and technical interventions in isolation from other measures would not result in the radical changes necessary to achieve improvements in health. In addition to technical interventions, there needed to be an emphasis on social justice, community participation, intersectoral action, and prevention if the health needs of the whole population were to be addressed. This was first articulated in the Alma Ata declaration of 1978, and picked up again in the Ottawa Charter.

Despite these statements from WHO, few health systems have managed to deliver on this agenda, with strong emphasis remaining on technical interventions, and education now taking the form of social marketing. The gap between the rhetoric and everyday activity of the health sector is a reality that remains a challenge for all public health practitioners.

What's the difference?

The Ottawa Charter emphasizes that health promotion works through concrete and effective community action in:

- setting priorities
- making decisions
- planning strategies and
- implementing them.

At the heart of this process is the empowerment of communities, their ownership and control of their own destinies. Endorsing this implies at the very least:

- acknowledging inequalities in power, ownership, and control, and vested interests in maintaining inequalities
- challenging professional control of health promotion and health service planning

• validating and supporting community health initiatives that are seeking to transform the distribution of power, ownership and control.[3]

What approach to a programme of work is suggested?

While there is no single method for putting the Ottawa Charter into action, a community development approach is consistent with the principles and has been tested in many environments. Community development as a public health practice has been defined as 'the process of organising and/or supporting community groups in identifying their health issues, planning and acting upon their strategies for social action/change and gaining increased self-reliance and decision making power as a result of their activities'.[4] There are many examples of such community development projects.[5]

What are the pitfalls of a community development approach?

Community empowerment challenges the concepts of expertise that are now dominant. It also runs counter to the structures and time frames for decision-making of most bureaucracies. It takes a long-term view of health gain and does not fit neatly with single-issue programmes, with contracts that tightly specify outputs or with an annual business cycle.

Given the difficulty of addressing disparities in health status between privileged and deprived groups, many health systems and public health practitioners retreat to a reductionist, problem-based approach. However, this limited view of the possibilities for practice is not ethically sound. Sustainable health improvement comes from addressing the structural root causes of ill-health, rather than a targeted narrowly defined intervention.[2]

On the other hand, there is evidence that certain interventions such as providing smoking cessation programmes to pregnant women or fluoridation of water supplies can indeed reduce inequalities in particular health outcomes.[6] Such improvements, however, are unlikely to be sustained, unless the intervention has been developed in partnership with the community, with shared decision-making, and the potential to follow local rather than imposed priorities.

One way to visualize a comprehensive framework for action, consistent with the Ottawa Charter, is the 'Reducing inequalities intervention framework' developed in New Zealand.[7] This does not preclude the important question about who defines what the problem is and whether the process of intervening is empowering or imposed. However, it does provide a schema for mapping interventions and a framework for discussing possibilities and priorities with communities, with colleagues, funders, and managers in health and other relevant sectors.

Being a New Zealand framework, there is specific reference to Maori and the Treaty of Waitangi. This part of the framework can be adapted in any country to recognize the special rights of indigenous peoples and historical influences on current health issues. It is the responsibility of public health agencies to contextualize any difficulties 'reaching' indigenous people and think about how indigenous people are resourced to design and lead interventions (Figure 3.7.1).

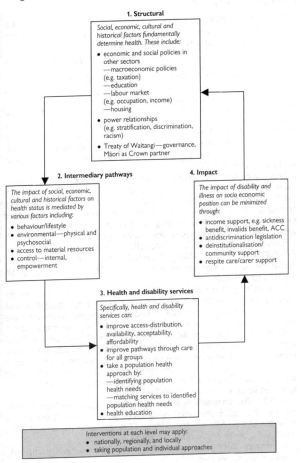

1. Structural

Social, economic, cultural and historical factors fundamentally determine health. These include:

- economic and social policies in other sectors
  —macroeconomic policies (e.g. taxation)
  —education
  —labour market (e.g. occupation, income)
  —housing
- power relationships (e.g. stratification, discrimination, racism)
- Treaty of Waitangi—governance, Māori as Crown partner

2. Intermediary pathways

The impact of social, economic, cultural and historical factors on health status is mediated by various factors including:

- behaviour/lifestyle
- environmental—physical and psychosocial
- access to material resources
- control—internal, empowerment

4. Impact

The impact of disability and illness on socio economic position can be minimized through:

- income support, e.g. sickness benefit, invalids benefit, ACC
- antidiscrimination legislation
- deinstitutionalisation/ community support
- respite care/carer support

3. Health and disability services

Specifically, health and disability services can:

- improve access-distribution, availability, acceptability, affordability
- improve pathways through care for all groups
- take a population health approach by:
  —identifying population health needs
  —matching services to identified population health needs
- health education

Interventions at each level may apply:
- nationally, regionally, and locally
- taking population and individual approaches

Figure 3.7.1. Intervention framework to improve health and reduce inequalitites

Examples of success and failure

Two striking examples of the effectiveness of different approaches are provided by steps taken to address sudden infant death syndrome (SIDS) in New Zealand and the approach adopted to control the spread of HIV/AIDS.

SIDS in New Zealand

> SIDS, by its tragically and uniquely quantifiable outcome, has provided an unprecedented opportunity to observe how Maori health outcomes are influenced by the strategic approach taken.
>
> David Tipene-Leach

In the early 1980s New Zealand had a higher rate of SIDS than comparable countries, with a particularly high rate among the indigenous Maori population. By 1991, there was published evidence that SIDS was a syndrome having multiple risk factors, with three significant 'modifiable' risk factors—prone sleeping position, lack of breastfeeding, and maternal cigarette smoking. Other significant risk factors like low socio-economic status, young motherhood, young maternal school leaving age, low birth weight, prematurity, and admission to neonatal intensive care were not postulated to be modifiable.[8]

This conceptual dichotomy led to the development in 1991 of a national SIDS prevention campaign comprising intensive publicity about the three risk factors. Subsequent SIDS prevention activities were based around a minimal intervention, risk reduction approach that provided simple health information, relying on individual change of behaviour without any form of personal or community support.

Between 1988 and 1992 national SIDS mortality fell by 48% (from 4.4/1000 live births to 2.3/1000). Maori SIDS rates were twice as high, and during the same period a more modest fall of 24% was observed (from 9.1/1000 to 6.9/1000).[9]

It seems that Maori mothers readily adopted the 'easy to do' prone sleeping position for their babies, although there is some contention that because of the high prevalence of bed sharing in this community, the prone sleeping position was a less significant risk. The impersonal 'educative' approach, however, did not foster a commitment among Maori women or communities to deal with the 'difficult to do' risk factor: cigarette smoking. In addition, there was no strategy and no specific funding to address this particular Maori health need. There was certainly no planning that allowed a Maori community-based consideration of the identified so-called 'non-modifiable' risk factors.

In 1994, after considerable advocacy by Maori public health professionals, the Maori SIDS prevention programme was launched, based on the provision of a support service to Maori SIDS families at the time of infant death and a health promotion programme that included:

- information sharing and consultation in Maori communities, particularly with influential women elders
- consistently utilizing Maori protocols

- promotional messages couched within a Maori world view
- development of resources for smoking cessation and breastfeeding promotion that Maori women 'owned'
- identification of disempowering factors in the lives of Maori mothers and work with communities for change
- attempts to induce structural change within maternal and child health care to provide accessible and acceptable services.

There has been no sudden drop in Maori SIDS to the low 0.4/1000 rate enjoyed by the non-Maori community in 2000. Indeed, a subsequent change of the official definition of Maori ethnicity in 1995 makes interpretation of decreasing rates since the start of the prevention programme very difficult. Suffice to say that since 1996 the Maori SIDS rates dropped from 4.6/1000 to 2.6/1000 by 2000. The Maori SIDS prevention programme continues to seek structural or political change in the New Zealand health environment that might ameliorate the Maori deprivation at the heart of the Maori SIDS phenomenon.

HIV/AIDS in New Zealand

Early in the AIDS campaign, it was recognised that the groups most 'at risk' from HIV/AIDS, men who have sex with men, sex workers and intravenous drug users, were engaging in activities that were all, at that time, illegal. This meant that conventional approaches to AIDS prevention were unlikely to be successful.

Warren Lindberg (personal communication, 2000)

The response of the gay community to HIV/AIDS in New Zealand illustrates many aspects of the Ottawa Charter in action. The AIDS campaign has been effective in limiting the spread of HIV/AIDS in gay men and extensive spread into other groups has not occurred.

The initial response to news of the AIDS epidemic was informal networking and counselling provision within the gay community itself. It is not possible to detail the complexity of the developments over the early 1980s, but key points are:

- recognition of the potential health problem came from within the group most 'at risk' and leadership came from within that community
- capacity building started early with significant mobilization of the gay community and organization building
- partnerships with key people in the health sector and influential people outside the gay community were developed to assist in meeting the demands of the corporate health sector and political environment
- affected communities gained representation at government advisory level—the original council included two people with HIV infection and representatives of gays, sex workers, intravenous drug users, and Maori and Pacific communities
- a multilevel approach was adopted.

In addition to publicity and promotion of safe sex practices, the AIDS prevention campaign included actions as diverse as:

- establishment of a needle exchange scheme
- a human rights campaign to include sexual orientation and HIV status in the Human Rights Commission Act

- the HERO project, a direct attempt (beginning with a dance party) to strengthen the gay community's identification with and involvement in the epidemic and raise the profile of the issues in the wider community.[10]

This multi-faceted, participatory strategy has been effective in limiting the spread of HIV in New Zealand.

Alternative approaches

Some of the most effective interventions may be at a structural or environmental level:

- Adolescent smoking may be decreased by legislation limiting retail practices, taxation policy and advertising bans.
- Fluoridation of water supplies to improve dental health is a classic 'environmental' approach.
- Road engineering changes in response to accidents is another.

With 'upstream' interventions, input from affected communities is still essential. Consultation and information sharing provide insights that might otherwise be missed and creates 'buy-in' to support the approach if it makes sense to the leaders in that community.

What are the competencies needed to achieve health gains in marginalized groups?

This chapter has attempted to illustrate that 'hard to reach' groups are a construct of a 'top-down' public health perspective that fails to acknowledge the historic, social, and economic forces that have denied certain sectors of society the choices available to others.

As public health workers, we can be part of the problem or part of the solution. Taking an issue by issue approach to population health without addressing disparities between population groups and supporting 'quick-fix' solutions without questioning the context in which health problems are generated contributes to the perpetuation of inequality. We can contribute by:

- legitimizing and promoting approaches that are rooted in community health action
- stimulating debate about the structural barriers to achieving health for all
- monitoring the gap between rhetoric and reality
- challenging the monopolization of health promotion by health professionals
- constantly raising and setting up mechanisms for participation by marginalized people in decision-making.[3]

A key role for public health professionals is to influence the distribution of health resources. There are a variety of mechanisms for matching resources to need both at a population level (through population-based funding formulae that include variables such as deprivation indices, ethnicity, etc.) or at provider level. Marginalized communities often express amusement at being labelled 'hard to reach' when, in their experience, they feel 'locked out' of meaningful participation in decisions about resource allocation.

How do decisions about existing or new resources (including funding, recruitment, 'pilots', research grants) reflect the needs of marginalized groups within your agency?

Partnerships

Formal planning or project partnership can be used to build constructive relationships with traditionally disempowered communities or to tackle particular issues. Partnerships inevitably raise issues of power and control.[11] It is helpful to be clear about the type of partnership you are intending. Shared expectations are a constructive starting point. Types of partnerships include:

- *Community action partnerships* in which the partnership forms to address a specific issue or pursue a specific opportunity.
- *Community organization partnerships* in which a set of organizations in a similar service sector agree to collaborate for mutually agreed goals.
- *Community development partnerships* in which a partnership attempts to increase participation by people and organizations in collaborative activities on multiple fronts or contribute to community assets and services in multiple areas.[12]

What are the key determinants of success in working with marginalized communities?

- Good analysis of the 'problem' and whose problem it is—this means having time to debate the issues before approaching a community.
- Open-ended meetings with communities to determine what their priorities are and how the public health perspective fits or does not fit with these.
- Development of partnership and sharing of knowledge and research.
- Participation and ownership by the community.
- Capacity building within the community and support for locally generated solutions—information, funding, training, people resources, evaluation tools.
- Ongoing communication in an atmosphere that supports critical analysis, honesty, and flexibility.

Although these points look self-evident, in practice it takes patience and a high level of commitment. The temptation is to submit to pressures to adopt faster methods.

Many communities have a legacy of mistrust based on experience of health agencies or state institutions and this has to be overcome. Failure of health services to meet immediate curative needs may lead to skepticism about initiatives in other areas. Securing better links between health services and a marginalized community can help future work. Primary health care, where this is accessible and has a strong community connection, can be an effective partner for engagement on population health issues. Youth health services with high levels of youth participation and broad networks are one example but there are many other 'niche' services with credibility and long-term relationships with marginalized groups.

Lay knowledge is often not valued by health professionals. These attitudes are readily internalized by communities themselves so that they may appear reluctant to make suggestions or take leadership roles initially. Such challenges are common and it is wise to identify mentors or experienced people from the communities involved to provide supervision and support.

How will you know when or if you are successful?

The community will be owning and driving a strategy and will have the information, confidence, and resources to implement it. The institutions of power will feel challenged and those within them may be making themselves hard to reach.

Further resources

Sanders D, Carver R (1985). *The struggle for health: medicine and the politics of underdevelopment.* Macmillan Education, Oxford.

References

1 LeBlanc R (1997). Definitions of oppression. *Nurs Inq*, **4**, 257–61.
2 Adams L, Pintus S (1994). A challenge to prevailing theory and practice. *Crit Public Health*, **5**, 17–29.
3 Farrant W (1994). Addressing the contradictions: health promotion and community health action in the United Kingdom. *Crit Public Health*, **5**, 5–17.
4 Labonte R (1993). Community development and partnerships. *Can J Public Health*, **84**, 237–40.
5 Voyle J, Simmons D (1999). Community development through partnership: promoting health in an urban indigenous community in New Zealand. *Soc Sci Med*, **49**, 1035–50.
6 Arblaster L, Lambert M, Entwistle V et al. (1996). A systematic review of the effectiveness of health service interventions aimed at reducing inequalities in health. *J Health Serv Res Policy*, **1**, 93–103.
7 New Zealand Ministry of Health (2002). *Reducing inequalities intervention framework in reducing inequalities in health.* Ministry of Health, Wellington.
8 Mitchell E, Scragg R, Stewart A et al. (1991). Results from the first year of the New Zealand Cot Death Study. *NZ Med J*, **104**, 71–6.

9 New Zealand Health Information Service. Ministry of Health, Wellington, 1993.
10 Lindberg W, McMorland J (1996). From grassroots to business suits: the gay community response to AIDS. In: Davis P (ed.) *Intimate details and vital statistics. Aids, sexuality and the social order in New Zealand*, pp.102–20. Auckland University Press, Auckland.
11 Popay J, Williams G (1998). Partnership in health: beyond the rhetoric. *J Epidemiol Commun Health*, **52**, 410–11.
12 Gamm L (1998). Advancing community health through community health partnerships. *J Healthc Manag*, **43**, 51–67.

3.8 Genetics in disease prevention

Ron Zimmern and Alison Stewart

Objectives

By the end of this chapter you should:
- understand the principal associations between genetics and disease
- be able to discuss their implications for the prevention and treatment of disease
- be aware of the public health strategy for achieving effective translation of genome-based knowledge and technologies into benefits for population health.

Introduction

All human variation and all disease processes are, with few exceptions, determined both by environmental and by genetic factors. These often interact, and individuals with a particular set of genes may either be more or less likely, if exposed, to be at risk of developing a particular disease. These effects may be measured by showing that the relative risk of exposure to the environmental factor is significantly greater (or lesser) for the subgroup with the abnormal gene than the risk in those without.

Genetic variation exists in all populations. Clinically relevant polymorphisms, as these genetic changes are known, will be identified and associated with different diseases over the next few decades. While classical epidemiology presupposes that the genetic features of populations under study are homogeneous, and compares groups of people exposed to with those not exposed to the environmental factor under study, the new genetic paradigm will seek to compare two genetically different populations under similar environmental conditions for disease outcomes.

It is the appreciation that gene and environment interact that will allow greater effectiveness and efficiency in the use of preventive and public health strategies. Preventive strategies which rely on an understanding of genetics are not about genetic manipulation, nor do they embrace eugenic processes such as attempts to prevent couples from exercising their own choice to reproduce, nor put pressure on them to abort affected fetuses. Public health interventions will continue to be directed at environmental or behavioural factors, but greater genetic knowledge will allow interventions to be focused on those subgroups of individuals whose genes make them particularly susceptible, rather than on the general population.

The extent to which genes contribute to disease forms a continuum, but it is useful in practice to distinguish three types of situation. First, where the presence of the genetic abnormality accurately predicts whether the individual has or will develop the disease. These diseases are usually caused by a single gene defect and transmitted from generation to generation in a Mendelian fashion, and are conventionally referred to as genetic diseases (Box 3.8.1). Second where, in complex common disorders such as breast or colorectal cancer, Alzheimer's disease or hypertension, rare genetic subgroups which behave in a similar way to conventional genetic diseases can be defined (Box 3.8.2). Third, where the presence of known genetic abnormalities increases the risk of disease in an individual, but does not predict it with any degree of certainty. These changes, often referred to as polymorphisms, are found much more frequently than the gene mutations in conventional genetic disorders, but their penetrance, or the probability of developing the disease in question given the presence of the abnormality, will be much less. Knowledge of the status of genetic polymorphisms will be akin to knowledge about biological markers such as cholesterol levels or blood pressure in individuals. They define a risk, or probability, of developing (in this example) heart disease or stroke, but whether the disease actually develops or not will be the consequence of unidentified multitudinous interactions between the genetic abnormality in question, other genes, and environmental factors.

Box 3.8.1 Examples of conventional genetic diseases

- Duchenne muscular dystrophy
- Cystic fibrosis
- Huntington's disease
- Phenylketonuria
- Adult polycystic disease of the kidney
- Neurofibromatosis

Box 3.8.2 Examples of rare, genetic subtypes of common complex diseases

- Familial polyposis coli
- Hereditary non-polyposis colorectal cancer (HNPCC)
- *BRCA1* and *BRCA2* in breast cancer
- *PSEN1* and *PSEN2* in Alzheimer's disease

Public health skills

Public health practitioners should appreciate the growing influence of knowledge about the genetic contribution to disease, and the potential of using that knowledge for more efficient and effective disease prevention. 'Prevention' in this context encompasses primary, secondary, and tertiary interventions that respectively bring about environmental or lifestyle change, early detection and intervention, and the prevention of complications and deterioration.

If involved in research the public health practitioner should:
- be aware of the genetic heterogeneity of population groups
- question proposals for large-scale epidemiological studies which do not measure relevant genetic factors
- think not just in terms of the greater risk of disease posed by an environmental exposure but also of the genetic factors that might determine why some exposed individuals develop the disease and others do not.

In relation to conventional genetic diseases the public health practitioner should appreciate that:
- their total burden is quite considerable, even though each disorder is comparatively rare
- many service issues remain to be addressed, including those of service quality, of antenatal and neonatal screening programmes, of the development and evaluation of new genetic tests, and of commissioning and funding.

In relation to the rare, genetic subtypes of common complex diseases, the public health practitioner should:
- seek to establish a minimum level of knowledge about the clinical epidemiology of the genetic determinant (Box 3.8.3)
- be aware of familial aggregation in these subgroups, and the importance of family history as a means of assessing risk
- question the utility of making the genetic diagnosis and ask if there are proxy criteria, such as clinical manifestations, that might lead to the genetic diagnosis without the use of molecular genetic tests
- be aware not only of the relative risk of possessing the genetic defect, but its absolute risk over a defined period of time
- question how individual patients in these subgroups should be managed in order to prevent the disease from developing or to improve survival (Box 3.8.4).

Box 3.8.3 Epidemiological characteristics of a genetic determinant

- The gene and its chromosomal location
- Its known allelic variants
- Their prevalence in the population at risk
- The relative and attributable risk of the variant in the diseased population
- The positive predictive value, or penetrance, of the variant
- The population-attributable risk and population-attributable fraction
- The potential for molecular genetic tests
- The sensitivity, specificity, and predictive value of the test
- The nature of any know interaction with other genes or with environmental exposures

Box 3.8.4 Intervention strategies for prevention or
reducing mortality

- Early detection: colonoscopy for colorectal cancer (HNPCC),
  mammography for breast cancer (*BRCA1* and *BRCA2*)
- Chemoprophylaxis: tamoxifen for breast cancer (*BRCA1* and *BRCA2*),
  statins for familial hypercholesterolemia (FH)
- Removal of target organs: oophorectomy for ovarian cancer
  (*BRCA1*), mastectomy for breast cancer (*BRCA1* and *BRCA2*)

In relation to low-penetrance susceptibility genetic influences on common complex disorders the public health practitioner should:
- realize that the examples of susceptibility genes of clinical relevance
  are as yet few, but that in the coming decades these are likely to
  multiply
- endorse the principle that, in most situations, the use of genetic tests
  for detection and diagnosis should be avoided where there are no
  effective preventive or therapeutic interventions
- appreciate that there are significant ethical implications in relation to
  privacy and confidentiality of genetic information
- assess the positive predictive value of carrying a genetic polymorphism,
  appreciating that it is identical to the concept of penetrance as used by
  geneticists
- understand that there will also be many examples where the
  possession of the abnormal gene protects against disease in the
  context of specific environmental factors
- be aware that much research will be needed before these concepts
  result in interventions which will change significantly the incidence and
  prevalence of common diseases
- understand that high-penetrance genes are rarely implicated in
  complex, common disorders and are unlikely to contribute to a
  significant population risk, but will be of crucial importance to the
  individual and the family
- be aware that the more common polymorphisms, responsible for
  susceptibility, have yet to be identified, but that their penetrance and
  population prevalence will together determine the population-
  attributable fraction, an indicator of the significance of their
  contribution to the burden of disease.
In general the public health practitioner should:
- be sensitive to the ethical, legal, and social issues surrounding all
  aspects of genetics and genetic testing
- be aware of the importance of taking into account the views of the
  public, which, if mishandled, may hinder the translation of basic
  research into technologies that will benefit the patient in the clinic and
  the public health.

A strategy for public health action

The volume of new knowledge and technologies stemming from genetic and genomic research is such that a concerted effort is needed to ensure the effective translation of these scientific advances into benefits for population health. International consensus has been achieved on a public health strategy for achieving this goal.

This strategy recognizes the central importance of an explicit process of knowledge integration, both within and between disciplines. The knowledge and methodologies of the population sciences must be applied to the outputs of genomic research in order to validate proposed relationships between genetic variants, environmental factors, and disease risk in different populations. Input from the humanities and social sciences is needed to assess the ethical and social acceptability of new genome-based treatments or preventive interventions.

This integrated and interdisciplinary knowledge base is used to underpin four core sets of activities: informing public policy, developing new health services (both preventive and clinical), communication and stakeholder engagement, and education and training of health professionals. The method of working to accomplish these activities relies on the well-established cycle of public health practice: analysis–strategy–action–evaluation.

A new initiative, GRAPH *Int* (Genome-based Research And Population Health International) has been established to promote this strategy for public health action in the genomics era. GRAPH *Int* is an international collaboration that facilitates the responsible and effective integration of genome-based knowledge and technologies into public policies, programmes and services for improving the health of populations. Its goals are to provide an international forum for dialogue and collaboration, to promote relevant research, to support the development of an integrated knowledge base, to promote education and training, to encourage communication and engagement with the public and other stakeholders, and to inform public policy.

Practitioners of public health must contribute to this endeavour, remaining aware of the growing importance of our understanding of genetic mechanisms in disease, and of the potential to utilize the new genetic knowledge for the benefit of both individuals and society.

Further resources

Burke W, Zimmern R (2004). Ensuring the appropriate use of genetic tests. *Nat Rev Genet*, **5**, 955–9.

Coughlin SJ (1999). The intersection of genetics, public health and preventive medicine. *Am J Prev Med*, **16**, 89–90.

Haga SB, Khoury MJ, Burke W (2003). Genomic profiling to promote a healthy lifestyle: not ready for prime time. *Nat Genet*, **34**, 347–50.

Halliday JL, Collins VR, Aitken MA, Richards MPM, Olsson CA (2004). Genetics and public health—evolution, or revolution? *J Epidemiol Commun Health*, **58**, 894–9.

Khoury MJ, Little J, Burke W (2004). *Human genome epidemiology*. Oxford University Press, Oxford.

Khoury MJ, Thomson E (eds) (2000). *Genetics and public health in the 21st century.* Oxford University Press, Oxford.

Khoury MJ, Yang Q, Gwinn M, Little J, Dana Flanders W (2004). An epidemiologic assessment of genomic profiling for measuring susceptibility to common diseases and targeting interventions. *Genet Med,* **6**, 38–47.

Zimmern R, Cook C (2000). *Genetics and health: policy issues for genetic science and their implications for health and health services.* The Stationery Office, London.

Zimmern RL (1999). Genetics. In: Griffiths S, Hunter DJ (eds) *Perspectives in public health,* pp. 131–40. Radcliffe Medical Press, Oxford.

3.9 The practice of public health in primary care

Steve Gillam

The central importance of primary care for public health has long been acknowledged. In 1978 at Alma Ata, primary health care was declared to be the key to delivering 'health for all' by the year 2000.

Objectives

After reading this chapter you should be able to:
- understand why effective systems of primary care are integral to delivering public health objectives
- know those public health interventions that primary care professionals provide
- define those elements of primary care that need strengthening in order to deliver public health objectives.

Definitions

Primary health care 'based on practical, scientifically sound and socially acceptable methods and technology made universally accessible through people's full participation and at a cost that the community and country can afford' was carefully distinguished from primary medical care.[1] The social and political goals of this epoch-making declaration, acknowledging as it did the social and economic determinants of health, were subsequently diluted. So-called 'selective primary health care' and packages of low-cost interventions such as GOBI-FFF (growth monitoring, oral rehydration, breastfeeding, immunization; female education, family spacing, food supplements) in some respects distorted the spirit of Alma Ata.[2] Nevertheless a central justification for universal primary care is ethical: the public health preoccupation with equity.

Primary care is often defined in terms of 'four Cs': it is continuous, comprehensive, the point of first contact, and coordinates other care. This coordinating function underlines a second set of arguments in support of primary care concerning efficiency and cost-effectiveness. International comparisons of the extent to which health systems are oriented to primary care suggest that those countries with more generalist family doctors with registered lists acting as gatekeepers are more likely to deliver better health outcomes, lower costs, and greater public satisfaction.[3] The association between constrained health spending and the presence of gatekeepers is complex; the latter indeed could be a consequence rather than cause of the former.[4] The World Health Organization (WHO) continues to extol the central place of primary care in delivering the millennium development goals.[4]

Bridging the divide

Primary care professionals and public health specialists improve health by different means:

- general practitioners concentrate on personal, continuing health care
- public health physicians focus on the population through changes in the environment, society, and health service provision.[5]

At the heart of the relationship between general practice and public health is an ethical conflict between individual and collective freedom.[6,7] The utilitarian values underpinning population-oriented care are at odds with the individualistic nature of the traditional doctor–patient relationship. For primary care professionals, the roles of carer, advocate, and enabler may overlap and conflict with one another.[8]

Clinical generalists develops a unique understanding of the personal and social determinants of their patients' health.[9] However, traditional primary care based on the perspective of the clinician exposed exclusively to individual patients presenting for care has evident limitations. Knowledge about the distribution of health problems in the community cannot be derived from experience in the practice alone, for most episodes of ill-health do not lead to a medical consultation. An understanding of how disease presents is not obtainable without a population focus. Doctors overestimate their role in the provision of care, although primary health care is not synonymous with medical general practice and is provided by a range of other health personnel. Finally, professional knowledge about disease does not necessarily reflect people's illness experiences and needs to be supplemented with the insights of the community.

Several international trends in the delivery of health services are facilitating community-oriented approaches to primary care. Public health competencies, especially as they relate to the management of chronic disease, are of increasing importance to the 21st century primary care workforce.[10] More training is now taking place in community settings. An emphasis on more effective and more efficient health care will entrench community-oriented approaches if they prevent disease and encourage more discriminating use of medical technologies. In many countries, a 'secondary to primary shift' is relocating specialist care closer to patients. Primary health care teams have always been pivotally placed to combine high-risk and population approaches to disease prevention.[11]

How does primary care deliver public health?

With the decline in infectious diseases and ageing of the population, an increasing proportion of the workload in general practice deals with the consequences of chronic disease. This has required the development of new services and changing systems of care. Many diseases, such as diabetes, that were once the exclusive preserve of hospital specialists are now managed by teams in the community.[12] If the 1970s saw the birth of a 'new public health', the first years of the millennium have seen the emergence of a 'new primary care' in the UK (Box 3.9.1). How each of these five elements contributes to public health is considered below.

Box 3.9.1 Elements of today's primary care

- Self-care
- First contact care
- Management of chronic disease
- Health promotion in primary care
- Primary care management

Self-care

Less than one in ten ailments experienced are brought into contact with the formal system of health care. Most are self-managed using whatever knowledge and support is available to the sufferer. Increasingly, many patients are more knowledgeable than their doctors about the management of their chronic disease. Nevertheless, they sometimes need help in making sense of the surfeit of information available. The computer screen threatens the personal nature of the consultation but new tools are changing clinicians from being repositories of facts to being managers of knowledge.[13] Some clinicians are nervous of giving patients better information, and not all patients want it. However, most people want to be in charge of decisions about their health—for the default approach to be empowerment rather than paternalism. Giving patients more knowledge or a consultation style that facilitates shared decision-making improves not only patient satisfaction but also clinical outcomes.[14] Indeed, as people gain access to information about risk, a higher proportion may choose not to accept the offer of screening or treatment.[15]

First contact care

If the bulk of first contact care is provided by friends and relatives, the next port of call has traditionally been general practice. However, there is an increasing plurality of routes through which primary care can be obtained (Figure 3.9.1), including telephone helplines and community pharmacies. Experience in many countries has suggested that multiple access points with poorly coordinated record-keeping may result in fragmented care.[16] Questions over the cost efficiency of these services remain. Nevertheless, they have exposed the limitations of conventional medically orientated general practice in providing basic care for populations who have not, for reasons of culture or convenience, gained satisfactory access to primary care in the past.

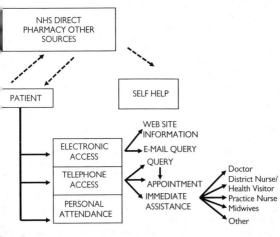

Figure 3.9.1 Routes of access into primary care in England.

Management of chronic disease

Numerous studies attest to the variable quality of care provided to people with chronic diseases. The new GP contract in the UK provides financial incentives for practices to enhance the quality of their care in 10 specific areas (Box 3.9.2). Much infrastructural investment is required to develop registers and call–recall systems, but the benefits in terms of public health are potentially significant. Much routine disease monitoring is undertaken by practice nurses with extended training. Disease management is becoming more complicated as pharmaceutical advances allow more care to be shifted from secondary to primary care. There is growing interest once more in North American techniques of managed care—risk stratification, targeting the heaviest consumers of care, and utilization review—but little clear-cut evidence to guide policymakers.[17]

Box 3.9.2 Ten chronic diseases

- Coronary heart disease
- Stroke
- Hypertension
- Hypothyroidism
- Diabetes
- Mental health problems
- Chronic obstructive pulmonary disease
- Asthma
- Epilepsy
- Cancer

Health promotion in primary care

General practitioners have always understood the importance of social factors such as housing, employment, and education as influences on their patients' health. The registered list, which defines the practice population, provides the basis for effective health promotion programmes in primary care in the UK. Preventive activities within primary care can be divided into individual, organizational, and community interventions.[18–20] Individual interventions take place between health professionals and patients, often classified into primary, secondary, and tertiary prevention (Box 3.9.3).

The public health approach to screening focuses on maximizing participation in screening rather than on informed participation. For example, current recommendations for the primary prevention of coronary heart disease in groups at high risk depend on screening through primary care and provision of risk-related advice or treatment. However, we lack evidence for the cost-effectiveness of multiple risk factor interventions delivered through primary care.[21] Presenting the uncertainties associated with the assessment and reduction of cardiovascular risk has the potential to be more cost-effective than screening conducted in a traditional public health paradigm if it results in participants who are more motivated to reduce their risks.[22]

Organizational interventions are concerned with improving the management of care and access to services for disadvantaged groups. Such interventions may take place at the level of the practice or the whole health system. An example of the former might be changes to make cervical screening more accessible to certain ethnic groups by providing information in different languages and increasing the availability of female health professionals. More wide-ranging organizational changes could include the provision of nurse-led primary health care to address previously unmet needs in deprived, under-doctored locations.[23]

Box 3.9.3 Primary, secondary, and tertiary prevention

Primary prevention
- Health education and behavioural change, e.g. dietary, smoking cessation, exercise
- Immunization, for an ever-increasing range of infections
- Welfare benefits advice
- Community development

Secondary prevention
- Detection and management of ischemic heart disease
- Screening, e.g. for cervical cancer, breast cancer, and colon cancer

Tertiary prevention
- Management of chronic disease, e.g. diabetes mellitus

The third category of interventions is community-wide. For example, in their roles as employers, users of resources, procurers, producers of waste, deployers, and vendors of land, primary care professionals and organizations have opportunities to enhance community health.[24] Community development has a stronger pedigree in developing countries

Every year 530,000 women die from maternal causes, 4 million infants die in the neonatal period, and a similar number are stillborn. If the millennium development goals to reduce maternal and child mortality are to be achieved, public health programmes need to reach the poorest house-holds. Most maternal and neonatal deaths take place at home, beyond the reach of health facilities. Evidence is growing that primary care strate-gies centred on community-based interventions are effective in reducing maternal and neonatal deaths in countries with high mortality rates, even if institutional approaches are necessary to reduce them further.[25] Randomized controlled trials of the community effectiveness of such interventions are urgently required.

Primary care management

New styles of public management with their emphasis on targets and objec-tive-setting have permeated all parts of the health service. One important consequence of the growth of large practice-based teams has been the differentiation of administrative functions. Increasingly, primary care teams need to accept responsibility for auditing the health status of their patients, publicizing the results, monitoring and controling environmentally deter-mined disease, auditing the effectiveness of preventative programmes, and evaluating the effect of medical interventions. Public health specialists still have an important role in supporting these functions.

What challenges should public health practitioners address?

What kind of primary care?

The difficulty of transposing health systems across international bounda-ries is universally acknowledged. Care at the level of the community within any system reflects different histories and cultural contexts. No single model of primary health care will be universally applicable. For example, community-oriented primary care (COPC) seeks to integrate public health practice by delivering primary care to defined communities on the basis of its assessed health needs.[26] COPC remains a powerful, enduring concept but its protagonists have made little mark beyond developing countries. In part, this reflects the lack of financial incentives within hospital-oriented health systems.

How should the public and patients be involved?

There is a fundamental difference between health care that is multisec-toral, preventive, participatory, and decentralized and low-cost (low-quality) curative treatment aimed at the poorest and most marginalized segments of the population, particularly if that care is provided through programmes that are parallel to the rest of the health-care system without active participation of the full population. Julian Tudor Hart, an eloquent exponent of COPC in the Welsh mining village where he practiced, has argued for the need to look in a new way at the relationship between doctors and patients as 'co-producers of health' and develop alliances between health workers and the public in defence of health.[27]

What information systems are needed?

The creation of a single, longitudinal electronic patient record should create a powerful new means of monitoring and improving care. An easily accessible, portable record ought to increase the involvement of users in their own management.

How should services be evaluated?

Assessing the health impact at the level of the organization or individual health worker is challenging. Even large UK general practices serve populations that are usually too small to compare health outcomes such as all-cause or disease-specific mortality rates. The focus is on intermediate outcomes: changes in established markers of quality care. The Quality and Outcomes Framework provides an example of an evidence-based approach to measuring (and rewarding) improvements in the management of common chronic diseases. Public health practitioners will be familiar with the measurement challenges listed in Box 3.9.4.

> **Box 3.9.4 Factors complicating the assessment of primary care**
>
> - Small denominators and the play of chance
> - 'Street lamp effect'— focusing on what is measured (paid for), ignoring the penumbra
> - Measuring the easily measurable but unimportant…
> - while ignoring the difficult to measure (e.g. communication skills, continuity of care)

How can equity be ensured?

One well-attested form of differential access to care is the so-called 'inverse prevention' effect whereby communities most at risk of ill-health tend to experience the least satisfactory access to the full range of preventive services.[28] Access may be affected in more material ways, e.g. through the provision of aids for wheelchair users or translated materials for people for whom English is not their first language. User charges for primary care have been repeatedly shown to deter those most likely to benefit from preventive activities.[29] Ethnic monitoring can allow disease management activities to be analyzed in terms of their impact on different practice subpopulations.

What continuing professional development is needed?

Primary care like public health is a multidisciplinary endeavour. At present, labor is being divided in new ways between many different health workers. A new cadre of primary care nurses is taking responsibility for minor illness management, triage, and routine care of common chronic diseases. The particular skills of others such as community pharmacists are being recognized. Beyond strengthening appraisal and revalidation mechanisms within different disciplines, there lies the challenge of ensuring that professional development activities are congruent and coordinated across teams.

How can effectiveness be maximized?

The dearth of evidence in support of many preventive interventions highlights the need for further research. Reasons for the failure to implement best practice go beyond the quality of the research, and accumulating further technical evidence may not be the most useful response. Barriers to implementation include a consistent failure to address the opportunity costs of new or different activities in primary care. For example, increasing the public health role of primary care means doing less of something else. Related to this is a failure to address adequately, and with all relevant stakeholders, the question of the role of primary care. This is not a technical agenda but one of achieving shared values as a starting point for any changes in professional roles.

Table 3.9.1 Public health and primary care practitioners—core competencies contrasted

Public health practitioners	Primary care practitioners
Care for populations	Care for individuals on practice lists
Use of environmental, social, organizational, and legislative interventions	Use of predominantly medical and technical interventions
Prevention through the organized efforts of society	Care of the sick as their prime function with the consultation as central
Application of public health sciences (e.g. epidemiology/medical statistics)	Application of broad clinical training and knowledge about local patterns of disease
Skills in health services research and report and policy writing	Skills in clinical management and communicating with individuals
Analysis of information on populations and their health in large areas	Analysis of detailed practice/disease registers and information on individuals
Use of networks that are administrative: health and social care authorities, voluntary organizations	Use of networks that are less bureaucratic: frontline health and social care providers, other primary care teams

Conclusions

Health systems are in constant flux, and everywhere the generalist seems to be under threat. What were once seen as strengths of general practice or family medicine are now regarded as liabilities—the registered list is seen as restricting choice, gate-keeping can be seen as rationing. Accordingly there has been a move to increase access points and choice. Public health practitioners should, however, be mindful of the law of unintended consequences. For example, one result of increasing access points may be discontinuous, poorly coordinated services for those most in need. Paying practitioners by results may create disincentives to practice where care is already weakest.

Fragmented primary care will yield poorer public health. But public health practitioners who understand the complementary nature of these disciplines (Table 3.9.1) will mobilize the resources of primary care more effectively.

References

1 World Health Organization (1978). *Primary health care.* Report of the International Conference on Primary Health Care, Alma-Ata, USSR, 6–12 September 1978. World Health Organization, Geneva.

2 Tejada de Rivero D (2003). Alma-Ata revisited. *Perspect Health*, **8**, 1–6.

3 Starfield B (1994). Is primary care essential? *Lancet*, **344**, 1129–33.

4 Forrest C (2003). Primary care in the United States. Primary care gatekeeping and referrals: effective filter or failed experiment? *BMJ*, **326**, 692–5.

5 Bhopal RJ (1995). Public health medicine and primary health care: convergent, divergent, or parallel paths? *J Epidemiol Commun Health*, **49**, 113–16.

6 Pratt J (1995). *Practitioners and practices. A conflict of values?* Radcliffe Medical Press, Oxford.

7 Fitzpatrick M (2001). *The tyranny of health—doctors and the regulation of lifestyle.* Routledge, London.

8 Gillam S, Meads G (2001). *Modernisation and the future of general practice.* King's Fund, London.

9 Heath I (1995). *The mystery of general practice*, pp. 5–14. Nuffield Provincial Hospitals Trust, London.

10 World Health Organization (2005). *Preparing a workforce for the 21st century: the challenge of chronic conditions.* World Health Organization, Geneva. Available at http://www.who.int/chronic_conditions/resources/workforce_report.pdf (accessed 24 January 2006).

11 Rose G (1992). *The strategy of preventive medicine.* Oxford University Press, Oxford.

12 Moore G (2000). *Managing to do better. General practice for the twenty-first century.* Office of Health Economics, London.

13 Muir Gray JA (1999). Post-modern medicine. *Lancet*, **354**, 1550–2.

14 Florin D, Coulter A (2001). Partnership in the primary care consultation. In: Gillam S, Brooks F (eds.) *New beginnings—towards patient and public involvement in primary health care.* King's Fund, London.

15 Barry MJ, Fowler FJ Jr, Mulley AG Jr, Henderson JV Jr, Wennberg JE (1995). Patient reactions to a programme designed to facilitate patient participation in treatment decisions for benign prostatic hyperplasia. *Med Care*, **33**(8), 771–82.

16 Jones M (2000). Walk-in primary care centres: lessons from Canada. *BMJ*, **321**, 928–31.

17 Gillam S (2004). What can we learn about quality of care from US health maintenance organisations? *Qual Primary Care*, **12**, 3–4.

18 Ebrahim S, Davey Smith G (2001). Multiple risk factor interventions for primary prevention of coronary heart disease (Cochrane review). In: The Cochrane library, issue 1. Update Software, Oxford.

19 Hulscher MEJL, Wensing M, van der Weijden T, Grol R (2001). Interventions to implement prevention in primary care (Cochrane review). In: The Cochrane library, Issue 1. Update Software, Oxford.

20 Ashenden R, Silagy C, Weller D (1997). A systematic review of the effectiveness of promoting lifestyle change in general practice. *Fam Pract*, **14**(2), 160–75.

21 Rouse A, Adab P (2001). Is population coronary heart disease risk screening justified? A discussion of the national service framework for coronary heart disease (standard 4). *Br J Gen Pract*, **51**, 834–7.

22 Kinmonth A-L, Marteau T (2002). Screening for cardiovascular risk: public health imperative or matter for individual informed choice? *BMJ*, **325**, 78–80.

23 Lewis R, Gillam S (eds) (1999). *Transforming primary care. Personal medical services in* the new NHS. King's Fund, London.

24 Coote A (ed) (2002). *Claiming the health dividend.* King's Fund, London.

25 Costello A, Osrin D, Manandhar D (2004). Reducing maternal and neonatal mortality in the poorest communities. *BMJ*, **329**, 1166–8.

26 Mullan F, Epstein L (2002). Community-oriented primary care: new relevance in a changing world. *Am J Public Health*, **92**, 1748–55.

27 Tudor Hart J (1988). *A new kind of doctor.* Merlin Press, London.

28 *Independent inquiry into inequalities in health.* (The Acheson report.) (1998). The Stationery Office, London.

29 NHS Centre for Reviews and Dissemination (2000). *Evidence from systematic reviews of the research relevant to implementing the 'wider public health' agenda.* NHS Centre for Reviews and Dissemination, University of York, York.

3.10 Public health in poorer countries

Nicholas Banatvala and Jenny Amery

More than a quarter of the developing world's people still live in poverty as measured by the human poverty index (a composite measure including life expectancy, basic education, and access to public and private resources).[1] Around 2.5 billion people live on less than $2 a day (40% of the world's population) and 1 billion live on less than $1 a day.[1] This chapter looks at the broader determinants of health and the links to other sectors.

Objectives

After reading this chapter you will be able to understand the major public health issues among the poor populations of the world and the approaches used to tackle them.

This chapter is based on the approach of the UK Government's Department for International Development, drawing extensively from its policy papers.[2,3]

Why is this an important public health issue?

Not only is health a long recognized human right, but improving health is associated with a decrease in poverty by securing better livelihoods. This is so at both a micro (family) level—less time caring for the sick means more time to earn and learn—and at a macro level—less sickness leads to regional and national economic growth.

Communicable diseases are the most important reason for the existence of the 'poor–rich' gap (world's poorest 20% to richest 20%) accounting for 77% of deaths and 79% of disability-adjusted life years (DALYs). WHO estimates that in 2015 in low-income countries, the burden of disease (DALYs) and death rates will be slightly higher for chronic diseases (including smoking-related disorders) than for communicable, maternal, and nutritional disorders combined.[4] The prevention of chronic diseases in low and middle income countries is now a priority. Heart disease, diabetes, and cancers are increasingly affecting poor people in developing countries. The costs of treating them are high and contribute to household poverty.

There is huge variation in health not only between the poor and the rich globally but also within developing countries:

- The poorest 20% of the world's population are 10 times more likely to die before they are aged 14 years than the richest 20%, and the greatest burden of ill-health is in sub-Saharan Africa.[1]
- If all children in developing counties had the same life chances, 11 million fewer children would die each year.[3]
- In Guinea there is a 10-fold variation in the percentage of richest and poorest fifths benefiting from public subsidy for health.[5]

There have been a number of attempts to quantify the costs of essential health care. The Commission for Macroeconomics and Health[6] estimated that a minimum of $34 per person per year is needed to introduce a set of essential health interventions. Currently many developing countries spend less than $10 per person per year and these funds are often not distributed equitably within countries.[6]

What are the approaches to subdividing a programme of work around this issue into defined tasks?

To tackle this massive agenda clear targets are required to provide milestones against which progress towards the goal of eliminating poverty can be measured. These are based on recent UN Conventions and Resolutions. The Millennium Development Goals (MDGs) and their targets are given in the section 'key determinants of success' below. MDGs will only be successful if there is the political will to address international development in both poorer and richer countries.

Objectives for eliminating poverty

Four primary objectives can be considered when poverty elimination is the objective in poorer countries:

1. policies and actions which promote sustainable livelihoods (pro-poor policies, development of efficient and well-regulated markets, access of poor people to land, resources, and markets, prevention and resolution of conflicts)
2. better opportunities for poor people to get health, education, water, and sanitation services[7]
3. empowerment of women[1,8]
4. protection and better management of the natural and physical environment (sustainable management of physical and natural resources, efficient use of productive capacity, protection of the global environment).

What are the tasks needed to address these objectives and key areas?

The four key areas for *health gain* are:
- infant and child mortality
- maternal mortality
- reproductive health
- HIV, TB, malaria, and other communicable diseases.

HIV remains a continual threat to global development and, in some areas, is overturning many decades of development investment. The epidemic is affecting both rich and poor countries economically, socially, politically, and culturally. More recently, poorer countries have had access to increased resources to tackle HIV and AIDS.

In order to achieve these objectives, there are key areas where intervention is likely to be more effective (most of which relate to a primary aim of elimination of poverty):
- the support of local and self-sustaining economic growth
- water and food
- education
- essential health care
- population growth
- income and employment opportunities
- good governance, elimination of corruption, and the rule of law
- gender inequalities
- rights of the child
- disasters and emergencies (see Chapter 3.5).

There are four key responses that, taken together and vigorously pursued at national and international levels, would impact on the health and wealth of poor populations (Table 3.10.1).

Table 3.10.1 Response and action to improve the health of the poor

Priority response	Specific priorities	Examples of actions
Addressing the priority problems of the poorest billion, strengthening access to care, services, and products	Making pregnancy safer and improving reproductive and sexual services	Developing appropriate local policies and strategies, empowering communities, improving access to essential obstetric care including abortion services, promoting availability of contraceptives, generating school-based programmes
	Reducing child mortality and improving child health	Introducing programmes for the integrated management of childhood illnesses (e.g. immunization, malaria, diarrhoea, and acute respiratory illness management) access to safe water and sanitation, female education
	Controlling communicable diseases	Controlling malaria, tuberculosis, HIV/AIDS. Eradication of polio, onchocerciasis, and lymphatic filariasis. Responding to emerging infections (e.g. SARS)
	Preventing injuries and non-communicable diseases	WHO Tobacco-Free Initiative. Understanding the impact of mental illness[9]
Investment in strong, efficient, and effective health systems (public, private and informal)	Supporting coherent systems rather than fracturing effort	Developing institutional and financially sustainable health systems, promotion of intersectoral actions towards health improvement, utilizing public subsidies to assure equal access to health service for equal need
Creating conducive social, political, and physical environments that enable poor people		Increasing safe shelters, road and vehicle safety. Minimizing environmental hazards, violence, pollution, and waste
A more effective global response to HIV/AIDS	Raising the profile	Advocacy at local national and international levels
	Enabling environment for HIV prevention and control	Improving gender equity, programmes to reduce stigma and discrimination
	Caring for people living with HIV/AIDS	Improving access of poor to HIV care and support
	Improving knowledge and technology	Vaccine and microbiocide development, understanding social and behavioural issues such as risk behaviour

What is the best way to work?

No one single player is able to transfer the above policies into action. Those involved in developing strategies to implement international policy need to work in four ways.

Work in partnership

Partnerships with poor countries can involve private and voluntary sectors, the research community, multilateral development organizations, and donors. To avoid the burden of multiple initiatives and projects, donors increasingly work with governments and other stakeholders in poor countries in a sector-wide approach so that all efforts are focused on agreed priorities. Examples of public-private partnerships include: the Global Fund to Fight AIDS, TB, and Malaria; the Global Alliance for Vaccines and Immunisation; and Roll-Back Malaria. Many of the programmes developed by international non-governmental organizations (NGOs) have focused on generating programmes sustained by host government, private organizations, or local NGOs.

Use both multilateral and bilateral initiatives effectively

Examples of this include strengthening the technical and operational arms of UN agencies such as WHO and UNICEF and working directly on projects with governments and other partners in poor countries. The World Bank, Regional Development Banks, and the International Monetary Fund (IMF) are key partners for development work.

Ensuring local ownership of initiatives

Ensure local ownership of initiatives, local capacity development, and where an evidence base exists base activities on this. The sustainable livelihoods approaches encourage a holistic view rather than just focusing on a few factors (e.g. economic issues, communicable disease, food security). The principles of sustainable livelihoods are that activities should be people- centred, responsive and participatory, multilevel, conducted in partnership, sustainable, and dynamic.[10]

Match political commitment with funding and debt relief

2005 was crucial for garnering political support. There were initiatives such as the G8 summit, Live 8, the Commission for Africa and the UN Millennium Review Summit. These have resulted in faster and deeper debt relief, more money for development, and commitment from poor countries to use aid better.

How can the risk of failure be reduced?

The agenda above is more likely to succeed if a number of fundamental principles are adhered to. Success is unlikely where there is failure to:
- address the causes rather than just the symptoms of ill-health
- remove barriers that prevent the poor accessing services
- assure standards, accountability, and responsiveness to health service users

- strengthen the state in policy-making, regulation, and providing services
- encourage the private sector to deliver appropriate services to poor people
- recognize that the UN system needs support in order to provide the necessary leadership for health
- fully committing to achieving the MDGs.

Nine fallacies

International public health policy is as prone to dogma as any area of domestic public health.

Fallacy 1: Models concentrating on one particular discipline are most effective in tackling the public health problems in developing countries

Approaches to international health have changed over time with bio-medical, economic, and institutional approaches each promulgated at varying times. The present consensus is that poverty reduction should be at the core of international health policy and addressed through a range of different disciplines.

Fallacy 2: Either vertical or horizontal public health programmes are always better

Vertical programmes have been successful in areas such as immunization and useful in introducing new concepts (e.g. directly observed therapy, short course for tuberculosis (DOTS)). In the longer term, however, sustainable services need health systems that integrate into national health systems rather than focusing on a few specific interventions and services.

Fallacy 3: The cost of action and attaining the MDGs cannot be met

The targets are not easy but can be met through international cooperation (the harnessing of private and public sectors, global alliances including governments, NGOs, and philanthropists), increased funding for programme activity as well as R&D, and employing principles of sustainable livelihoods.

Fallacy 4: Models of health-care delivery developed in Western settings can be effectively transferred to other situations

Enthusiasm for health sector reform based on new management trends in Europe (decentralization, managerial autonomy, contracting, and internal market mechanisms) has been dampened by a realization that reforms must be closely tailored to local circumstances.

Fallacy 5: Cost-recovery systems are an effective approach to providing long-term delivery of health services

Cost-recovery systems (self-sustaining systems financed by the local community) have rapidly fallen out of favour with concern about consequences for equity, with poorer patients excluded and subsidies benefiting the non-poor. In any event, revenue yields have often been minimal.

Fallacy 6: In developing countries there is no place for anything other than publically funded and run services

The private sector is to be encouraged and valued in areas of service delivery, support of health systems, research and development, and as a policy-maker and donor. Indeed in some of the most desperate countries such as Afghanistan, private health care will form a greater component of overall health delivery than government-funded health care. The private sector cannot therefore be ignored.

Fallacy 7: There are too many players in international health with policies muddled through the competing agendas of UN agencies, NGOs, and others

While there has been a proliferation in agencies responding to global health needs over the last 20 or so years, the challenge is to coordinate these actors. Compared with the number of agencies in developed countries the number of agencies in development projects in resource-poor countries is often small. It is fair to say, however, that high-profile relief events (e.g. Rwanda 1994, Kosovo, 1999) often result in a number of competing agencies searching for financial and media opportunities. Governments and other institutional donors have a responsibility to distribute funds to agencies with proven track records in the field of work and geographic region.

Fallacy 8: The real threat to development is globalization

Globalization is far from detrimental—there are plenty of opportunities, if harnessed appropriately, that come from a global community: economic, trade agreements and a international response to debt relief, communication and rapid transfer of information, maximizing flows of finance and capital, and investment, competition and the private sector.

Fallacy 9: Funding development activities is more effective than the funding of relief

Disaster preparedness and prevention are an essential component of development assistance. Disasters, natural and of human origin, including war, are more common in poor countries. The 'relief–development continuum' (cycles of relief and development) with agencies cooperating in different areas of expertise and 'developmental relief' (development models being used in chronic relief efforts often seen in complex emergencies) are both increasingly accepted approaches.

Examples of successes, failures, and lessons learnt

Readers interested in specific geographic or sector initiatives are best referred to either a health database search or are advised to contact donors and implementers in these areas (see Chapter 4.9). Almost all donors and implementing agencies will produce annual reports which often identify recent programmes. Examples include those produced by the bilateral agencies (e.g. DFID), World Bank, WHO, and NGOs. These are widely available on the Internet.

What are the most valued criteria for measuring success?

The MDGs are the measures of success. There are 8 MDGs and 18 targets relating to poverty, human development, environmental sustainability, and partnership working (Box 3.10.1).

Box 3.10.1 Four of the Eight Millennium Development Goals (MDGs) and associated targets

Goal 1: Eradicate extreme poverty and hunger
- Halve, between 1990 and 2015, the proportion of people whose income is less than $1 a day
- Halve, between 1990 and 2015, the proportion of people who suffer from hunger

Goal 4: Reduce child mortality
- Reduce by $2/3$, between 1990 and 2015, the under-five mortality rate.

Goal 5: Reduce maternal mortality
- Reduce by ¾, between 1990 and 2015, the maternal mortality rate

Goal 6: Combat HIV/AIDS, malaria and other diseases
- Have halted by 2015 and begun to reverse the spread of HIV/AIDS
- Have halted by 2015 and begun to reverse the incidence of malaria and other major diseases

How will we know if we have been successful?

Forty-eight indicators measure the progress of the 8 MDGs. These were reviewed at the 2005 Millenium Summit. Developing countries and UN agencies collect data to track their poverty reduction strategies. It is important that the development community supports improved data collection.

Acknowledgement

The authors are based at the UK Department for International Development (DFID). Views expressed are not necessarily those of the DFID.

Further resources
Department for International Development (UK). http://www.dfid.gov.uk/ (accessed 29 June 2005).

MDG links:

The MDGs. http://www.un.org/millenniumgoals/ (accessed 22 December 2005).

The 2005 MDG Report. http://unstats.un.org/unsd/mi/pdf/MDG%20Book.pdf (accessed 24 July 2006).

Médecins sans Frontières. http://www.msf.org/ (accessed 29 June 2005).

Oxfam UK. http://www.oxfam.org.uk/ (accessed 29 June 2005).

United Nations Development Programme. http://www.undp.org/ (accessed 29 June 2005) (see also Human Development Reports http://hdr.undp.org/ (accessed 29 June 2005)).

World Bank Group. World Development Reports. http://econ.worldbank.org/wdr/ (accessed 29 June 2005).

World Health Organization. http://www.who.int/en/ (accessed 29 June 2005).

Wroe M, Doney, M (2004). *The rough guide to a better world.* http://www.dfid.gov.uk/pubs/files/rough-guide/better-world.pdf (accessed 21 December 2005).

References

1 United Nations Development Programme (1997). *Human development report 2005: International cooperation at a crossroads—aid, trade, and security in an unequal world.* Oxford University Press, Oxford.

2 Department for International Development (1997). *Eliminating world poverty: a challenge for the 21st century.* HMSO, London.

3 Department for International Development (1999). *International development strategy, better health for poor people: target strategy paper* (consultation document). Department for International Development, London.

4 Strong K, Mathers C, Leeder S, Beaglehole R (2005). Preventing chronic diseases: how many lives can we save? *Lancet*, **266**, 1578–82.

5 United Nations Development Programme (2000). *Human development report 2000.* Oxford University Press, Oxford.

6 The Commission on Macroeconomics and Health (2001). *Macroeconomics and health: investing in health for economic development.* WHO, Geneva. Available at: http://www.cmhealth.org (accessed 20 may 2006)

7 World Bank (2004). *Making services work for poor people.* World Development Report, The World Bank, Washington, DC.

8 Department for International Development (2000). *Poverty eradication and the empowerment of women.* Department for International Development, London.

9 Summerfield D (2000). Conflict and health: war and mental health: a brief overview *BMJ*, **321**, 232–5.

10 Livelihoods Connect. *Creating sustainable livelihood to eliminate poverty.* Available at: http://www.livelihoods.org/ (accessed 29 June 2005).

Part 4

Making policy

Introduction

According to the *Oxford English Dictionary*, policy is 'a course of action or principle adopted or proposed by a government, party, individual, etc., or any course of action adopted as advantageous or expedient'. In this part we consider approaches to influencing policy at various levels. We start with an overall framework at government level, move 'down' to the micro-environment of the public health practitioner's own team or organization, and up again to the international arena. At each of these levels policies can have powerful effects on health, and public health practitioners need to be armed with the skills and insights necessary to safeguard and improve health by improving policy. Without the coherent framework that good policy offers, the actions of organizations can become fragmented and different initiatives can easily undermine each other.

Science and logic may help to identify public health problems and potential solutions, but emotion and power relationships determine whether anything is done about them. Turning analysis into policy requires a range of specific skills. In Chapter 4.1 Anderson and Hussey provide a guide to understanding policy and policy-making at governmental level, with examples from the USA and UK. The US political system at federal level is characterized by a relatively weak executive branch of government, often in policy-making competition with different groupings in Congress. With expensive and frequent elections, interest groups, the media, and public opinion are openly acknowledged as central to the policy-making agenda. Anderson and Hussey also emphasize how much policy can change during the implementation process, and how important evaluation of the end results of policy is to making further progress.

Public policy-making is, of course, 'political' and seldom driven by public health evidence. To achieve healthy public policy, Nutbeam (Chapter 4.2) suggests that timing and the relevance of evidence to policy are crucial. Evidence needs to support a practical programme of actions, but much public health research can be criticized for providing elaborate descriptions of problems rather than possible solutions. Nutbeam also points to the need for public servants who are equipped with critical appraisal skills to use evidence in policy development.

One of the most powerful instruments of policy is law, and Gostin (Chapter 4.3) points out that most of the 10 great public health achievements in the 20th century in the USA were realized in part through law reform or litigation. In many countries, public health law is so old that it reflects historical rather than modern realities. Gostin identifies seven models of legal intervention, from tax and spend, through changing the built and socio-economic environment, to regulation in one form or another. The increasing use of legal instruments in international public health is also explored.

Most policies require local action to be successful, and Koh (Chapter 4.4) addresses the development of policy at the local organizational level.

In addition to external influences, including government policy, many internal factors come into play. Relationships, both organizational and personal, are often crucial and values, habits, pressure groups, and pragmatics all shape action, often more strongly than evidence.

Good policy is designed for successful implementation, and one approach to focusing attention on the progress of policy implementation is to set targets. In Chapters 4.5 and 4.6, Battersby and Jenkin et al. provide overviews and examples, highlighting the methodological skills, local knowledge, communication skills, and understanding of the process of government that is needed to translate centrally set targets into local action.

Much of the public discourse on health issues is abbreviated by the media into simplified notions of what each issue is really about. To public health practitioners, gun control is about saving lives, but to the gun lobby, opposing gun control is about limiting the power of the state and preserving the freedom of the individual. As Chapman points out (Chapter 4.7), such framing of issues in the media is critical to how they are dealt with, and understanding this process, and responding directly to an adverse framing of an issue, can be critical to influencing policy and politicians.

While local action is often essential, developments at levels above the nation state are increasingly important in a world with a globalizing economy. All too often, influencing supranational institutions is perceived as extremely difficult, and public health organizations have some way to go to catch up with international commerce in being effective at these levels. For many readers, the European Union is perceived as just such a distant supranational body, but McKee (Chapter 4.8) has provided an overview of institutions and relevant responsibilities. He points out that there are several entry points for public health advocates.

Global companies and global organizations can now have major influences on 'local' public health problems, and practitioners must now both think and act locally and globally, as Lang and Caraher explain in Chapter 4.9. They point to the rich public health tradition of global action, including the eradication of smallpox. Appreciating the full international picture behind modern public health challenges can help us focus on causes rather than symptoms.

In an age in which people are encouraged to think of themselves as individuals and consumers, the collective institutions of government and business influence ever more aspects of health. These institutions are themselves held together by links at every level from the local to the global. In the global village, public opinion and the media can be critical to getting public health issues onto the policy agenda, and keeping them there. In analyzing the opportunities to influence policy at the various levels, our contributors have returned to the same major themes: the importance of recognizing the task of influencing policy as a specific challenge of public health practice, as a challenge that requires an understanding of the policy-making process and the adoption of specific attitudes and skills. At most levels above the local, getting public health issues into the mainstream of public debate and influencing public opinion is seen as a major challenge to public health practitioners.

DM

4.1 Influencing government policy: a framework

Gerard Anderson and
Peter Sotir Hussey

Introduction

Influencing government policy requires an understanding of what public policy is, how public policy is developed, and what levers are available to influence the policy-making process. While countries differ in the details of their policy-making arrangements, the broad themes set out below are relevant in most Western democracies.

The national policy process is important to public health professionals because much of the funding of public health activities comes from national sources. In addition, policy makers establish regulations, administer programmes, and influence many activities relevant to the health of their populations.

Objectives

This chapter will help you:
- understand the nature and steps involved in the policy process
- understand the available levers and skills needed to influence policy.

Public policy and the policy-making process

Box 4.1.1

Public policy is what the government chooses to do or not to do about perceived problems, and **policy-making** is the process by which the government decides what will be done about perceived problems.

Political scientists have summarized the policy-making process in four stages, as shown in Figure 4.1.1.

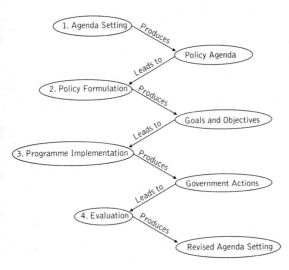

Fig. 4.1.1 The policy making progress

Agenda setting

Agenda setting occurs when policy makers identify a problem and develop broad goals to address it. In health care, examples of potential problems include rising health expenditures, an unexpected increase in infant mortality, or an unexpected increase in the prevalence of a disease (e.g. AIDS). Health-care issues such as these must compete against other policy issues (such as national defence) to become national priorities, and specific health issues must compete for attention with other health issues. Policy makers can focus on only a limited number of problems at any one time.

A considerable amount of effort is required to place an issue at the forefront of the policy-making agenda. The following factors can help place an issue on the political agenda:
• the greater the number of people who perceive that the problem exists
• the greater the perceived severity of the problem
• the more immediate and novel the problem is perceived to be
• the more likely it is to affect an individual personally.

Public interest alone does not guarantee that an issue will be placed on the public agenda, however. To be placed on the public agenda, policy makers must *consider the issue within the purview of government action* and deserving of public attention. Many policy issues that have long-term consequences or only minor consequences for an individual are unlikely to become one of the two or three most pressing health-care policy concerns. Unfortunately, many traditional public health issues fall into this category.

Many different approaches are used to place an issue at the forefront of the public policy agenda. One method is to try to influence public opinion. This can be done through the media (see Chapter 4.7), personal appeals by public officials and celebrities, advertising to raise public awareness, and many other approaches. Public opinion has its greatest impact on government decision-making when people feel strongly about clear-cut preferences. Although government policy tends to coincide with public opinion, this may not always be the case, particularly when a well-organized interest group intervenes or public apathy is evident. Special interests can have a particularly important role in technical issues or issues that involve only a few people.

In health care, there is an unequal distribution of information; doctors and other health professionals have specialized knowledge. As a result, individuals must often place their trust in health-care professionals. These health-care professionals who hold and control information have considerable leverage over public opinion.

The *media* can have a strong influence on public opinion. Interest groups, politicians, and others are all trying to influence how the media frame issues and report the news. Political leaders and news people are often mutually dependent. Politicians rely on the media to provide them with information and to convey their messages to the public. The media, in turn, rely heavily on public officials for information they use as the basis for their reporting (see Chapters 4.7 and 7.4).

Box 4.1.2

As a major source of political information, *the media* help shape the public's perception of reality. These perceptions, in turn, constitute a basis for the public's political activity.

Interest groups attempt to influence the agenda-setting process to foster their own particular interests. They provide information and financial resources, mobilize voters, and use other techniques to influence the agenda-setting process. The influence of individual interest groups depends on such factors as the nature of the group's membership, its financial and leadership resources, its prestige and status, and government structure, rules, and procedures.

Political parties serve as linkages or intermediaries between the citizens and their government. 'A Party is a body of men united, for promoting by their endeavours the national interest, upon some particular principle in which they are all agreed.' (Edmund Burke, 1770).

Officially and unofficially political parties have a major role in agenda setting. Party leaders have major roles in determining the agenda of the party in advance of an election and then balancing the conflicting priorities of various interest groups between elections.

Policy formulation

Once it is widely recognized that a problem requires government attention, policy makers must develop a broad policy agenda into specific policy options. Policy formulation involves developing alternative proposals and then collecting, analyzing, and communicating the information necessary to assess the alternatives and begin to persuade people to support one proposal or another. Policy formulation involves compromising and bargaining in order to satisfy various interests and build a coalition of support.

Next, specific policies have to be adopted. Known by political scientists as legitimization, government policy must conform to the public's perception of the proper way to do things. Frequently, previous policies of the government are good predictors of future policies, since people tend to prefer incremental changes over major changes.

Box 4.1.3

In the United States, the benefits of *incrementalism* were most apparent in the Clinton administration's proposal to reform the health-care system. Introduced as a fundamental reform with numerous provisions that altered nearly every aspect of the health-care financing and delivery system, it alienated nearly every constituency on some issue. Following its defeat, the Clinton administration emphasized incremental health-care reform. Hillary Rodham Clinton, one of the major architects of the proposal, later declared herself a member of the 'school of smaller steps' in the area of health-care policy (*Washington Post*, 9 July 1999, p. A4). In the 2004 presidential election campaign, both George Bush and John Kerry proposed only incremental reforms to the health-care system.

In policy formulation, information is assembled, arguments developed, and alternatives shaped towards winning the approval of policy makers. Sometimes this is accomplished through rational analyses of the pros and cons of various alternatives. At other times, policy formulation is a more fluid process that is highly influenced by which participants are involved at specific times and unexpected opportunities to affect change that arise suddenly.

Once the policy has been formulated, statements of government policies and programmes are promulgated. These can be laws, regulations, decisions on resource allocation, court decisions, etc. Equally important, the government can decide that the best alternative is inaction.

Implementation

Few government policies are self-implementing. Once a policy has been formulated and promulgated, it must be *implemented*. Even the most brilliantly crafted law, executive order, or court decision will fail to meet the designer's goals if it is poorly implemented.

Implementation involves three activities directed towards putting a policy into effect. The three activities required for implementation are:

- interpretation
- organization
- application.

Interpretation requires the translation of the programmatic language into acceptable and feasible administrative directives. Administrators need to discern the policy-makers' intent and fill in the details about how the goals will be accomplished. In many instances, legislation or court decisions are purposefully left somewhat vague to allow administrators wide latitude to respond to changing conditions and conflicting demands.

An example of how implementation can affect the outcome is the 1990 reform of the UK National Health Service. This reform attempted to create an 'internal market' by separating the purchasing and provision of health services. The Secretary of State for Health held the ultimate responsibility for the implementation of the policy, and a wide range of political and bureaucratic actors had a role in decision-making. The parties affected by restructuring appealed to political officials to delay or cancel implementation of elements of the reform that ran counter to their interests. In the end, the desired effects of the 'internal market' were tempered by government control.

Organization requires the establishment of administrative units and methods necessary to put a programme into effect. Resources (money, buildings, staff, equipment) are required to implement a programme. Implementers may choose to organize a new policy through an existing agency, or create a new agency to administer the policy.

Application requires the services to be routinely administered. As described here, interpretation, organization, and application may appear to be rather dull and routine. However, the manner in which policies are implemented can dramatically affect the success or failure of a programme.

The process of interpreting policy and designing the organization to implement it is often termed *strategic planning* (see Chapter 5.2), which focuses on setting out the broad approaches and methods for achieving the policy gaols in practice, over the medium term. Strategy must then be followed by *operational planning and management*, in the application phase of the implementation.

Policy evaluation

The last step is *evaluation*. The policy is evaluated to determine how well it was implemented, whether its goals were achieved, and what impact was achieved. The results of these assessments can result in a programme being maintained, expanded, changed, or even terminated. The general public, providers, and special interests provide input into the evaluation process. Sometimes the input is anecdotal, while in other instances it is a formal evaluation of a government programme. After the formal or informal evaluation, the policy-making process is repeated, beginning with the formulation of a revised policy agenda based upon the evaluation.

Policy makers do not always encourage evaluation of their policies. For example, Tony Blair's Labour government has not (at the time of writing) sponsored an evaluation of his NHS plan to increase health-care funding.

What are the key determinants of success and what are the pitfalls?

As described above, incremental change is easier to bring about than major change. Two pre-conditions for major health-care policy change are:

- the timing of policy initiatives, which is critical. Many factors, including those outside the health-care arena, can add up to create a 'window of opportunity' for new policy
- the factors favouring policy change, which must be sufficient to overcome or temper resistance by the affected parties.

There are potential pitfalls at every point in the policy-making process. The more 'clearance points' that must be passed, the greater the chance that a policy will be derailed. Different political systems have different 'clearance points', but at some point in the process affected interests must be accommodated.

Opposition to policies can come in different forms. Interest groups are one form, but other forms of opposition may be more subtle. For example, implementation of a new policy could be delegated to an agency opposed to it, an interest group in opposition could be granted a formal role in the implementation process, or officials involved in implementation could delay process or make token efforts at implementation.

Health policy and the policy-making process: an example

This chapter concludes with an example of a health policy issue that has been prominent on the health policy agenda in the US and several other countries—disease management (see Chapter 6.3). Disease management is 'a system of co-ordinated health care interventions and communications for populations with conditions in which patient self-care efforts are significant'.[1] These interventions aim to improve the cost-effectiveness of care by promoting adherence to evidence-based practices. This example describes the path disease management took through the four stages of the policy process.

Agenda setting

Health-care spending has been growing rapidly in most industrialized countries. These costs get onto the policy agenda because they affect large numbers of people, are felt by individuals, and are perceived as a severe problem.

The number of people with chronic conditions has been increasing as people live longer and treatments for previously lethal diseases are discovered. Health systems, on the other hand, have not changed and are still organized to treat acute illnesses.

Studies on the quality of health care have consistently shown that evidence-based treatment guidelines for chronic conditions are frequently not followed. As a result, spending is higher and outcomes are poorer than they could be.

Policy formulation

Several policy alternatives have been promoted to increase the cost-effectiveness of treating people with chronic conditions. Several of these have been wrapped up into the disease management model, including:

- emphasis on primary care and prevention to limit the number of acute episodes resulting from chronic conditions
- coordination of care among the many different providers that treat people with chronic conditions
- increasing compliance with evidence-based guidelines.

Disease management programmes were first developed in the private sector. Some programmes were developed by pharmaceutical companies as a way to encourage the recommended use of their drugs for chronic conditions. Other disease management models were adopted by insurance companies and eventually the public sector became involved.

Implementation

Disease management has been implemented in several settings:

- In Germany, disease management was implemented as an incremental change to the way insurance funds ('sickness funds') operate. Previous policies had increased competition between sickness funds, but funds with more beneficiaries with chronic conditions were at a competitive disadvantage. Disease management allowed funds to be reimbursed for the additional costs of chronic care, while at the same time improving the quality of care for people with chronic conditions. Implementation required cooperation and compromise between the sickness funds and physicians over what evidence-based guidelines would be used in the disease management programmes.
- In the US, disease management programmes began in the private sector as a way to improve compliance with practice guidelines. The stand-alone disease management firms as well as subsidiaries of pharmaceutical companies operate most programmes. Recently, the Medicare programme has funded a series of disease management demonstrations.
- In the UK, there is an ongoing demonstration of disease management operated by the pharmaceutical company Pfizer.

Evaluation

Because the disease management programmes are so new, few rigorous evaluations have been completed. As a result, most evaluations have been conducted internally and the findings have emphasized the positive aspects of disease management.

Conclusion

Understanding the policy-making process is a prerequisite to influencing it. To achieve policy change, a wide range of skills is needed, usually necessitating cooperation between groups of individuals or organizations. Both political and technical skills are needed to pass the 'clearance points' on the way to policy change.

Further resources

Downs A (1957). *An economic theory of democracy.* Harper and Row, New York.

Kingdon J (1995). *Agendas, alternatives, and public policies.* Harper Collins, New York.

Redman E (2001). *The dance of legislation.* University of Washington Press, Seattle, WA.

Walt G (1994). *Health policy.* Zed Books and Witwatersrand University Press, London.

Reference

1 Disease Management Association of America. http://www.dmaa.org/ (accessed 11 January 2006).

4.2 Developing healthy public policy

Don Nutbeam

Objectives

This chapter aims to provide readers with a better understanding of:
- the process of policy-making and the role of public health information and evidence in shaping policy
- the role of public health practitioners in influencing the policy process through the provision of evidence and advocacy.

Definition of key terms

- *Public policy* (see Chapter 4.1) comprises public issues identified for attention by the government, and the courses of action that are taken to address them.
- *Public policy-making.* Policy is often enacted through legislation or other forms of rule-making that define regulations and incentives, and enable the provision of resources, programmes and services to address public issues.
- *Healthy public policy* is a concept promoted by the World Health Organization to highlight the potential impact that all government policies can have on health. Healthy public policy is policy that makes explicit the impact it may have on health. The World Health Organization's Ottawa Charter emphasizes that health should be on the policy agenda in all sectors and at all levels of government and that governments should be held to account for the health consequences of their policies.[1]
- *Evidence* is simply defined as 'proof of an unknown or disputed fact', and is generally derived from research. In public policy-making, 'evidence' is derived from information gathered from a wide variety of sources other than traditional research. These include expert knowledge; stakeholder consultation; as well as the experience of frontline health workers in departments, agencies, and local authorities to whom policy is directed.[2]

Why is it important to be able to inform/influence policy with evidence?

Public health practitioners are often frustrated that public health evidence and a population-based perspective do not adequately influence public policy, particularly in sectors other than health. An improved understanding of the policy-making process by public health practitioners and researchers will enable a more effective transfer of knowledge into the policy arena and lead to greater influence on the development of healthy public policy.

How is healthy public policy made?

Policy develops and changes on the basis of underlying beliefs about both the cause of a problem and the potential effect of proposed interventions. These beliefs contribute to the policy-making process and final policy direction along with the social and political context in which the decision is made. The ability to interpret the causes of a problem, and to identify effective solutions are critical skills that can enable public health practitioners more effectively to influence policy decisions. These basic skills will be enhanced by an understanding of the social and political context of the problem and its possible policy solutions.[3]

Policy-making is rarely an 'event', or even an explicit set of decisions. Policy tends to evolve iteratively, subject to continuous review and incremental change. Policy-making is an inherently 'political' process, and the timing of decisions is usually dictated as much by political considerations as the state of the evidence. As such, policy-making requires a point in time appraisal of:
- what is scientifically plausible (evidence-based interventions or policy options)
- what is politically acceptable (policy option fits with political vision), and
- what is practical for implementation.[4]

What are the theoretical models that help explain the relationship between public health evidence and the policy-making process

Evidence will be used in a variety of ways to lead, justify, or support policy development. Carol Weiss has developed a set of models to explain the different ways in which evidence has been used to guide the policy-making process.[5] These include:
- *The knowledge-driven model* where the emergence of new knowledge from research will automatically create pressure for its application in policy. In public health, the development of new vaccines often leads

to public pressure for their immediate adoption, often regardless of their cost relative to benefit.

- *The problem-solving model* where evidence derived from a variety of sources is gathered and applied as a starting point for the development of policy, and used as part of a rational process with a clear beginning and end. For example, in The Netherlands, the government resolved to introduce a limited range of interventions to tackle health inequalities for which there was good evidence, and an established system for monitoring progress.[6]
- *The interactive model* where research knowledge is only one input in the decision-making process, along with experience, social pressures, and political considerations. The current approach taken to tackling health inequalities in the UK[4], reflects this more complex process and mix of influences.
- *The political model* where evidence is selectively used to justify a pre-determined position. The exclusive use of mass media campaigns and/or school-based interventions to address complex problems such as drug misuse and antisocial behaviour can be seen as examples of this model.
- *The tactical model* where the normal uncertainty of research findings is exploited to delay a decision or where weak evidence is used to justify an unpopular decision. The early responses of some governments to the rise of HIV/AIDS in the 1980s provides an example of this model.

In reality, it is most likely that evidence will be used in policy development in ways that correspond to the interactive, political, and tactical models described above. In order to better influence public policy, public health practitioners need to understand the place of evidence in the political processes that occur during policy development.

Who is involved in developing healthy public policy?

Four key players have been identified in the development of healthy public policy. These include:

- *policy makers* (usually politicians and bureaucracies) who have initiated or hold a mandate for a specific policy and move the policy at a pace that meets their interests
- *policy influencers* (who can be groups inside or outside government) who have an interest in the issue and may try to influence the content of the policy and the speed and way in which it is implemented—public health practitioners form part of this group, both from inside and outside government
- *the public* (audiences, consumers, taxpayers, and voters) whose opinion will ultimately affect the adoption of the policy—public health practitioners can play an important role as community leaders and opinion makers with the public, especially by making effective use of the media (see Chapter 4.7)
- *the media* (print and electronic) influence both the policy makers' and public's understanding of, and attitude towards, an issue.

The ways in which evidence is used in the policy-making process will vary according to the beliefs of those who create and influence policy. 'Evidence' can be used internally to monitor, analyze, and critique policy options, or externally to persuade or mobilize others into action. The media have a particularly important role in creating public opinion, not only by what they report, but by choosing who is allowed to speak, how much prominence the issue is given, and the way in which an issue is framed.[3]

Public health practitioners and academics often complain that their evidence is ignored by policy makers. However, our choice of research, methods of communication, and general dislocation from the policy process contribute to this situation. From a policy-making perspective, a large amount of public health research appears to be devoted to ever more elaborate descriptions of public health problems, in ways that offer no practical way forward or suggest solutions to the problems that were examined. Evidence will be better able to inform policy if there is a shift from the mostly descriptive research currently undertaken to more intervention, outcome, and implementation-focused research.

What determines success in developing healthy public policy?

Policy-making is inherently 'political', and decisions are usually dictated as much by political considerations as the state of the evidence. Policy is most likely to reflect public health priorities and the evidence that determines them if:

- the evidence is available and accessible at the time it is needed
- the evidence is presented in a way that fits with the political vision of the government (or can be made to fit)
- the evidence points to feasible actions, i.e. powers and resources are (or could be) available, and the systems, structures, and capacity for action exist
- there is successful public health advocacy within and outside of the political system
- public servants have critical appraisal skills and support in using evidence in policy development.

While there are many obstacles to the use of public health evidence in developing healthy public policy, there are real signs of progress in many countries, including:

- overt commitments by governments to use evidence in policy-making
- the growth of active public health communities and a strengthened voice in public debate
- modest changes to research funding to better align research with policy needs
- investments in institutions to build the public health evidence base.

What are the potential pitfalls?

Public health researchers and practitioners often fail to understand the intensely political nature of policy-making. They need a better understanding of how policy is made and must be more realistic about the possible contribution of their evidence. We also need to be aware of rare 'windows of opportunity' for the uptake of evidence into policy, when the policy makers' interests and the social climate coincide to support public health evidence in policy-making. Timing is everything.

Public health practitioners need to develop advocacy skills. This may involve building relationships with civil servants and policy makers within government departments, establishing partnerships and alliances with organizations and individuals with similar objectives, and effectively engaging with the media. Importantly, researchers need to develop closer working relationships with policy makers, from the earliest stages of research design through to programme implementation and beyond (see the case study below).

The transfer of evidence into policy is further hampered by a lack of knowledge and skill in handling research evidence among policy makers. The ability to critically appraise the quality of research, interpret results, and draw wider conclusions from the research findings are skills that would enable policy makers to competently and comfortably consider research evidence in their decisions.

Myths and misconceptions

The emergence of evidence-based medicine in the early 1990s has placed pressure on policy makers to become more evidence-based in their decision-making. In the scientific and medical communities, where evidence-based practice is highly regarded, there is a common misconception that policy-making is and should be a purely evidence-based and rational process. Nick Black suggests that policy makers often have other valid and competing concerns when formulating policy. Political survival, financial constraints, and public opinion are strong motivators in policy decisions. Tapping into these motivators will greatly increase the chances of influencing policy.[7]

A case study showing implementation of methods, consequences and lessons learned: physical activity in New South Wales (NSW) schools

Research and the policy process
The NSW Schools Fitness and Physical Activity Survey was undertaken to provide reliable scientific evidence in response to growing professional

and community concern around reduced physical activity and rising levels of obesity in Australian children.

The study measured the body composition, health-related fitness, physical activity habits, and fundamental motor skills of primary and high-school students in NSW. It also studied the school facilities, policies, and practices relevant to students' participation in physical activity.

Fundamental movement skills include running, jumping, catching, throwing, kicking, and forehand strike and are essential prerequisites for participation in and enjoyment of sports and other forms of physical activity. The results from the study showed that only about 30% of students had completely mastered running and jumping, with another 30% close to mastery. Girls in particular scored poorly on some skills, with less than 20% showing mastery or near mastery of kicking and forehand strike. As most of these skills should be mastered by Year 4, the results showed that NSW school children had surprisingly poor physical skills.

Two relatively small and achievable recommendations were made to policy makers. It was recommended that 2 hours per week be allocated to physical education in primary schools, 1 hour of which should be on developing fundamental movement skills. These recommendations were taken by contacts within the department to higher levels in the organization, until they reached the relevant minister and were accepted.

The resulting skills development programme in primary schools was very well supported. Resources were developed to support the teachers in implementing the programme and included videos, workbooks, phone support, and face-to-face training.

Subsequent research showed a dramatic improvement in the fundamental movement skills of NSW primary school children, along with an association between skill proficiency and higher levels of physical activity and lower levels of obesity.

Lessons learned

Several conditions assisted this transfer of evidence into education policy:

- Public health researchers engaged in a sustained media advocacy campaign, using their evidence to portray the lack of physical skills in Australian children as an important problem for society. This created the social and political climate needed for the adoption of healthy policy change.
- Public health researchers worked collaboratively with contacts in the Department of School Education throughout the process, from the design and implementation of the study, through to the evaluation of the subsequent skills development programme.
- The involvement of policy makers in the design phase of the survey meant that factors amenable to policy change and implementation were also measured. For example, school facilities, sports equipment, and time allocated to physical education were measured.
- Lastly, the policy changes were consistent with the Department of School Education's broader goals and within their capability to implement.

Further resources

Booth M, Macaskill P, McLellan L et al. (1997). *NSW Schools Fitness and Physical Activity Survey 1997*. NSW Department of School Education, Sydney.

References

1 World Health Organization (1986). *Ottawa Charter for Health Promotion*. WHO, Geneva.
2 UK Cabinet Office (1999). *Professional policy-making for the 21st century*. The Cabinet Office, London. Available at: http://www.policyhub.gov.uk/docs/profpolicymaking.pdf (accessed 11 January 2006).
3 Milio N (1987). Making healthy public policy: developing the science by learning the art. *Health Promotion Int*, **2**, 263–74.
4 Nutbeam D (2003). How does evidence influence public health policy? Tackling health inequalities in England. *Health Promotion J Aust*, **14**(3), 154–8.
5 Weiss CH (1979).The many meanings of research utilisation. *Public Admin Rev*, **39**, 426–31.
6 Mackenbach J, Stronks K (2002). A strategy for tackling health inequalities in the Netherlands. *BMJ*, **325**, 1029–32.
7 Black N (2001). Evidence-based policy: proceed with care. *BMJ*, **323**, 275–9.

4.3 Law in public health practice

Lawrence O. Gostin

Introduction

Public health practitioners often regard law as arcane, indecipherable, and not at all helpful in pursuing their objective of improving the public's health. Certainly, law can obfuscate rather than clarify, impede rather than facilitate. But even when the law stands as an obstacle, practitioners must understand it; they may even seek to circumvent legal barriers provided it is lawful and ethical to do so. More important, the law can be empowering, providing innovative solutions to the most implacable health problems. Of the 10 great public health achievements of the 20th century, most were realized, in part, through law reform or litigation:

- vaccinations
- safer workplaces
- safer and healthier foods
- motor vehicle safety
- control of infectious diseases
- tobacco control
- fluoridation of drinking water.

Only three did not involve law reform (family planning, healthier mothers and babies, and decline in deaths from coronary heat disease and stroke).[1]

The law is far more important in public health than usually acknowledged. Law creates a mission for public health authorities, assigns their functions, and specifies the manner in which they may exercise their power. The law is a tool that is used to influence norms for healthy bahaviour, identify and respond to health threats, and set and enforce health and safety standards. The most important social debates about public health take place in legal forums—legislatures, courts, and administrative agencies—and in the law's language of rights, duties, and justice. It is no exaggeration to say that 'the field of public health...could no longer exist in the manner in which we know it today except for its sound legal basis'.[2]

Box 4.3.1

'Health officers must be familiar not only with the extent of their powers and duties, but also with the limitations imposed upon them by law. With such knowledge available and widely applied by health authorities, public health will not remain static, but will progress.'

Tobey (1926)[3]

Objectives

The objectives of this chapter are to help readers understand:

- the impact of legislation, regulations, and litigation on the public's health
- the powers, duties, and restraints imposed by the law on public health officials
- the potential of legal change to improve the public's health, and
- the role of international law in securing public health in the face of increasing globalization.

Definitions

There is a subtle difference between 'public health law' and 'law and the public's health'. The former is the body of primary and secondary legislation that creates governmental public health agencies and enables them to carry out their activities. The latter is the wider body of law that can be used in a variety of ways to safeguard and promote the public's health.

Public health law can be defined as the legislation and administrative rules that delineate a public health agency's mission, duties, and powers to assure the conditions for people to be healthy and the limits on an agency's power to constrain the autonomy, privacy, liberty, or proprietary interests of individuals.

The *law and the public's health* can be defined as the legislation, regulations, and case law that can be used as a tool to safeguard and promote the public's health including altering the socio-economic, informational, natural, and built environments.

The law for public health practitioners

Public health practitioners should understand and obey the law. This means that they must act within the scope of their legal authority, never abuse their power, treat persons with respect, and consult with community leaders. If the law is unclear, practitioners should seek the guidance of public health lawyers. Since few lawyers have a specialized knowledge of population health, education and training programmes in public health law should be established.

Public health law: deficiencies and opportunities

Inadequacy of existing legislation

In many countries, public health legislation is so old that it tells the story of health threats through time, with new layers of regulation with each page in history—from plague and smallpox to tuberculosis and polio, and now HIV/AIDS and SARS. Legislation often pre-dates modern public health science and practice and does not conform to modern ideas relating to the mission, functions, and services of agencies. Existing laws also often pre-date advances in human rights, failing to safeguard civil liberties. These deficiencies become particularly apparent in times of crisis such as terrorism or emerging infectious diseases.

The purposes of sound public health legislation

Sound public health legislation should provide agencies with a clear and modern mission to create the conditions in which people can be healthy.[4] The statute should enable agencies to exercise a full range of necessary functions, services, and powers. It should similarly provide funding and other structures necessary to carry out the agency's mission. At the same time, public health legislation should protect individual rights to privacy, autonomy, liberty, and non-discrimination. In particular, it should enunciate clear standards for the exercise of powers, due process, and fair treatment.

Box 4.3.2 Model public health legislation

In response to the attacks on the World Trade Centre and subsequent dispersal of anthrax in the US, the Centre for Law and the Public's Health at Georgetown and Johns Hopkins universities drafted the Model State Emergency Health Powers Act (MSEHPA). The MSEHPA was structured to reflect five basic public health functions to be facilitated by law: [5]
- preparedness
- surveillance
- management of property
- protection of persons, and
- public information and communication.

In 2003, the 'turning point' Public Health Statute Modernization Collaborative drafted a comprehensive public health act focusing on the organization, delivery, and funding of essential public health services, together with a full set of powers and safeguards.[6] Currently, the World Health Organization is developing a model national public health law that can be used as a template by countries with different legal traditions.

Public health law: power, duty, and restraint

Public health law creates public health agencies and grants them specific powers. These powers include:
- surveillance and monitoring
- vaccination and treatment
- partner notification and contact tracing, and
- isolation and quarantine.

The effective and careful use of these powers allows public health officials to protect and improve the public's health. The law, however, also constrains the exercise of these powers. Public health officials should be conscious of how the exercise of these powers impacts on the enjoyment of liberties (e.g. the right to privacy and freedom of movement) and should implement appropriate limits and procedural safeguards to ensure that a proper balance between individual liberties and the public's health is reached.

Law and the public's health: regulation and litigation as a tool

If government has an obligation to promote the conditions for people to be healthy, what tools are at its disposal? There are at least seven models for legal intervention designed to prevent injury and disease, encourage healthful bahaviours, and generally promote the public's health. Although legal interventions can be effective, they often raise critical social, ethical, or constitutional concerns that warrant careful consideration.[7]

Model 1: the power to tax and spend

The power to tax and spend is ubiquitous in national constitutions, providing government with an important regulatory technique. The power to spend supports the public health infrastructure consisting of: a well-trained workforce, electronic information and communications systems, rapid disease surveillance, laboratory capacity, and response capability. The state can also set health-related conditions for the receipt of public funds. The power to tax provides inducements to engage in beneficial bahaviour and disincentives to engage in risk activities. Tax relief can be offered for health-producing activities such as medical services, childcare, and charitable contributions. At the same time, tax burdens can be placed on the sale of hazardous products such as cigarettes, alcoholic beverages, and firearms.

Model 2: the power to alter the informational environment

The public is bombarded with information that influences their life choices, and this undoubtedly affects health and bahaviour. The government has several tools at its disposal to alter the informational environment, encouraging people to make more healthful choices about diet, exercise, cigarette smoking, and other bahaviours:

- use communication campaigns as a major public health strategy (e.g. educate the public about safe driving, safe sex, and nutritious diets)
- require businesses to label their products to include instructions for safe use, disclosure of contents or ingredients, and health warnings
- limit harmful or misleading information in private advertising (e.g. ban or regulate advertising of potentially harmful products, including cigarettes, firearms, and even high-fat foods).

Model 3: the power to alter the built environment

Public health has a long history in designing the built environment to reduce injury (e.g. workplace safety, traffic calming, and fire codes), infectious diseases (e.g. sanitation, zoning, and housing codes), and environmentally associated harms (e.g. lead paint and toxic emissions). Many developed countries are now facing an epidemiological transition from infectious to chronic diseases. Environments can be designed to promote liveable cities and facilitate health-affirming behaviour by, for example:

- encouraging more active lifestyles (walking, cycling, and playing)
- improving nutrition (fruits, vegetables, and avoidance of high-fat, high-caloric foods)
- decreasing use of harmful products (cigarettes and alcoholic beverages)
- reducing violence (domestic abuse, street crime, and firearm use), and
- increasing social interactions (helping neighbours and building social capital).

Model 4: the power to alter the socio-economic environment

A strong and consistent finding of epidemiological research is that socio-economic status (SES) is correlated with morbidity, mortality, and functioning.[8] SES is a complex phenomenon based on income, education, and occupation. Some scholars have even suggested that 'Justice is good for our health'.[9] By narrowing socio-economic disparities, the state seeks to reduce inequities and improve the population's health.

Model 5: direct regulation of persons, professionals, and businesses

Government has the power to directly regulate individuals, professionals, and businesses:

- regulation of individual bahaviour (e.g. use of seatbelts and motorcycle helmets) reduces injuries and deaths
- licences and permits enable government to monitor and control the standards and practices of professionals and institutions (e.g. doctors, hospitals, and nursing homes)
- inspection and regulation of businesses helps to assure humane conditions of work, reduction in toxic emissions, and safer consumer products.

Model 6: indirect regulation through the tort system

Attorneys general, public health authorities, and private citizens possess a powerful means of indirect regulation through the tort system. Civil litigation can redress many different kinds of public health harms:

- environmental damage (e.g. air pollution or groundwater contamination)
- exposure to toxic substances (e.g. pesticides, radiation, or chemicals)
- hazardous products (e.g. tobacco or firearms), and
- defective consumer products (e.g. children's toys, recreational equipment, or household goods).

For example, in 1998 tobacco companies negotiated a master settlement agreement with American states that required compensation in perpetuity, with payments totaling $206 billion through to the year 2025.

Model 7: deregulation—law as a barrier to health

Sometimes laws are harmful to the public's health and stand as an obstacle to effective action. In such cases, the best remedy is deregulation. Consider laws that penalize exchanges or pharmacy sales of syringes and needles. Restricting access to sterile drug injection equipment can fuel the transmission of HIV infection. Similarly, the closure of bathhouses to prevent the spread of sexually transmitted infections can drive the epidemic underground, making it more difficult to reach sexually-active gay men with condoms and safe sex literature.

World health law: comparative and international perspectives

The use of the law to improve the public's health is also important at the international level. Health hazards—biological, chemical, and radionuclear—have profound global implications. Whether the threat's origin is natural, accidental, or intentional, the harms transcend national frontiers and warrant a transnational response. The potential scope of international public health law is vast,[10] ranging from communicable (e.g. global surveillance and border control) and non-communicable diseases (e.g. occupational health and narcotics) to trade, environmental, and human rights concerns.[11] This section briefly discusses three important international legal instruments.

The International Health Regulations (IHR)

The World Health Assembly adopted the IHR in 2005.[12] The IHR had been critiqued because of its narrow scope (applying only to cholera, plague, and yellow fever); lack of enforcement; failure to set minimum national public health capacities; and failure to provide sufficient financial and technical assistance to poor countries.[13] The main improvements in the new IHR are:

- *expanded jurisdiction* covering 'all events which may constitute a public health emergency of international concern'
- *national focal points* for official WHO communications in each country
- *core capacities* for public health preparedness in order to detect, report, and respond to public health risks
- *global surveillance* by using official and unofficial sources of information and modern data systems
- *recommended measures* to reduce health risks on a standing or temporary basis.

The Framework Convention on Tobacco Control (FCTC)

The WHO has turned to international law solutions in the area of chronic diseases as well as infectious diseases. Particularly remarkable is the FCTC, adopted by the World Health Assembly in 2003.[14] As of 2005,

168 states had signed the convention, 118 states had ratified, and the FCTC had come into force. The FCTC establishes a 'framework' for ongoing diplomacy to reduce the global health threat posed by tobacco.

Conclusion

The law is a much under-appreciated tool for health improvement. Many public health practitioners distrust the law and the law-making process; they are often not skilled in using, or reforming, the law to improve the public's health. Yet law at the national and international level can have profound effects in changing attitudes and bahaviours of individuals and businesses with remarkable benefits for the health of populations.

Further resources

Books and articles

Fidler D (1999). *International law and infectious diseases*. Oxford University Press, Oxford.

Gostin LO (2000). *Public health law: power, duty, restraint*. University of California Press and Milbank Memorial Fund, Berkeley and New York.

Gostin LO (2002). *Public health law and ethics: a reader*. University of California Press and Milbank Memorial Fund, Berkeley and New York.

Luca Burci G, Vignes CH (2004). *World Health Organization*. Kluwer Law International, The Hague.

Martin R, Johnson L (2001). *Law and the public dimension of health*. Cavendish Publishing, London.

Monaghan S (2002). *The state of communicable disease law*. Nuffield Trust, London.

Monaghan S, Huws D, Navarro M (2003). *The case for a new UK Health of the People Act*. Nuffield Trust, London.

Reynolds C (2004). *Public health law and regulation*. Federation Press, Sydney.

Websites on public health law

The Centre for Law and the Public's Health (Georgetown and Johns Hopkins universities). http://www.publichealthlaw.net/ (accessed 28 June 2005).

US Department of Health and Human Services Centres for Disease Control and Prevention. Public health law programme. http://www2a. cdc.gov/ phlp/ (accessed 28 June 2005).

Australian Government Department of Health and Ageing. Public Health Education and Research Programme (PHERP) innovations project. Centre for Public Health Law. http://www.health.gov.au/internet/wcms/ publishing.nsf/Content/pherp-innovations-6.htm (accessed 28 June 2005).

World Health Organization. http://www.who.int/en/ (accessed 28 June 2005).

References

1 Centre's for Disease Control and Prevention (1999). Ten great public health achievements—United States, 1900–1999 (1999). *Morb Mortal Wkly Rep*, **48**(12), 241–8.

2 Grad FP (1990). *Public health law manual*. American Public Health Association, Washington, DC.

3 Tobey TA (1926). *Public health law: a manual of law for sanitarians*. The Commonwealth Fund, New York.

4 Institute of Medicine (2003). *The future of the public's health in the 21st century*. National Academies Press, Washington, DC.

5 Gostin LO, Sapsin JW, Teret SP *et al.* (2002). The Model State Emergency Health Powers Act: planning and response to bioterrorism and naturally occurring infectious diseases. *J Am Med Assoc*, **288**, 622–8.

6 Turning Point Model State Public Health Act. Available at: http://www.publichealthlaw.net/Resources/Modellaws.htm (accessed 27 October 2004).

7 Gostin LO (2004). Law and ethics in population health. *Aust NZ J Public Health*, **28**, 7–12.

8 Marmot M (2004). *Status syndrome: how your social standing affects your health and life expectancy*. Bloomsbury, London.

9 Daniels N, Kennedy B, Kawachi I (2000). Justice is good for our health. *Boston Rev*, **25**(1), 6–15.

10 Taylor AL, Bettcher DW, Fluss SS, Deland K, Yach D (2002). International health instruments: an overview. In: Detels R (ed.) *Oxford textbook of public health*, 4th edn, pp. 359–86. Oxford University Press, Oxford.

11 Fidler DP (2002). *Global health governance: overview of the role of international law in protecting and promoting global public health*, discussion paper No. 3. World Health Organization/London School of Hygiene and Tropical Medicine, Geneva/London. Available at: http://www.lshtm.ac.uk/cgch/Reports.htm (accessed 27 October 2004).

12 World Health Assembly (2005). *Revision of the International Health Regulations:*. Available at: http://www.who.int/csr/ihr/en/ (accessed 27 December 2005).

13 Gostin LO (2004). International infectious disease law: revision of the World Health Organization's International Health Regulations. *J Am Med Assoc*, **291**, 2623–7.

14 World Health Organization (2005). *Framework Convention on Tobacco Control*, WHO doc. A56/VR/4 (2003). Available at: http://www.who.int/tobacco/framework/WHO_FCTC_english.pdf (accessed 11 January 2006).

4.4 Shaping your organization's policy

Yi Mien Koh

Introduction

Public health professionals often have to influence and help shape policy decisions at all levels for the benefit of public health. At the local level, policy development could take a number of forms: implementation of national policies, adapting national policies to local situations, developing local policies to meet local population health needs and internal organizational policies. This chapter is about what you can do to help shape the public health policies of your organization.

Objectives

After studying this chapter, you will be better able to:
- appreciate the policy-making cycle
- understand what evidence-based policy is
- analyze the factors influencing policy-making in organizations
- apply the evidence-based policy approach to policy-making
- examine the role of power in organizations
- improve your skills in managing conflict
- develop your own ability to influence policy-making.

Organizations and policies

A policy is a plan or course of action that a person, team, or organization takes, or proposes to take. It sets out the rules or principles that will apply when faced with a given problem or situation.

In order to shape policy in your organization, you need to understand both the current situation and the preceding events. In particular you need to understand:
- the rationale of the prevailing policies—what they set out to achieve
- the actual consequences of the policies—what they actually achieved
- the origins of these policies—both in terms of organizations and people
- the forces that have shaped and encouraged (and inhibited) both their ratification and implementation.

The policy-making cycle

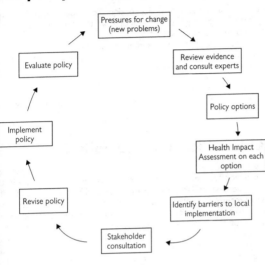

Figure 4.4.1 The policy formulation cycle

The model in Figure 4.4.1 adopts the excellent policy-making model proposed by the Cabinet Office (1999)[1] and applies the 'plan, do, study, act' cycles of quality improvement (NHS Modernisation Agency 2002)[2] to the policy-making process.

The cycle presents a single sequence. In reality, lots of the activities go on in parallel, with short cuts and backward steps round the loop. For example:
- assessing 'barriers to local implementation' may make one go back to the 'policy options' stage again
- almost any of the boxes may/should lead to consultation/dialogue with stakeholders; and conversely
- 'stakeholder consultation' may force re-entry into another box, e.g. 'examine evidence' (if presented with new evidence sources) or health impact assessment (HIA) or barriers.

The model has the following features that have been identified for successful policy-making:[1]
- a focus on a specific topic
- using evidence-based policy
- testing change of ideas (e.g. using a 'plan, do, study, act' approach)
- continuous improvement
- being time limited
- adopting a project management approach
- engaging wider stakeholders (see 'How to do consultation'), and
- having measurement systems in place.

How to do consultation

Consultation is a key part of policy-making. You would normally have taken informal soundings from key people at the earliest stages. The formal consultation process should be:

- done early enough to influence, and not be a sham
- clear and open about the parameters of the possible (on a spectrum from 'blue sky' to being heavily constrained)
- a listening exercise but not necessarily agreeing (e.g. with lobby groups) so that people feel they have been heard
- providing your organization with an opportunity to communicate with key stakeholders and to prevent unwanted surprises.

What is evidence-based policy?

Evidence-based policy has been defined as an approach that helps people make well-informed decisions about policies, programmes, and projects by putting the best available evidence from research at the heart of policy development and implementation.[3] This approach stands in contrast to opinion-based policy, which relies heavily on either the selective use of evidence or on the untested views of individuals or groups, often inspired by ideological standpoints, prejudices, or speculation.[4] Grey[5] proposed a new dynamic to decision-making in health care and other areas of public policy, replacing opinion-based policy with evidence-based policy.

Evidence–based policy approach to policy-making

The push behind the evidence-based policy movement is the growing demand for rational and effective policy interventions based on an informed understanding of 'what works'. Systematic literature reviews play an essential part in the process, with greater emphasis on explicit consideration of the quality of evidence used to support policy development (see 'Further resources' for examples of sources of evidence for policy).

If evidence-based policy becomes a major part of many governments' approaches to policy-making and the machinery of government, local organizations would be more likely to buy in to policies that are evidence based, properly evaluated, and based on best practice.

Factors (other than evidence) influencing policy-making in organizations

New policies can be triggered by internal or external factors. You need to develop your skills to get to know the key factors in your own and other organizations:

- internal factors include leadership changes, the introduction of new systems, changes in organizational structures, e.g. mergers, or the identification of problems leading to action being needed
- external factors can include new government policies cascading down for local implementation, changes in technology, and changes in local, national, or global economic or political conditions.

Key relationships, both organizational and personal, are important influences. There are also key influential people to win over. Lobby and staff groups also play important roles.

The evidence-based policy and practice approach takes time and resources. It also requires sounds research evidence to be there. There are many areas of public health practice where there is still little or no valid social scientific evidence. In reality, unless there is strong evidence available, the policy process should integrate the other factors that influence policy-making and policy implementation. The following, adapted from Davies[4], serves as a useful checklist:

- *Experience, expertise, and judgement*: judgement based on the experience and expertise of decision makers may be of critical significance in those situations where the existing evidence is equivocal, imperfect, or non-existent.
- *Resources*: policy-making is not just a matter of 'what works' but what works at what cost and with what outcomes (both positive and negative). Economists have well-developed methods for appraising, analyzing, and evaluating the cost-effectiveness, cost–benefit, and cost–utility of different courses of action. (see Box 1.4.2)
- *Values*: policy-making takes place within the context of values, including ideology and political beliefs. You should consider the values of key decision makers, the organizations involved, the local communities, and stakeholders. The attitudes, values, and understanding of ordinary people is important, especially in sensitive policy areas, and are best addressed by consultation at early stages of policy development.
- *Habit and tradition*: changing traditional and habitual ways of doing things in order to modernize may cause resistance.
- *Pressure/lobby groups and experts*: pressure groups and experts may compete with evidence to influence policy-making. Opinion leaders and local media are other major influences. It is not that these groups fail to use evidence to promote particular policies. Rather the evidence is often less systematic and more selective, and may be biased.
- *Pragmatics and contingencies*: agreeing a timetable for the process is helpful to everyone. Some things such as the parliamentary terms and key meeting dates could be planned for. You also need to build in

flexibility to enable you to respond to unanticipated events, e.g. disease outbreaks. Should they arise, start by identifying what is already known about the problem and what is not.

Any significant change in policy, or revision of old policies, implies changes to the ways people and organizations work. Change is rarely universally welcomed; some people are likely to resist it, often for personal reasons as much as for more ideological reasons. Conflict is not unusual, but if managed well, could lead to more effective policy development and implementation.

Managing conflict

Conflicts are bound to arise when new policies are being developed or implemented. Conflicts arise because we all want different things, both in terms of process and outcomes, especially at times of change.

Successful conflict management skills require you to be flexible and capable of switching between styles. You also need to present your arguments clearly, listen actively, question effectively and read other people's bahaviour accurately.

Power as a source of influence

Policy changes are heavily influenced by power relationships between and within groups of people. Power can be defined as the capacity to get others to do things they might not otherwise do. Maintaining and increasing your power in an organization in order to let you shape policy means being highly attuned to your organization's objectives and to the objectives of other influential people within it. As power is relative, the degree of power you have depends on how much power others have.

Understanding who has which types of power bases would help you to identify who you need to influence to get their support for the new policy, as well as help you manage those negative sources of power. It also helps you to identify your own sources of power which you may be under-using.

Conclusions

Few public health practitioners hold formal positions that come with great power to shape the policies of their organization, but most have potential for considerable influence. By improving your conflict management skills and understanding the policy-making cycle and how policies could be influenced, will enable you to contribute to policy-making in a positive and more effective way.

Further resources

Davies P (1999). What is evidence based education? Br J Educ Stud, 47(2), 108–21.

National Institute for Health and Clinical Excellence (NICE) (UK). http://www.nice.org.uk/ (accessed 28 June 2005). Produces evidence-based guidelines on public health and other clinical interventions.

UK Economic and Social Research Council (ESRC) Network for Evidence Based Policy and Practice (Evidence Network). http://www.evidencenetwork.org/ (accessed 28 June 2005).

References
1 Cabinet Office (1999). *Professional policy making for the 21st century.* Cabinet Office, London.
2 NHS Modernisation Agency (2002). *Improvement leaders guide to setting up a collaborative programme.* Department of Health, London.
3 Davies HTO, Nutley S, Smith PC (2000). *What works? Evidence-based policy and practice in public services.* The Policy Press, Bristol.
4 Davies PL (2004). *Is evidence based government possible? Jerry Lee Lecture 2004,* presented at the 4th Annual Campbell Collaboration Colloquium, Washington, DC, 19 February 2004. Government Chief Social Researcher's Office, Prime Minister Strategy Unit, Cabinet Office, London.
5 Gray JAM (1997). *Evidence-based healthcare: how to make health policy and management decisions.* Churchill Livingstone, London.

4.5 Translating policy into indicators and targets

John Battersby

Introduction

Like them or not, indicators and targets have become a fact of life. They have been used in some sectors of industry for many years and, increasingly, they are now being used to measure and manage health systems. Certainly it is difficult to read a newspaper article without finding reference to government targets.

An understanding of what indicators are and how indicators and targets are constructed is essential for public health practitioners. You will be called upon to interpret indicators, you will be expected to meet targets, and you may well have to construct indicators and set targets for others.

Objectives

After reading this chapter you will have a better understanding of:
- what targets and indicators are
- what they can be used for
- how to go about constructing a good indicator
- when not to use indicators and targets.

Definitions

There are a number of definitions used for the terms indicator and target. For the purposes of this chapter the following definitions have been used:
- *indicator*—a proxy measure, which indicates the condition or performance of a system (implies a *direction*).
- *target*—a specific, time bound, *destination*.

In other words an indicator suggests what you are trying to achieve, whilst a target shows you how close you are to achieving it.

Why do indicators and targets matter?

Turkey farmers in Norfolk, UK know the old saying 'You can't fatten a turkey by weighing it'. What applies to turkeys also applies to health systems; measuring performance doesn't necessarily improve it. There are two reasons for measuring performance:

- So that you know when things are going wrong. For example if you don't measure infection rates following surgery you won't know when they are getting worse.
- So that you know when things are going right. If you redesign a care pathway you need to measure one of its outcomes to know whether you have improved care or not.

What can be measured with indicators?

Indicators can be used to measure various elements of health and health care. What a particular indicator measures will be determined by how that indicator is constructed but it will measure either health status (inequality), the provision of health services (equity), or the performance of the system itself.

Performance can be measured in several ways:

- at different places, either geographic or organizational
- at different stages in a pathway, for example
  structure → process → output → outcome
- at different times (e.g. the same measure repeated annually).

(Output is the immediate effect of an intervention or process, e.g. the number of quitters in a smoking cessation programme, whereas outcome is the longer-term effect, e.g. the reduction in lung cancer mortality as a result of the smoking cessation programme.)

Performance indicators usually include an element of comparison. Is an organization getting worse or better? How does one organization compare with another?

Properties of indicators and targets

Indicators are *always*:

- proxy measures (although the relationship should be *clear*, *plausible*, and *valid*)
- objectively quantifiable
- constructs (because performance is not *directly* measurable).

Indicators are *often*:

- complex composite or summary measures (and it should therefore be possible to de-construct them and explain them).

Indicators are *ideally* constructed so that:

- they measure parts of causal pathways that are understood
- they identify parts of the pathway that are amenable to change.

Targets should always be SMART:

- Specific
- Measurable
- Achievable
- Relevant/Realistic
- Time bound.

Some measures can act as both targets and indicators depending on how they are used. For example, life expectancy is commonly used as an indicator of the health of a population and to compare the health of different populations. Life expectancy has many of the properties of an indicator, it is objectively quantifiable and it is a proxy measure, as health itself cannot readily be measured. Life expectancy can also be used as a target, and indeed the UK government has recently set a target to increase life expectancy in England to 78.6 years for men and 82.5 years for women by 2010.[1] Using it in this way it is clearly specific and time bound, and fulfils the other SMART criteria.

What makes a good indicator?

There is probably no such thing as a perfect indicator. However, there are several criteria that can be used to judge the quality of an indicator and these are listed below; most of them apply equally well to targets. You must remember that at times there will be a trade-off between two or more of these criteria. If you are developing indicators you need to be explicit about what trade-offs have been made, and if you are using them you need to understand those trade-offs. For example indicators should:

- have a clear purpose and be rational
- be valid
- be deconstructable
- be comparable
- be statistically robust
- be scalable
- be balanced *within* and *between* sets
- not induce perverse incentives or unintentional consequences
- be sensitive and responsive
- be linked to other organizational and policy-driven initiatives
- be easily explained and communicated.

In addition to these criteria there are a number of more technical issues that you need to consider when constructing an indicator or a target. The first of these is whether the data that you need are actually available or, if not, whether they could be collected. More often than not data are available but are of poor quality, possibly incomplete or poorly coded. This needn't be a bar to using such data in an indicator as the completeness and quality of data collection usually improve with time, especially when the data are used and fed back to those responsible for data collection. (Box 4.5.1 gives an example of the need for good timely data.)

Box 4.5.1 The need for good timely data

The 2004 contract for primary care doctors in the UK is a good example of data quality as a barrier to effective use of indicators.[2] The contract includes the collection of large numbers of primary care data that will be used to assess the quality of primary care services and also measure disease prevalence. Because this process currently relies on a variety of data collection systems it is likely to take at least 3 years before the quality of those data are consistent across the UK. Until data collection is consistent, the resulting indicators must be interpreted with great caution.

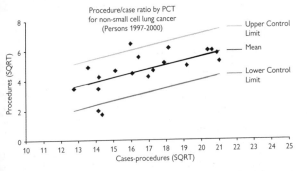

Figure 4.5.1 A process control chart plotting lung cancer cases not receiving surgical treatment (x-axis) against cases receiving surgical treatment (y-axis). The plot shows health districts in the east of England. Districts falling outside the control limits show more than the expected degree of variation.[6]

Many indicators rely on the underlying measurement of rare events, for instance measurement of suicide at a subnational level, or measurement of death rates following surgery at a hospital or even practitioner level. The inherent variability associated with measurement of rare events needs to be handled carefully. There are a number of tools that you can consider to help you with this such as funnel plots,[3] process control charts,[4] and, particularly for measuring individual performance, CUSUM monitoring.[5] Figure 4.5.1 shows an example of a process control chart.

These techniques are all methods of separating out the inherent variation of measurement from the variation that occurs when something is going wrong. Such techniques, which have been used in industry for many years, are increasingly being used as the basis for indicators and targets in health care. The Further resources section at the end of this chapter points towards further information on these topics.

What are the potential pitfalls of indicators and targets?

There are several problems associated with the use of indicators. These include:

- Their appeal. Indicators and targets appeal to busy people who exercise authority (e.g. managers and politicians); however, that appeal may not be matched by an understanding of how the indicator or target has been constructed
- They can make people feel very threatened and if performance is judged to be poor or a target is missed can be very demoralizing
- They can divert resources from other areas of health care. They do this in two ways, firstly because it requires resources to both construct and particularly to collect the necessary data to populate indicators or to assess the achievement of a target. Secondly, if they are not used correctly they may lead to the diversion of resources away from the real problems
- The final pitfall is associated with not using them. Failure to use indicators and targets correctly can result in wasted resources and potentially it can result in harm to patients.

The key to avoiding most of these pitfalls is for those who are measuring (often managers) and those who are being measured (often clinicians) to have a shared understanding of how the indicator or target has been developed and how it is going to be used.

If you are asked to develop a local indicator or target involve the clinicians who will be generating the data and make sure that both you and they understand:

- what is being measured
- why it is being measured
- how it is being measured.

One particular area that deserves mention is that of partnerships. Much public health work rightly involves public health practitioners and health services working in partnership with other organizations such as local government, voluntary organizations, education authorities, and social care organizations. Like other aspects of health care, partnership work is often measured and work is often focused on reaching targets. It is vitally important in this context to be clear on what the contribution of each organization is to a particular target or indicator. There is nothing more demotivating or unfair than being held accountable for something over which you have no control.

National or local targets, does it matter?

Indicators and targets are not always geographically scalable. Imagine two local health districts in a country working to reduce health inequalities. Both districts have to achieve a national target of a 4% improvement in life expectancy over a given time period. District A is in an affluent rural area and district B is in a deprived urban area and so life expectancy in district A is better than in district B. If both districts manage to achieve the 4% target, because they started off at different levels, the gap between them will actually have increased. So applying the same national target to different local situations is not always a good idea.

In this example a better approach would have been for district A to have a different local target of reducing the gap in life expectancy within its area. That way the national target could be achieved without increasing health inequalities.

How will you know when you have identified the perfect indicator?

You will know you have got it about right when:
- clinical colleagues feel motivated and encouraged
- nobody complains about it
- managers can use it to demonstrate how much a service has improved
- politicians ask you to develop some more!

Further resources

Battersby J, Williams C (2003). *Quantifying performance: using performance indicators*. Briefing papers on topical public health issues, 4. Eastern Region Public Health Observatory, INpho, Cambridge.

Fitzpatrick J, Jacobson B (2003). *Local basket of inequalities indicators*. Association of Public Health Observatories and Health Development Agency, London.

Flowers J, Bailey K, Streather M, Walrond S, Wilkinson J (2004). *Regional indications 2. Main report*. APHO, Cambridge.

References

1 Department of Health (2004). *National standards, local action health and social care standards and planning framework*. Department of Health, London.

2 Department of Health (2003). *Delivering investment in general practice: implementing the new GMS contract*. Department of Health, London.

3 Spiegelhalter D (2002). Funnel plots for institutional comparison [comment]. *Qual Saf Health Care*, **11**(4), 390–1.

4 Mohammed MA, Cheng KK, Rouse A, Marshall T (2001). Use of Shewhart's technique. *Lancet*, **358**(9280), 512.

5 Bolsin S, Colson M (2000). The use of the Cusum technique in the assessment of trainee competence in new procedures. *Int J Qual Health Care*, **12**(5), 433–8.

6 Battersby J, Flowers J, Harvey I (2004). An alternative approach to quantifying and addressing inequity in healthcare provision: access to surgery for lung cancer in the east of England. *J Epidemiol Commun Health*, **58**(7), 623–5.

4.6 Translating indicators and targets into public health action

Rebekah A. Jenkin, Michael S. Frommer, and George L. Rubin

Introduction

Indicators and targets serve two purposes in public health. First, they enable governments and health agencies to specify their responsibilities for the health of populations and communities. Second, they provide objective means of reviewing programmes and policies, and assessing their effectiveness.

The purpose of this chapter is to examine how such targets and indicators can be used to guide and inform the choice, implementation, and evaluation of public health action. Box 4.6.1 contains a glossary of the terms used.

Box 4.6.1 Explanation of terms

- *Goal.* A goal is a general statement of intent or aspiration. It refers to outcomes that are considered to be achievable with current knowledge and resources.[1] A health goal may refer to health status; prevalence or incidence of, or mortality from, a particular condition; diagnostic or treatment processes; social, personal, or environmental risk factors; processes to modify risk factors or outcomes; or any other social dimension connected with health. Goals may be relevant to a whole population or to particular groups within it.
- *Target.* A public health target specifies a measurable change in a health-related phenomenon that can be expected to occur within a given time in a particular population. Targets usually express the intended occurrence of the phenomenon at a future date, and this future value is often published together with a baseline figure. A goal may be related to or expressed in terms of one or more targets.
- *Indicator.* A public health indicator is a measure that reflects, directly or indirectly, the occurrence of a health-related phenomenon, some aspect of a health-related phenomenon, or a process which could influence the occurrence of a health-related phenomenon. Health indicators may be classified as reflecting health status; the outcomes of particular interventions; risk factors; or processes. Targets are usually expressed in terms of indicators.

Global perspective

There is a global impetus to define targets and indicators for measuring progress in health. A bold example was the United Nations' adoption of the eight Millennium Development Goals (MDGs)[2] in 2000, aiming to halve abject poverty by 2015. However, such high-level goals often fail to take a sufficiently broad approach, ignore sustainability and disadvantaged groups, or fail to refer to public health requirements that involve cross-sectoral issues such as water supply, or political considerations such as human rights. The MDGs have been similarly criticised.

Despite these (and other) reservations, many nations and aid agencies have adopted MDGs to orient their policy and work, and to define accountabilities.

National goals may be expressed using targets and indicators. For example, the US Government's Healthy People 2010[3] policy defines two overarching goals: increased years of healthy life and elimination of health disparities. These will be attained using *developmental and measurable* objectives. *Developmental* objectives identify areas for improvement in health outcomes or status, with a need for data monitoring to provide evidence for intervention programmes.

Measurable objectives provide explicit targets for action, using data from existing representative datasets as baselines for measuring improvements. Most developed countries have frameworks or policy statements that outline planning cycles or steps (see Chapter 5.2). Australia's *Planning framework for public health practice*[4] and the US *Framework for environmental health risk management,*[5] are examples.

Scenario: A large regional Australian health service is preparing as Action Plan for local implementation of a State Government initiative for the prevention of obesity in children and young people. The Action Plan will draw on evidence-based clinical guidelines for the management of obesity and must address national priorities to attract funding. The plan will be implemented using existing resources, already stretched by the health needs of a population spread across large towns with advanced secondary health services and isolated remote areas. The region has a large proportion of younger people and a relatively large number of indigenous people, both groups identified as being at risk of high rates of obesity. The priority areas for action include: improving the nutritional value of food and drinks sold in school canteens; promotion of breastfeeding; increasing community awareness of overweight and obesity, nutrition and physical activity; improving knowledge of the prevalence of overweight and obesity in minority groups and disadvantaged people; and, improving early childhood services for disadvantaged and remote communities.

The following questions may be helpful in formulating a local action plan.

What are the principles upon which any public health action plan should be based?

▸ Any action plan should reflect the ethos of the national and regional health systems. For example, the New South Wales Department of Health *Strategic Directions for Health 2000–2005*[6] has four key aspirations—healthier people, fairer access, quality health care, and better value. The regional plan should reflect these aspirations, and also address the targets and indicators outlined in the action plan.

- The primary task of the health service is to reconcile the broad national (or regional) goals and targets with the health needs of the region's population. This will include both identification of local problems and problem solving. It will entail making local plans that reflect the national and/or regional approach, identify priority health problems, and balance investment across different areas of public health. The health service will take responsibility for implementing the plans through coordinated local action.
- Both national and regional systems have a commitment to accountability, reporting, and continuous quality improvement. Monitoring systems that can track locally important health indicators, as well as progress towards national and state targets, is an essential part of the response. The information and data needs for reporting and for indicators should be considered at the start of the development of an action plan.
- The health service should be opportunistic and creative in pursuing additional resources national and state political commitment to goals and targets. These resources (available in association with funds or intellectual capacity) can be used for regional priorities that mirror the national priorities. The resources can also often provide spin-off support for other regional priorities.
- Regional efforts to contribute to national goals and targets should select interventions, both new and existing, for which there is evidence of effectiveness. Guidelines on levels of evidence for public health and public health interventions have been developed and are helpful in appraising the evidence base for potential public health interventions.[7]
- The health service should be committed to local community values and culture.

  Box 4.6.2 details some generic principles for public health planning.

Box 4.6.2 Generic principles of public health planning

- Each community or population subgroup should have access to strategies, services, and activities that optimize their health.
- Each community or population subgroup should have access to a healthy and safe environment including clean air and water and adequate food and housing.
- Public health efforts must proceed in partnership with non-health sectors and in collaboration with international partners.
- A supportive legal and political environment is integral to the public health effort.
- Improvements in knowledge about current and emerging health determinants and risks are vital to effective public health efforts.
- Priority setting and decision-making should be based on scientific evidence as far as possible and on criteria that are open to public scrutiny and debate.
- Optimizing population health outcomes requires effective linkage between public health and health system planning.
- An ongoing capacity to scan and monitor the social and environmental trends likely to affect future health status is essential for long-term planning to prevent ill health.

Extracted from memorandum of understanding between members of the National Public Health Partnership.[4]

What are the core public health activities or functions that are encompassed by the health issue and need to be addressed in implementing the national strategy and regional action plan?

Public health is a broad field, but some core public health functions can be identified. Box 4.6.3 lists those identified by the National Public Health Partnership in Australia. (compare these to the list in the main introduction from the US Health and Human Services Public Health Service; p. xxxi.)

Box 4.6.3 Core public health functions

1. Assess, analyze, and communicate population health needs and community expectations.
2. Prevent and control communicable and non-communicable diseases and injuries through risk factor reduction, education, screening, immunization, and other interventions.
3. Promote and support healthy lifestyles and bahaviours through action with individuals, families, communities, and wider society.
4. Promote, develop, and support public health policy, including legislation, regulation, and fiscal measures.
5. Plan, fund, manage, and evaluate health gain and capacity-building programmes designed to achieve measurable improvements in health status, and to strengthen skills, competencies, systems, and infrastructure.
6. Strengthen communities and build social capital through consultation, participation, and empowerment.
7. Promote, develop, support, and initiate actions that ensure safe and healthy environments.
8. Promote, develop, and support healthy growth and development throughout all life stages.
9. Promote, develop, and support actions to improve the health status of Aboriginal and Torres Strait islander people and other vulnerable groups.[8]

Specific action plans are likely to refer to combinations of these functions. For example, a plan to reduce the prevalence of overweight and obesity could propose the introduction of school-based exercise and nutrition interventions, such as the provision of free exercise and breakfast programmes in targeted high-risk local communities. The interventions could be coupled with research designed to assess and record the health status and diets of children and their families, thereby providing up-to-date information. Such interventions would encompass core functions 2, 3, and 6–9.

What information is required to develop an action plan?

Development of a plan for local implementation of a national strategy and regional action plan requires information from several sources. One approach to gathering this information is given below.

Situation analysis

This entails:

- getting a clear and detailed understanding of national and regional level expectations associated with the national strategy and regional action plan

- identifying the determinants of the health problem and the context in which they operate, including the population groups or subgroups most at risk
- reviewing the epidemiology of the health problem at a local level in relation to the determinants, national and regionwide goals and targets, and the availability of data on the problem
- setting priorities among the determinants, taking account of the risks and benefits, and of national and regionwide priorities for action
- reviewing the existence, effectiveness, and cost of current local objectives and programmes relevant to the national strategy, and
- identifying aspects of the health problem at a local level that are not covered by the national strategy and/or regional action plan.

Consultation

Effective consultation is crucial for the validity of the plan, its acceptability to local communities and health practitioners, and its subsequent implementation. Consultation should be wide-ranging and inclusive, and run from the development of the plan, through to implementation and evaluation. The consultation process should identify barriers to the implementation of the plan and lay the groundwork for lowering or removing them. The consultation process is critical to ensuring that the needs and preferences of disadvantaged and high-risk population groups are recognized and addressed in the action plan.

Review of published and unpublished ('grey') literature and information

The purpose of this review is to find and/or evaluate intervention options that are likely to work in solving the problems identified in the situation analysis. The review should include an appraisal of the level of evidence for each intervention.[7]

How should decisions about interventions be made?

Guidelines are available for deciding on interventions, for example *Deciding and specifying an intervention portfolio*.[9] In addition to the preferences of those likely to be affected, criteria for the selection of interventions may include the following:

- *Assessment of the feasibility* of the interventions if they were applied locally, including estimates of the resources needed to carry out the interventions, both financial and human. Are the necessary infrastructure and human resources available, or do they need to be procured?
- *Assessment of the effectiveness* of the interventions: whether they will provide short, medium or longer-term solutions to the health problem; the likely magnitude of their effect in a given time period; their sustainability; and any other effects on the current services (positive or negative).
- *Consideration of the ethics, acceptability and distribution of the interventions.* Are the expected benefits likely to reach all groups? Are they evenly distributed? Do they particularly affect some groups to the detriment of others? Are the proposed interventions appropriate and acceptable, politically, socially, and culturally, to the communities that

they target? Are the resources required to implement the interventions equitable given the burden of the problem for different population groups or subgroups?

- *Assessment of the costs associated with the potential interventions.* Has an economic evaluation of the potential interventions been conducted?
- *Timing.* How soon can the potential interventions be introduced? How soon will the benefits be realized? For example, any intervention aimed at community-wide weight reduction is unlikely to achieve quick results, and a measure of success is the sustainability of the weight reduction.
- *Risk management.* Risks to the successful implementation of the preferred interventions should be identified, along with options for managing them. Risks include changes in the political and policy environment, shifts in priorities, escalation of costs, and unanticipated effects.

All available objective evidence and information about the relative costs, benefits, risks, and effectiveness of potential interventions should be examined in deciding upon an intervention portfolio. However, the final decision will be based on a combination of objective and subjective factors, as well as findings from the situation analysis.

What are the elements of a local action plan?

Prior to implementation, the selected interventions must be formulated into a local action plan for endorsement by the regional executive. This plan must articulate the specific agreed goals that will be pursued. Some goals may be broad (e.g. improve community knowledge about the benefits of an active lifestyle), and some may be very narrow (e.g. increase the rates of breastfeeding in infants aged 0–6 months). The plan must also detail how the baseline rates of activity in relation to these goals are measured and how they will be measured during and after the interventions.

The local action plan will include:

- a list of new actions to be started
- a list of existing interventions or programmes to be stopped (because there is evidence that they do not work or are not effective enough)
- a list of existing interventions to be maintained, either at their current level or with some enhancement or diminution.

In addition, the local action plan will identify local goals and targets in relation to the health problem. These targets are important because they help to set appropriate local expectations, taking account of baseline rates of health problems (the initial situation analysis will show whether and by how much local rates differ from national rates). Local targets may differ substantially from national or regional targets because of characteristics unique to the locality and translation of interventions and problems into a local context. For example, if overweight and obesity rates are greatly elevated in a particular subgroup of a local community, the target rates may be modified.

In setting local targets, it is also important to recognize the heterogeneity of the population, not only because of variations in baseline occurrence of diseases or risk factors but also because of the varying responsiveness of particular groups to specific interventions. For some conditions, variations in baseline rates are enormous. For example, the prevalence of type 2 diabetes in many Australian indigenous communities is up to seven times that of the rest of the Australian population.[10] The setting of targets for diabetes control in these communities requires both knowledge of the medical interventions and an understanding of indigenous social values and community processes.

How will the action plan be implemented?

Implementation requires the translation of knowledge on interventions into the particular local context. It takes into account:
- local resources, including human resources and infrastructure
- specific characteristics of the population
- baseline incidence of the health problem
- the latency period before an effect of the intervention will be observed
- a balance between achieving targets that reflect process change and those that reflect risk factor change
- local variations in the likely effectiveness of particular interventions.

It is valuable to make use of the skills and expertise of local public health practitioners in the development and implementation of local action plans. They bring expertise and knowledge in the following areas.

Methodological skills
- The ability to search literature databases and appraise published evidence for and against particular interventions.
- Methodological skills and experience in epidemiology, population health surveillance, health needs assessment, public health programme development, implementation and evaluation, and health economics.

Local knowledge
- First-hand personal and epidemiological knowledge of the local population and the local environment (political, social, and physical).
- Knowledge of, and possible responsibility for, local programmes (existing, planned, and possible) which are likely to influence the goals and targets.

Communication skills
These include advocacy skills, that can be used in persuading decision makers and fund holders to initiate and sustain effective programmes, or cease ineffective interventions.

Understanding of government processes
Many public health practitioners have a well-developed understanding of government processes. They recognize when and how to persist with well-argued public health recommendations in the face of varying budget cycles and the continuous structural changes that affect all health systems. They know how to identify opportunities, and are ready to adjust recommendations in response to new opportunities.

Further resources

Child and Youth Health Intergovernmental Partnership (2004). *Healthy children—strengthening promotion and prevention across Australia;*

developing a national public health action plan for children 2005–2008. National Public Health Partnership, Melbourne.

Commission on Macroeconomics and Health (2001). *Macroeconomics and health: investing in health for economic development.* World Health Organization, Geneva.

Jenkin R. Frommer M (2005). *A framework for developing or analyzing health policy.* The University of Sydney, Sydney, Australia.

Leeder SR, Raymond S, Greenberg H, Liu H, Esson K (2004). *A race against time—the challenge of cardiovascular disease in developing economies.* Columbia University, New York.

Nutbeam D, Wise M, Bauman A, Harris E, Leeder S (1993). *Goals and targets for Australia's health in the year 2000 and beyond.* Australian Government Publishing Service, Canberra.

United Nations (2000). *United Nations millennium declaration.* United Nations, New York.

References

1 Commonwealth Department of Human Services and Health (1994). *Better health outcomes for Australians. national goals, targets and strategies for better health outcomes into the next century.* Australian Government Publishing Service, Canberra.

2 World Health Organization (2003). *The world health report.* World Health Organization, Geneva.

3 United States Government (2000). *Healthy people 2010.* Available at: http://www.healthypeople.gov/ (accessed 6 February 2006).

4 National Public Health Partnership (2000). *A planning framework for public health practice. National Public Health Partnership,* Melbourne, Australia.

5 United States Presidential Congressional Commission on Risk Management (1997). *A framework for environmental health risk management.* US Government, New York.

6 New South Wales Department of Health (2000). *Strategic directions for health.* NSW Health Department, Sydney, Australia.

7 Rychetnik L, Frommer M (2002). *A schema for evaluating evidence on public health interventions, version 4.* National Public Health Partnership, Melbourne. Available at: http://www.nphp.gov.au/publications/phpractice/ schemaV4.pdf (accessed 6 February 2006).

8 National Public Health Partnership (2000). *Public health practice in Australia today: a statement of core functions.* National Public Health Partnership, Melbourne. Available at: http://www.nphp.gov.au/publications/phpractice/phprac.pdf (accessed 6 February 2006).

9 National Public Health Partnership (2000). *Deciding and specifying an intervention portfolio.* National Public Health Partnership, Melbourne.

10 Commonwealth Department of Health and Aged Care and Australian Institute of Health and Welfare (1999). *National health priority areas report: diabetes mellitus 1998* (AIHW cat. No PHE 10). AusInfo, Canberra.

4.7 Influencing governments via media advocacy

Simon Chapman

Introduction

The media are peerless as a means of engaging large numbers of people, including those with influence, in public health debates. If a public health issue is ignored by the news media, or if the media choose to frame its meaning from the perspectives of those working against the interests of public health, it is highly unlikely that sought after political, public, or funding support will follow. There are few, if any, examples of robust public health policy or well-funded programmes that have not been preceded and sustained by widespread and supportive news coverage. As a veteran reporter of 40 years' experience with the *Wall Street Journal* said:

> Well-done investigative reporting produces public outrage (or policy maker outrage) that forces new regulations and laws or tougher enforcement of existing ones. Ten-thousand-watt klieg lights turned on a situation focuses the minds of policy makers very fast.[1]

Objective

The objective of this chapter is to help readers understand:
- how public health issues are dealt with by the media
- how framing of an issue can be crucial to its success in changing policy
- how practitioners can prepare themselves to deal with the adverse framing of a public health issue.

In most areas of public health, proposed interventions are controversial and frequently attract bitter opposition. Public health advocacy, particularly through media advocacy, is the strategic use of the news media to advance a public policy initiative.[2]

Framing

A core skill found in effective media advocates is that they appear to audiences to have an instinct for framing their concerns in ways that make their issues instantly comprehensible in terms of wider discourses that reach beyond the manifest or overt subject of their concerns. For example, while few people may comprehend the complexities of the tobacco litigation now rampant in the US, people do understand from years of negative press reportage about the tobacco industry[3] that the cases are being fought about allegations of negligence, cover-up, and deceit. Such dimensions or subtexts allow audiences who may not have detailed knowledge or awareness about the particulars of a given issue to identify that here is something similar to an issue they *do* understand. Subtexts serve to link topics to familiar, wider socio-political discourses so that coverage of particular events is decoded by audiences as instances of more general themes or types of story. In this way, much news is not instructively seen as news, but as 'olds'—essentially the retelling of age-old stories, only with new casts, circumstances, infectious agents, and so on. For example, the on-going news saga about doping in sport and use of anabolic steroids is essentially the retelling of the myth of Narcissus—a moral tale about the dangers of vanity, inflected to involve another widely understood subtext: that cheats should not prosper. Effective public health advocates must learn to think about their issues in such terms, rather than assume that news media have intrinsic interest in specific issues like cancer, infection, injury, and so on.[4,5]

There is no 'objective reality' that any platform of public health policy can be said to be *really* about. The often heated nature of news discourse about public health issues testifies to the essentially contested nature of advocacy. To injury prevention specialists, compulsory bicycle helmets might mean reduced brain injury and deaths; to indifferent parents their meaning might be framed more in terms of additional expense; and to fashion-conscious youth, the intrusion of a paternalistic state on their ability to dress as they please and thumb their nose at danger. Reality is always a socially constructed notion.

The emphasis or 'framing' that is placed around particular events or issues that seek to define *what this issue is really about* will represent but one of many competing meanings that jostle for public dominance. While health interests may frame the meaning of a bill to introduce proof of immunization in terms of the protection of children's health, anti-immunizationists may choose to describe the bill in terms of the encroachment of the 'nanny state', 'compulsory medication', and other negative metaphors.[6]

Box 4.7.1

Politics is largely about the problem of competing interest groups seeking to advance multiple definitions of the same events.

Politics, and therefore the progression of public health policy, is largely about the problem of competing interest groups seeking to advance multiple definitions of the same events. In public health, policy advocacy is ultimately the process by which advocates for different positions and values seek to define what is at issue for the public, media gatekeepers, and policy makers and legislators. For example, are compulsory fences for backyard swimming pools:[7]

- a blight on garden aesthetics and evidence of Big Brother, regulatory bureaucracy stepping ever closer into our personal lives?
- the use of a sledgehammer to crack a walnut (i.e. with any given pool having a very low probability of 'hosting' a drowning, should every pool owner—particularly those with no children—bear the cost of installing a fence?)
- a safety net to prevent drowning, the leading cause of death in 1–5-year-olds in Australia?

An example: gun deaths

Gun control provides a good example of the role of 'framing' in the media handling of an issue, and in the progress of efforts to change policy.

Are gun deaths:

- the occasional, unfortunate 'blood price' communities with liberal gun laws pay for the freedom to defend their homes from malevolent intruders?
- perpetrated by criminals and the mentally ill who are beyond the reach of law?
- preventable carnage, capable of reduction as with any other public health problem?

When a lone gunman shot 35 people dead at Port Arthur, Australia, in April 1996, within a month, all political parties united in support of the Australian Prime Minister's call for semiautomatic rifles and shotguns to be banned, for all guns to be registered, for self-defence to be explicitly excluded as a legitimate reason to own a gun, and for gun ownership to be limited only to those who satisfied a limited number of reasons to own a gun. Australian gun control advocates had promoted these policies for years and Port Arthur was a watershed event that overnight made reform of gun law politically compelling.

Both before and after Port Arthur, the gun lobby sought to define gun control in ways that would minimize political interest in its implementation. The task for gun control advocates, of course, was to do the opposite.

Over the years, we had collected many examples of their key arguments and, in hindsight, came to see that we had subjected these to a process of analysis amenable for use in media advocacy planning. Rather than responding off-the-cuff to gun lobby efforts to frame gun control as misguided folly, hundreds of media opportunities were disciplined by strategic attempts at framing and reframing the debate[8] to achieve particular objectives.

Planning attempts to reframe debates

A prepared and disciplined response to debates of public health issues depends on dealing with the following questions:

- what was our public health objective?
- what frame put around this objective would most neatly and clearly define what was at issue?
- what symbols, metaphors, or visual images could be referenced that would trigger this frame in audiences?
- what 'sound bites' (typically, about 7 s of speech or two to three sentences in newsprint) could encapsulate the essence of the frame?

Table 4.7.1 Two worked examples using a matrix for framing media advocacy

Public health objective	Frame	Symbol, visual image, or metaphor	Sound bite
Gun lobby position (1): 'Why don't you ban knives, axes, and baseball bats too?'			
To communicate that guns are especially dangerous because they are so effective at killing. They kill and injure many more than other weapons, so they merit special restrictions	Guns as ultra-lethal	When a gun is available during an argument, it's like throwing petrol on a fire. Fist fight versus gun fight. With guns, minor altercations can lead to death	Gun + criminal intent = 17 dead (Dunblane). Gun + criminal intent = 35 dead (Port Arthur) but machete + criminal intent = 7 injured (Wolverhampton). 'Guns are a permanent solution to a temporary problem'. 'I've never heard of a drive-by stabbing'
Gun lobby position (2): 'Guns don't kill people, people kill people'.			
To refocus on the lethality of guns	To pull guns back inside the frame defining directions for solutions. Guns as controllable, people as less controllable	A violent/disturbed/ upset person with an ultra-lethal means of expressing anger	People kill—guns make it possible. This is like saying...bare wires don't kill, electricians do. Guns don't die—people do!

Table 4.7.1 illustrates two examples of how this process is an adaptation of an approach suggested by Charlotte Ryan[9] and subsequently applied by the Berkeley Media Studies Group to the study of the way that gun control is debated in the US press. Gun lobby 'definitions' of what was at issue are shown, together with a reframing strategy encompassing the four questions listed above.

Strategic planning of effective advocacy

Developing effective advocacy requires careful strategic planning, in the same way as other sorts of public health interventions (see Chapter 5.2). Box 4.7.2 summarizes the questions that need to be addressed in developing your strategy. As always, clarifying objectives at each stage is essential, and understanding the politics and respective strengths and weaknesses of others' positions is very helpful.

Unfortunately many public health organizations are inhibited from developing advocacy, often fearing a loss of support from the governments they seek to influence. Advocacy is therefore often limited to small grass-roots groups. Developing public health advocacy from professional organizations is a high priority.

> **Box 4.7.2 Ten questions for public health advocates**
>
> 1. What are your public health objectives for this issue?
> 2. Can a 'win–win' outcome be first engineered with decision makers?
> 3. Who do the key decision makers answer to, and how can these people be influenced?
> 4. What are the strengths and weaknesses of your and the opposition's position?
> 5. What are your media objectives?
> 6. How will you frame what is at issue here?
> 7. What symbols or word pictures can be brought into this frame?
> 8. What sound bites can be used to convey 6 and 7?
> 9. Can the issue be personalized?
> 10. How can large numbers of people be quickly organized to express their concerns?
>
> From Chapman[2]

Conclusions

Media debates of public health and other issues are characterized by the use of simplified 'subtexts' of what the issues are 'really' about. This 'framing' of issues provides opposing sides in debates with metaphors and images to use, to advance their own views, and to oppose the views of others. Politics, and therefore the progression of public health policy, is largely about competing interest groups seeking to advance multiple definitions of the same events.

A prepared and disciplined response to debates of public health issues is possible and depends on identifying and using the symbols that would trigger the desired 'frame' in audiences and using the right 'sound bite' to encapsulate the essence of that frame.

References

1 Otten AL (1992). The influence of the mass media on health policy. *Health Affairs*, winter, 111–18.
2 Chapman S (2004). Advocacy for public health: a primer. *J Epidemiol Commun Health*, **58**(5), 361–5.
3 Christophides N, Dominello A, Chapman S (1999). The new pariahs: how the tobacco industry are depicted in the Australian press. *Aust NZ J Public Health*, **23**, 233–9.
4 Wallack L, Dorfman L, Jernigan D, Themba M (1993). *Media advocacy and public health: power for prevention.* Sage, Newbury Park, CA.
5 Chapman S, Lupton D (1994). *The fight for public health: principles and practice of media advocacy.* BMJ Books, London.
6 Leask J, Chapman S (1998). 'An attempt to swindle nature': press reportage of anti immunisation, Australia 1993–97. *Aust NZ J Public Health*, **22**, 17–26.
7 Carey V, Chapman S, Gaffney D (1994). Children's lives or garden aesthetics? A case study in public health advocacy. *Aust J Public Health*, **18**, 25–32.
8 Chapman S (1998). *Over our dead bodies: Port Arthur and Australia's fight for gun control.* Pluto, Sydney.
9 Ryan C (1991). *Prime time activism.* South End Press, Boston, MA.

4.8 Public health policy at a European level

Martin McKee

Background

For those living and working in the countries of Europe, decisions that influence health are increasingly made at a European rather than a national or local level. It is important to understand the process by which decisions are made and how you might influence them. There is also much that can be learned by taking a European perspective. There are large differences in life expectancy and in rates of individual diseases in the different countries of Europe. While public health professionals have often looked at where their locality lies in relation to the country in which it is situated, it can be helpful to see how it compares with neighbouring countries. This can sometimes shake one's complacency! Finally, many public health professionals are already taking advantage of the opportunities presented by closer European integration, joining in networks and collaborative research projects.

Objectives

This chapter will help you to:
- understand the diversity of health within Europe and so help you to think of ways in which things might be done differently
- understand the decision-making process in the European Union and how you can influence it
- be aware of the scope for European collaboration and how you can participate in it.

The public health geography of Europe

From a political, and therefore a public health perspective, 'Europe' has many different boundaries:
- The European Union although expanded to 25 countries in 2004 still excludes many countries that are unambiguously European but includes some territories that lie far beyond the continent of Europe, such as French Guiana, on the coast of South America, or La Reunion, in the Indian Ocean, both overseas departments of France (these are the outlines that appear in the lower left corner of Euro notes).
- In 2007, the European Union is expected to expand further, to include Bulgaria and Romania, and possibly Croatia.

- The European Economic Area—a wider grouping, bringing together the European Union member states with Liechtenstein, Norway, and Iceland; although in western Europe, Switzerland remains outside while continuing to participate in many European Union activities.
- The European region of the World Health Organization—52 countries, including the countries in central Asia that were once part of the USSR.

The health of Europeans

At the risk of simplification, the countries of Europe can be divided into three broad groupings in terms of patterns of health:
- Western Europe—sustained improvements in life expectancy since the Second World War.
- The former communist countries of central and eastern Europe—stagnation in life expectancy in the late 1970s and 1980s driven by rising adult mortality, partially compensated by a continuing decline in child mortality.[1]
- The former Soviet Union—a distinct pattern, with stagnation in life expectancy between the mid-1960s and mid-1980s, followed by a series of large fluctuations driven mainly by changing death rates from cardiovascular diseases and injuries, and linked to socio-economic changes and alcohol consumption.[2]

However, within these broad categories, there is also considerable diversity. This diversity provides a large number of natural experiments that can shed light on the determinants of population health:
- the 'Mediterranean diet', linked to low rates of cardiovascular disease,[3] has helped understanding of the benefits of olive oil rather than animal fats, and of fruit and vegetable consumption
- research in Russia has revealed the adverse cardiovascular effects of binge drinking[4]
- sustained increase in deaths from tobacco- and alcohol-related diseases in Denmark, in contrast to the situation in Sweden, shed light on the health effects of different approaches to regulation.[5]

In several cases, comparisons have stimulated action:
- research showing that if Scotland was an independent country it would have among the worst health statistics in Europe[6] helped persuade politicians of the need for policies including a ban on smoking in public places
- evidence that cancer survival in the UK lagged behind that in other European countries stimulated a major reform of the provision of cancer services[7]
- recognition of the high toll from road traffic injuries in France led to a major initiative on road safety.

There are many more so far untapped opportunities to learn from the experiences of other countries and while Europeans (and particularly the British) have traditionally looked for inspiration across the Atlantic, there is much to be gained by studying the diversity among one's neighbours.

European organizations

The European Union

The impact of European Union law on issues related to health is increasing steadily. It is important to understand something about how this body of law comes about.

The European Economic Community was created in 1957 as a free trade area linking six continental European countries. It has expanded progressively over time, both in the number of countries that are members and in the scope of its powers. In 1992, with the Treaty of Maastricht, it became the European Union. The powers of the European Union are agreed by the governments of its member states and have been set out in successive treaties.

The policies of the European Union are based on the *four freedoms*, of movement of goods, persons, capital, and services. Traditionally, health has featured only where it relates specifically to these issues, for example the mobility of patients (in their role as workers) or health-care providers, or trade in pharmaceuticals. As the health dimensions of trade have increasingly been recognized, and as the European Union has developed a social dimension to complement its previous economic focus (reflecting concerns about the need to counter the excesses of the market), its activities in the field of health have steadily grown, as illustrated by its action to ban tobacco advertising in media that potentially cross borders.

The European Union can, however, only act in areas where it has been given competence to do so by the treaties and, in acting, it is bound by the principle of *subsidiarity*, so that it can only take action if the objective being pursued cannot be achieved by the member states acting alone. It must also do no more than is necessary to achieve that objective.

Once a need for action has been identified, new European legislation is proposed by the European Commission. It is then considered by the Council of Ministers and by the European Parliament. If the council and the parliament cannot agree on legislation they enter into a process of reconciliation (Box 4.8.1).

There are several possible products of this legislative process (Box 4.8.2). Where there is a conflict, European law takes precedence over national law, and where a member state fails to give force to a directive within 2 years, then the original directive has force of law in the country concerned.

Inevitably, there are often situations in which the precise application of a legal measure is unclear. In these cases the European Court of Justice will make a decision.

Box 4.8.1 The institutions of the European Union

- European Commission—the European Union's civil service. It is responsible for initiating legislation, implementing policies at a European level, and taking enforcement action where member states or others subject to European law are thought to be in breach of it.
- Council of Ministers—this is the forum at which the ministers in national governments come together to discuss policies. Every 6 months there will be a series of councils, each attended by the relevant ministers, such as the Health Council. The Council of Ministers must agree legislation jointly with the European Parliament. Depending on the topic, the Council of Ministers may determine their support or otherwise by unanimity or by qualified majority voting, where each country is allocated a particular quota of votes reflecting its size. For some issues and in some countries, where a subject is the responsibility of regional government, the council will be attended by representatives of the regions (e.g. health in Germany, Austria, and Italy). An exception is the UK, where responsibility for health is devolved to the four constituent territories but the English Department of Health speaks on behalf of the UK.
- European Parliament—this is the body that represents the people of Europe and is made up of democratically elected members representing constituencies from each member state. Members sit in groupings based on their political perspectives, rather than in national groupings.
- European Council—this brings together the heads of government in regular summit meetings that provide direction and political impetus for EU policies.
- European Court of Justice—this court is the guardian of the treaties and has assumed political significance through its exercise of judicial review.

Box 4.8.2 European legal instruments

- *Regulations*—specific measures that have immediate and direct force of law, so that, as with the treaty provisions, an individual can seek redress in a national court. They do not need to be adapted to take account of national circumstances, so they are typically used in areas such as external trade.
- *Directives*—these set out goals to be achieved but allow each member state to draft legislation in a manner appropriate to its circumstances. The national legislation must be in place within a fixed time period and, if not, an individual can seek redress against the state in question or any public authority within it, in which case the national court is obliged to rule on the basis of the earlier directive as long as its provisions are sufficiently clear to do so.
- *Decision*—these have direct force of law, like regulations, but do not relate to all member states. For example, they may be used in relation to a ferry service linking two countries.
- *Recommendations and opinions*—these set out goals that it would be desirable to achieve but do not have force of law.

As the treaties specify that health care is a matter for national governments, while European legislation covers almost all aspects of the provision of care, such as mobility of patients and providers or trade in pharmaceuticals, many key decisions about health care have been made by the court, acting in the absence of any clear guidance from the legislative process.[8] In doing so it has to balance issues of health with those of trade and competitiveness, a role that is widely viewed as one that should be dealt with by the legislative process rather than the court, to avoid the situation in which case law evolves based on the particular features of often highly unrepresentative cases.[9]

The responsibilities of the European Union in the field of health, if not in health care, have been growing. Since 1992, the European Union has been required by the treaties to promote a high level of human health. Over the past decade, activities have been stimulated by evidence of failure to act in some situations such as the emergence of bovine spongiform encephalopathy (BSE) and, more recently, by a political imperative to respond to the perceived threat from bioterrorism. Consequently, the focus of much of its policy has been on communicable disease. During the 1990s a series of networks were created in which national surveillance programmes collaborated to exchange information, recognizing how, with increased mobility, many outbreaks, for example of *Legionella* in a holiday hotel, could affect people from many countries.[10]

Within the European Commission, responsibility for health is widely dispersed. Although the Directorate General for Health and Consumer Affairs (DG Sanco) plays a key role, with responsibility for the European Union's public health programme, health features in the work of many other directorate generals. For example:

- DG Social Affairs—responsibility for many issues relating to health care
- DG Research—manages a major framework programme conducting health-related research
- DG Agriculture—the health implications of the Common Agricultural Policy.

There is a requirement that the health consequences of the policies promulgated throughout the European Union should be assessed but this is an area that is widely recognized to be weak.[11]

Public health is a key element of several of the new EU specialized agencies:

- The European Centre for Disease Control (Stockholm)
- The European Food Safety Authority (Parma)
- The European Drugs Monitoring Centre (Lisbon).

Beyond the European Union

The European Union has recognized that its interests extend beyond its own borders and has created several mechanisms for cooperation in a variety of sectors, including health, with its neighbours. These include its European Neighbourhood Policy, which supports participation in European Union structures by countries in the western part of the former

Soviet Union, such as Belarus, Russia and Ukraine, as well as countries in the Middle East and North Africa.[12] Another mechanism is the Stabilisation and Association Process, which includes Albania and the remaining countries of the former Yugoslavia.[13]

How to influence European Union policy

National governments guard jealously their role in European decision-making through the Council of Ministers and, with a few exceptions such as Sweden, have resisted efforts to make the process more transparent. However, there are several entry points for public health advocates:

- The European Parliament—either your local MEP or members of the parliament's Committee on Environment, Public Health and Food Safety.
- The European Commission—although it has a very small staff in relation to the tasks it must undertake, especially in relation to public health, and it must depend extensively on external advisers, operating through its various advisory committees or by undertaking the targeted research that it commissions.
- The Council of Ministers—in larger countries this may be more difficult, simply because ministers are less accessible. However, all countries have a voice, regardless of size, and several of the smaller countries have been especially active in promoting public health.
- European non-governmental organizations—many of these have well-developed chains of communication to the commission and parliament. The European Public Health Alliance (www.epha.org) plays a leading role but there are many others dealing with more specific issues.
- The annual European Health Policy Forum, held each autumn in Bad Gastein, in Austria (www.ehfg.org), bringing together academics and policy makers from the European institutions, member states, and private industry.

Much of the European legislation that affects health has been developed to address other issues so the impact on health is often not realized by legislators. In other cases, policies that might promote health are the target of efforts by powerful vested interests to water them down. In both cases public health advocates can play a role:

- identify the issue at an early stage, ideally when draft legislation is still under consideration
- make a very clear case about why there is a problem, and if possible that there is an alternative, practical solution
- work with colleagues in other member states to build a Europe-wide coalition
- make sure that your case enters into the policy arena, using as many as possible of the entry points listed above
- make full use of the media—MEPs, ministers, and European Commission officials read newspapers and watch television too!

The World Health Organization (WHO)

The World Health Organization Regional Office for Europe (http://www.euro.who.int/) is based in Copenhagen but has offices in several other parts of Europe (Box 4.8.3).

Box 4.8.3 WHO offices in Europe

- European Centre for Environment and Health—Bonn, Germany
- European Office for Integrated Health Care Services—Barcelona, Spain
- European Office for Investment for Health and Development— Venice, Italy
- European Centre for Environment and Health—Rome, Italy
- International Agency for Research on Cancer—Lyons, France (accountable to WHO Headquarters)

The WHO has two main roles, the provision of technical advice and support to countries. In pursuing these roles it has established a series of networks that enable individuals and organizations to come together to exchange experience. Examples include:
- the Healthy Cities network
- the Healthy Regions network
- the Health Evidence Network.

The Council of Europe

The Council of Europe is a body that pre-dates and is separate from the European Union. It consists of 46 countries, including all those of the enlarged European Union as well as many from the former Soviet Union. Its main goals are to preserve human rights, democracy, and the rule of law, while supporting a shared European identity. It hosts the European Court of Human Rights, which is the guardian of the European Convention on Human Rights. Although health forms only a small part of its activities, the Council of Europe is involved in several important health-related areas:
- medical ethics
- policy on illicit drugs (the Pompidou Group)
- promoting social cohesion
- the European Pharmacopoeia.

Other networks

There are many other networks that enable public health professionals to come together to exchange experience in Europe. Many focus on specific areas, such as tobacco or alcohol, or health-promoting hospitals. There are also some more broadly based organizations (Box 4.8.4).

Box 4.8.4 Selected European organizations in the field of public health

- European Public Health Association (EUPHA)—brings together national scientific associations. It publishes the *European Journal of Public Health*.
- European Public Health Alliance (EPHA)—brings together non-governmental organizations working to improve health.
- Association of Schools of Public Health in the European Region (ASPHER)—brings together schools of public health. It has developed a system of peer-review that facilitates exchange of experience.
- European Health Management Association—primarily made up of organizations with a managerial focus, but with a strong health focus.

Further resources

Health for All Database. This is a valuable resource produced by the European Regional Office of the WHO that includes data on a wide range of health-related variable from the 52 member states of the European region. Available at http://www.who.dk/hfadb (accessed 28 June 2005).

The European Observatory on Health Systems and Policies. The European Observatory brings together international agencies (such as the WHO and the World Bank), governments, NGOs, and universities. It functions as a knowledge broker, publishing detailed analyses of countries' health systems (*Health Systems in Transition* reports) and studies on a range of issues related to the financing and delivery of health care in Europe as a whole and in subregions. Available at http://www.euro.who.int/observatory (accessed 27 June 2005).

OECD Health Database. This covers the entire OECD (western Europe, North America, Australasia, Japan, Korea) and contains detailed information on health-care structures and processes. Available at http://www.oecd.org (accessed 28 June 2005).

References

1 Chenet L, McKee M, Fulop N *et al.* (1996). Changing life expectancy in central Europe: is there a single reason? *J Publ Health Med*, **18**, 329–36.

2 Shkolnikov V, McKee M, Leon DA (2001). Changes in life expectancy in Russia in the 1990s. *Lancet*, **357**, 917–21.

3 de Lorgeril M, Renaud S, Mamelle N *et al.* (1996). Mediterranean alpha-linolenic acid-rich diet in secondary prevention of coronary heart disease. *Lancet*, **343**, 1454–9.

4 Chenet L, McKee M, Leon D, Shkolnikov V, Vassin S (1998). Alcohol and cardiovascular mortality in Moscow, new evidence of a causal association. *J Epidemiol Comm Health*, **52**, 772–4.

5 Chenet L, Osler M, McKee M, Krasnik A (1996). Changing life expectancy in the 1980s: why was Denmark different from Sweden? *J Epidemiol Comm Health*, **50**, 404–7.

6 Leon DA, Morton S, Cannegieter S, McKee M (2003). *Understanding the health of Scotland's population in an international context*. London School of Hygiene and Tropical Medicine, London.

7 Berrino F, Gatta G, Chessa E, Valente F, Capocaccia R (1998). The EUROCARE II study. *Eur J Cancer*, **34**, 2139–53.

8 McKee M, Mossialos E, Baeten R (eds) (2002). *The impact of EU law on health care systems*. Peter Lang, Brussels.

9 Kanavos PG, McKee M (2000). Cross-border issues in the provision of health services: Are we moving towards a European Health Policy. *J Health Serv Res Policy*, **5**, 231–6.

10 MacLehose L, McKee M, Weinberg J (2002). Responding to the challenge of communicable disease in Europe. *Science*, **295**, 2047–50.

11 Mossialos E, McKee M (2002). *EU law and the social character of health care*. Peter Lang, Brussels.

12 McKee M, Rechel B, Schwalbe N. (2004). Health and the wider European neighbourhood. *EuroHealth*, **10** (3–4), 7–9.

13 Rechel B, Schwalbe N, McKee M (2004). Health in South Eastern Europe: a troubled past, an uncertain future. *Bull WHO*, **82**, 539–46.

4.9 Influencing international policy

Tim Lang and Martin Caraher

Introduction

Why bother about the international view when public health and ill-health are manifest locally? Addressing the international dimensions of public health might arguably be a luxury—something one would like to do if only there was enough time. One could argue that international affairs are best left to bodies such as the World Health Organization (WHO) or UNICEF, the UN Children's Fund. This chapter argues that these views may be common but are flawed.

Far from being an optional extra, it is now essential in public health to always ask the international questions. This might have been a luxury in the past, though we doubt it, but it is definitely essential in the modern age. Environmentalists have long subscribed to the view that citizens have to 'think globally and act locally'. Now, even this is inadequate: 21st-century public health professionals not only have to think but act internationally, even as we think and work locally.

Objectives

This chapter aims to help readers:
- identify the reasons why public health practitioners should think and work both globally and locally
- understand what can be done to advance public health at the international level
- understand the available levers for influencing international public health policy and its translation to local action.

What are the reasons for needing an international focus?

There are at least five reasons for needing an international focus:
1. Diseases are not confined by national boundaries.
2. Social and lifestyle causes of disease spread internationally.
3. Increasing numbers of people are travelling internationally.
4. Goods are travelling internationally.
5. The institutions for addressing trans-national problems are often poorly resourced and/or poorly organized to cope with the new public health challenges.

Firstly, avian flu is just the latest disease to know no boundaries. Communicable diseases have a tendency to travel, both within and between countries.

Secondly, non-communicable diseases also cross borders. For example, diet-related diseases are spreading globally due to lifestyle and social changes. Obesity and coronary heart disease (CHD) and some food-related cancers (e.g. bowel cancer)[1] are on the increase in developing countries in affluent groups with Western patterns of food consumption and health risks.

Thirdly, people are travelling increasing distances (and more rapidly) out of choice. An estimated 600 million people are international tourists each year, and they run an estimated 20–50% risk of contracting a food-borne illness.[2]

Fourthly, goods, too, are travelling increasingly, as a result of the removal of barriers to trade (e.g. through the General Agreement on Tariffs and Trade (GATT)). Generally, a revolution in the food trade has meant that more food comes longer distances: the so-called 'food miles' effect.[3] An industrial food system increases the chance of problems through breakdowns in health controls and an increase in processed food which is generally high in fat, salt and sugar.

Fifthly, political and institutional frameworks for addressing 'health trans-nationalization' are often under-resourced or not modernized to cope with economic, social, and cultural changes. Public health institutions tend to be locally and nationally based, while economic and social changes tend to be driven internationally. Risk to health is a 'threat' while trade is perceived as an 'opportunity'.[4] Despite spending most of the 1980s and 1990s dismantling public health trade barriers, the BSE crisis taught the European Union the need for stronger public health measures, resulting in the rapid alert system.[5]

In summary, the internationalization of life and culture means that health professionals also have to think and work internationally. This does not mean dropping local or national work. Whatever the work, public health protection and promotion require action on four levels simultaneously: the local, national, regional, and global. If any one is missing, the health jigsaw is incomplete.

Can anything be done about the international dimension of public health?

Achieving health-promoting change at the international level requires:
- identifying the underlying causes of ill-health
- identifying the necessary public health interventions
- arguing for action and winning policy support and resources, while dealing with ideological and other barriers.

Identifying the causes

The traditional public health response to isolate sources of ill-health and to control them is difficult if a problem is international. The modern world is highly complex and isolating causes of changing health patterns takes time and skill. The impact of economic restructuring can take decades to betray a health effect. 'Westernization' of diets and lifestyles, for instance, has shown up in new patterns of diabetes in India[6] and cancers in the developing world.[7]

It is easy to focus on symptoms rather than causes, as can happen in the case of obesity or the treatment of communicable diseases such as HIV/AIDS. There is a need to refocus on what Wilkinson[8] calls the determinants of health. For example, the food system (combined with a reduction in levels of exercise) and the type of food we eat contributes to obesity. Concentrating on altering individual behaviour ought to be accompanied, perhaps pre-empted, by a refocus 'upstream'.[9] What forces promote excessive consumption? What stops people taking exercise?

Identifying and promoting public health interventions

The use of regulation to protect public health has been politically unfashionable within the dominant neo-liberal model of economics. Regulation has been demoted in favour of a consumer-driven model, where individuals are encouraged to make their own decisions and to take responsibility for their own health. In this respect, 20th-century globalization has highlighted a choice of approaches for public health, one primarily focused on the individual and the other population oriented.[10]

Table 4.9.1 Two approaches to public health action

Policy agenda	Neo-liberal model	'New' public health or ecologic model
Relationship to general economy (health/wealth nexus)	Trickle down theory; allow for inequalities; based on markets	Reduction of inequality by state action provides health safety net
Economic direction for health policy	Individual risk insurance	Social insurance including primary care and public health services
Morality	Individual responsibility/ self-protection	Societal responsibility based on a citizenship model
Health accountancy/ costs	Costs of ill-health not included in price of goods	Costs internalized where possible
Approach to the state	Keep it minimal; avoid 'nannyism'	Potential corrective lever on the imbalance between individual and social forces
Consultation with the end user	As consumer	As citizen having a stake in the public health
Approach to problems	Target 'at risk' groups; focus on the end consumer	Population-wide; review entire chain of creation of ill-health

Food policy is a good example of where these public policy choices for health have become clear in recent years. Tensions over food standards and information given to consumers have led to questions about whether market mechanisms can be relied upon to protect public health. The social and moral questions stem directly from changes in the food economy. Health costs are 'externalized' and not reflected in the cost paid for food by consumers across the counter. This is represented schematically in Table 4.9.1, where the economic neo-liberal model based on free trade and choice is contrasted with an ecologic model of public health.

In practice it is hard to develop appropriate public health responses to global phenomena, especially at a local or regional level. Changes may seem sweeping and overwhelming. For instance, the WHO predicts that from 1997 to 2020 there will be a rapid growth of obesity and diabetes.[11] How are local and national public health approaches supposed to deal with such global phenomena? It means tackling powerful food interests, advertising and lifestyle aspects, governments, and much more. Can public health proponents really take this on? Or must they just deal with the symptoms?

Arguing for action

Once an international problem is recognized, public health professions can argue for action. This does not mean, necessarily, that they will win policy or political support for their work, but it helps. The global campaign to address HIV/AIDS is an illustration. Even governments that adopted a censorious moral stance (blaming 'lax' social mores for the spread of sexually transmitted diseases) were ultimately persuaded of the need to act. Global health action can be naked self-interest.[12]

What global policy levers do we have?

There are several institutions that operate on a global level. Table 4.9.2 summarizes these. Some are official governmental institutions, others are non-governmental and yet others commercial.

The world bodies concerned with health have adopted a number of conventions and agreements. The Convention on the Rights of the Child was adopted on 20 November 1989 and was based upon Article 49 of the UN Charter. It provides a basis for international action to ensure, for example, good food and education, both precursors to health. The WHO Code on Breastfeeding, agreed by UNICEF and the WHO in 1990 has the goal that 'all women should be enabled to practice exclusive breastfeeding and all infants should be fed exclusively on breast-milk from birth to 4–6 months'. It committed national governments to implementing a wide range of policies such as taking action on the marketing of breastfeeding supplements and to promote breastfeeding for instance in hospitals.[13] Although agreed, it has met difficulty in practice, in part due to the failure of governments, hospitals, and services to implement it, and in part due to systematic attacks by business. Companies making breast-milk substitutes have looked to developing countries as new markets, subject to fewer controls than developed economies.[14]

Table 4.9.2 Global institutions involved in health

Remit	Examples of organization/bodies
Public health	World Health Organization (WHO), Food and Agriculture Organization (FAO)
Children and health	UNICEF—UN Children's Fund, UNESCO
Global economic bodies with health impact	World Bank, International Monetary Fund, UN Conference on Trade and Development (UNCTAD), World Trade Organization (WTO), World Intellectual Property Organization (WIPO), Organisation for Economic Co-operation and Development (OECD)
Intergovernmental agreements with a health impact	Bio-safety Convention, International Conference on Nutrition, Basel Convention on hazardous waste
Emergency aid	World Food Programme, International Committee of the Red Cross/Crescent
Environmental health	Global Panel on Climate Change, UN Conference on Environment and Development (UNCED), International Maritime Organization
Commercial interests	International Chamber of Commerce, trans-national corporations, International Federation of Pharmaceutical Manufacturers Associations
Regional bodies with a health role	European Union, regional offices of WHO and FAO
Trade associations	International Hospitals Federation
Networks to promote public health ([ ] indicates UN support)	Healthy Cities Network [WHO], International Baby Food Action Network (IBFAN), Local Agenda 21 Network, Pesticides Action Network, Tobacco Free Initiative [WHO]
Professional associations	International Union for Health Promotion and Education
Non-governmental organizations	Greenpeace, Friends of the Earth, Oxfam, Médecins sans Frontières, Médecins du Monde, World Federation of Public Health Associations

The International Conference on Nutrition provides an example of a global commitment, this time by national governments, to monitor the food security of 'at risk' social groups.[15] Another is the WHO European Region's (then) 51 member states who by signing the Health for All 21 programme have committed themselves to a regional policy approach to public health. Twenty-one targets are set for the 21st century.[16] Such actions build on the 1978 Alma-Ata Declaration on Primary Health Care.[17] This committed governments to strengthen and reorient health services towards primary care and 'to respond to current and anticipated health conditions, socio-economic circumstances and needs of the people…'.[18]

In other words, there are conventions and international agreements that can justify public health action. The problem, however, is that they often seem remote and practitioners may not know about them. A health visitor trying to promote breastfeeding in the face of a local hospital flouting the WHO/UNICEF code on marketing of breast-milk substitutes might get personal satisfaction from knowing that she is right to do so, but lacks levers to get her management to put their own house in order.

Considerable education within the public health world may be needed to shake up local complacencies. Vested interests and power blocs are always strong. So alliances are needed, inside and outside the place of work. Health impact assessments (see Chapter 1.5) offer a way forward for public health workers at a local level to include a global public health perspective.

What all this entails is a need to move beyond health education and health promotion to adopting a global population perspective and a view of health that acknowledges trans-national influences on health.

Too often an international perspective in health is no more than an appeal to campaign. The work of NGOs shows how effective this can be. Campaigns about genetically modified foods or pesticides have been highly effective in encouraging debate and preventive action. Public health requires material and political, not just attitudinal, change. Policy development should be premised on the notion of consultation and alliances but there has to be action, not just promises.

Conclusion

If a global perspective teaches us that the cause of problems may be complex, it also shows us that public health cannot be achieved by individual action. Alliances are essential, across sectors as well as regions.

The international dimension to public health teaches the following:

- good public health combines the local, national, regional, and global approaches
- the international dimension makes action more complex but realistic
- health impact is never local or global but both
- international health institutions exist but need strengthening
- partnerships and alliances are essential in tackling the forces of ill-health.

Further resources

Bradshaw YW, Wallace M (1996). *Global inequalities*. Pine Forge Press, Thousand Oaks, CA.

British Medical Association (1998). *Health and environmental impact assessment*. British Medical Association, London.

Commission of the European Communities (1995). *Proposal for adopting a programme of community action on health promotion, information, education and training within the framework for action in the field of public health*. COM(95) 633 Final. Office for Official Publications of the European Communities, Luxembourg.

Commission of the European Communities (1996). *Second report from the Commission to the Council, the European Parliament, the Economic and*

Social Committee and the Committee of the Regions on the integration of health protection requirement in Community policies. COM(96) 407 Final. Commission of the European Communities, Brussels.

Drewnowski A, Popkin BM (1997). The nutrition transition: new trends in the global diet. *Nutr Rev*, **55**(2), 31–43.

Egger G, Swinburn B (1997). An 'ecological' approach to the obesity pandemic, *BMJ*, **315**, 477–80.

Environmental Health Commission (1997). *Agendas for change.* Chartered Institute of Environmental Health, London.

Howson CP, Fineberg HV, Bloom BR (1998). The pursuit of global health: the relevance of engagement for developed countries. *Lancet*, 21 February, 586–90.

Labonte R (1998). Healthy public policy and the World Trade Organisation: a proposal for an international health presence in future world trade/investment talks, *Health Promot Int*, **13**(3), 245–56.

Lang T, Heasman M (2000). *Food wars.* Earthscan, London.

Soros G (1998). *The crisis of global capitalism: open society endangered.* Little, Brown and Company, London.

Townsend P (1995). Poverty in eastern Europe: the latest manifestation of global polarisation. In: Rodgers AG, Der Hoeven V (eds) *New approaches to poverty analysis and policy III: The poverty agenda: trends and policy options,* pp. 129–52. International Institute for Labour Studies, Geneva.

Weil O, McKee M, Brodin M, Oberlé D (1999). *Priorities for public health action in the European Union.* Société Francaise de Santé Publique, Vandoeuvre-les-Nancy.

World Health Organization (1999). *Health for all in the 21st century.* World Health Organization, Copenhagen.

References

1 World Cancer Research Fund (1997). *Food, nutrition and the prevention of cancer,* Ch. 9. World Cancer Research Fund/American Institute for Cancer Research, Washington, DC.

2 Kaeferstein FK, Motarjemi Y, Bettcher DW (1997). Foodborne disease control: a transnational challenge. *Emerg Infect Dis*, **3**, 503–10.

3 Department for the Environment, Food and Rural Affairs (DEFRA) (2005). *The validity of food miles as an indicator.* DEFRA, London.

4 Unwin N, Alberti G, Aspray T et al. (1998). Economic globalisation and its effect on health. *BMJ*, **316**, 1401–2.

5 Commission of the European Communities (2000). *White Paper on food safety.* Brussels 12 January 2000, COM(1999) 719 Final. Commission of the European Communities, Brussels.

6 Ramachandran A (1998). Epidemiology of non-insulin-dependent diabetes mellitus in India. In: Shetty P, Gopalan C (eds) *Nutrition and chronic disease: an Asian perspective,* pp. 38–41. Smith-Gordon, London.

7 World Health Organization/Food and Agricultural Organization (2003). *Diet, Nutrition and the Prevention of Chronic Diseases: report of the Joint WHO/FAO consultation. Technical Report Series 916.* World Health Organization, Geneva.

8 Wilkinson R (1996). *Unhealthy societies: the afflictions of inequality.* Routledge, London.

9 McKinlay JB (1993). The promotion of health through planned socio-political change: challenges for research and policy. *Soc Sci Med,* **36**(2), 109–17.

10 Sram I, Ashton J (1998). Millennium report to Sir Edwin Chadwick. *BMJ,* **317**, 592–5.

11 World Health Organization (1999). *World Health Report 1998.* World Health Organization, Geneva.

12 Navarro V (1999). Health and equity in the world in the era of 'globalisation'. *Int J Health Serv,* **29**(2), 215–26.

13 World Health Organization/UNICEF (1990). *Breastfeeding in the 1990s: a global initiative (The Innocenti Declaration).* World Health Organization, Geneva.

14 Palmer G (1993). *The politics of breast-feeding.* Pandora, London.

15 Food and Agriculture Organization/World Health Organization (1992). *International conference on nutrition.* Food and Agriculture Organization, Rome.

16 World Health Organization Regional Office for Europe (1998). *21 targets for the 21st century—a public health guide to the targets to the Health for All policy for the European region.* European Health for All Series No. 5, World Health Organization, Copenhagen.

17 World Health Organization (1978). *Alma-Ata: primary health care,* Health for All series No 1. World Health Organization, Geneva.

18 World Health Organization (1998). *World health declaration,* paragraph III. World Health Organization, Geneva.

Part 5

Developing health system strategy

Introduction

Policies set out grand principles or courses of action, frequently with scant detail and occasionally with little apparent thought as to how they will be implemented. In this part we deal with approaches to translating health-care policies into practice. Traditionally two major steps are identified—developing strategy and making detailed plans. While using the traditional policy (strategy) planning terminology we acknowledge that many governments and organizations deploy these terms loosely and sometimes interchangeably.

Developing strategy, i.e. defining a practical means of implementing policy, is a crucial step. The World Health Organization's (WHO) early policy aspirations of eradicating smallpox failed until a new strategy, the Global Intensified Eradication Programme was adopted in the late 1960s. This new strategy maintained the same policy aim as previously but included the new methods of mass vaccination and containment of infection by vaccinating close contacts: a change in strategy that was key to delivered a great public health success.

Strategy needs to be seen both as a process (making strategy) and a product (a strategy document). As Pencheon points out (Chapter 5.1), strategy-making must involve communicating and engaging people, so that policies are properly implemented in practice. Public health practitioners should be involved in strategy because of their skills in seeing the big picture, commitment to equity and efficiency at the population level, and their technical know-how. Often public health practitioners are involved in strategy development as consultants, and in Chapter 7.6 Guest explores this role, pointing to pitfalls including self-censorship—telling clients what they want to hear rather than what they need to know.

After the policy aspirations and the strategy process or document, the third step in the chain to implementation is planning. Planning sets out the details of specific developments, allocating resources to specific actions usually over a relatively short time period. Experienced practitioners will know that policy is often confounded during the planning and implementation steps, with resources mysteriously used for unintended purposes by competing policy, managerial, or staff priorities.

In developing strategies and plans, a number of practical tools can be used and Lawrence describes the key ones in Chapter 5.2. However, the technical contributions of building an accurate picture of the problems and solutions through good information, and developing practical options and appraising them in a systematic way, are necessary but not sufficient. The most difficult task in planning is the process of changing perceptions and cultures—without this, planning documents will be just documents.

Modern health services face many common challenges, including ageing populations and the obesity epidemic. Comparing local health-care strategies with those in other countries has become popular, but Dixon (Chapter 5.3) points out the many pitfalls of crude comparisons. Transferability is often limited, with policy contexts differing in surprising ways. In addition, systems tend to be more complex than they appear and many of the popular comparison measures are crude and difficult to nterpret. Nevertheless, looking outside your own setting is always stimu-lating and sometimes salutary.

In all health-care systems resources are limited and all systems have tactics to say 'no' to some people while benefiting others. Whether the tools for prioritizing are based on ability to pay or some notion of 'need', health-care priorities should be examined and debated rather than being hidden or 'accidental'. In Chapter 5.4 Griffiths *et al.* present a framework for ensuring that the process of deciding priorities is open and fair. This chapter also points to the complexities and puts tools such as economic appraisals into a practical context: as always, technical analyses are insuf-ficient on their own to build support and legitimacy for positive action.

The poorer health status of the less privileged in most societies is well known but health services are unlikely to play a major role in creating these inequalities. Nevertheless health systems do play some role, and Donald (Chapter 5.5) identifies two basic problems: inequalities in the distribution of health-care resources and discriminatory treatment. A prescription of measurement, addressing causes and monitoring progress, is set out.

In many health-care systems, budgets and commissioning of 'blocks' of care or whole services is used as a financial and management tool in place of reimbursement of individual items of activity. While this approach controls total costs, efforts are needed to ensure that the commissioned services achieve health and equity goals. Richards (Chapter 5.6) identifies six basic elements of a commissioning agreement, including definition of the nature of services to be provided, the quantity (e.g. number of patients to be seen), the quality standards, and the price.

Throughout this part it is clear that the terms policy, strategy and planning are seen as being part of a hierarchy of time-scale, but definitely not a hierarchy of challenge or importance in achieving aims. It is clear across this part that, in many ways, the real work only starts after policy is agreed. To implement policy involves a cascade of technical steps as well as inclusion of those affected: these tasks provide many opportuni-ties for public health practitioners to protect and promote health.

DM

5.1 An introduction to health-care strategy

David Pencheon

What is strategy?

Strategy is about where you want to be in 5 years. Strategy is both a process and a product (although a common pitfall is to over-emphasize the latter)—a methodological framework for achieving a vision. A good strategy should identify those key steps that need to be taken (that wouldn't happen anyway) that are critical to achieving the changes needed over 5 years. The key to this is to identify what would happen if you did nothing; this should help identify the important parts of the strategy. Although strategy is quite distinct from short-term (tactical) planning, strategy must inform the detailed planning process, indeed it should be one of the most important pieces of guidance for the planning process. Planning that ignores strategy suggests a poor strategic process. Conversely, strategy should be informed, although not dominated, by the same sort of intelligence that feeds the planning processes. Similarly strategy that ignores the policy context will result in poor strategy. Hence there is an important relationship between the policy process, strategy, and planners.

Why have strategies?

We have strategies like we have most other tools—in order to help us do things better. Strategies provide a vision and a framework. In the world of health this helps a wide range of partners contribute to understanding, appreciating, and addressing key issues in ways that are similarly prioritized and articulated.

Why should public health practitioners be involved with strategy?

- Public health and strategy are both concerned with the big picture.
- Public health potentially affects a lot of people.
- Public health can consume a lot of resources.
- If public health practitioners don't get involved with strategy, it is unlikely that other population perspectives such as need, equity, effectiveness, etc. will get the attention they deserve.

- Strategy development is an uncertain process that requires people who can cope with uncertainty without descending into vagueness.
- As a public health practitioner you will almost undoubtedly get involved with strategy both in terms of technical public health and epidemiological input, and in terms of management and leadership.

The relationship with planning

Strategies are about broad visions and directions, not specific plans. Strategy development is about communication, involving and engaging people in the key issues, and developing a shared framework for addressing such issues.

A 'strategy' consists of more of a journey and a process (reaching a consensus, understanding, being creative, developing, etc.) rather than being simply a product (the documentation) of a specific agenda for action. Strategies are about visions and the key steps necessary; plans are about *all* the tasks necessary. Planning needs to be guided by strategies. The reverse is also true; planners may feed into the strategy process by providing guidance on whether some of the assumptions made are supported or refuted by data, evidence, and opinion. That doesn't mean that the content of any strategy must be exclusively material for which there is a strong and traditional evidence base, although equally it does not mean that the those who are responsible for developing a strategy have a licence to ignore the facts. The domination of strategies by quantitative evidence is a threat to creativity and lateral thought in identifying the best ways of achieving the vision or goal.

Table 5.1.1 Planning compared with strategy development

Planning	Strategy development
Data should focus thought and action	Data should broaden thought and action
Progression in small incremental and predictable steps	Progression in a less predictable time and direction due to novel and creative possibilities
Concentrates on systematic aggregated information	Depends on synthesizing themes from a wide perspective involving intuition, creativities, and spontaneity
Analysis through the planning process may feed into strategy development	The articulation and elaboration of a strategy helps formulate operational plans

The key question for *planners* is: 'what are the most important issues to address now in order to ensure the strategy is most likely to be delivered'. In summary, don't confuse strategy development with planning (see Table 5.1.1).

Relationship with policy

Policy is 'a course of action or principle adopted or proposed by a government, party, business, or individual'. Good strategy is both informed by the principles inherent in relevant policies and, in turn, informs the practicalities of putting policy into action. Both policy and strategy offer sound frameworks. The practical difference is that policy is often articulated in more general terms; giving substance to the philosophy and ethics of the rules of the organization. Strategy, when developed, is an altogether more practical road map, informed by practical considerations of opportunities and obstacles in order to make a vision real. Planning concerns the day-to-day details of how the key steps to strategy are achieved over months and years.

Table 5.1.2 The relationships between policy, strategy, and planning: with examples

Policy	Strategy	Planning
Specific principles adopted by organizations, teams etc. often based as much on politics as information. Heavily influenced by objective information, politics, public opinion, and the media (but not necessarily in that order)	The key steps that need to be taken (that wouldn't happen anyway) that are critical to achieving the changes needed over 5 years. Needs to be supported by good intelligence. However, such input should not unduly constrain creative thinking	All the steps that need to be taken to achieve the key steps of the strategy. Progression takes place in small, incremental, and predictable steps. Logistic exercise
Example: It is the policy of the ambulance service to take severely injured people to trauma centres not necessarily the nearest emergency department	Example: the strategic intent of the local health department is to ensure that within 5 years nowhere in the area is more than 30 min ambulance travel time from a trauma centre	Example: the detailed day-by-day project plan of how the local trauma service will be developed over the next year

Whilst strategies are about the long-term vision, policy is about specific principles (we have a policy of only providing services in secondary care that cannot safely be delivered in primary care; we have a policy of not providing social care to people who . . .) on which such strategies are both designed and then subsequently implemented (see Table 5.1.2).

What factors are associated with successful strategies?

- *Shared values and vision.* A strategy needs to incorporate the shared values and vision of a critical mass of the people who will carry it through and actually implement it.
- *Direction and priorities.* Any strategy to which the reader's response is: 'I now have a much better idea of where this organization, initiative, etc., is going' is likely to be successful. The converse is true. A strategy should set out clearly a jargon-free vision and provide a long-term framework for planning where the key issues can be identified in such a way that they can be addressed by planners.
- *Iterative process not polished products.* Involving the right people and organizations in the right way is crucial for successful strategy development. This is not about participation for the sake of it. Strategies have uncertain directions initially, and cannot look over the horizon. The likelihood of aiming at the right part of the horizon is increased by broad but judicious early involvement of key people.
- *Link to policy, planning, and other strategies.* Strategy development that does not acknowledge the policy context nor the needs of planners in taking forward the key issues will fail.
- *Continuous reflection.* Strategic planning is an uncertain process, especially early on. Reflection and restating of recorded objectives, issues, processes, and direction is important to keep people focused without constraining lateral thinking.

Pitfalls in strategy

- *Over-emphasizing the product rather than the process.* Both are important, but there is no shortage of impressive strategy documents gathering dust. This is usually due to lack of clarity, engagement (with both the right people and the relevant policy context), evaluation, and implementation.
- *Getting bogged down with complexity.* Strategy development can quickly get highly complex. To minimize the complications, first ensure you are constantly reminded of the broad objectives of the strategy. This must be done with care, as too much focus can really constrain creative thought. Second, try and be as practical and simple as possible, again without constraining thought. Keeping focused is important, but ensure you keep people more focused on the objectives/possible destination and not on the minutiae of the route.

Further resources

Mintzberg H (1994). The rise and fall of strategic planning. *Harvard Business Rev*, Jan–Feb, 107–14.

Mintzberg H, Ahlstrand B, Lampel J (1998). *Strategy safari: a guided tour through the wilds of strategic management*. Prentice-Hall, London.

Mintzberg H, Quinn JB (1991). *The strategy process: concepts, contexts, cases*, 2nd edn. Prentice-Hall, Englewood Cliffs, NJ.

Porter M (1996). What is strategy? *Harvard Business Rev*, Nov–Dec, 61–78.

Whittington R (1993). *What is strategy and does it matter?* Routledge, London. (Reviewed in the *Journal for Management Learning*, **25**(1), 1994.)

'It is a mistake to look too far ahead. Only one link of the chain of destiny can be handled at a time.'

Winston Spencer Churchill

'Most people overestimate what they can accomplish in one year and underestimate what they can achieve in a decade.'

Anthony Robbins

'Be bold in strategy and careful in tactics.'

Anon.

'A vision without a task is a dream, a task without a vision is drudgery.'
Black Elk, Holy Man of the Oglala Sioux

5.2 Strategic approaches to planning health services

David Lawrence

Objectives

This chapter shows you how to contribute to successful planning of health services at the strategic level.

What is health services planning?

Planning converts policy aspirations into practical efforts to change patterns of health (and social) service provision. It aims to deliver specified objectives by examining options for change and choosing a desired course. The result should be the mapping out of an efficient and effective way forward.[1]

A health service is a system—a set of interconnected elements, where what happens in one part of the system affects the rest, so that they act together as a whole.[2] System approaches to planning are therefore useful.[2]

Health services systems

A health service is a complex economic input–output system. Patients with a need for care, demand (in economics usage) to use a service and, together with professionals and plant, are the inputs. The primary outputs are health outcomes: changes in patients' health status and quality of life. Health services differ from most other economic systems in important ways which will affect your ability to plan successfully:

- The usual pyramidal power hierarchy is inverted: doctors and other frontline health-care professionals are numerous, wield political and managerial power, and effectively control resource use in the system.
- Most users of health care have relatively little health knowledge and so consumer sovereignty and choice are limited.
- Health care has a special political and social position in most societies.

Conceptual frameworks for planning

One framework for health-care planning, e.g. Guy[3] and Box 5.2.1, is a rational system framework:

- identify a future desired state
- compare it with the present state

- identify possible pathways from one to the other (options)
- implement the most cost-effective pathway.

This so-called 'hard system' approach works best where there are well-defined, material-based and structured systems, with easily identifiable objectives, for example in car production. Health services are 'soft' systems: people-based, with complex difficult-to-define objectives. Here, 'soft' systems planning is likely to be more successful. This approach includes:

- intervention in a continual, iterative, cycle
- recognition of cultural constraints
- participation in planning by all those involved in the system
- approaching the problem using both systems and 'real world' (pragmatic or 'corporate') thinking.[2]

Table 5.2.1 shows various conceptual frameworks summarizing a health-care 'soft' system and a commodity 'hard' system (car manufacture).

Table 5.2.1 Models and examples of input–output systems

'Input–output' model	Input	Input	Output 1	Output 2	Output 3
'Medical care' model	Need	Demand	Activity	Outcome 1	Outcome 2
Donabedian model[a]	Structure	Process	Process	Outcome 1	Outcome 2
Health services example: ophthalmology	Cataract patients, doctors, optometrists etc., managers, plant	Appointments requested for eye examination	Cataract extractions/ lens implants performed	Change in visual functioning	Vision-related quality of life. Patient utility
Commodity production example: car manufacture	Workers, managers, materials, plant	Producers' decisions to manufacture	Cars produced	Cars sold	Cars used. User utility

[a]See Chapter 6.1.

Box 5.2.1* Rational system planning case study: planning cleft lip and palate services in England[4]

In 1998 the UK Clinical Standards Advisory Group (CSAG) report on cleft lip and palate services recommended replacing the 57 centres in England with 8–15 cleft centres, because of good evidence that better clinical outcomes would be achieved in well-staffed centres with higher case-loads.[5] The recommendations were accepted by government and professional organizations. The Cleft Implementation Group (CIG) was set up to help implement these recommendations, which were expected to take a year. The final site in England was finally designated in 2005.

Factors which influenced the implementation of changes in cleft care were:

- the sound evidence base for the changes, derived from the CSAG research
- the broad support for the CSAG recommendations from government, clinicians, and patients
- the close involvement of the patients' and parents' support group, the Cleft Lip and Palate Association.

Factors which hindered implementation were:

- lack of clarity about the role of the CIG, which was advisory, with no managerial powers
- dealing with the service changes on an England-wide, rather than a UK-wide basis, following devolution of powers to other UK countries
- unrealistic estimates of the time necessary to achieve service changes that needed resource allocation, negotiation between multiple existing providers, consultants and other appointments to new centres, sometimes capital developments and frequently public consultation, with subsequent referral to Ministers for decisions
- changes in NHS structures during the process, with consequent alterations in responsibility for service commissioning and monitoring
- changes in civil service staffing at the Department of Health which resulted in fragmented support to the group
- lack of clarity in some of the guidance that was issued to the NHS about the process
- difficulties in reaching agreement with representative and professional bodies about the process of appointment to the new teams.

Decisions have now been reached about the sites of the new centres in England, but concerns remain:

- strategic planning structures are still diffuse: will they have the capacity to deal adequately with detailed planning and monitoring of the services?
- it is not clear whether enforceable arrangements to deal with disagreements about funding are in place.

(See also the UK Department of Health website.[6])

* by kind permission of Dr. June Crown

Strategic planning

Strategic planning sets out overall approaches or methods for achieving policy objectives. It typically involves whole or large parts of health service systems and time-scales of years. Operational or management planning details the specific tasks which will deliver the policy and strategy; usually these plans are shorter term and cover smaller units and individual departments.

In order to ensure that your planning efforts yield net benefits, it is necessary to understand both how a health-care system operates and its external environment. Planning the external environment is usually on a whole country or state scale and is the subject of health policy.[7]

The planning process will vary depending on health-care funding arrangements. The system may be funded:

• publicly, by taxes or by regulated socially-based insurance
• privately, by commercial risk-based insurance or fees for services
• a mixture of these.

Publicly funded services are sometimes needs based, with a needs-based planning process. Conversely, private funding and provision usually have a demand-based market planning process.[8] In many countries there is a mixture of the two. Though these two approaches may differ fundamentally at the whole-country level, the practical planning processes at the local level often have common elements.

What are the approaches to subdividing planning into defined tasks?

'Rational satisficing' policy-making[7] is akin to 'hard' systems planning, whereas pragmatic, incrementalist policy-making[7] is akin to 'soft' systems planning. In practice, planning is usually a mixture of 'rational' and 'pragmatic' processes.

One key public health skill is to judge for any given planning situation how much the rational and pragmatic strands are going to influence the outcomes (see Table 5.2.2).

The order of tasks in effective strategic planning

The first type of task is organizational: working with the people responsible for planning health care in such a way that they ask you to help achieve their planning imperatives. You can achieve this by showing them how you and the tools you use will support and improve their planning decisions.

The most important and difficult part of the planning process is coming across changed perceptions, understanding, knowledge, and cultures, especially in 'soft' systems. Here, knowing why and how people have the views and behaviour that they do, is paramount.

Table 5.2.2 'Rational satisficing' or 'incremental' planning—which approach will work?

	Favourable to rational evidence-based planning	Favourable to pragmatic, incremental or 'corporate' planning
Use of technical information and quantitative modelling	Available, understood, believed, and used	Missing, not believed, and not used
Degree of concern to, or opposition to change from, powerful pressure groups in society	Not controversial, little concern	Controversial, great concern
Degree of consensus between most pluralist groups in the society	High consensus	Low consensus
Local or central control	Local flexibility	Central, target-driven
Type of system: nature of objectives	'Hard' well-understood system with well-defined objectives	'Soft' difficult-to-understand system with difficult-to-define objectives

You will need to work with:

- Managers and clinicians in organizations who are involved in purchasing (or commissioning) and providing health care.
- Patients and users. They will have experienced most of the good and bad aspects of any system, but to be most effective patients need training in the planning role, just as professionals do. Citizens' panels can be a good way to do this,[9,10] but are time-consuming and expensive.
- There are likely to be existing planning groups and you will need to work with these to be effective, but to be useful these planning groups need to be part of the power structure, with authority over budgets (see Box 5.2.1).

The second type of task you will usually need to carry out is to help develop specific options for implementing policy, including new 'models of clinical care', involving changes to inputs or processes (see Box 5.2.1 for example). Your role is to present to commissioners and providers research evidence on the effectiveness of relevant clinical interventions, organizing clinical work, and knowledge of the way health-care systems work.

The third type of task you will do is provide information for planning.[11] This includes quantifying how the new models of care will affect health service patterns of provision, activity, budgets, and outcomes. Models can be useful for this, including 'whole systems' models, such as the 'balance of care' model. Though this was developed for planning continuing care of older people,[1,12] it is in fact a universal tool. This model involves defining the need for care, specifying the mix and amount of professional and technical resources needed to meet that need, and, crucially, estimating the costs of those resources. It provides 'what ifs', rather than definitive answers, and helps to look at the outcomes and resource and budget implications of possible changes.

The output from the above tasks is usually an implementation plan for a strategy or project proposal, using an agreed work plan.

The final type of task, dissemination and supporting decision-making, is to work through the implications of the policy options produced in earlier tasks. The planning cycle then begins again with the monitoring and evaluation tasks, to determine what effect implemented changes are having on the health system.

Potential pitfalls in health planning

Completing the implementation of planning decisions usually takes years. Often you will not have that time, but the framework presented here can help produce the most benefit in the time you have.

To save time you may, for example, have to use estimates from others rather than undertake your own needs survey. The aim of using information in planning is to give planners an understanding of how changing resources will affect how the system works. That is, it is a marginal process in the health economics sense.

Planning rarely goes 'according to plan' as circumstances and personnel change.

The intended objectives in planning are usually only partially attained and there are often unintended consequences. Therefore monitoring the effects of planning and making adjustment are crucial.

Myths and fallacies about health planning

- *Planning is rational and evidence based*: it is usually a mix of pragmatic and rational.
- *Planning is a one-off*: planning is continual and evolves.
- *Planning stifles creativity*: planning can help creativity by allowing an orderly process.
- *Planning is trying to predict the future: to give the 'right' answer*: planning is providing intelligence on what might happen in complex systems so as to allow more effective decision-making.

Examples of success and failure in health planning and lessons learnt

The planning of the specialist cleft lip and palate services for England (Box 5.2.1) is a very good example of the reality of planning. The report[4] is essential reading for all would-be planners, showing the difficulties in implementing an evidence-based clinical care model.[5]

One successful planning example is the development and implementation of a business planning model at a hospital in England.[13]

Key determinants of success
- As in many areas, a key skill is to know what is feasible and to work well with people.
- Do the technical homework, especially presenting information and evidence in a way which politicians, managers, and clinicians will understand and find useful.
- Be useful, for example find information on the most pressing concerns managers and clinicians have.

How will you know if you have been successful?

- *Monitoring and evaluation.* Success is usually not absolute. Obviously there should be specific objectives and measurement of their attainment. But success, like the planning process, is iterative, it comes little-by-little. That implies that monitoring and evaluation are essential to successful planning.
- *Feedback.* Discussions with colleagues and formal evaluations, including workshops, are important.

Further resources

Brownson RC, Baker EA, Leet TL, Gillespie KN (2003). *Evidence based public health.* Oxford University Press, New York.

Department of Health. Available at: http://www.dh.gov.uk/Home/fs/en (accessed 28 June 2005; search 'health care planning').

Hunter D (2002). Management and public health. In Detels R, McEwen J, Beaglehole R, Tanaka H (eds) *Oxford textbook of public health, pp. 921–35.* Oxford University Press, Oxford.

Thai KV, Wimberley ET, McManus SM (2003). *Handbook of international health care systems.* Marcel Dekker, New York.

References

1 McCallion G (1993). Planning care for elderly people. *Health Serv Manage Sci,* **6**(4), 218–28.

2 Van Wyk G (2003). *A systems approach to social and organizational planning.* Trafford Publishing, Victoria, BC.

3 Guy M (2001). Diabetes: developing a local strategy. In: Pencheon D, Guest C, Melzer D, Gray JAM (eds) *Oxford handbook of public health practice,* 1st edn, p. 559. Oxford University Press, Oxford.

4 Crown J (2003). *Cleft lip and palate services.* Report from the Cleft Implementation Group and Cleft Monitoring Group. Available at: http://ehims.org.uk/phlearningwiki/index.php?title=Health_care_strategic_management (accessed January 13, 2006).

5 Clinical Standards Advisory Group (1998). *Cleft lip and/or palate: report of the CSAG Committee.* The Stationery Office, London.

6 Department of Health website. Available at: http://www.dh.gov.uk/ (accessed 4 June 2006).

7 Walt G (1994). *Health policy: an introduction to process and power.* Zed Books, London.

8 Green A (1999). *An introduction to health planning in developing countries.* Oxford University Press, Oxford.

9 Abelson J, Eyles J, McLeod CB, Collins P, McMullan C, Forest-Pierre G (2003). Does deliberation make a difference? Results from a citizens panel study of health goals priority setting. *Health Policy*, **66**(1), 95–106.

10 Church J, Saunders D, Wanke M, Pong R, Spooner C, Dorgan M (2002). Citizen participation in health decision-making: past experience and future prospects *J Public Health Pol*, **23**(1), 12–32.

11 Bullas S, Ariotti D (2002). *Information for managing healthcare resources.* Radcliffe Medical Press, Abingdon.

12 Forte P, Bowen T (1997). Improving the balance of elderly care services. In: Cropper S, Forte P (eds) *Enhancing health services management*, pp. 71–85. Open University Press, Buckingham.

13 Bowen T, Forte P (1997). Activity and capacity planning in an acute hospital. In: Cropper S, Forte P (eds) *Enhancing health services management*, pp. 86–102. Open University Press, Buckingham.

'Planning is an unnatural process. It is much more fun to just do something. That way failure comes as a complete surprise, rather than being preceded by a period of worry and depression.'

John Harvey-Jones

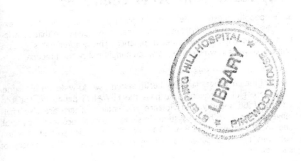

5.3 Learning from international models of funding and delivering health care

Anna Dixon

Selective perception is the original sin of comparative studies

Klein (1991, p. 278)[1]

Introduction and objectives

This chapter will help you appreciate the benefits and pitfalls of learning from other health systems, familiarize you with different models of funding and delivering health care, and give you some analytical tools to enable you to critically review health system policies in other countries and apply learning to your own context.

Why learn from other countries?

Some people question the value of participation in international exchanges and cross-national research. It seems an indulgence that contributes little to national public health practice. This chapter will suggest a number of ways in which such work can benefit policy and practice.

Common challenges

Many of the challenges faced by health systems world-wide are the same. There are global challenges such as the HIV/AIDS pandemic, tobacco control, food security, and violence and conflict. There are also challenges common to health systems in similar political, economic, cultural, and social contexts (see Box 5.3.1). Working together to find common solutions prevents duplication of effort and increases the chances of success.

Box 5.3.1 Examples of common challenges to health systems

- Political legacy: restructuring large hospital sectors in the former Soviet Union.
- Economic development: allocating limited public resources to health care in low-income countries.
- Social and cultural norms: changing alcohol consumption patterns in Scandinavia.
- Population profiles: meeting the health-care needs of indigenous populations in Australia and Canada.
- Demographic trends: funding long-term care for a rapidly ageing population in many countries.
- Epidemiologic trends: combating childhood obesity in the USA and other industrialized countries.

International agencies

International agencies are playing an increasingly important role in the development of health systems (see Box 5.3.2 and Chapters 4.8 and 4.9). It is only through cooperation that their impact can be evaluated and through multilateral action that policies can be changed.

Box 5.3.2 International agencies and health systems

The World Health Organization has strengthened its focus on health systems.[2] New public–private partnerships have been established such as the Global Fund to Fight AIDS, TB and Malaria. The World Bank directly shapes health system reforms in countries where it lends and influences global debate. Despite the limited public health remit of the European Union, through the European Working Time Directive, internal market policies and decisions of the European Court of Justice, the EU is having a profound effect on health systems in member states.[3] There is growing concern that the liberalization of trade in services under the General Agreement on Trade in Services (GATS) of the World Trade Organization has the potential to undermine public health systems.

Benchmarking

By comparing health systems across a range of indicators you can highlight areas where improvements may be needed. League tables and rankings of health systems, hospitals, and individual clinical performance have been criticized.[4] Indeed crude comparisons of inputs can be misleading (more below). Comparing process indicators can highlight inefficiencies (see Box 5.3.3). Outcomes are the most useful but care needs to be taken to adjust for case mix (see Box 5.3.4).

Avoid mistakes

Other countries have experience from which you can learn. Evaluating their policies and practices can ensure mistakes are not repeated.

Policy transfer

Looking at how another country organizes its health services may give rise to new policy ideas. Sometimes it is difficult to think creatively because of the constraints of how things have always been done.

Box 5.3.3 Comparing the length of stay in hospitals

A number of studies have compared the performance of the NHS in England with Kaiser Permanente (KP), a managed care organization based in California, USA. One prompted much debate about the validity of the comparison, the standardization and adjustments made to the data, and the conclusions drawn.[5] However, another study comparing hospital utilization in the over-65s by procedure has led to some interesting insights[6]. It found that the standardized length of stay for some procedures was five to six times higher in the NHS than in KP. Length of stay was consistent across age ranges in KP, whereas within the NHS length of stay increased with age. This has prompted further investigation into the use of intermediate care and intensive home-care services which enable older patients to be discharged promptly when they no longer have a need for medical care.

Box 5.3.4 Comparing cancer outcomes in Europe

The EUROCARE project (http://www.eurocare.it) (accessed 12 January 2006) is an international collaborative study on the survival of cancer patients in Europe. It uses population-based cancer registries in 22 European countries to compare survival rates of different cancers. These data, which showed England had lower survival rates in comparison with other European countries, were cited by Wanless[7] to highlight the need for increased investment in the NHS to improve cancer care.

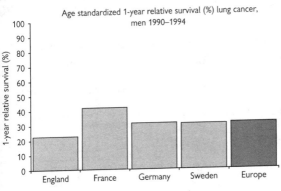

Age standardized 1-year relative survival (%) lung cancer, men 1990–1994

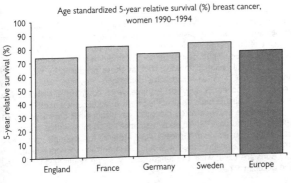

Age standardized 5-year relative survival (%) breast cancer, women 1990–1994

Potential pitfalls in learning from other systems abroad

Despite the benefits of cross-national research it can easily be misused or misinterpreted.

Transferability

Even if you were to identify an apparently successful public health policy or practice in another setting, will it work in the same way? Probably not. The context in which a policy is implemented is often as critical to its success as the content of the policy. Try and be systematic about analyzing context. Table 5.3.1 sets out some of the dimensions to consider.

Table 5.3.1 Dimensions of the context of policy (based on Leichter)[9]

Dimensions of context	Definition	Examples
Situational factors	Major but transient events	New Minister of Health appointed
Structural factors	Constant features of the political and economic system	Decentralized health-care system
Cultural factors	Values and norms	Preference for professional paternalism
Environmental factors	External to the specific policy arena	Accession to the European Union

Comparability

Arguments such as 'We have too many/too few hospital beds/ nurses/doctors' or 'We spend too much/too little on health compared with the rest of Europe/the world' tend to dominate policy debates. Such comparisons of crude inputs do not support informed decision-making.

International health databases, such as those produced by the OECD and the WHO, try to standardize definitions. However, national data collection procedures vary. For example, when counting beds should you include all available beds or all staffed beds or all occupied beds?

Even where a standardized measure is available what does Figure 5.3.1 tell you? If you have fewer beds than another country is that a good or bad thing? On its own it means very little. If, for example, you were interested in efficiency then it would be important to understand how the beds are used, what the length of stay is, the readmission rate, and the occupancy rate.

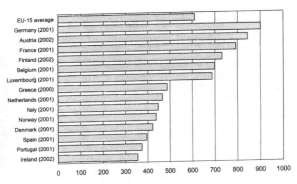

Figure 5.3.1 Number of hospital beds per 100,000 population in selected European countries. (Source: WHO Health for All database, June 2004 http://www.who.dk/hfadb (accessed 28 June 2005))

Complexity

A danger of cross-national learning is to isolate one element of the health system without understanding the complex interactions with other parts of the system. For example, the policy to give patients the choice of going to any hospital has been credited with a reduction in surgical waiting times in Denmark. However, factors such as spare capacity in other hospitals, patients' willingness to travel, and a sufficiently generous payment transfer between county councils were also critical to its success. (See Box 5.3.5 and Chapter 6.9.)

Box 5.3.5 Questions to ask when engaging in cross-national learning

- What is the problem I face? Which other countries are facing a similar problem?
- What solutions have other countries tried? Have they worked? Why?
- What data would help me find out? Are they available?
- Are the data comparable, up-to-date, and accurate?
- What factors contributed to the success of the policy? Are these factors present here? What adaptations or changes would be needed?
- What else was going on? How important were contextual factors?

Different models of health-care funding and delivery

From Bismarck to Beveridge and beyond?

Since the 19th century, western European welfare states have been dominated by two models of health-care financing and delivery: Bismarck and Beveridge (see Table 5.3.2). Chancellor Bismarck introduced national health insurance to Germany in 1883. Aneurin Bevan, the British Minister of Health in 1948, is usually honoured as the founder of the National Health Service (NHS). However, it was the Beveridge Report which laid the foundations for the NHS. Other countries introduced similar models later in the 20th century. The Soviet Union and eastern bloc countries had a centrally-planned and state-funded system of health care called the Semashko model named after the Minister for Health of the Russian Republic. Subsequent reforms in most countries mean these models no longer exist in practice. In order to analyze modern health systems you need to understand the decisions that health policy-makers have made about how to finance and deliver health-care services.

Table 5.3.2 Key features of the Bismarck and Beveridge models of health care

	Bismarck	Beveridge
Entitlement based on…	Contribution status	Citizenship/residence
Revenues from…	Wage deductions, employees and employers pay half each	General taxation
Benefits covered are…	Defined (explicit rationing)	Comprehensive (implicit rationing)
Insurance provided by…	Occupational sickness fund managed by joint boards of workers' representatives (usually the trade unions) and the business representatives	State
Relationship with providers	Contracts or patient reimbursement	Integrated

Strategic choices

There are a series of strategic choices that determine the organization of funding and delivery of health care in any country. Understanding how different countries have answered these questions will give you a good basis for assessing the health system.

Box 5.3.6 Questions to ask when assessing health-care systems

- How much money is collected, and who decides this?
- Who collects the money, and from whom?
- Who and what is covered?
- How are resources pooled?
- How are resources allocated to purchasers?
- Is there choice between insurers/purchasers?
- From whom are services bought and how?
- At what price are services bought and how are services paid for?
- Where are the services delivered and by whom?

Collecting the money

Ultimately all the money that is spent on health care comes from individuals and households. There are a number of different methods of raising revenues: general taxation (through direct or indirect taxes), social insurance contributions (compulsory levies on wages), private health insurance premiums, direct charges to patients, or charitable donations. As Figure 5.3.2 shows, most OECD countries fund the majority of health care from either taxation or social health insurance contributions, with the exception of the USA where only 44% of total expenditure on health is publicly funded.

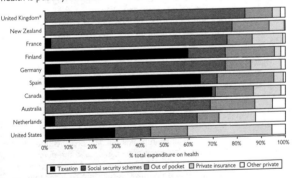

Figure 5.3.2 Breakdown of expenditure on health by source of revenues, selected OECD countries 2000. (Source: OECD Health Data 2003 and *private data 1996.)

To make or buy?

The third party agent, such as the state or insurance fund, responsible for providing services to patients, has several choices about how to provide health-care services:

- reimburse the patient for costs incurred
- reimburse the providers for costs incurred
- contract with providers and set out agreed terms and conditions

● directly employ or own providers.

Each of these options has advantages and disadvantages, some of which are discussed elsewhere in this volume (see Chapter 5.6).

Getting value for money

How producers of services are financially rewarded has implications for efficiency (see Box 5.3.7). Financial incentives are, however, not the only factors that drive provider behaviour. Other rules and sanctions, professional ethics, and personal goals and objectives also play a role.

Box 5.3.7 Options for paying health-care providers

● *Capitation*: a fixed sum per head over a defined period of time. Commonly used in general practice where doctors are responsible for a registered population.
● *Salary*: a fixed sum for working a set amount of time unrelated to activity. Used in hospitals and for non-physician staff. Increasingly combined with performance-related pay.
● *Fee for service*: an amount per item of service. Occasionally used to pay hospitals and hospital doctors, more common in ambulatory care. Often pre-negotiated rates.
● *Budgets*: fixed sum for a fixed period unrelated to activity. Calculated on the basis of historical allocations or historical or predicted levels of activity. May be hard (any overrun or underspend is borne by the provider) or soft (an indicative budget).
● *Per diem*: a fixed amount per day. Used extensively in the past for hospital care but incentives for excessive lengths of stay. Still used for hotel costs.
● *Per case or episode payments*: a fixed amount for each admitted patient or spell of activity. Diagnosis-related groups (DRGs) are the most commonly used. Payment associated with primary diagnosis on admission, often with case-mix adjustment for severity.

Public or private providers?

The ownership status of hospitals has become more complex with the increasing role of private finance in capital building projects, the franchising of hospital management to private companies, and the outsourcing of a number of non-clinical and clinical services. The dichotomy between public and private ownership is no longer a sufficient basis for the evaluation of hospital performance.[10] An assessment of the level of state control versus provider control over aspects of the organization such as pay and conditions, private capital, disposal of assets, and scope of services, can give a fuller picture (see Figure 5.3.3).

Integration

Another important dimension of health-care delivery is the extent to which providers are integrated. The organizational relationships will influence the level of cooperation, coordination, and incentives. Horizontal integration is where groups of providers at the same level form a single organization. For example, a cooperative of general practitioners or a single company which owns a chain of acute hospitals. Vertical integration

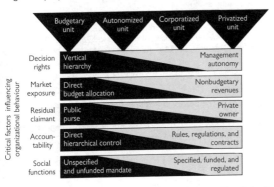

Figure 5.3.3 Factors influencing the organizational behaviour of hospital units. (Based on Preker and Harding[10] p. 49.)

is where a single organization provides care at different levels. For example a health maintenance organization which employs family doctors and runs its own hospitals and home-care services. Virtual integration describes providers that work together without being part of a single organization. For example, a tertiary cancer centre may be virtually integrated with oncologists and radiologists working in general hospitals and palliative care facilities as part of a cancer network.

Summary

Armed with some of the basic concepts about the organization of health-care systems set out in this chapter, you should be able to:

- more effectively critique published comparative studies
- participate more effectively in cross-national learning
- begin to appreciate the diversity of policy options for funding and delivering health care
- contribute more confidently to wider policy debates on health-care reform.

This chapter is only a starting point. For those with an appetite for more, there are many sources of written information (see Further resources), but nothing beats visiting a country and finding out for yourself how things really work in practice.

Further resources

Useful websites

European Observatory on Health Systems and Policies. http://www.euro.who.int/observatory (accessed 28 June 2005).
European Union. http://europa.eu.int/ (accessed 28 June 2005).

Global Fund. http://www.theglobalfund.org/en/ (accessed 28 June 2005).

Health Policy Monitor. http://www.healthpolicymonitor.org/index.jsp (accessed 28 June 2005).

Organisation for Economic Co-operation and Development (OECD). http://www.oecd.org (accessed 28 June 2005).

World Bank. http://www.worldbank.org/ (accessed 28 June 2005).

World Health Organization. http://www.who.int/en/ (accessed 28 June 2005).

World Trade Organization. http://www.wto.org/ (accessed 28 June 2005).

Further reading

Freeman R (2000). *The politics of health in Europe*. Manchester University Press, New York.

McKee M, Healy J (eds) (2002). *Hospitals in a changing Europe*. European Observatory on Health Care Systems, Open University Press, Buckingham.

Mossialos E, Dixon A, Figueras J et al. (eds) (2002). *Funding health care: options for Europe*. European Observatory on Health Care Systems, Open University Press, Buckingham.

References

1 Klein R (1991). Risk and benefits of comparative studies: notes from another shore. *Milbank Q*, **69**(2), 275–91.

2 World Health Organization (2000). *The World Health Report 2000: health systems: improving performance*. World Health Organization, Geneva.

3 Mossialos E, McKee M (2002). Health care and the European Union. *BMJ*, **324**(7344), 991–2.

4 Marshall MN, Shekelle PG, Leatherman S, Brook RH (2000). The public release of performance data: what do we expect to gain? A review of the evidence. *J Am Med Assoc*, **283**(14), 1866–74.

5 Feachem RG, Sekhri NK, White KL (2002). Getting more for their dollar: a comparison of the NHS with California's Kaiser Permanente. *BMJ*, **324**(7330), 135–41.

6 Ham C, York N, Sutch S, Shaw R (2003). Hospital bed utilisation in the NHS, Kaiser Permanente, and the US Medicare programme: analysis of routine data. *BMJ*, **327**(7426), 1257.

7 Wanless D (2001). *Securing our future health: taking a long-term view. An interim report*. HM Treasury, London.

8 Benedict R (1935). *Patterns of culture*. Routledge and Kegan Paul, London.

9 Leichter HM (1979). *A comparative approach to policy analysis: health care policy in four nations*. Cambridge University Press, Cambridge.

10 Preker AS, Harding A (2003). *Innovations in health service delivery: the corporatization of public hospitals*. World Bank, Washington, DC.

'Experience is the name everyone gives to their mistakes.'

Oscar Wilde

'Comparative studies release us from boundaries of our habits of thought, and show us the wide gamut of pattern possible in human interaction.'

Benedict[8]

5.4 Setting priorities in health care

Siân Griffiths, Tony Jewell, and Tony Hope

Introduction

Making the best use of limited resources in a health-care system depends on:
- adopting the most efficient care processes
- optimizing the allocation of limited care resources between potential beneficiaries.

All health-care systems have limited resources, and effectively exclude categories of treatment or groups of people: scarcity of resources is a fact of life everywhere. Saying 'no' to some people whilst others benefit is not a comfortable thing to do, but is a thing in which many people in public health are necessarily involved.

In private insurance systems, specific exclusions and co-payments are commonly used rationing tactics. These systems vary in the efforts they make to act with fairness or to limit the negative health effects of their rationing strategies.

Government funded systems based on reimbursement (e.g. US Medicare) ration through refusing to reimburse certain types of activities, as well as undertaking some strategic planning and control of health facilities.

Needs-based health-care systems (run by government or health maintenance organizations) often have empowered stakeholder groups, and rationing or priority setting comes under intense scrutiny.

Competition for resources is often driven by new technologies becoming available, or growing demand for treatment due to increased awareness or increased need. The pressures of innovation, public participation/expectation, patient-focused care, political policies, and demography (ageing) make the setting of priorities a vital part of public health practice.

Objectives

This chapter provides practical advice on setting up a robust process for making difficult allocation choices by exploring the example of the Priorities Forum developed in Oxfordshire, England.[1] This model dates from the 1990s, but the underlying principles remain, despite changing structural and organizational arrangements.

The Priorities Forum provided a whole-systems approach, which involved all partners in the making of difficult decisions. As a subcommittee of the board of the local health system it provided the opportunity to debate the merits of competing priorities for limited resources.

The UK process for determining which services will be provided to a local population depends on the Primary Care Trusts (PCTs)/local health boards commissioning those services. Typically a host of competing options are available (see Box 5.4.1)

Box 5.4.1 Example of competing demands for limited funding

At the year end there was an additional £100,000 available for commissioning. The hospital identified three competing areas for the resource available:

- The waiting list for cataract operations. One cataract operation costs £715. Investment here would mean that 140 operations could be done, which would improve the vision of that number of older people, enabling them to live independently in the community.
- Adults waiting for cochlear implant operations. Investment here would mean that four hard-of-hearing or deaf adults could be helped to hear at a cost of £25,000 per implant with maintenance.
- Dementia. Twenty patients with dementia could attend the memory clinic and be given the drug donepezil. Thirty per cent of those taking the drug are thought to benefit, with variable improvements in their quality of life.

Which would you choose?

The key questions that arise are:
- How can we be fair when making rationing decisions?
- How do we account for our decisions?

The key elements in making these decisions are:
- an ethical framework (see below)
- open processes
- involvement of clinicians and other stakeholders.

Using a framework of ethics in making difficult choices

What is an ethics framework and how does it help?

An ethics framework is structured around three main components:
- evidence of effectiveness
- equity
- patient choice.

An ethical framework helps to:
- Structure discussion and ensure that the important points are properly considered.
- Ensure consistent decision-making, over time and with respect to decisions concerning different clinical settings.

- Enable articulation of the reasons for the decisions that are made. This is particularly important for the support of any appeals procedure and in the event of a decision coming under legal scrutiny. In such circumstances the courts are likely to consider whether the process and the grounds for making the decision were reasonable. An ethics framework is particularly important in judging the reasonableness of the grounds on which the decision was made.

Evidence of effectiveness

In deciding the priority of a health-care intervention it was considered that the evidence of effectiveness is of major importance. As there are commonly too many 'effective' interventions to fund completely, cost-effectiveness must also be considered.

Public health has a key role in providing practical advice to local health-care economies based on this guidance. This evidence can fall broadly within three categories:

- There is good evidence that the treatment is not effective.
- There is good evidence that the treatment is effective (for a specific patient group and indication).
- The evidence either way is not good.

Clearly treatment which falls into the first category should not be funded. Treatments that fall into the second category may or may not be funded—dependent on their relative health impact on the population. Many treatments (or other health-care interventions) fall into the third category. In such cases, many clinicians (and lobby groups) may believe that the treatment is valuable but large well-designed trials have not been carried out. It could be said for treatments in this third category that there is no good evidence for effectiveness. However, they should not be confused with the first category. It is desirable to obtain good-quality evidence about effectiveness, and research aimed at obtaining such evidence should be encouraged. However, when evidence is poor, then a judgement about the likely effectiveness has to be made in the knowledge that good-quality evidence is not available (see Chapter 2.11).

Box 5.4.2 Beta-interferon

Beta-interferon is a drug which has received its licence for use in the relapsing–remitting form of multiple sclerosis (MS), which is the commonest cause of disability for young people. Its impact is to reduce the relapse rate, thereby slowing the disease for 30% of those who are treated appropriately. The cost for a year is around £10,000. The estimated quality adjusted life years (QALYs) gained per patient range from £750,000 to £5.5 million—with a cost per exacerbation prevented of £61,000.

Thus the drug is efficacious but its impact small. Is it worth funding? The Oxfordshire Priorities Forum believed not and gave available resources to increase quality of care for all patients with MS: more doctor/nurse time and counselling.

Equity

The basic principle of equity (fairness) is that people in similar situations should be treated similarly. For this simple reason it is important that there is consistency in the way in which decisions are reached at different times and in different settings (see Chapters 2.10 and 5.5). This principle of equity also requires that there is no discrimination on grounds irrelevant to priority for health care such as gender or ethnicity.

In developing the principles on which equity is based, two broad approaches can be taken:
- maximizing the welfare of patients within the budget available (a utilitarian approach—the greatest good to the greatest number)
- giving priority to those in most need.

Neither approach by itself is adequate. The maximization of welfare takes no direct account of how that welfare is distributed between different people. Equity would seem to require giving some priority to those in most need even if this does not produce the greatest level of welfare overall.

These approaches can be balanced using a two-step process:
1. Consider the cost-effectiveness of the intervention under consideration, e.g. on the basis of QALYs (see Chapter 1.4).
2. If the intervention is less cost-effective than those normally funded, are there nevertheless reasons for funding it?

Having considered the approaches, into which category does a treatment fall? It may be:
- urgent need (e.g. immediate life-saving treatment)
- need for treatment for those whose quality of life is severely affected by chronic illness (e.g. due to a severely incapacitating neurological condition)
- need due to characteristics of the patient, which adds to the cost—these characteristics should not affect the priority. An example of what we mean is that the same level of dental care should be available to people with learning disabilities as to the normal population, even if it is more costly (less cost-effective) because more specialized services are needed.

Box 5.4.3

Beta-interferon prevents relapse rates in some patients with MS. In our population there are 25 patients who would potentially benefit but only enough money for 15 to receive the drug. How should the patients be selected? On a first-come, first-served basis? Using a lottery? Using criteria such as age or other patient-specific features?

In our experience we would say there is no perfect way to do this. We would reject the use of personal characteristics as unethical. We would not accept a lottery because it would be unacceptable within our population. We would accept a first-come, first-served approach within the limited resources if all patients being referred met the criteria laid out in the guidelines.

Patient choice

Respecting patients' wishes and enabling patients to have control over their health care are important values (see Chapter 8.4) The initial work in Oxfordshire stressed the value of patient choice, with three implications:

- In assessing research on the effectiveness of a treatment it is important that the outcome measures used in the research include those which matter to patients
- Within those health-care interventions that are purchased, patients should be enabled to make their own choices about which they want
- Each patient is unique. Good-quality evidence about the effectiveness of an intervention normally addresses outcomes in a large group of people. There may be a good reason to believe that a particular patient stands to gain significantly more from the intervention than most of those who formed the study group in the relevant research. This may justify a particular patient receiving treatment which is not normally provided.

Within a resource-limited system, the dilemma continues to exist that the benefit of choice for one patient may deprive another patient. Difficult decisions about the context and limits of choice need to be made.

Ensuring that the process of setting priorities is open and fair

To be fair in setting priorities, processes need to be robust and explicit. Using the Priorities Forum as a model, we would suggest the following:

Who needs to be involved?

- those responsible for funding and commissioning
- representative clinical groups from primary care and family medicine
- hospital-based specialist clinicians, clinician managers, and managers
- members of the public and representatives of patient groups.

What is discussed?

- implications of policy
- introduction of new drugs not covered by decisions at a higher level
- innovative treatments
- individual exceptional needs.

What is the outcome?

- statements summarizing the debate and decisions go to all general practices and primary care organizations as well as hospital trusts
- public reports go to the board meetings
- appeals are heard by the chairman and chief executive of the board, who do not attend the meetings
- discussions are fed into commissioning discussions.

Involving clinicians

Involvement of clinicians in presenting the evidence for their case is important to enable informed discussion. Discussion needs to take place with reference to a defined *envelope of resource*, a notional amount spent on each particular service which is often based on historic spend not empirical need. Any change or development needs to consider making the envelope bigger (or smaller!) or alternatively changing the components within the existing envelope (see Chapter 1.4).

Guidelines to clinicians ask them to consider three questions:

1. If you want something outside your current fixed envelope of resource can it be done by substituting a treatment of less value?
2. If demand for your service is increasing, what criteria are you using to agree the threshold of treatment?
3. If you do not believe that it is possible to either substitute or agree thresholds, from where would you withdraw resource in order to enlarge/increase your own?

These are not easy questions, and the debate is often less structured than this approach may imply, but it is used consistently so members of the Priorities Forum can attempt to be fair.

Box 5.4.4 Substitution

Dermatologists wished to prescribe isotretinoin for acne. There was no capacity to increase the size of the envelope of resource. They agreed to stop treating hirsutism on public funding—deemed to be of lower priority—and resources were thereby made available for acne sufferers.

Improving the process

The process described is not meant to be a blueprint but reflects development over a period of time. Issues that could be addressed include:

- more health economics input (see Chapter 1.4)
- greater public involvement (see Chapter 8.4)
- adapting to changing policies, resources, and expectations (see Chapter 5.2).

The role of public health practitioners and teams

Within health economies and organizations, public health can provide an overview across the community and balance the external needs of local communities. The skills of needs assessment, critical appraisal, application of evidence-based care, and management of risk which are key to public health are all needed to develop this role.

Whatever changes occur to the structure of health services, local clinicians will continue to make decisions on a patient by patient basis, guided by many factors including accepted good practice guidelines and reimbursement rules. The difficulty of balancing resources can be assisted by clear processes and common ethical values, with the development of appropriate decision-making frameworks within which trade-offs can be made. This requires open and mature debate.

Further resources

Coulter A, Ham C (eds) (2000). *The global challenge of health care rationing.* Open University Press, Buckingham.

Hunter D (1998). *Desperately seeking solutions.* Longman, Harlow.

Klein R (1995). Priorities and rationing: pragmatism or principles? *BMJ*, **311**, 761–2.

Klein R, Day P, Redmayne S (1998). *Managing scarcity: priority setting and rationing in the NHS.* Open University Press, Buckingham.

Mechanic D (1995). Dilemmas in rationing health care services: the case for implicit rationing. *BMJ*, **310**, 1655–9.

New B (1999). *A good enough service—values, trade-offs and the NHS.* King's Fund and IPPR, London.

New B, LeGrand J (1996). *Rationing in the NHS: principles and pragmatism.* King's Fund, London.

Smith R (1995). Rationing: the debate we have to have. *BMJ*, **310**(6981), 686.

Wennberg JE (1990). Outcomes research, cost containment, and the fear of health care rationing. *N Engl J Med*, **323**(17), 1202–4.

Reference

1 Hope T, Hicks N, Reynolds DJ, Crisp R, Griffiths S (1998). Rationing and the health authority. *BMJ*, **317**, 1067–9.

5.5 Improving equity in health care

Anna Donald

Definitions

This chapter is concerned with minimizing unfair or unacceptable inequalities in quality and access to health care for people with the same health needs. Note that:

- As 'supply-side' issues, inequalities in access and quality of health care lie within the control of health professionals. They are distinct from the larger issues of inequalities in health outcomes and health-care utilization, which are beyond the control of most health professionals and, therefore, the scope of this chapter
- The words 'inequality' and 'inequity' are often used interchangeably. However, *inequality* is a broader term, meaning 'unequal' or a 'difference in size, degree or circumstances'[1] while *inequity* is a more specific and moral term, meaning 'lack of fairness or justice'.[1]

Why are inequalities in health care an important public health issue?

Inequalities in health care are important because they cause excess suffering and death and impede social justice. In general, deprived and socially marginal groups have the greatest need for care, but, in the absence of strong public policy measures are the least able to obtain it (the 'inverse care law', Box 5.5.1). For example, children's access to physicians varied by almost 200% if they were from low-income families, depending on which US state they lived in.[2] Factors such as age, sex, ethnicity, and geographic remoteness can also increase people's need for care while impeding access and quality.

Box 5.5.1 The inverse care law

The availability of good medical care tends to vary inversely with the need for it in the population served.

Tudor Hart[3]

What are the main causes of unequal access and quality of health care?

The main inequalities in health care result from two problems: unequal distribution of money and services and discriminatory treatment of groups with the same health needs.

Unequal distribution of money and services—macro and micro

The main cause of inequalities in health care is the way in which health systems are financed and regulated.[4] At a macro level, unequal distribution of finances for health care can result either from unequal insurance coverage (more typical of multipayer systems) or unequal central planning (more typical in single-payer systems, i.e. health systems in which one actor, usually the government, purchases health care on behalf of the whole population). Not surprisingly, health systems that cover everyone, regardless of income, have more equal health care in all respects than those that do not. Even in health systems with universal coverage, however, health care tends to become unequally distributed if policies to safeguard quality and access in less desirable areas are not strictly enforced. For example, Australia and the UK have not always sufficiently enforced policies to ensure access to doctors and specialist services in rural and deprived areas.[5]

At a micro level, inequalities in access and quality of care usually result from poor design of services and insufficient local planning to take into account the special needs of marginal groups. For example, services that can be reached only by car, in English, or by filling in lengthy forms are usually less accessible to more deprived groups.

Different treatment of groups with the same health need

This may result from:
- ignorance and poor training (for example under-treating women with heart disease)[6]
- conscious or unconscious discrimination against a particular group, either due to individual prejudice or embedded in policy (for example, non-white groups in the US[4,7])
- different perceptions of and preferences for care by different social groups[8] (for example, some groups' preferences for complementary medicines over Western ones).

Identifying and assessing inequalities in health care

To identify and assess inequalities in health care, compare the expected versus actual use of health care based on health needs. The steps of assessing health inequality are:
- measuring health need
- measuring access to health care

- measuring quality of health care
- measuring overall supply of health care.

Measuring health need (demand for health care)

There are different ways to define need for health care[9] (see Chapter 1.3). Once you have decided the most appropriate definition for your assessment, you can assess people's need for health care with routine or specialized survey instruments. Further measures that may help to define these include measures of patient preferences and perceptions of treatment.[10]

Measuring quality of health care

Many countries have their own indicators of health-care quality. The recent US-based National Health Disparities Report identified four factors affecting quality of care: effectiveness/appropriateness for key conditions, such as diabetes, cancer, and maternal health; safety; timeliness; and patient- centredness. Statistics often need to be reformulated (or even re-collected) to reflect service use per capita of defined populations: service use per clinic statistics can obscure inequalities. Linking care to social groups of interest (for example, people with low income) may need additional data or routinely collected proxy measures, such as zipcode/postcode.[11] If resources are scarce, it may be possible to confine assessment to a few key goods and services.

Measuring access to health care

Access to health care can be measured in several ways, including routine statistics, specialized surveys, and stratified sampling of a common 'basket' of procedures. Access measures can include measures of entry into the health-care system (for example, insurance coverage); structural barriers within the system (for example, waiting times); patient perceptions of providers' ability to help them (for example, quality of communication and cultural competency), and health-care utilization, where this is amenable to control by health professionals (for example, avoidable hospitalizations).[12]

Measuring the supply of health care: the Gini coefficient

A simple graphic overview of roughly who gets how much health care can help assess equality in supply of health care in a particular region or country. The curve in Figure 5.5.1 helps to measure equity of supply of health care. The straight line represents an equal health-care expenditure across the five quintiles of the population (e.g. quintiles by income) (see sample data in Table 5.5.1). The degree of unequal distribution of health-care expenditure can be represented by the size of area A. A health-related 'Gini' coefficient can be calculated as the proportion of the total area $A + B$ made up by area A. The larger $A/(A + B)$ (a value between 0 and 1), the more unequal the resource distribution. (This technique can be extended to control for the greater need that is associated with poorer income groups; see Goddard and Smith,[13] p.7). More details concerning Lorenz curves can be found in Chapter 2.10 and Stilgitz.[14]

Table 5.5.1 Example of data needed to draw a Lorenz curve and calculate a Gini coefficient. A Gini coefficient (after Corrado Gini, Italian demographer and economist, 1884–1965) is a measure of how dispersed (or unequal) a set of values is (e.g. income distribution, health-care expenditure, etc.) in a specified population. The value is derived from a Lorenz curve (Figure 5.5.1)

Quintile	Income (as a percentage of total population income)	Cumulative population	Cumulative income
1st	5	20	5
2nd	10	40	15
3rd	18	60	33
4th	26	80	59
5th	41	100	100
	100		

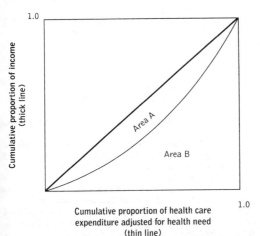

Figure 5.5.1 A Lorenz curve for displaying the distribution of health care expenditure by income group. A Lorenz curve (after Max Lorenz, American statistician, 1876–1959) is a graph on which the cumulative percentage of some variable (e.g. income or health-care expenditure) is plotted against the cumulative percentage of the corresponding population (ranked in increasing size of share). The extent to which the curve sags below a straight diagonal line indicates the degree of inequality of distribution. See Chapter 2.10 for more applications of Gini coefficients and Lorenz curves.

Addressing inequalities in health care

General measures

Generic steps in planning include:

- Identifying the size and nature of the problem and what might be causing it (see above)
- Prioritizing potential solutions according to the severity of the inequality and disease burden it places on the under-served population, the resources available, and the feasibility of solutions
- Setting realistic time-scales. Some may involve staggered programmes or policies which take years or even generations to see to fruition, particularly if the programme's immediate impact is on children or young health professionals (for example, see Rabinowitz et al.[15])
- Identifying potential political (and other) barriers. If reform is politically contentious then it can help to make it more palatable by presenting it differently. For example, fluoridating water (a good way to improve poorer people's dental care) can be presented as 'clean teeth for all' (which is, of course, true—just more true for poorer groups!)
- Appreciating that addressing inequalities in health outcomes usually requires measures beyond health-care reform, such as educational and taxation reforms. Trying to address these larger, income- and opportunity-based inequalities purely through health-care measures may even result in creating further unacceptable inequalities.[16]

Specific measures

Specific strategies are likely to vary depending on the level at which you are working. Often, solutions to address unequal distribution of regional or national resources lie at a macro-policy level, but more piecemeal solutions can be effective in addressing inequalities arising from biases in particular services:

- Whatever level you are working at, *make equality of care according to need an explicit policy criterion*. For example, against such a criterion, hospital closure policies would need to be assessed for how they affect overall equality of access to services
- Replace political 'horse-trading' arrangements (whereby political representatives vie for health resources for their area) with explicit allocation formulae that weight resource allocation according to health need (for example, by age, sex, geography, particularly for expensive conditions such as HIV infection)[17,18]
- Develop measurable outcomes of equitable health-care distribution and access and monitor them (either continuously or sporadically) on a population basis (rather than on a service basis), and use them to manage health services
- Identify and address individual or systematic prejudice against particular groups. This may involve changes to legislation, guidelines, political mobilization, helplines, simple anonymous feedback forms, ombudsmen, media, or educational programmes
- Provide policies, incentives, and regulations to ensure that health workers and services are distributed according to health need. For example, ensure that health commissioners for different areas (who

tend to serve different social groups) are required to purchase care according to health need rather than according to other criteria that will tend to bias care away from those who need it most . Design services to maximize access for those who need them most
* Similarly, ensure that the treatment at point of use is the same for people with similar health needs. For example, alert health workers to under-served groups or adapt treatments for easier use (for example, providing tablets in easy-to-open bottles)
* Empower under-served groups to demand the care they need. Empowerment can involve media campaigns to ensure that under-served populations are aware of services and their rights of access (for example antenatal and immunization services); collaboration with advocacy groups and distribution of health information with routine information (for example local council leaflets, electricity bills, supermarket receipts, or newspapers).

Measuring success in addressing inequalities in health care

There are many ways of measuring the gap and how it might be changing. Ideally, use several measures at the same time ('triangulate'), ensuring they make sense in the context in which you are working. They do not all need to be quantitative; qualitative data can reveal a lot about how health care is distributed. Examples of measurement include:
* mapping the distribution of health-care activity (for example clinics, doctors, or procedures for conditions that are more common in poorer groups, such as coronary bypass surgery) against a map of income distribution
* comparing quality of care indicators for different groups. What is the distribution of failed hip replacements?
* describing and comparing premises in different areas. What are waiting rooms and building maintenance like in different sectors of the community?
* critical incident/exception reporting. How often do rare, serious events, such as maternal mortality happen in different sections of the community?

If some of these measures are designated important criteria, measured and followed over time, then you are performing an 'equity audit', like any other audit. This can help you communicate what you are doing to others as well as keep track of how the situation is changing around you. Clearly the change and your interventions may be unrelated, but the importance of serial measurements should not be underestimated. If nothing else, the high profile you give this can keep it high on the political agenda, an important outcome in itself.

Health and health care

Unfair inequality in health outcomes is a much larger problem than inequalities in health care. It results largely from inequalities in income, employment, education, transport, and housing. These factors usually have much larger effects on health outcomes because they dramatically affect the incidence of disease onset and death rather than affecting the course of disease once it has begun.[19,20] Although inequalities in health outcomes lie beyond the immediate control of most health professionals, public health professionals can powerfully influence local and central policies by demonstrating how they damage health.

Further resources

Acheson D (1998). *Independent inquiry into inequalities in health report*. The Stationery Office, London.

Bulletin of the World Health Organization (2000), **78**(1), 1–152. (Special theme issue on 'Inequalities in health'.)

National Healthcare Quality Report. Fact sheet. http://www.ahrq.gov/qual/nhqrfact.htm (accessed 28 June 2005).

Improving health and reducing inequality. In: *The NHS plan: a plan for investment; a plan for reform*, ch 13, Cm. 4818-I, July 2000. HMSO, London.

Oliver A, Mossialos E (2004). Equity of access to health care: outlining the foundations for action. *J Epidemiol Commun Health*, **58**, 655–8.

Povertynet. World Bank resources on inequality, poverty, and socio-economic performance. http://www.worldbank.org/poverty/inequal/index.htm (accessed 30 December 2004).

References

1 *The new Oxford dictionary of English* (1998). Oxford University Press, Oxford.

2 Long SH, Marquis MS (1999). Geographic variation in physician visits for uninsured children. *J Am Med Assoc*, **281**, 2035–40.

3 Tudor Hart J (1971). The inverse care law. *Lancet*, **696**, 405–12.

4 Smedley BD, Stith AY, Nelson AR (eds) (2003). *Unequal treatment: confronting racial and ethnic disparities in healthcare*. National Academies Press, Washington, DC.

5 Benzeval M, Judge K (1996). Access to health care in England: continuing inequalities in the distribution of GPs. *J Publ Health Med*, **18**, 33–44.

6 Raine R, Hutchings A, Black N (2003). Is publicly funded health care really distributed according to need? The example of cardiac rehabilitation in the UK. *Health Policy*, **63**, 63–72.

7 Schulman KA, Berlin JA, Harless W et al. (1999). The effect of race and sex on physicians' recommendations for cardiac catheterization. *N Engl J Med*, **340**, 618–26.

8 Le Grand J (1984). Equity as an economic objective. *J Appl Phil*, **1**, 39–51.

9 Goddard M, Smith P (2001). Equity of access to health care services: theory and evidence from the UK. *Soc Sci Med*, **53**, 1149–62.

10 Pencheon D (1998). Matching demand and supply fairly and efficiently. *BMJ*, **316**, 1665–7.
11 Danesh J, Gault S, Semmence J, Appleby P, Peto R (1999). Postcodes as useful markers of social class: population based study in 26000 British households. *BMJ*, **318**, 843–5.
12 National Healthcare Disparities Report. Available at: http://www.ahrq.gov/qual/nhdr02/prenhdr.htm (accessed 28 June 2005).
13 Goddard M, Smith P (1998). *Equity of access to health care*. University of York, Centre for Health Economics, York.
14 Stiglitz JE (1993). *Economics*. W.W. Norton and Co., New York.
15 Rabinowitz HK, Diamond JJ, Markham FW, Hazelwood CE (1999). A programme to increase the number of family physicians in rural and underserved areas. *J Am Med Assoc*, **281**, 255–60.
16 Hauck K, Shaw R, Smith PC (2002). Reducing avoidable inequalities in health: a new criterion for setting health care capitation payments. *Health Econ*, **11**, 667–77.
17 Resource Allocation Working Party (1976). *Sharing resources for health in England*. HMSO, London.
18 Rice N, Smith PC (2001). Capitation and risk adjustment in health care financing: an international progress report. *Milbank Q*, **79**, 81–113, IV.
19 Marmot M, Wilkinson RG (eds) (1999). *Social determinants of health*. Oxford University Press, Oxford.
20 The Copenhagen Declaration on Reducing Social Inequalities in Health (2002). *Scand J Publ Health*, **30**(Suppl. 59), 78–9.

5.6 Commissioning health care

Richard Richards

Introduction

This chapter is concerned with the use of contracts and payments as a means of ensuring that care maximizes health at minimum cost. The chapter aims to cover the full range of health-care commissioning from the simplest form, an individual patient making a private payment to an individual practitioner, through to the most complex, tax funded, social medicine 'free at the point of delivery'.

In all health-care commissioning a common set of concerns arise:
- the nature of the need, including an assessment of the (cost-)effectiveness of the relevant interventions
- examination of the services available, including inputs, quality of care, and outcomes
- the costs and efficiency of the care on offer
- the development of formal commissioning agreements.

Assessing need

For the individual, assessing need will usually require a diagnosis and often an assessment of the severity of the disease and associated co-morbidities. Often, there is a much uncertainty about the patient's condition, introducing risk, and limiting rational behaviour in the health-care 'market'.

At the population level, a variety of approaches exist to assess need (see Chapter 1.3). A centrally planned health-care system requires information on the numbers of people with each type of need, to plan the extent of provision. Even entrepreneurial market systems, considered more able to change and willing to accept mistakes and failures, would first use market research to help determine the level of provision required.

Need, by definition, involves the presence of an undesirable health state plus the existence of effective interventions. In most circumstances resources are limited, so the goal is to buy the most cost-effective care to improve health.

Inputs

The resources needed to deliver health care are of crucial interest both to the provider and consumer/commissioner as they determine the *costs* to the former and *price* to the latter. In the situation of the private consultation, an unaffordable price represents an inaccessible treatment; in the situation of a third-party payer this situation is referred to, pejoratively, as rationing. To the consumer, be they patient or third-party payer, the input needs to be affordable and to maximize the outcomes for the available funds.

Cost containment is an inevitable goal of commissioning systems. Approaches vary from the prospective payment systems used in the US Medicare system, through removing incentives to unproductive overactivity, e.g. by placing physicians on salaries rather than fees for service payments and placing contracts with managed care providers. The socialized health providers in several European countries operate cost containment through direct control and annual budget setting.

Inputs come in a variety of standards, quality, and availability (scarcity), which will be reflected in differences in costs and thus price. This applies to facilities, diagnostic and treatment equipment, drugs and staff.

Quality and outcomes

The quality of health care has many dimensions, including the structures (staff, equipment, etc.), processes and outcomes. Commissioning should clearly state the quality expected in whatever dimensions seem necessary.

Whilst health technology assessments can show what treatments should be given, audit will indicate whether a unit is actually providing those treatments as intended. Often units are too small and case mixes too complex to yield definitive indications of quality of care. The lack of good information on providers' quality and outcome often means that the patient/commissioner faces significant uncertainties and cannot choose rationally between providers in the way suggested by advocates of idealized market systems.

Efficiency, the ratio of costs to outcomes, provides a measure of value for money. Commissioners seek to maximize the efficiency of services, maximizing the output for the funding they give. Providers seek to maximize funding whilst minimizing costs: where there is a relationship between quality and higher costs, this can drive down quality for the individual patient. The profit motive can further distort incentives.

Coping with risk in health-care commissioning

Risks take different forms. Ask a bank manager for a loan and the manager will assess the risk compared to the likelihood of profit for the bank. From the public health perspective the 'bottom line' is not financial profit but health gain. Each commissioning decision carries a risk that the funding will not result in health gain.

Small organizations, be they commissioners or providers, can face significant financial risks from high-cost, low-volume interventions. These occur unpredictably in any given year. Ways for commissioners to handle that risk are all based on increasing these numbers to predictable levels by:

- grouping many low-volume, high-cost interventions together in one 'basket'
- collaborating with other small organizations to increase numbers, sharing costs on a weighted capitation basis
- creating a 'higher' tier (dictated by rarity of the intervention) responsible for commissioning
- any combination of these.

Commissioners and providers can share financial risk. A provider may serve a number of small commissioners and will therefore see a larger number of the rarer interventions, which will allow risks to be shared or spread.

An agreement that includes 'floors' and 'ceilings' can also be used to share risk. A range of activity around a central estimate is commissioned and paid for: no change in funding occurs within those limits. Should activity fall below the 'floor' the provider returns funding to the commissioner and should the activity exceed the 'ceiling' the commissioner pays extra.

Agreeing costs

The amount of funding involved in commissioning a whole service depends on the concept of 'marginal' and 'step-up' cost, two sides of the same coin. Some costs to a provider are 'fixed', independent of activity levels (staff salaries, equipment, buildings, etc.). If the activity increases, these fixed costs can be spread across larger numbers of cases; the number of cases agreed determines the 'full cost' (per case) that will cover all of the fixed costs.

Once fixed costs are covered, extra activity will cost marginally less, due to the use of consumables and other non-fixed costs. Conversely, lower activity will return amounts smaller than the 'full cost'.

'Step-up' costs occur when activity exceeds the capacity of the provider, despite efficient use of facilities, requiring that extra capacity be introduced. Such capacity cannot be introduced in small amounts; it is not practicable to build a one-bedded hospital ward! It is these problems that work against change in some systems, making change very expensive for commissioners.

The chosen mechanism for sharing risk will depend on circumstances and the type of commissioning arrangement in use. There are generally four types:

- *block*: a global sum of money in exchange for a loosely defined set of services; the provider moves money between departmental budgets; the commissioner and provider negotiate differences towards the end of the financial year
- *cost and volume*: specified activity levels and funding at various levels of detail (e.g. surgical, medical etc.; by specialty; by procedure type, or groupings of procedures such as healthcare resource groups); monthly plans are agreed and monitored against targets

- *cost per case*: each episode of care is paid for; cost may vary depending on the level of activity or be fixed, independent of activity levels
- *fee for service*: costs for individual inputs, diagnostic, or treatment activities are separately reimbursed. This system is typically used in private insurance and parts of the US health system, and is usually combined with a range of instruments to contain costs and limit coverage.

A cost per case system based on a set price ('tariff') for any provider can facilitate choice, and change through choice, but it can also stifle the creation of new capacity as providers have to carry the risk of additional marginal costs before activity levels use enough of the new capacity to generate the income needed. Despite a supposedly fixed cost, a commissioner may be forced to agree a higher price per case if extra capacity is needed.

In free markets for consumer products, increased sales typically result in lower costs, generating greater consumption as goods become more affordable, although the total amount of money spent in the market increases. In health care, higher volumes can also generate lower costs. However, extra consumers (patients) can only be generated by reducing treatment thresholds (to lesser severities) or treating a different condition. This will change benefit/risk and cost/effectiveness ratios, especially at the margins of this extra activity. The funding needed to cover this activity might be more effectively directed elsewhere. Commissioners need to understand the total cost and benefits, and resist simplistic claims of reduced treatment costs making a treatment more widely available.

The six basic elements of a commissioning agreement

So what would a contract or service level agreement look like? It should have at least six elements:
- *Parties* to the contract. Typically one or more commissioners and a provider. A complex pathway may require several providers but this could be addressed by requiring the main provider to subcontract.
- *What treatments and services are to be provided?* Ideally this should be described by the patient pathway and encompass 'hotel services' (nutrition, shelter, and comforts) as well as details of the diagnostic and treatment processes based on evidence of effectiveness. A good contract should be composed of many such pathways relating to the many diseases to be treated (though there are examples of providers doing a single procedure) covering both emergency care and planned care. What is excluded may also be specified.
- *Quantity of care*. The number of patients to be treated within the contract. This may be just one or in the case of block contracts undetermined except by historical patterns. Ideally each pathway should have a number established by the epidemiology of incidence/prevalence and treatment thresholds. The provider will be expected to report activity levels regularly to the commissioner.

- *Standards to be achieved.* The quality of care must be clearly specified along with the mechanisms of monitoring. Such standards could and should include nutrition ('five portions of fresh fruit or vegetables a day', free access to fluids), the environment (clean; non-smoking; access to 'entertainments' and access for visitors, especially important in paediatrics), as well as the skills and knowledge of staff, equipment, devices, and drugs. For some conditions or treatments an individual clinician and team may be designated (even named), e.g. for breast cancer, and minimum activity levels specified to maintain skills. Standards may be specified by reference to recognized clinical guidelines and protocols such as those produced in the UK by the National Institute for Health and Clinical Excellence (NICE) in England and Wales or the Scottish Intercollegiate Guidelines Network (SIGN). Clinical governance (including audit) will be specified as the mechanism for maintaining standards within the provider. In some reimbursement systems detailed standards are set for individual patient diagnosis and treatment planning. Often there are formal requirements on providers to seek permission from payers prior to starting specified forms of care. Permission procedures may involve the reporting of detailed clinical data to the payer to prove the presence of a health-care need that is covered by the patient's insurance coverage.
- *Price.* No commissioning or purchasing agreement is complete without agreement of the price. Prices may be agreed locally or fixed by the commissioner so as to allow providers to compete on quality over and above that specified.
- *Arbitration arrangements.* Things rarely go to plan, contracts are rarely exactly met as specified. Contracts should therefore specify how the parties would reach agreement should, for example, the contract not be met, demand fail to reach, or exceed, the contract, the case mix differ in terms of severities or conditions from that anticipated, new treatment become available or if events occur not covered within the contract, such as a major disaster.

Who should be involved in commissioning?

The commissioning process requires a broad range of skills and experience. Genuine team work is essential (see Chapter 8.1). Sometimes these can all be embodied in one person but this is rare and usually a team-based multidisciplinary process works best.

Table 5.6.1 identifies the skills, people and tasks needed in commissioning health-care services.

Table 5.6.1 Skills, people, and tasks needed in commissioning health-care services

	Person or discipline	Tasks
Epidemiology	Epidemiologist, public health practitioner	To use data (e.g. mortality, demographic, surveys, case registers). To analyze these data to determine the actual and potential health problems in the population
Health technology assessment	Health economist, public health practitioner	To evaluate critically the (cost)-effectiveness of health-care interventions. To highlight gaps in information where further research is needed
Negotiation and conflict management	NHS manager, all members	To negotiate skilfully matching what the commissioner believes is required and the provider wishes to offer
Financial	Accountant, NHS manager	To handle complex finances (services are rarely costed comprehensively and in a way that readily allows comparison)
Clinical	Public health clinician, GP, specialist clinician, nurse	To understand the specialist clinical aspects of the services being offered and provided. (Beware: like any input, specialist clinical advice can be biased—more general clinical advice, for example from primary care practitioners, is often equally or more important; 'experts' are almost always enthusiasts, not disinterested observers)
Experience of the wider health system	NHS manager, public health practitioner	To appreciate how the individual services fit in with the wider health-care provision of the locality or region—experience and understanding of the wider health service is essential
Information	Information specialist, operational researcher, epidemiologist	To understand health information systems. (Information systems are complex and not always designed specifically to serve the commissioning process.) To understand issues such as case mix measurement, relationships between case mix, costs, and prices. To understand how the provision of health care should be matched to predictions of need
Informing and supporting patient choice	Any clinician but also anyone appropriately trained	To provide and explain information on outcomes and quality issues to patients in a way they can understand that will permit them to make choices that are best suited to their conditions and circumstances

Specialized services

There is no one agreed definition of specialized services; most of what has been described above applies to specialized services, but to reiterate some important aspects, specialized services typically involve rarer conditions, thus patient numbers are *small* and *often unpredictable*.

To ensure optimum outcomes for patients (e.g. sustained training and clinical competence for specialized staff) and optimum use of resources (e.g. to ensure cost-effectiveness of provision, making the best use of scarce resources including clinical expertise, high-technology equipment, donor organs etc.) a *critical service mass* is required at each centre and patients from a wide area must be referred to these centres to achieve minimum activity levels. As a result, the population on behalf of which services are commissioned is much larger than that of a single commissioning organization.

Specialized services may have some characteristics different from mainstream health care, one of which is *rapidly developing high technology services*. Services can develop very quickly and often involve high technology, where research and development need to be supported and where the introduction of new technologies needs to be managed. In these situations note that the evidence for effectiveness is often emerging rather than established, making commissioning decisions on the basis of complete evidence difficult. As the new technology becomes more widely adopted, additional clinicians can be properly trained in those centres initially established.

Commissioning services with prominent ethical dimensions

Difficult ethical issues can arise, for example, around equity of access (see Chapters 2.10 and 5.5), requiring commissioners of health care to balance the high cost needs of the minority against the needs of the majority. Examples are treatment of a variety of genetically determined diseases requiring extremely expensive genetically engineered replacement therapies, and the commissioning of very expensive secure psychiatric facilities to protect society (see Chapter 1.7).

Nonetheless, the general 'rules' of commissioning can and should be applied to specialized services. There is a danger that issues of cost-effectiveness are set aside. Whilst larger populations mean that costs are a smaller proportion of the total budget and thus appear affordable, opportunity costs remain the same: the opportunity to treat the same number of patients is lost, irrespective of the population level at which services are commissioned. There remains a reluctance to address explicitly the issues of distributive justice in these cases and costs are rising exponentially: lifetime costs for one individual can reach £10,000,000 yet deliver only marginal benefits. The principles of distributive justice must be addressed.

Part 6

Improving quality in health care

Introduction

Poor quality in health care is easily recognized, with regular scandals drawing attention to unexpected deaths and treatment mishaps. When the scandals do arise the immediate political reaction is generally to look round for someone to blame—a 'bad apple'. Bad apples do exist and dealing with them is important. It is far more important, however, to focus on the bigger picture of harm from poor quality—the harm generated from the everyday actions of staff doing their best within flawed systems.

The first step in improving quality is to define and measure it. As Shekelle *et al.* point out in Chapter 6.1, quality is only definable against set standards. At least in the clinical dimensions of quality those standards must be evidence based. Systematic methods of standard setting have been developed, with several packages of quality criteria now available for local adaptation.

After measurement, action to improve quality must follow, and Tomson and Massoud (Chapter 6.2) introduce us to the systems approaches. The 'central law' of improvement is that 'every system is perfectly designed to achieve the results it achieves'. To change systems a process of building 'will', the right ideas, and the support of seniors is needed. A good quality improvement team can often share ideas and build on successful projects elsewhere.

Professional roles in health care developed in the age of acute illness, and are ill-suited to managing many chronic conditions. Davis (Chapter 6.3) identifies seven components of renewed systems, including collaborative practice models incorporating physician and support-service providers, patient self-management education, and routine reporting/feedback loops.

To the newcomer to health care, the idea that large variations exist in the rates of surgical operations from area to area and clinician to clinician is often rather shocking. A structured approach to analyzing these variations is described by Steel and Melzer in Chapter 6.4 (based on two key ideas from Wennberg). The first is a clear definition of unwarranted variation: care that is not consistent with a patient's preference or related to a patient's underlying illness. The second is the categorization of unwarranted variations into effective, preference-sensitive, and supply-sensitive care. There is at least one more critical idea in this chapter: that higher rates of activity are not generally associated with better quality.

One area of promise in improving care is the use of information technology, with programmed reminders and electronic prescribing as prominent examples. In an overview of the IT agenda, Detmer (Chapter 6.5) points to the potential of the new generation of systems to support more ambitious uses, including surveillance and decision support. He warns, however, that public policy on privacy, often fashioned with a disproportionate emphasis on personal autonomy, may undermine use of data for quality improvement and research.

Recent decades have seen an extraordinary explosion of scientific output in medicine and a wonderful inventiveness on the part of pharmaceutical, imaging, and test companies. Unfortunately some of that inventiveness has gone into hype. Health technology assessment (Stevens and Milne, Chapter 6.6) provides a structured approach to sifting through tests and treatments, be they new or old. Four deceptively simple questions must be answered: does the technology work? For whom? At what cost? How does this technology compare with alternatives?

Busy jobs and the vast scale of the literature mean that few can keep up with research. Troubling delays in implementing some key findings have resulted. Ward et al. (Chapter 6.7) point out that that interventions that address specific barriers or hurdles are more likely to succeed: for example, audit and feedback may be useful when professionals are unaware of suboptimal practice, but reminders can work when barriers relate to information processing within consultations. Effectiveness guidelines can also be useful tools describing appropriate treatment and Feder and Griffiths (Chapter 6.8) similarly identify that great care is needed in planning implementation, with a need for a good project plan, including piloting to identify barriers.

Many public health practitioners work for bodies with funding or auditing responsibilities, and have to evaluate whole services. Hicks (Chapter 6.9) explores the challenges and advises that clarity is key, including clarity of purpose and dimensions of outcomes to be considered. Good outcome data are rare, however, but health services do generate large amounts of process data. Jessop (Chapter 6.10) cuts through the noise and suggests that process data are only useful if they monitor effective care.

It is clear from the previous chapters that quality improvement has grown into a very complex set of activities, at various levels. These activities need to be pulled together into an effective system of their own. Hall and Scally (Chapter 6.11) explore the British model, under the banner of clinical governance. They point out that public health practitioners have key roles to play, technically in understanding health data but also in engaging stakeholders and promoting a population view. Perhaps most importantly, public health practitioners can help build an environment in which skilled quality improvement can flourish and apportioning blame can be minimized.

DM

6.1 Understanding health-care quality

Paul Shekelle, David Pencheon, and David Melzer

Scoping quality in health care

Lack of quality in health care can be easy to recognize, when for example the wrong kidney is removed, the wrong drug prescribed, or where communication between different professionals breaks down. Being systematic about defining, measuring, and improving it is far more challenging. This chapter concentrates on defining the dimensions of quality, approaches to setting standards, and measuring quality.

Defining and measuring the quality of health care

According to the US Institute of Medicine (IOM) 'Quality of care is the degree to which health services for individuals and populations increase the likelihood of desired health outcomes and are consistent with current professional knowledge'.[1]

This definition explicitly acknowledges that:

- quality is measured as a scale or *degree* rather than as a binary phenomenon
- quality encompasses all aspects of care by referring to *health services*
- quality of health-care provision can be observed from an *individual* as well as a *population* perspective
- quality outcomes are *desired* without specifying for whom, thus allowing the possibility of differing perspectives on which aspects of quality are most important (professional, patient, public, political…)
- the link between the quality of care and outcomes is rarely causal by stating that what is measured is a *likelihood* or probability
- the phrase 'consistency *with current professional knowledge*' indicates that quality of care can only be judged relative to what is known at that moment in time.

However, despite quality often being perceived as difficult to define, Donabedian constantly stresses that the quality of a service is the degree to which it conforms to preset *standards* of good care. (See Chapters 1.8, 3.6, and 5.2.)

An important dimension of measuring (and thus defining) quality is to make the standards against which one is assessing quality explicit and preset. The importance of words such as 'standards' and 'right' is that they emphasize and make explicit the *subjective nature of quality* (i.e. 'quality is in the eye of the beholder or begetter').

Dimensions of quality

The first step toward assessing or measuring quality is to deconstruct it into its core dimensions.

Maxwell (in the UK context) suggested six dimensions which form the basis of quality of care.[2,3] This classification has the advantage of making it easier to operationalize the definition, i.e. to measure these dimensions individually (see Box 6.1.1).

Box 6.1.1 Maxwell's original dimensions of quality

- *Effectiveness*: Does the intervention in question produce the desired effect?
- *Efficiency*: Is the output (e.g. health) maximized for a given input or (conversely) is the input minimized for a given level of output? How does the unit cost compare with the unit cost elsewhere for the same treatment/service?
- *Acceptability*: How humanely and considerately is this treatment/service delivered? What does the patient think of it? What would/does an observant third party think of it? (How would I feel if it were my nearest and dearest?) What is the setting like? Are privacy and confidentiality safeguarded? (i.e. to what extent does the service conform to patient/public expectations?)
- *Access*: Can people get this treatment/service when they need it? Are there identifiable barriers to service—for example, lack of information, large distances to travel, inability to pay, and waiting times—or straightforward breakdowns in supply?
- *Equity*: Is this patient or group of patients being fairly treated relative to others? Are there any identifiable failings in equity, for example, are some people (perceived as) being dealt with less favourably than others?
- *Relevance*: Is the overall pattern and balance of services the best that could be achieved, taking account of needs and wants of the population as a whole?

Adapted from Maxwell[3]

Table 6.1.1 Three areas of quality

1. **Effectiveness/efficacy/appropriateness/safety.** Whether the service actually delivers in the way it is claimed (either under ideal conditions (efficacy) or in practice (effectiveness))	**Appropriate[a] and safe.** Can it work? (efficacy). Does it work? Does it do more good than harm? (effectiveness)
2. **Cost/efficiency.** Are there more efficient ways to deliver this service or are there other services that would be a better use of the resources? (Eliminating waste, and improving efficiency are integral to quality)	**Cost.** Is it worth it? (efficiency, e.g. cost–benefit). Is it wasteful?
3. **Equity/acceptability/access/ownership/relevance/legitimacy/responsiveness.** How is the service received by those who (might) receive it? Is it relevant, fair, flexible, responsive to demand? Is it what patients want? Is it what professionals judge what the public 'need'?	**Ownership.** Is the system fair? (equity). Can people use it? (accessible). Is it what individuals/society wants, and if not, can the system be changed accordingly? (acceptability, legitimacy, and responsiveness)

[a]Some definitions of appropriateness will include the issue of resources (see The appropriateness of clinical interventions below).

There are many variants of the six dimensions mentioned in Box 6.1.1. They all have in common three broad areas, shown in Table 6.1.1.

Whose quality is it?

The IOM definition of quality recognizes that the link between care and outcomes is rarely deterministic, and also qualifies outcomes as having to be desirable. But for whom should they be desirable? This perspective on quality, and the priority given to particular *aspects* of quality, can depend on who is the interested party. Table 6.1.2 gives a summary of the different perspectives of quality depending on who is considering it.

Table 6.1.2 Differing perspectives of quality

Interested party	High-priority elements of quality
Consumers/patients/public (i.e. those who demand and receive the care)	Responsiveness to perceived care needs. Level of communication, concern and courtesy. Degree of symptom relief. Level of functional improvement
Practitioners/clinicians (i.e. those who deliver the care)	Degree to which care meets the current technical state of the art. Freedom to act in the full interest of the patient. Accountability to 'professional standards'
Commissioners/funders/purchasers (i.e. those who sanction and pay for the health care)	Efficient use of funds available for health care. Appropriate use of health-care resources. Maximum possible contribution of health care to reduction in lost productivity. Accountability to politically set philosophy, objectives, targets, goals

Structure, process, or outcomes?

The quality of health care can be measured using structure, process, or outcomes. *Structure* refers to the elements of the health-care system such as the presence of a hospital, the number of beds in the hospital, the ratio of the number of nurses to the number of beds in a hospital, the presence of a trauma centre, and the like.

The *processes* of health care are those things delivered to individual patients in specific clinical circumstances, such as prescription of certain medications, the delivery of surgical procedures, diagnostic tests, etc.

Outcomes refer to health states such as death, having a stroke, improvements in functional status, etc.

While measuring outcomes has an intuitive appeal, there are serious limitations to widespread use of outcomes as measures of health-care quality:

- many determinants of outcome are poorly understood or not under the control of the health-care system
- for many chronic conditions, the time between the key processes of care and the outcomes may be very long. For example, untreated hypertension may be asymptomatic for years before leading to stroke or kidney failure.

Consequently, outcome measures of quality are usually restricted to areas where these problems are not present: mortality and morbidity following major surgical procedures and some acute hospital stays are examples.

The advantages of processes as measures of quality, covering what is delivered to patients under specific clinical circumstances, include:

- processes are likely to be seen by physicians as core to quality of care
- process measures directly identify potential areas for quality improvement (unlike many outcomes)
- process measures tend to be more sensitive to differences in quality (see, for example, Mant and Hicks[4]).

In order for processes to be the basis of valid measures of quality they must be strongly linked to subsequent outcomes, preferably by good evidence from, for example, randomized clinical trials, or professional consensus (see The appropriateness of clinical interventions below).

For all of these reasons, measures of health-care quality, whether in the USA, the new general practitioner contract in the UK National Health Service (NHS), or in other countries, are dominated by process measures rather than outcome measures.

Measuring quality of care

In order to assess and improve quality, it first must be measured.

A *quality indicator* is a statement about a specific health-care process that should be delivered under specific clinical circumstances—such as, if a patient has diabetes and is over the age of 55 and is at increased risk for cardiovascular disease then they should be offered treatment with an ACE inhibitor.

A *quality measure* is the operationalization of this quality indicator to a specific population and data sources and spells out precisely how patients with diabetes are to be identified, what factors and how they are measured are considered to be evidence of increased cardiovascular risk, and what efforts count in terms of offering ACE inhibitor therapy.

Criticisms of the use of quality indicators or measures include that the selected items aren't necessarily related to improved health outcomes and that focusing attention on certain measures will lead to decreasing attention on other aspects of health care, which may be as or more important. Therefore, development of measures should aim to:

- be as rigorous as possible
- cover a broad array of aspects of health care, to better represent care and minimize the ability to distort or game the measurement system.

The appropriateness of clinical interventions

Investigators at RAND Health and the University of California, Los Angeles, have defined 'appropriateness' of health-care interventions as the *degree to which benefit of care exceeds the expected negative consequences.* Through this concept it is possible to establish a set of rules or standards of care based on identifying appropriate interventions which should be used (or not used) in specific clinical situations.

The 'appropriateness method' was developed as a pragmatic solution to the problem of trying to assess for which patients certain surgical and medical procedures are 'appropriate'. Attempts were made to determine 'appropriateness' with a thorough literature review, but this proved insufficient for developing comprehensive, clinically detailed measures of appropriateness.

Several fundamental concepts helped shape the solution:

- clinical judgement is required to 'fill in the gaps': the medical literature alone is insufficient
- all relevant clinical disciplines must be involved
- indicators must be specific, and described in sufficient clinical detail that each description is relatively homogeneous with respect to risks and benefits of the procedure: a clear labelling of appropriate or not must be possible in practice
- the definitions of appropriate care should be comprehensive and applicable to most clinical situations relevant to the procedure; ergo, a very large number of clinical situations need to be considered
- applying the method must be feasible in terms of resources.

To apply these concepts, methods such as the Delphi and the Nominal Group Technique are used (for more details of the RAND-UCLA appropriateness method, see Fitch et al[5]). In short, clinical panelists are asked to rate many hundreds of possible indicators in a first round, with a moderator seeking to identify agreement and resolve differences, using highly defined procedures. The second, final ratings by the panel are used for the analysis. A good example of this approach is the development of the ACOVE quality standards (see Box 6.1.2).

Box 6.1.2 An example of quality standards and measures

One example of the development of quality indicators and measures is the 'Assessing Care of Vulnerable Elders' (ACOVE) project in the USA. This project targeted people over the age of 65 years who, because of advanced age or functional limitations, are at greatly increased risk for death and disability in 2 years. Fig 6.1.1 shows a flow chart summarizing the steps in the development of the ACOVE indicators.[6,7]

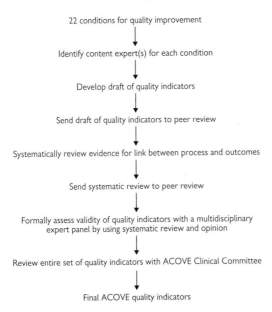

22 conditions for quality improvement

↓

Identify content expert(s) for each condition

↓

Develop draft of quality indicators

↓

Send draft of quality indicators to peer review

↓

Systematically review evidence for link between process and outcomes

↓

Send systematic review to peer review

↓

Formally assess validity of quality indicators with a multidisciplinary expert panel by using systematic review and opinion

↓

Review entire set of quality indicators with ACOVE Clinical Committee

↓

Final ACOVE quality indicators

Figure 6.1.1 Flowchart showing development of ACOVE indicators

As key elements of the method are somewhat arbitrary, the appropriateness method has been criticized[8–10] mainly for:

- the potential variability in the process due to the composition of the panel or the actual panel members themselves
- the role of the moderator
- the possibility of misclassification bias of individual scenarios
- a lack of specificity about what outcomes are being considered for individual scenarios
- a worry that the ratings reflect nothing more than codifying existing clinical dogma.

A substantial amount of methodological research has been done to try and assess these concerns. The results are very sensitive to the composition of the panel, in that clinicians who perform the procedure are more enthusiastic about its use.[11] If composition in terms of disciplines is held constant, the results are about as reproducible as some common diagnostic tests.[12,13]

Favourable predictive validity for appropriateness ratings have been reported for several procedures, including coronary angiography,[14,15] carotid endarterectomy,[16] and coronary revascularization.[17,18]

Other studies comparing the results of appropriateness method panels with decision analysis have reported mixed results.[19,20] The sensitivity and specificity of the method for identifying inappropriate over use and under use has been estimated at varying between 68% and 99%, and 94% and 97%, respectively.[21]

Comparative approaches to setting quality standards

In contrast to the appropriateness-based indicators for specific patients and interventions, a variety of standards have been set by comparing performance between clinicians or services. Imagine, for example, that there are a hundred orthopaedic services in a country. The case-mix-adjusted unplanned readmission rate after surgery (a measure of certain adverse short-term outcomes) across units varies from 1% to 20% and the range of readmission rates can be plotted as a distribution curve. What rate of unplanned readmission should we adopt as an indicator of high-quality care? If we adopt the lowest, we may be ignoring avoidable problems even in the best units. On the other hand, we may be setting impossible targets that cannot be achieved. Similar questions arise in setting process- or structure-based standards.

Should the benchmark be the average or the best possible?

It is important to decide the principles underlying the standards adopted. For instance, there has been a long tradition of considering and adopting the status quo as the standard; rather than aiming at better practice for local use.[22]

Different levels of standards are typically used:

- *Excellent standards*: these are typically standards achieved by the 'best' services, for example based on the lowest 5% of unit readmission rates. Such standards can identify what's possible and challenge excuses.
- *Minimal acceptable standards*: are those below which no service should fall; for example, again it could be deemed (somewhat arbitrarily) that the maximum acceptable readmission rate is 15%, because 90% of units are achieving better.
- *Achievable standards*: although setting standards at the top end of distributions can be appealing, in practice many services will view them as unattainable. Sometimes, therefore, standard setters adopt more modest standards: in the UK breast cancer screening programme

standards were based on a cut-off point between the top quartile and the rest.

In practice, standards must fulfil two criteria to be useful:[23]

- it must be clear what *individuals* need to do to achieve them (the link between individual activity and achievement is important)
- the standards must be attainable, i.e. a balance needs to be struck between standards of excellence and achievable standards.

Local or (inter)national standards?

Like guidelines, in order to get standards agreed to, implemented, and achieved, there has to be local ownership. However, if standards vary greatly depending on geography, then they are probably not good standards.

Because the process of setting standards for clinical care includes evidence, values, and resources, standards developed in one country may not necessarily be applied in another. Nevertheless, standards developed in the US have been helpful in developing standards in the UK, but often require a process of adaptation to reflect local realities.[24,25]

Trading off dimensions of quality

Rather than being independent, different dimensions of quality can sometimes be in conflict with each other, requiring trade-offs. For instance having a trauma unit on the corner of every block may maximize accessibility but it is clearly not the best overall use of resources. Some trade-offs relate to the value of *longer-term versus shorter-term outcomes* (e.g. eventual functional improvement versus comfort and short waits). Not only do different people value different dimensions but the same individual may value different dimensions over time or depending on the condition that needs attention.

Costs and quality

The perspective held by those who commission health care, for whom efficiency is a high-priority element of quality, can create uneasy tensions.[26] The economic notion of an 'opportunity cost' can apply where improving, for example, access or responsiveness of services conflicts with improving efficiency (see Chapter 1.4).

Including economic efficiency in the definition of quality is controversial. The US IOM definition does not explicitly include any mention of efficiency, in contrast to the Maxwell dimensions of quality from the UK. Of course, maximizing quality for those whose care is paid for can result in unsustainable spending, which often results in indefensible exclusions of individuals or procedures from coverage, in subsequent attempts to control overall costs. On the other hand, Wennberg's work on activity variations has shown that there is little relationship between high quality and high cost in services across the US (see Chapter 1.6): often quality can be improved for the same amount or even less money.

Separating systems aimed at improving value for money and quality can help to avoid unrealistic expectations.

Perspectives on improving quality: 'bad apples' or system improvements

No one would doubt that assessing quality through mechanisms such as monitoring, audit, and evaluation is essential. However, there are different philosophical and practical approaches to how a system's quality is maintained and improved. At their extremes they are characterized by the *'bad apple' approach* on the one hand and *continuous quality improvement* on the other.

In the 'bad apple' approach the *individual* whose quality of care is unacceptable is identified. Thus, performance tables comparing surgeons often aim to identify the worst performers. This has superficial political attractions in identifying 'the person responsible': it does little to drive up standards for most patients. In addition, punitive atmospheres lead to secrecy and conflict.

In the system improvement approach, emphasis is placed on learning from mistakes, and modifying the *system* of care to make mistakes less likely to happen again (see Chapter 6.2). Doing more clinical trials to identify the best treatments may also be the best response to wide variations in practice.

Both approaches require the measurement of quality, but in the first accountability, punishments, and awarding selective accreditation are emphasized. 'It is not possible to learn without measuring, but it is possible, and very wasteful, to measure without learning'.[22]

Summary: questions to ask when addressing 'quality'

Public health practitioners are often called on to measure quality of health care, or to help others with the process. Consider the following checklist. It should help scope the issues:

- *Why measure quality?* Ask people why they want to measure quality (There may be tangentially related issues at stake which may need addressing in completely different ways).
- *What do you actually plan to measure?* Agree a common definition. Enquire what would be considered good measures of quality of care: this will identify what subdimensions and approaches to quality are considered most important.
- *Who are you planning to involve in this whole process?* Consult those with a stake in this issue and consider their perspective on quality.
- *Which aspect(s) of quality are you planning to address?* Break quality of care down into measurable subdimensions and then agree which ones will be measured.
- *Whose perspectives are you going to consider most?* Each perspective has advantages and limitations. Are you going to concentrate on the society's approach to quality? If so, distinguish between:

- *population* appropriateness (effectiveness, modified by societal judgements and resources—a synthesis of a professional/technical perspective with a societal/political perspective)
- *individual* appropriateness (effectiveness, modified by patient characteristics and preferences).[27]

● *Which approach (or combination of approaches) are you planning to use?*
  Will you build:
  - A learning organization?
  - A measurement/audit system?
  - A simple care system—making it more difficult to make errors or be inefficient?
  - An educational model of quality improvement?
  - An evaluative and regulatory culture where all interventions are rigorously assessed and licenced, and all professionals are revalidated and reaccredited?

● *Which dimension: structure, process or outcome?*
  - Is the system/environment/organization right? (see Chapter 6.2).
  - Are the professionals competent? Do good information systems exist (clinical decision support, making good evidence available…) (see Chapter 6.5); are educational opportunities genuinely available? (to help professionals implement good evidence, and share and learn from practice…); what are the methods of improving professional practice? (regulation, continuing medical education (cme), continuing professional development (cpd), revalidation and relicensing…)
  - Are the interventions that are performed safe, rigorously evaluated, appropriate, the best use of available resources, fairly distributed and accessible?
  - When such errors and lapses in quality do happen: are they acknowledged? are they investigated? (confidential enquiries, critical incident analysis…), and is the learning fed back into the system? (Is this a genuinely learning organization nurturing life-long learners?)

Further resources

Deming WE (1993). *Out of the crisis.* Massachusetts Institute of Technology, Centre for Advanced Engineering Study, Cambridge, MA.

Donabedian A (2002). *An introduction to quality assurance in health care.* Oxford University Press. Oxford.

Enthoven AC (2000). In pursuit of an improving National Health Service. *Health Affairs*, **9**(3), 102–19.

Leape LL, Berwick DM (2000). Safe health care: are we up to it? *BMJ*, **320**, 725–6 (and the whole of the same special issue 'Errors in medicine' (18 March 2000)).

Øvretveit J (1992). *Health service quality.* Blackwell, Oxford.

Thomson R (1998). Quality to the fore in health policy—at last. *BMJ*, **317**, 95–6.

References

1 Lohr KN (1990). *Medicare: a strategy for quality assurance.* National Academy Press, Washington, DC.

2 Maxwell RJ (1992). Dimensions of quality revisited: from thought to action. *Qual Health Care*, **1**, 171–7.

3 Maxwell RJ (1984). Quality assessment in health. *BMJ*, **288**,1470–2.

4 Mant J, Hicks N (1995). Detecting differences in quality of care: the sensitivity of measures of process and outcome in treating acute myocardial infarction. *BMJ*, **311**(7008), 793–6.

5 Fitch K, Bernstein SJ, Aguilar MD et al. (2001). *The RAND/UCLA appropriateness method user's manual*. RAND, Santa Monica, CA.

6 Shekelle PG, MacLean CH, Morton SC, Wenger NS (2001). Acove quality indicators. *Ann Intern Med*, **135**(8, Pt 2), 653–67.

7 Wenger NS, Shekelle PG (2001). Assessing care of vulnerable elders: ACOVE project overview. *Ann Intern Med*, **135**(8, Pt 2), 642–6.

8 Phelps CE (1993). The methodological foundations of studies of the appropriateness of medical care. *N Engl J Med*, **329**(17), 1241–5.

9 Kassirer JP (1993). The quality of care and the quality of measuring it. *N Engl J Med*, **329**(17), 1263–5.

10 Hicks NR (1994). Some observations on attempts to measure appropriateness of care. *BMJ*, **309**(6956), 730–3.

11 Kahan JP, Park RE, Leape LL et al. (1996). Variations by specialty in physician ratings of the appropriateness and necessity of indications for procedures. *Med Care*, **34**(6), 512–23.

12 Shekelle PG, Kahan JP, Bernstein SJ, Leape LL, Kamberg CJ, Park RE (1998). The reproducibility of a method to identify the overuse and underuse of medical procedures. *N Engl J Med*, **338**(26), 1888–95.

13 Tobacman JK, Scott IU, Cyphert S, Zimmerman B (1999). Reproducibility of measures of overuse of cataract surgery by three physician panels. *Med Care*, **37**(9), 937–45.

14 Selby JV, Fireman BH, Lundstrom RJ et al. (1996). Variation among hospitals in coronary-angiography practices and outcomes after myocardial infarction in a large health maintenance organization. *N Engl J Med*, **335**(25), 1888–96.

15 Normand ST, Landrum MB, Guadagnoli E et al. (2001). Validating recommendations for coronary angiography following acute myocardial infarction in the elderly: a matched analysis using propensity scores. *J Clin Epidemiol*, **54**(4), 387–98.

16 Shekelle PG, Chassin MR, Park RE (1998). Assessing the predictive validity of the RAND/UCLA appropriateness method for performing carotid endarterectomy. *Int J Technol Assess Health Care*, **14**(4) 707–27.

17 Kravitz RL, Laouri M, Kahan JP et al. (1995). Validity of criteria used for detecting underuse of coronary revascularization. *J Am Med Assoc*, **274**(8), 632–8.

18 Hemingway H, Crook AM, Feder G et al. (2001). Underuse of coronary revascularisation procedures in patients considered appropriate candidates for revascularisation. *New Eng J Med*, **344**, 645–54.

19 McClellan M, Brook RH (1992). Appropriateness of care. A comparison of global and outcome methods to set standards. *Med Care*, **30**(7), 565–86.

20 Silverstein MD, Ballard DJ (1998). Expert panel assessment of appropriateness of abdominal aortic aneurysm surgery: global judgement versus probability estimation. *J Health Serv Res Policy*, **3**(3), 134–40.

21 Shekelle PG, Park RE, Kahan JP, Leape LL, Kamberg CJ, Bernstein SJ (2001). Sensitivity and specificity of the RAND/UCLA Appropriateness Method to identify the overuse and underuse of coronary revascularization and hysterectomy. *J Clin Epidemiol*, **54**(10), 1004–10.

22 Berwick DM (1998). The NHS's 50 anniversary. Looking forward. The NHS: feeling well and thriving at 75. *BMJ*, **317**, 57–61.

23 Jewell D (1992). Setting standards: from passing fashion to essential clinical activity. *Qual Health Care*, **1**(4), 217–18.

24 Steel N, Melzer D, Shekelle PG, Wenger NS. Forsyth D, McWilliams BC (2004). Developing quality indicators for older adults: transfer from the USA to the UK is feasible. *Qual Saf Health Care*, **13**(4), 260–4.

25 Marshall MN, Shekelle PG, McGlynn EA, Campbell S, Brook RH, Roland MO (2003). Can health care quality indicators be transferred between countries. *Qual Saf Health Care*, **12**(1), 8–12.

26 Schwartz WB, Joskow PL (1978). Medical efficacy versus economic efficiency: a conflict of values. *N Engl J Med*, **299**, 1462–4.

27 What do we mean by appropriate health care? Report of a working group prepared for the Director of Research and Development of the UK NHS Management Executive. (1993) *Qual Health Care*, **2**(2), 117–23.

6.2 Taking action to improve quality

Charlie Tomson and Rashad Massoud

Objectives

By reading this chapter you will learn how to organize and complete a quality improvement project in health care, you will understand the key determinants of success or failure of an improvement project, and you will understand how best to sustain the improvement within the organization and to spread the successful changes to other organizations.

Definition

A quality improvement project is a clearly articulated plan to improve the quality of health care. It is useful to consider quality in one of these six areas (the acronym STEEEP can be used to remember these):

- Safety
- Timeliness
- Effectiveness
- Efficiency
- Equity
- Patient-centredness.

The need for systems thinking

Lucian Leape, a leader in safety and prevention of medical errors, has described the concept that medical errors are caused by bad systems as a 'transforming concept'.[1] Berwick has described the central law of improvement: 'every system is perfectly designed to achieve the results it achieves'.[2] Systems thinking is second nature to engineers, but can be difficult for doctors who are focused on the individual patient–doctor relationship.

How should a quality improvement project be organized?

To run a successful improvement project you will need to build will, have good ideas, and have a carefully thought out strategy for execution. Building 'will' has two critical aspects: the support of senior leaders and

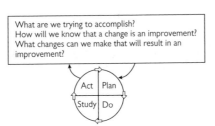

Figure 6.2.1 The 'model for improvement'[3,4]

clinicians and the formation of a quality improvement team that will see the project through. The 'ideas', or 'change package', may be a strategy for implementing clinical practice guidelines that has already been tested and is ready for local adoption and adaptation, or may require innovation if no one has achieved quality improvement in a similar setting before. 'Execution' requires a clearly articulated plan to keep the team motivated and on track; we recommend the 'model for improvement' (Figure 6.2.1).

Obtaining the support of senior leaders and clinicians

Senior leaders and clinicians may not be directly involved in the day-to-day work of your improvement project, but their support is crucial to your success. 'Not all change is improvement, but all improvement is change',[2] and big organizations tend to resist change. Getting leadership 'on board' will help remove obstacles to change, for instance enlisting the Forms Committee if your change package involves tests of changes in the way you collect clinical information. There are several strategies that you might use to obtain support:

- Use data to demonstrate the opportunities for improvement—the 'chasm' between current practice in your organization and best practice, or between your results and those of other organizations.
- Build a business case for improvement. The details of this will depend on the setting of the project. Perverse financial incentives (e.g. payment per hospital admission for patients with chronic disease) occur in all systems, but the details may vary. Despite these problems, it is possible to build a persuasive case for quality improvement.[5,6] (See Box 6.2.1.)
- Press to get reports on safety and quality onto the governing board's agenda as a regular item for discussion, equal in importance to the finance report (presenting a 'balanced scorecard' view of the organization).
- Use stories about real patients to bring the issue of quality alive; if possible, invite patients to participate in your improvement team.

Box 6.2.1 The business case for improvement

Payment by results:
- Direct payments based on quality of care
- Increased revenue due to increased efficiency (e.g. as a result of reduced length of stay due to improved flow)

Direct costs of defective care:
- Increased length of stay due to hospital-acquired infection

Indirect costs of defective care:
- Insurance premiums
- Litigation costs

Improvements in staff retention (e.g. reduced costs of agency nursing)
Reduction in waste within the system:
- Repeated tests due to missing results
- Reduced length of stay

Forming your quality improvement team

The team should include representatives from all disciplines and departments involved in the improvement work. Don't hesitate to 'pick winners' who you know will be enthusiastic; once you have demonstrated success, others will follow until the tipping point is reached and even the late adopters start asking to make the change. Ignore hierarchy: a team designed to improve out-patient waiting times will fail if it doesn't include the receptionist, as will a team wanting to reduce MRSA transmission if it doesn't include a representative from the housekeeping staff. Use the support you have obtained from your leaders to allocate time for the team to meet regularly.

Once your team has formed, encourage them to spend time studying the existing process that they want to improve by making a flowchart of the existing process. For example, the process of urgent care at a hospital starts with the patient arriving at the hospital emergency department with acute pain, going through a registration step, being seen by a triage nurse, undergoing a medical examination (with or without laboratory or radiological investigations), and ending with the possible administration of treatment and either discharge home or admission to the hospital. If you map this process carefully using a flowchart you will find that multiple smaller steps exist within each of the major process steps. This will help identify opportunities for improvement. Work on reducing the number of steps required: this will improve the reliability of your system and smooth the flow through the system, for instance, the flow of patients through the hospital.

Collaborating and sharing ideas

The Institute for Healthcare Improvement's Breakthrough Series collaborative model[7] is based on the 'all teach, all learn' philosophy. Typically, members of improvement teams focusing on a particular topic meet face-to-face for a learning session, keep in touch with each other using E-mail and phone conferences, post their tests of change and results for all other teams to see, and reconvene for one or two further learning sessions over a 10–12-month period. The collaborative model approach is most useful when you are trying to disseminate changes that are already known to work—for instance better implementation of evidence-based prevention of wound infection after surgery—rather than when you are trying to find totally new solutions to a problem.

Planning and executing your quality improvement project

The model for improvement (Figure 6.2.1) is an extremely useful framework for planning a quality improvement project. This model was developed by a group of quality improvement consultants and statisticians who observed that failure to ask any one of these three questions was nearly always associated with failure of quality improvement projects in industry.[3] It has now been widely adopted in health-care quality improvement work, although it is not the only model in use.

What are you trying to accomplish?

Setting clear, measurable goals is important in focusing the efforts of your team. A team asked to 'improve central line care' is less likely to succeed than one that is given the target to 'reduce central line-related bloodstream infections by 50% over 6 months'.

How will you know that a change is an improvement?

All improvement requires change, but not all change results in improvement. It is therefore essential that you plan to measure the results of your improvement project, not just at the beginning and end but regularly as part of the project itself. Graphical display of results, often in the form of a simple annotated run chart, allows your team to chart their progress and see the impact of the changes they have tested (Figure 6.2.2).[8]

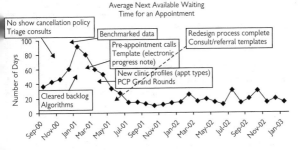

Figure 6.2.2 Run chart showing improvement in access to specialist care, annotated with the tests of change used. The changes used are described in the paper. (From Schall et al.[8])

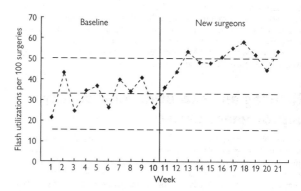

Figure 6.2.3 Statistical process control chart for the flash sterilization rate: the baseline compared with the period following the arrival of a new surgical group, showing that this procedure (traditionally only used in emergencies) became more common shortly after a new group of surgeons joined the hospital staff. Statistical process control is widely used in industry, and is a branch of statistics that combines rigorous time-series analysis with graphical presentation of data. The upper and lower lines are control limits, set at three standard deviations from the mean (centre line). (From Benneyan et al.[9])

Sometimes your team will want to know whether changes in their measurements are due to random variation or to a real change in the system. In this instance, a statistical process control chart (Shewhart chart) is appropriate (Figure 6.2.3).[9]

What changes can you make that will result in improvement?

Many quality improvement projects in health care are focused around improving the implementation of evidence-based care. Clinical practice guidelines are available that summarize the evidence. In this situation you know what you want to achieve: how to implement the specific guidelines of care in your institution effectively and reliably. For an example see Box 6.2.2.

What skills and competencies are needed to succeed in a quality improvement project?

Recognize that improvement requires skills that are seldom taught in medical school. Quality improvement requires not only knowledge of subject matter but also an understanding of psychology, variation, the theory of knowledge, and systems thinking, among other things.

Use lessons from industries outside health care

You will encounter stiff resistance to any suggestion that you might be able to improve your system by learning how other industries have improved theirs, but it's worth persevering. Although patients are not cars on an assembly line, the lessons learned in redesigning assembly lines by companies like Toyota[10] can be applied to any process where patients move through a system, for example a hospital admission, a request for an out-patient visit, or a surgical operation.

Box 6.2.2 Example of improving the implementation of evidence-based care

AIM. To reduce the rate of ventilator-associated pneumonia in the adult intensive care unit to zero within 4 months.

MEASURE. The rate of ventilator-associated pneumonia (requires a careful definition of how the condition is diagnosed and how the denominator is calculated).

CHANGES. Implement a 'bundle' of evidence-based interventions that, when implemented together, improve outcomes in ventilated adults. Measure compliance with this process as an 'all or nothing' score rather then measuring implementation of each intervention separately. The interventions are:
- Elevation of the head of the bed to between 30 and 45 degrees
- Daily 'sedation vacation' irrespective of physician's opinion on readiness to wean
- Daily formal assessment of readiness to wean
- Prophylaxis against stress ulceration
- Prophylaxis against deep venous thrombosis

Achieving 100% compliance with each of these interventions will require numerous small tests of change, with measurement of compliance for each intervention as well as for the composite 'bundle'. For instance, the team may test the impact of computer screensavers reminding nurses about the new policy on elevation of the head of the bed. Before doing the test they predict the outcome. They then activate the screensavers and study the rate of compliance with the policy over the next week. Once the test is complete they study the results, identify what led to the failures, and plan the next test, which might be a new sign attached to the mechanism that allows the head of the bed to be elevated.

Even if the specifics don't translate well, the underlying principle of continuous quality improvement in manufacturing is that people want to do a 'good job', that everyone is an expert on their own job, and that we all gain motivation if we are continually encouraged to find more efficient ways of working. If this has been shown to be true on a production line (where shaving a second off a standardized task like fitting screws into a seat is a major achievement), one would expect it to be even truer in health care.

Promoting innovation

Sometimes you will want to achieve improvement in a new clinical or topic area in which no one has established a proven change package. In this situation you will need to promote innovative thinking. You will need

specific skills to persuade workers to think about how to change a pattern of work they have become so accustomed to that they cannot
imagine any alternative to 'trying harder'. In routine clinical practice,
habits and patterns are safety features—indeed, standardization is one
important way to achieve high reliability in health care. These patterns
need to be purposely put aside to enable innovative thinking about how
to rework the system. There is evidence that creativity is not a 'gift' and
that anyone can be taught to come up with creative ideas.[11,12]

Determinants of success

A study of five national quality improvement collaboratives in the Veterans Health Administration System[13] identified three factors associated
with success:

- strong organizational support
- strong team leadership
- high levels of interpersonal team skills.

A similar study of collaboratives in seven countries[14] identified the following as predictive of success: sponsorship, topic, ideas for improvements,
participants, senior leadership support, preliminary work and learning,
and strategies for learning about and making improvements.

Can quality improvement projects be assessed using the same scientific model as drug treatments?

Many of the quality improvement concepts you have been introduced to
in this chapter come from outside medicine and involve very different
concepts from those required for evaluating medical interventions.[15]
Whether quality improvement projects that address system-level changes
in health-care delivery can or should be tested by randomized controlled
trial remains uncertain[16] and may require complex design.[17] A comprehensive review of the collaborative approach to health-care improvement
in chronic disease management is under way.[18]

Conclusions

Improving health care is hard work and requires commitment and support from the leadership, but it is extremely rewarding and important.
Using the model for improvement will help you focus your quality
improvement efforts. Sharing ideas, whether about a change package or
how to get the package adopted locally, is vital: someone, somewhere
will be trying to achieve improvements in the same area as your project,
and you will achieve improvement faster if you share your experiences.

Further resources

Clinical Microsystems. http://www.clinicalmicrosystem.org/ (accessed
29 July 2005). Resources on how to analyze and improve clinical microsystems, including a workbook that can be downloaded and adapted.

Directed Creativity. http://www.directedcreativity.com/ (accessed 29 July 2005). Advice on using specific psychological techniques to encourage people accustomed to working in fixed patterns to think differently and identify innovative ideas.

Improving Chronic Illness Care. http://www.improvingchroniccare.org/ (accessed 29 July 2005). Relates specifically to chronic conditions.

Improvement Leaders Guides. http://www.wise.nhs.uk/cmsWISE/Tools+and+Techniques/ILG/ILG.htm (accessed 29 July 2005). These guides from the NHS Modernisation Agency give detailed advice on all aspects of improvement projects.

Institute for Healthcare Improvement website. http://www.ihi.org/ihi (accessed 29 July 2005). Contains numerous examples of successful improvement projects, change packages, tools and resources (see 'Topics'), including an 'improvement tracker' that can be used to track your own progress (see 'Workspace').

US Agency for Healthcare Research and Quality. http://www.ahrq.gov/clinic/epc/qgapfact.pdf (accessed 29 July 2005). A comprehensive report entitled 'Closing the quality gap: a critical analysis of quality improvement strategies'.

References

1 Leape LL (2000). Institute of Medicine medical error figures are not exaggerated. *J Am Med Assoc*, **284**(1), 95–7.

2 Berwick DM (1996). A primer on leading the improvement of systems. *BMJ*, **312**(7031), 619–22.

3 Langley GJ, Nolan KM, Nolan TW *et al*. (1996). *The improvement guide: a practical approach to enhancing organizational performance*, 1st edn. Jossey-Bass, San Francisco, CA.

4 Berwick DM, Nolan TW (1998). Physicians as leaders in improving health care: a new series in *Annals of Internal Medicine*. *Ann Intern Med*, **128**(4), 289–92.

5 Bailit M, Dyer MB (2004). *Beyond bankable dollars; establishing a business case for improving healthcare*, Commonwealth Fund publication no 754. Available at: http://www.cmwf.org/usr_doc/Bailit_beyond_bankable_dollars_business_case.pdf (accessed 20 January 2005).

6 Blumenthal D, Ferris T (2004). *The business case for quality: ending business as usual in American health care*. Available at: http://www.cmwf.org/usr_doc/715_Blumenthal_business_case.pdf (accessed 20 January 2005).

7 Institute for Healthcare Improvement (2003). *The Breakthrough Series: IHI's collaborative model for achieving breakthrough improvement*, IHI Innovation Series. Institute for Healthcare Improvement, Boston, MA.

8 Schall MW, Duffy T, Krishnamurthy A, *et al*. (2004). Improving patient access to the Veterans Health Administration's primary care and specialty clinics. *Jt Comm J Qual Saf*, **30**(8), 415–23.

9 Benneyan JC, Lloyd RC, Plsek PE (2003). Statistical process control as a tool for research and healthcare improvement. *Qual Saf Health Care*, **12**(6), 458–64.

10 Spear S (1999). Decoding the DNA of the Toyota production system. *Harvard Business Rev*, Sept–Oct, 95–106.

11 de Bono E (1994). Creativity and quality. *Qual Manag Health Care*, **2**(3), 1–4.

12 Plsek PE (1994). Tutorial: directed creativity. *Qual Manag Health Care*, **2**(3), 62–76.

13 Mills PD, Weeks WB (2004). Characteristics of successful quality improvement teams: lessons from five collaborative projects in the VHA. *Jt Comm J Qual Saf*, **30**(3), 152–62.

14 Wilson T, Berwick DM, Cleary PD (2003). What do collaborative improvement projects do? Experience from seven countries. *Jt Comm J Qual Saf*, **29**(2), 85–93.

15 Greenhalgh T, Robert G, Macfarlane F, *et al.* (2004). Diffusion of innovations in service organizations: systematic review and recommendations. *Milbank Q*, **82**(4), 581–629.

16 Grol R, Baker R, Moss F (2002). Quality improvement research: understanding the science of change in health care. *Qual Saf Health Care*, **11**(2), 110–11.

17 Verstappen WH, van der Weijden T, Sijbrandij J, *et al.* (2004). Block design allowed for control of the Hawthorne effect in a randomized controlled trial of test ordering. *J Clin Epidemiol*, **57**(11), 1119–23.

18 Cretin S, Shortell SM, Keeler EB (2004). An evaluation of collaborative interventions to improve chronic illness care: framework and study design. *Eval Rev*, **28**(1), 28–51.

6.3 Quality improvement through chronic disease management

Ronald M. Davis

Introduction and objectives

Chronic diseases have become the most common cause of death and disability world-wide. According to the World Health Organization, non-communicable conditions—including cardiovascular and respiratory diseases, cancer, and diabetes—are responsible for 59% of the 57 million deaths annually and 46% of the global burden of disease.[1] Furthermore, there are considerable resource implications of managing people with chronic diseases/long-term conditions. In 2002, diabetes required $92 billion in direct medical expenditures in the US.[2]

The purpose of this chapter is to identify and describe the major components of chronic disease management programmes.

As chronic illnesses impose an increasing burden on health-care systems and providers, chronic disease management (CDM) (in the US) or long-term conditions (LTC) (in the UK) have become recognized fields in health-care delivery in these and many other countries. Many companies with disease management programmes have appeared in the US, and this development is now emerging in the UK and other countries.[3,4] An important component of CDM is proactive upstream care which improves quality of life whilst simultaneously reducing the risk of a patient's condition deteriorating to an extent where an acute admission is necessary. Investing in upstream care is designed to deliver:

- a net financial benefit to the health-care system as a whole (e.g. from fewer acute admissions)
- better disease markers (e.g. glycaemic control)
- better therapeutic concordance and
- improvements in the quality of patients' lives.

In its report 'Crossing the quality chasm: a new health system for the 21st century',[5] the US Institute of Medicine (IOM) wrote:

> The committee [on the Quality of Health Care in America] recognizes the enormity of the change that will be required to achieve a substantial improvement in the nation's health care system...To initiate the process of change, the committee believes the health care system must focus greater attention on the development of care processes for the common conditions that afflict many people. A limited number of such conditions, about 15 to 25, account for the majority of health

care services [citations omitted].... Nearly all of these conditions are chronic. By focusing attention on a limited number of common conditions, the committee believes it will be possible to make sizable improvements in the quality of care received by many individuals within the coming decade.

Hospital usage appears to increase exponentially in patients who have more than one of these listed conditions (Box 6.3.1). For this reason, patients with multiple conditions are generally considered separately: they need carefully tailored care that takes into account how their diseases interact.

Box 6.3.1 Top 15 priority conditions

- Cancer
- Diabetes
- Emphysema
- High cholesterol
- HIV/AIDS
- Hypertension
- Ischemic heart disease
- Stroke
- Arthritis
- Asthma
- Gall bladder disease
- Stomach ulcers
- Back problems
- Alzheimer's disease and other dementias
- Depression and anxiety disorders

Source: Institute of Medicine,[5] based on the Medical Expenditure Panel Survey (2000).

Definition of disease management

The Disease Management Association of America has defined disease management as 'a system of coordinated healthcare interventions and communications for populations with conditions in which patient self-care efforts are significant'.[6]

Levels of chronic disease management

Chronic disease management is conventionally considered on three levels. The levels are usually illustrated by the risk stratification triangle that was developed by Kaiser Permanente (known as 'The Kaiser pyramid'). It is a triangle because there are many more patients on level 1 than on the higher levels.

Level 1: self-management—lower-risk patients (70–80% of patients)

Self-management is appropriate for population-wide interventions. Patients (e.g. all patients with asthma) might be offered information and support. They may also be enrolled into self-care programmes.

The remainder of this chapter will use the term disease management to address features common to all of these three groups.

Level 2: disease management—higher-risk patients

Disease management is designed to ensure that patients with a given disease receive the best care possible for that condition. In the UK this is being achieved through the family doctors (GPs) being offered strong financial incentives to compile disease registers and manage the disease with the use of evidence-based guidance.

Level 3: case management—patients with highly complex conditions

Case management focuses on small numbers of patients with very complex needs. These patients are offered a case manager who acts as a fixed point of contact for them and coordinates their care.

Components of disease management

The components of disease management include:
- population identification processes
- evidence-based practice guidelines
- collaborative practice models to include physician and support-service providers
- patient self-management education
- process and outcomes measurement, evaluation, and management.[6]

These strategies have been incorporated into a model developed by Edward Wagner for primary care of patients with chronic illness. The model identifies six essential elements of a health-care system that encourage high-quality chronic disease care:
- the community
- the health system
- self-management support
- delivery system design
- decision support
- clinical information systems.[7,8]

Population identification processes

Chronic disease management is wholly dependent upon effective population identification, so-called 'case finding'. Registers (see Chapter 2.7) can then be constructed which are designed to:
- contain information on personal health behaviours and risk factors, history of disease, and family history of disease, based on questionnaire responses, often supplemented by biomedical measurements such as height, weight, blood pressure, and blood chemistry tests

- estimate the individual's risk of death and/or other adverse health outcomes; and
- provide education or counselling to the individual on how to reduce health risks and improve health status.[9]

This process is often referred to as health risk appraisal (HRA). Methods of case finding range from using clinical knowledge to techniques such as predictive modelling.

Clinical knowledge

This employs professionals' clinical knowledge and health records of patients to identify patients with existing disease. This technique can be effective at identifying patients currently at risk, who are likely to be high service users in the future. However, it does not identify high risk persons who have yet to make contact with social or health-care services.

Predictive modelling

Predictive modelling can be highly sensitive and specific for future risk. It applies formulae to a range of historical data in order to make predictions. Relevant data sources include:

- hospital service use
- diagnostic codes
- socio-demographic data
- prescription data
- clinical data.

Evidence-based practice guidelines

Following clinical practice guidelines is an important component of high-quality care, evidence-based medicine, and disease management. Practice guidelines should be based on scientific evidence, or, in the absence of evidence, on explicit expert consensus (see Chapter 6.8). Practice guidelines have been developed by many professional medical associations for most chronic conditions, especially those imposing a substantial burden on the health-care system. (See examples at http://www.guideline.gov/ (accessed 28 July 2005), a comprehensive database of evidence-based clinical practice guidelines and related documents.)

Collaborative practice models to include physician and support-service providers

Patient care teams can improve clinical outcomes in the management of chronic diseases. The varied skills of the team can be used to improve the management of chronic disease through treatment planning, adherence to clinical management protocols, self-management support, group consultations, and close and sustained follow-up of patients.[10]

Patient self-management education

An important principle of chronic disease management is that patients play a central role in managing their health and health care. Disease management by the patient includes adhering to medication regimens, avoiding exacerbating factors, modifying health behaviours, self-monitoring the signs and symptoms of the illness (e.g. the blood glucose level in diabetics), following written action plans for managing symptoms, and attending classes. Studies have shown that these self-management strategies improve health outcomes, reduce symptoms, enhance physical functioning and psychological status, and lower health-care utilization.[11,12]

Process and outcomes measurement, evaluation, and management

The importance of measuring the impact of chronic disease programmes, and making any necessary refinements and improvements, is self-evident. One large measurement system addresses management of osteoporosis, hypertension control, medication and management of cholesterol after acute cardiovascular events, comprehensive diabetes care, use of medication by asthmatics, and management of antidepressant medication.[13]

Effectiveness of chronic disease management programmes

Several systematic reviews of studies evaluating chronic disease management programmes indicate that these programmes improve health outcomes. In a review of 24 studies of diabetes disease management (19 randomized clinical trials and four non-randomized controlled studies), Knight et al. found that the programmes 'can improve glycaemic control to a modest extent and can increase screening for retinopathy and foot complications'.[14] McAlister et al. reviewed 11 randomized clinical trials of disease management programmes for patients in heart failure, and they found that the programmes reduce hospitalizations and appear to be cost saving, but the data on mortality were inconclusive.[15] In a review of 24 studies of programmes to manage depression, Badamgarav and colleagues found that the programmes were associated with improvements in symptoms of depression, patient satisfaction with treatment, adherence of patients to the recommended treatment regimen, and the adequacy of prescribed treatment.[16]

The report from the Health Evidence Network (HEN) at the World Health Organization's Regional Office for Europe concluded that disease management programmes for diabetes, depression, chronic heart failure, and cardiovascular diseases have been shown to improve the management and control of these conditions, including the adherence of providers to evidence-based standards of care. However, the authors found no evidence linking disease management programmes to lower mortality or improved quality of life, nor did they find evidence about the cost-effectiveness of these programmes.[17] Similarly, the US Congressional Budget Office found that 'there is insufficient evidence to conclude that disease management programmes can generally reduce overall health spending'.[18]

Potential risks and pitfalls in disease management programmes

Several concerns have been raised about disease management programmes.[19]

Risk of fragmented services

Firstly, programmes operated without involving the patient's primary care physician may interfere with the doctor–patient relationship and, in some settings, risk creating fragmented and poorly coordinated care across multiple providers. Coordination and communication are critical. In the UK, community matrons seize the initiative to cancel unnecessary follow-up appointments, coordinate multiple out-patient appointments so that they take place on the same day, and facilitate communication between clinicians, especially across the primary/secondary care divide.

Cost versus quality

Secondly, disease management programmes that are driven more by cost considerations than quality improvement alienate physicians, who perceive the programmes as managing the utilization of services rather than the quality and appropriateness of the services. Such programmes can impair the quality of health care by reducing access to medically necessary treatments.

Over-rigidity in adherence to guidance

Thirdly, disease management programmes that are overly rigid in mandating adherence to practice guidelines and other care protocols may also compromise some patients' access to the treatments they need. Physicians argue that individual circumstances occasionally require a departure from clinical practice guidelines.

Conclusions

Much evidence indicates that chronic disease management programmes improve health outcomes, especially for persons with diabetes, cardiovascular disease, or depression. Several interventions used in disease management programmes—provider education, audit, feedback, and reminders; patient care teams including physicians and support-service providers; patient self-management; and reminders and financial incentives targeted to patients—all appear to contribute to the effectiveness of these programmes. It is less clear as to whether disease management programmes reduce mortality rates and overall health-care expenditure.

Further resources

Four *BMJ* theme issues devoted to managing chronic diseases:
19 March 2005: http://bmj.bmjjournals.com/content/vol330/issue7492/ (accessed 26 July 2005)
26 October 2002: http://bmj.bmjjournals.com/content/vol325/issue7370/ (accessed 26 July 2005)

27 October 2001: http://bmj.bmjjournals.com/content/vol323/issue7319/ (accessed 26 July 2005)

26 February 2000: http://bmj.bmjjournals.com/content/vol320/issue7234/ (accessed 26 July 2005)

References

1 World Health Organization. *Facts related to chronic diseases*. World Health Organization, Geneva. Available at: http://www.who.int/dietphysicalactivity/publications/facts/chronic/en/ (accessed 31 May 2005).

2 American Diabetes Association (2003). Economic costs of diabetes in the U.S. in 2002. *Diabetes care*, **26**, 917–32.

3 Bodenheimer T (2000). Disease management in the American market. *BMJ*, **320**, 563–6.

4 Greenhalgh T, Herxheimer A, Isaacs AJ, Beaman M, Morris J, Farrow S (2000). Commercial partnerships in chronic disease management: proceeding with caution. *BMJ*, **320**, 566–8.

5 Committee on the Quality of Health Care in America, Institute of Medicine (2001). *Crossing the quality chasm: a new health system for the 21st century*. National Academy Press, Washington, DC.

6 Disease Management Association of America (2005). *Definition of disease management*. Disease Management Association of America, Washington, DC. Available at: http://www.dmaa.org/definition.html (accessed 31 May 2005).

7 Bodenheimer T, Wagner EH, Grumbach K (2002). Improving primary care for patients with chronic illness. *J Am Med Assoc*, **288**, 1775–9.

8 Robert Wood Johnson Foundation and the Group Health Cooperative's MacColl Institute for Healthcare Innovation. *The chronic care model*. Robert Wood Johnson Foundation, Princeton, NJ. Available at: http://www.improvingchroniccare.org/change/index.html (accessed 5 June 2005).

9 DeFriese GH, Fielding JE (1990). Health risk appraisal in the 1990s: opportunities, challenges, and expectations. *Ann Rev Public Health*, **11**, 401–18.

10 Wagner EH (2000). The role of patient care teams in chronic disease management. *BMJ*, **320**, 569–72.

11 Clark NM (2003). Management of chronic disease by patients. *Ann Rev Public Health*, **24**, 289–313.

12 Warsi A, Wang PS, LaValley MP, Avorn J, Solomon DH (2004). Self-management education programmes in chronic disease: a systematic review and methodological critique of the literature. *Arch Intern Med*, **164**, 1641–9.

13 National Committee for Quality Assurance (2005). *The Health Plan Employer Data and Information Set (HEDIS®)*. National Committee for Quality Assurance, Washington, DC. Available at: http://www.ncqa.org/Programmes/HEDIS/ (accessed 6 June 2005).

14 Knight K, Badamgarav E, Henning JM et al. (2005). A systematic review of diabetes disease management programmes. *Am J Managed Care*, **11**, 242–50.

15 McAlister FA, Lawson FME, Teo KK, Armstrong PW (2001). A systematic review of randomized trials of disease management programmes in heart failure. *Am J Med*, **110**, 378–84.
16 Badamgarav E, Weingarten SR, Henning JM *et al.* (2003). Effectiveness of disease management programmes in depression: a systematic review. *Am J Psychiatry*, **160**, 2080–90.
17 Health Evidence Network, World Health Organization Regional Office for Europe (2003). *Are disease management programmes (DMPs) effective in improving quality of care for people with chronic conditions?* WHO Regional Office for Europe, Copenhagen. Available at: http://www.euro.who.int/eprise/main/WHO/Progs/HEN/Syntheses/DMP/20030820_1 (accessed 10 June 2005).
18 Congressional Budget Office (2004). *An analysis of the literature on disease management programmes.* Congressional Budget Office, Washington, DC. Available at: http://www.cbo.gov/showdoc.cfm?index= 5909 (accessed 10 June 2005).
19 American Medical Association Council on Medical Service (1997). *Disease management and demand management* (CMS Report 3, I-97). American Medical Association, Chicago. Available at: http://www.ama-assn.org/ama1/pub/upload/mm/372/i97-cms3.pdf (accessed 15 June 2005).

6.4 Variations in health-care activity and quality

Nick Steel and David Melzer

Objectives

After reading this chapter you should be better able to investigate the causes of variations in health-care activity and understand how to reduce inappropriate variations.

Well-documented inequalities in health exist between population groups determined by socio-economic status, race, and gender (see, for example, Wilkinson and Marmot[1]). This chapter is concerned with the analysis and reduction of variations in health-care practice which are evident at all levels, e.g. variations between individual physicians, between hospitals, geographic regions, and countries.

Why are variations in health care important?

From classic papers in the 1970s,[2,3] hundreds of articles have now been published on physical and geographic variations in health-care activity.

Physicians show important and often dramatic differences in the use of medical resources, hospital beds, surgery, diagnostic tests, and medical therapies: 'The variation phenomenon is so robust and consistently documented that it may be one of the most universal characteristics of modern medicine'.[4]

The US based 'Dartmouth Atlas' is the most systematic mapping of area variations. It has shown that Medicare spending per person in the US is over twice as high in some regions than others, even after correcting for differences in health (http://www.dartmouthatlas.org/current_atlases.php (accessed 7 February 2005)). This variation may reflect inadequate access to effective health care for people in some locations, and a considerable waste of public money in others.

Analyzing practice variations

Two key ideas allow health-care providers, policy makers, purchasers, and consumers to address variations in a logical and manageable fashion.

The first is a clearer definition of what unwarranted variation is: care that is not consistent with a patient's preference or related to a patient's underlying illness. This definition allows a fruitful debate about appropriate versus inappropriate care.

The second is the categorization of unwarranted variations into three categories of care: effective, preference-sensitive, and supply-sensitive (Box 6.4.1).[6]

Box 6.4.1 Categories of health care for analysis of unwanted variations

- **Effective care** is supported by strong evidence for improved health outcomes from clinical trials or valid cohort studies.
- **Preference-sensitive care** is where there are at least two valid alternative treatment options available. Variations in treatment are caused by differing choices about the risks and benefits of the options. These treatment choices could be made by informed patients, but in practice reflect local doctors' opinions, sometimes referred to as 'the surgical signature'. Examples are the use of lumpectomy or mastectomy for early breast cancer, and the treatment of prostatic hyperplasia.
- **Supply-sensitive care** is where medical theory is less well developed, and variations simply reflect the different availability of alternative treatment approaches. Examples are whether 3-month or 6-month intervals between visits for patients with diabetes or hypertension are best, or whether care is better provided in primary care, hospitals, or intensive care units. These variations can have a big impact on costs, particularly towards the end of life. For example, 50% of those who die in Miami spend time in intensive care compared with 14% in Sun City, Arizona. The local supply of medical specialists and acute care hospital capacity explains 41% of variation in end-of-life care intensity.[6]

Is more health care better?

It is for effective care, and internationally there is an undersupply of effective care. In the US, effective care is delivered to those who might benefit from it only about half of the time, and up to 30% may receive contraindicated care.[7–9] The quality of clinical care in general practice in the UK, Australia, and New Zealand almost never attained acceptable standards in one study.[10]

For preference-sensitive care, patients may receive more health care in many areas than they want. Patients and doctors value treatments differently, and patients tend to want less treatment than their doctors give them.[11,12] For supply-sensitive care, the variations are important economically, but do not usually affect health gains at the population level.

How can you reduce unwarranted variations in care?

The first priority is to provide effective care to all those who will benefit from it. This involves setting out what effective care will be provided to which population, providing the care, and then monitoring the population to determine the extent to which the care has been provided. Quality indicators are mainly used to describe effective treatment, but can also describe harmful and ineffective treatment to be prevented. Perhaps the largest quality improvement initiative anywhere is the contract entered into in April 2004 between family practitioners (GPs) and the government in the UK (Box 6.4.2).[13,14]

Box 6.4.2 A new contract to improve quality throughout UK general practice

A new contract between UK general practitioners and the government came into effect on 1 April 2004. Substantial financial rewards (more than £1 billion) are linked to performance against indicators of the quality of clinical and organizational care. The aims of the contract are to reduce variations in provision of effective care and to improve the quality of care provided to the population for 10 chronic conditions.

For each condition, quality indicators describe specific effective clinical interventions which will improve quality of care for that population. The practice receives a financial reward for achieving the indicators.

Example indicators for diabetes:

- The percentage of patients with diabetes whose notes record body mass index in the previous 15 months.
- The percentage of patients with diabetes in whom the last HbA1C is 7.4 or less in last 15 months.

Decision aids can be used to help patients make informed choices about preference-sensitive treatments.[15] For most preference-sensitive conditions, the choice between different treatment options is more important than the choice between different providers of the same treatment, although choice between providers receives more policy attention.

Supply-sensitive care needs to be critically evaluated and compared with practice in other regions. This requires a local infrastructure that can support a research agenda and respond to the results. The capacity of the local health-care system and follow-up rates can be compared with other regions, and costs if these are available. The frequency of use of supply-sensitive services by people with chronic illness is one of the major determinants of costs in a region, yet more frequent care does not generally improve population health. There is an increasing evidence base in this area which can be used as a starting point for local studies.[16]

Analysing local variations in health care

Box 6.4.3 summarizes the steps involved in analyzing local variations in activity.

Box 6.4.3 Questions to ask about activity variations

- Could the apparent variation be due to a data error, alternative classification, or other artefact?
- Could the variation reflect differences in medical need in the populations served?
- If the variation is unexplained, could it be unwarranted care: i.e. is it a pattern of care that could be inconsistent with patients' preferences or unrelated to patients' underlying illness?
- Is the variation due to scientific uncertainty, or medical errors and system failures?
- Is the variation due to differing preferences for treatment? If so, is this because of informed patient choice or because of physician-dominated decisions?
- Is supply of facilities driving the variation? Is there an unwarranted assumption that more activity is better?

It is important to consider data problems as a cause of variations. For example, coding practices for the same intervention may differ between institutions, or may just be much less accurate in some places than others. Similarly coded procedures may mean very different things, for example with surgical interventions that are done as day cases in some institutions but not in others.

Analysis of variations in health care requires a systems approach that accepts that clinicians are influenced by the capacity of the health-care system, and that supported patient choice in preference-sensitive conditions can lead to better outcomes. This approach has not been traditionally taught in medical schools, and may initially meet with resistance from those making policy decisions locally.

How will you know when/if you have been successful?

The part of the health-care system you are working with will redesign systems of care for chronic illness, incorporate shared decision-making into clinics, and use emerging research findings to continually improve health-care interventions. Compared with other regions, your costs will be lower and your achievement on quality indicators higher.

References

1 Wilkinson R, Marmot M (eds) (2003). *Social determinants of health: the solid facts*, 2nd edn. World Health Organization, Copenhagen.

2 Vayda E (1973). A comparision of surgical rates in Canada and in England and Wales. *N Engl J Med*, **289**, 1224–9.

3 Wennberg J, Gittelsohn A (1973). Small area variations in health care delivery: a population-based health information system can guide planning and regulatory decision-making. *Science*, **182**, 1102–8.

4 Margo CE (2004). Quality care and practice variation: the roles of practice guidelines and public profiles. *Surv Ophthalmol*, **49**, 359–71.

5 Wennberg DE, Wennberg JE (2003). *Addressing variations: is there hope for the future.* Health Affairs web exclusive. Available at: http://content.healthaffairs.org/cgi/content/full/hlthaff.w3.614v1/DC1 (accessed 22 July 2005).

6 Wennberg JE, Fisher ES, Skinner JS (2002). *Geography and the debate over medicare reform.* Health Affairs web exclusive. Available at: http://content.healthaffairs.org/cgi/content/full/hlthaff.w2.96v1/DC1 (accessed 22 July 2005).

7 McGlynn EA, Asch SM, Adams J et al. (2003). The quality of health care delivered to adults in the United States. *N Engl J Med*, **348**(26), 2635–45.

8 Wenger NS, Solomon DH, Roth CP et al. (2003). The quality of medical care provided to vulnerable community-dwelling older patients. *Ann Intern Med*, **139**(9), 740–7.

9 Schuster MA, McGlynn EA, Brook RH (1998). How good is the quality of health care in the United States? *Milbank Q*, **76**, 517–63.

10 Seddon ME, Marshall MN, Campbell SM, Roland MO (2001). Systematic review of studies of quality of clinical care in general practice in the UK, Australia, and New Zealand. *Qual Health Care*, **10**, 152–8.

11 Montgomery AA, Fahey T (2001). How do patients' treatment preferences compare with those of clinicians? *Qual Health Care*, **10** (Suppl I), i39–i43.

12 Steel N (2000). Thresholds for taking antihypertensive drugs in different professional and lay groups: questionnaire survey. *BMJ*, **320**, 1446–7.

13 Roland M (2004). Linking physicians' pay to the quality of care—a major experiment in the United Kingdom. *N Engl J Med*, **351**(14), 1448–54.

14 General Practitioners Committee BMA (2003), *The NHS Confederation. Investing in General Practice. The New General Medical Services Contract*. The NHS Confederation, London.

15 O'Connor AM, Stacey D, Rovner D et al. (2001). Decision aids for people facing health treatment or screening decisions. *Cochrane Database Syst Rev*, 3, CD001431.

16 Wennberg JE (2002). Unwarranted variations in healthcare delivery: implications for academic medical centres. *BMJ*, **325**(7370), 961–4.

6.5 Improving health and health care through informatics

Don Detmer

Introduction

The advent of the Internet, and more powerful and cheaper chips, means that informatics will become an essential technology for the ethical practice of the health professions in developed economies within 15 years. The growth in the knowledge base of medicine has outstripped the capacity of natural human memory to match the capacity of knowledge management linked to computer systems in order to bring sophisticated 'just in time' decision support to the point of care and the time of decision. Electronic health records of various types allow for adaptive evidence-based decision-support systems that will ensure far greater efficiency, effectiveness, quality, safety, and integration of new knowledge than would be possible without such support. This will develop to include primary prevention, health education, and computer-based diagnostics, therapies, and follow-ups.

Definitions

Informatics integrates the information sciences and related technology to enhance the use of the health sciences knowledge base to improve health care, biomedical and clinical research, education, management, and policy.

While there is no formally accepted nomenclature or taxonomy for informatics relating to health today, one can identify a number of overlapping yet somewhat distinct domains. These include:

- bioinformatics (computing for genomics, proteomics, epigenetics, and management of the knowledge bases these fields generate)
- clinical informatics, or informatics for use in patient care (electronic medical records of three types: patient, personal, and population)
- computer methods for health applications
- consumer health, or e-health informatics, especially those that link patients and professional caregivers
- health information policy
- health information networks (local, regional, national, and global)
- knowledge management utilizing structured databases such as results of randomized clinical drug trials

- adaptive evidence-based decision support systems (computer-based software that offers expert advice and the capacity to determine whether or not the advice proves to be good for the patient's health status).

Informatics integrates

Some fields with which informatics integrates include:
- computer science, information and telecommunication science, imaging, simulation, cognitive science, statistics, decision science, and management/organizational science
- library science
- bioscience and biomedicine
- knowledge management, decision support
- evidence-based medicine, knowledge bases such as Medline
- health evaluation sciences (biostatistics, epidemiology, health services research)
- health policy and management, organization behaviour, risk management, quality and safety, health values and bioethics.

Using informatics in health care

Robust systems are of necessity complex—they require a mixture of hardware, software, maintenance, relevant legal and policy infrastructure to handle such issues as authentication, security, and confidentiality, standards to enhance interoperability, and refinement of data emerging from biomedical, clinical, and public health research into relevant knowledge banks. Recently, a number of developed economies have embarked upon national health information infrastructures; global efforts to collaborate on standards are under way. The rise of the Internet linked to the above components is changing the practice of health care. For example, personal health records that allow patients to interact with their clinicians and the patient's own medical record whenever and wherever they wish offer the potential to greatly improve performance and outcomes of a variety of chronic illnesses including home monitoring. De-identified data from these records can then be used for indirect patient and public care and public health investigations including biosurveillance. Public policy relating to privacy can conflict with the need for access to person-specific data for a variety of types of biomedical and public health research.[1] Further, it has been argued that a disproportionate attention to personal autonomy is corrosive to social trust.[2]

Implementation of computer systems into clinical environments typically involves substantial change in work processes; management of change and an understanding of organizational behaviour as well as ongoing tailoring of software *programmes* to local circumstances is involved. Complex adaptive systems theory is particularly useful for supporting implementation and gaining major improvements in performance, particularly for safety and quality of care.[3]

Evidence that IT improves care processes and outcome

A growing body of evidence reveals that computer-based health records systems (incorporating decision support) can greatly improve the safety of care, particularly with respect to medications. Other reports reveal improvements in improving access, efficiency, effectiveness, timeliness, and greater patient involvement with better outcomes.[4] More cost–benefit studies are needed but some reports reveal a salutary return on investment.[5]

While more work is needed, the bulk of evidence today reveals that better-informed patients are less anxious, begin treatment earlier, are more satisfied with their care, follow advice better, opt for lower-risk interventions, and reduce health-care costs through greater self-management and a more efficient use of resources.[6]

What should you look for in a health-care IT system that will deliver better quality and outcomes?

Capabilities in IT systems that are likely to improve patient safety, quality, and outcomes include:
- electronic prescribing
- complete computer-based medical records plus continuity of care records that offer a concise summary of key patient data and can be accessed from a variety of clinical settings
- decision support for medications that incorporate capabilities such as clinical alerts
- reminders for preventive care
- dosage calculation support
- 'just-in-time' knowledge service
- integrated evidence-based clinical pathways that allow for over-riding by the clinician
- personal health records that capture records added by the patient that include alternative medications not typically listed by patients in ordinary paper-based settings
- the capacity to aggregate performance data on clinical practice for both clinician and statistical analysis.

If one is 'shopping' to purchase a clinical IT system for use in either a primary care or institutional setting, it is important to visit sites that are actively using the system to determine its functionality in the real world. The more complex the system the more important it is for a team to visit to ensure that all key users' needs will be met. The capacity of systems to interoperate with other systems outside the core setting is of increasing importance. Ease of implementation, cost, and built-in decision support are other factors worthy of evaluation. A key challenge for complex institutions is ensuring that the entire enterprise can cross-communicate. Dedicated systems for individual specialties may keep one set of consultants happy but greatly limit the capacity to achieve major gains in productivity across the institution.

IT and public health

The recent SARs epidemic offered real evidence that IT systems can be extremely important in determining both the spread of a new disease and in analyzing patient care data for clusters of symptoms to help understand the nature of a disease and how it spreads and acts. On-going biosurveillance is now critical for both emerging infections as well as management of potential and real bioterrorism.[7]

Further resources

There are far too many websites available to do justice to the issues raised here but what follows will give the reader some sense of the scope of issues involved.

Medical knowledge bases (all accessed 20 January 2006)

Medline Plus (http://medlineplus.gov/) is a website with range of consumer health information.

Public Library of Science (http://www.plos.org/) and BioMed Central (http://www.biomedcentral.com) are both open access web-based repositories for scientists and the public.

PubMed is a free continually updated source for access to the medical literature at the US National Library of Medicine (see http://www.ncbi.nlm.nih.gov/entrez/query.fcgi?).

Unbound Medicine (http://www.unboundmedicine.com/) and Up-to-Date (http://www.uptodate.com/index.asp) offer PDA and computer-based knowledge support for clinicians.

Standards, vocabulary, and terminology

Health Level 7 (see http://www.hl7.org/) is a major standards development group (accessed 22 July 2005).

SNOMED CT (see http://www.snomed.org/) is a systematized nomenclature of medicine (SNOMED) that incorporates universal health-care terminology (accessed 22 July 2005).

Unified Medical Language System (http://www.nlm.nih.gov/research/umls/) is a compendium of knowledge sources for medicine (accessed 22 July 2005).

National health information infrastructures

Australia: http://www.agimo.gov.au/publications/2005/04/enhancing_productivity/part1/health (accessed 22 July 2005).

Canada: http://www.hc-sc.gc.ca/ohih-bsi/chics/index_e.html (accessed 22 July 2005).

UK: UK National Health Service's National Project for Information Technology http://www.connectingforhealth.nhs.uk/ (accessed 22 July 2005).

USA: Office of the National Coordinator for Health Information Technology (ONCHIT) http://www.hhs.gov/onchit/framework/ (accessed

22 July 2005) and National Committee on Health and Vital Statistics (NCVHS) http://www.ncvhs.hhs.gov/ (accessed 22 July 2005).

General reading in medical informatics

Shortliffe EH, Perreault LE, Wiederhold G, Fagan LM (2000). *Medical informatics: computer applications in health care and biomedicine*, 2nd edn. Springer, New York.

References

1 Lowrance WW (2002). *Learning from experience: privacy and the secondary use of data in health research*. Nuffield Trust, London.
2 O'Neill O (2002). *The philosophy of trust. BBC Reith Lectures*, 2002. Available at: http://www.open2.net/trust/oneill_on_trust/oneill_on_trust1.htm (accessed 22 July 2005).
3 Crossing the Quality Chasm: The IOM Health Care Quality Initiative. Available at: http://www.iom.edu/focuson.asp?id=8089 (accessed 22 July 2005).
4 Henry SB, Lenert L, Middleton B, Partridge R (1993). *Linking process and outcome with an integrated clinical information system*. Knowledge Systems Laboratory, Stanford University, CA.
5 Zdon L, Middleton B (1999). Ambulatory electronic records implementation cost benefit: an enterprise case study. *Proc Health Inform Management Syst Soc*, **4**, 97–117.
6 Detmer D et al. (2003). *The informed patient: study report*. Judge Business School, Cambridge.
7 For example, The RODS Laboratory, Centre for Biomedical Informatics, University of Pittsburgh http://rods.health.pitt.edu/ (accessed 22 July 2005).

6.6 Evaluating health-care technologies

Andrew Stevens and Ruairidh Milne

Objectives

Reading this chapter will help you to:
- explain what health technology assessment (HTA) is
- understand what HTA has to do with public health
- make use of HTA
- know the basics of how to do HTA.

What is HTA?

Technology

'Health technology' is the established jargon for any element of health care. The term includes all treatments and tests used by those working in the health services to promote health, prevent and treat disease, and improve rehabilitation and long-term care.

The following are, therefore, all health technologies:
- drugs and devices
- diagnostic techniques
- surgical and other procedures
- *programmes* and settings of health care.

Assessment

Health technology assessment is health-care evaluation with an explicit purpose: that is, to improve the ability of health services to meet the objectives of decision makers. These decision makers may be patients, clinicians, managers, policy makers, or the public. Their objectives may be efficiency, humanity, choice, or equity—or whatever objectives those who make decisions seek to pursue. Health technology assessment asks four fundamental questions (Box 6.6.1).

> **Box 6.6.1 The four questions of HTA**
> - Does the technology work?
> - For whom?
> - At what cost?
> - How does it compare with alternatives?

Assessment and appraisal

It is useful to distinguish HTA from health technology appraisal. Assessment is the technical evaluation process. Appraisal is the political decision-making process. Appraisal is, of course, based on the assessment and on other considerations (such as local priorities). At a national level in the UK, assessment is undertaken by university research teams and appraisal by the National Institute for Health and Clinical Excellence (NICE) appraisal committee. At a local level, assessments are often undertaken by public health specialists, while appraisal is typically a function for local health authorities (Primary Care Trusts in England).[1]

The key steps of assessment are described in detail in Chapter 1.3 and in outline in the section 'Doing HTA: the key stages' later in this chapter. The main components are:

- a systematic review of evidence, typically using a hierarchy of evidence. (Where the issue is effectiveness, this places randomized controlled trials at the top and opinion at the bottom.)
- an economic assessment, typically using a decision model incorporating costs, relative effectiveness, and valuations of heath states (utilities) for different treatment modes.

A complete HTA often includes social and legal considerations too. Box 6.6.2 illustrates the argument so far with a real-life clinical issue.

Box 6.6.2 Growth hormone for growth-hormone deficient adults

- *The problem*: some adults become deficient in growth hormone, usually as a result of damage to the pituitary gland, for instance, after head injury.
- *The technology*: synthetic growth hormone is available. It is costly and requires daily injection.
- *The HTA question*: what is the cost-effectiveness of growth hormone replacement in improving the quality and length of life for people with growth hormone deficiency?
- *The appraisal question*: should a particular health system pay for growth hormone replacement?

Why HTA matters to public health

Health technology assessment is not something remote from or in opposition to public health. On the contrary, public health professionals need to understand HTA because:

- health technologies are the building blocks of health care and health care matters to the public
- health care is a major determinant of the health of the public, both for good (think of immunization) and for ill (MRSA in hospitals)
- investment in each element of health care means opportunity costs (foregone benefits) in other elements of health care
- as part of their job, they may have to contribute to the assessment and appraisal of health technologies.

Using HTA

Health technology assessment has become something of an industry in the last decade or so, and many of the assessments are complicated and lengthy. They are also often place-dependent and time-limited. So public health professionals using HTA need skills in three areas: finding the appropriate HTA; appraising what they find; and updating what they have appraised and adapting it to local use.

Finding the HTA

Medline is everyone's backstop in finding medical texts, but before going there, specialist HTA sources are more specific and often more complete:

- the INAHTA/CRD HTA database[2]
- the Cochrane library[3]
- NICE guidance.[4]

Appraising HTA

Critical appraisal is dealt with in detail in Chapter 2.11. In brief, the critical appraisal of HTA covers the focus of the question, the inclusion of the right studies and to ensure that they are quality assured and sensibly combined.

Updating and adapting to local use

Updating requires a Medline search but is usefully supplemented by a search on the National Electronic Library for Health[5] and/or a Google search of the key words.

Adaptation is important as local circumstances may well differ from those in a HTA report. You should particularly consider whether:

- the comparator technology is the one you really use locally
- the costs are applicable to local circumstances
- the social and policy backgrounds are comparable.

Doing HTA: the key steps

A comprehensive guide to HTA methods was published by NICE in 2004.[6] It builds on earlier guidance on systematic reviews,[7] extended to include elements of economic analysis and policy relevance.[8,9] The key steps are to:

- **Define the question to be addressed clearly, to include:**
  - the type of question (effectiveness? cost-effectiveness? cost-effectiveness and wider social, ethical, and legal implications?)
  - the precise technology under evaluation
  - the comparator (pre-existing) technology
  - the disease and client group for which it is being assessed
  - the outcome measures of interest. (Normally HTA looks for outcomes that are relevant to patients rather than surrogate or proxy outcomes.)
- **Search for background information.**

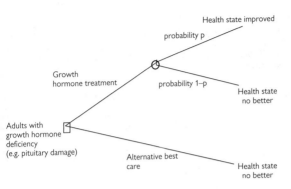

Figure 6.6.1 Decision tree for growth hormone treatment

- **Generate a rough 'decision tree'.** This is a diagram used to portray the alternative intervention plus outcome options for the chosen population. Figure 6.6.1 illustrates a simplified decision tree for the growth hormone example mentioned in Box 6.6.2. By convention, square boxes represent decision points and circles represent chance events. (Note that growth hormone treatment may last many years and it may have a wide range of impacts on health. The decision tree here is unavoidably a very crude over-simplification.)
- **Find the evidence.** Systematicity is vital. Comprehensiveness may not be.
- **Sort and appraise the evidence.** This includes the elimination of irrelevant material, the application of study inclusion and exclusion criteria, and a full appraisal of the quality of included studies.
- **Search for cost information.** This is often difficult as it can be in the 'grey' rather than the published literature. A starting point should be any current official lists of costs. Experts can often identify useful sources.
- **Extract the data.** This includes identifying and recording key features and results of included studies. Such data need to be summarized clearly, comparably, and consistently. Statistical summary estimates can be used to synthesize data where appropriate (meta-analysis).
- **Perform an economic evaluation.** The synthesis of effectiveness information is only half of a cost-effectiveness analysis: costs also need to be factored into the equation. And if HTA is to generate results which allow comparisons across different technologies in different areas of health care, a cost–utility analysis—in which effectiveness information is translated into generic units of health—will be needed (see Chapter 1.4).
- **Consider the wider ethical, social, and legal implications.** These can be gleaned from the literature, expert contacts, and common sense. The knock-on effects of the introduction of some new technologies may be among their most important aspects.
- **Write the report.**

Nobody is perfect but a team can be! It should be evident by now that undertaking a HTA requires skills in systematic review techniques (including information science), health economics, statistics and modelling, and clinical and public health expertise. It needs to be the work of a multidisciplinary team.

Lessons learnt and challenges

Health technology assessment is still a young discipline, having emerged first in the US less than 30 years ago.[10] It is closely linked with evidence-based health care and health economics, the other components of the revolution in effectiveness, and has great potential for improving public health. We suggest below two lessons learnt from this experience and two challenges for the future.

A colourful patchwork

In no health-care system in the world is HTA a single logical system: everywhere it is a multicoloured patchwork. Some of the pieces of this patchwork—the uses of HTA, as well as the funding, levels, and users of HTA—are outlined in Table 6.6.1. But they should all contribute to the essential goal of HTA: meeting the information needs of decision makers in health care.

Table 6.6.1 The patchwork of HTA

Dimension	Levels
Uses to which the HTA may be put	Licensing; coverage/funding; clinical decision-making; informed patient choice
Funding of HTA reports and systems	No explicit funding; publicly funded; privately funded.
Geographic areas at which the HTA is conducted	Local, regional, national, international (e.g. INAHTA)
The decision makers who use HTA reports	Patients, clinicians, managers, policy makers, the public

The sequence of HTA

Health technology assessment is part of a sequence of research-based information collection.[11] Typically, the sequence of HTA data gathering and synthesis looks like this:

- scanning the horizon for new technologies that are likely to emerge and diffuse within a year or so
- assembly of primary randomized trial data sufficient for licensing by a manufacturer/pharmaceutical company (typically phase II and phase III randomized trials)
- brief reports (such as bulletins, editorials, and vignettes) on the pros and cons of the new technology

- a mainstream HTA report—typically rapid systematic review and cost-effectiveness modelling (technology assessment reports produced for NICE are typical here)
- a longer term HTA or Cochrane systematic review (again mainstream HTA)
- pragmatic randomized controlled trials.
  Box 6.6.3 illustrates the sequence for HTAs of growth hormone.

Box 6.6.3 Growth hormone: the sequence of HTA

- A 'quick and clean' Development and Evaluation Committee report was produced in 1995[12] prior to licensing in 1996.
- A follow-up report that took account of new evidence was published in 1997.[13]
- Continuing concerns about the clinical and practical role of growth hormone continued and a NICE technology appraisal was set in train.
- This resulted in a published full technology assessment report[14] and guidance to the UK NHS.[15]
- A pragmatic randomized controlled trial assessing the cost-utility of growth hormone and its impact on long-term outcomes has yet to be undertaken.

Challenge 1: timeliness

Health technology assessment reports are a critically timely part of a research system for new technologies (particularly expensive pharmaceuticals). Decision makers need good, understandable information in weeks or at worst months, rather than years.

The challenge for the systems that produce HTA is to temper rigor with timeliness. Don't let the best become the enemy of the good.

Challenge 2: implementation

No matter how sophisticated the HTA process is, it won't on its own be enough to manage the introduction of new technologies. We also need some mechanism for ensuring knowledge of, and adherence to, its findings, given the evidence of slow uptake of research findings in clinical practice. In the UK the establishment of NICE and the National Screening Committee as two 'implementation arms' for HTA have been crucial in ensuring that HTA is of real value to health-care decision makers.

The challenge here is to find ways of bridging the worlds of assessment and implementation. The UK's experience is that a formal system of appraisal may be a useful approach to such a bridge.

Conclusion

Health technology assessment is not a panacea. Generating information that is useful and relevant to health service decision makers does not of itself ensure that that information is acted upon. But it is a necessary first step in the development of a health service that more closely meets the objectives of those who use, fund, direct, or provide that service.

References

1 Stevens A, Milne R (2004). Health technology assessment in England and Wales. *Int J Technol Assess Health Care*, **20**(1), 11–24.

2 Centre for Reviews and Dissemination, University of York. *Health technology assessment database* http://www.york.ac.uk/inst/crd/htahp.htm (accessed 28 December 2004).

3 The Cochrane Collaboration. http://www.cochrane.org/index0.htm (accessed 28 December 2004).

4 NICE guidance. http://www.nice.org.uk/page.aspx?o=cat.diseaseareas (accessed 28 December 2004).

5 NHS National electronic Library for Health. http://www.nelh.nhs.uk/ (accessed 28 December 2004).

6 NICE (2004). *Guide to the methods of technology appraisal*. National Institute for Clinical Excellence, London. Available at: http://www.nice.org.uk/pdf/TAP_Methods.pdf (accessed 28 December 2004).

7 NHS Centre for Reviews and Dissemination (1996). *Undertaking systematic reviews of research on effectiveness*, CRD Report no 4. University of York, York.

8 Liberati A, Sheldon T, Banta HD (1997). Eurassess project subgroup report on methodology—methodological guidance for the conduct of health technology assessment. *Int J Technol Assess Health Care*, **13**(2), 186–219.

9 Goodman C (1996). A basic methodology toolkit. In: Szczepura A, Kankaapaa J (eds) *Assessment of health care technologies*, pp. 29–65. Wiley, Chichester.

10 Stevens A, Milne R, Burls A (2003). Health technology assessment: history and demand. *J Public Health Med*, **25**(2), 98–101.

11 Milne R, Clegg A, Stevens A (2003). HTA responses and the classic HTA report. *J Public Health Med*, **25**(2), 102–6.

12 Anthony D (1995). *Growth hormone (somatotropin) for growth hormone deficient adults*, Development and Evaluation Committee Report No. 47. NHS, Bristol.

13 Anthony D, Milne R (1997). *Growth hormone for growth hormone deficient adults* (Development and Evaluation Committee report no 47). Wessex Institute for Health Research and Development, Southampton.

14 Bryant J, Loveman E, Chase D et al. (2002). Clinical effectiveness and cost-effectiveness of growth hormone in adults in relation to impact on quality of life: a systematic review and economic evaluation. *Health Technol Assess*, **6**(19), 1–106.

15 NICE (2003). *Full guidance on human growth hormone (somatropin) in adults with growth hormone deficiency*, no 64. National Institute for Clinical Excellence, London. Available at: http://www.nice.org.uk/page.aspx?o=83428 (accessed 28 December 2004).

6.7 Getting research into practice

Jeanette Ward, Jeremy Grimshaw, and Martin Eccles

Objectives

After reading this chapter, you will be able to:
- identify opportunities for research transfer in clinical and public health settings
- apply a systematic approach to research transfer, including the selection of evidence-based strategies to promote professional behaviour change.

Key concepts

- Public health practitioners are well placed to facilitate implementation of research findings in both clinical and public health practice.
- Implementation strategies are intended to encourage practitioners to change their own practice in line with research evidence.
- 'Implementation research' is that academic discipline which generates knowledge about strategies effective in getting research into practice.
- Evidence from implementation research should inform research transfer (Box 6.7.1).

Box 6.7.1

Evidence-based medicine should be complemented by evidence-based implementation

Grol[1]

Why is research transfer an important public health responsibility?

There is an increasing evidence base to inform specific clinical and public health practices. However, compelling results from clinical or public health research will not change population outcomes unless health services and health-care professionals adopt them in practice. Information overload, pressures of work in health-care systems, and other factors can result in troubling lag times between research findings and their delivery in practice (Box 6.7.2). As a result, population outcomes are compromised. The population health gain inherent in more effective and efficient research transfer affords public health a unique leadership role in getting research into practice wherever aspects of the health system are underperforming.

Box 6.7.2 Examples of failure in research transfer

Clinical[2,3]

A range of different interventions have been shown to improve survival following myocardial infarction; however, the median proportion of eligible patients in 11 European countries receiving appropriate management was:
- thrombolysis 36% (range 13–52%)
- beta blockers 46% (range 31–77%)
- aspirin 87% (range 72–94%)

Public health[4,5]

- Rates of participation in cervical screening can be as low as 55% in subpopulation groups. However, it is well established that a population age-adjusted rate of cervical cancer of no more than 3 per 10 000 women is achievable if evidence-based screening guidelines were implemented equitably.
- Studies of the frequency and quality of the provision to smokers of evidence-based cessation advice by primary care providers repeatedly show poor preventive practice. An applied research agenda has been recommended to prioritize research that rigorously tests strategies designed to change physician behaviour.

A systematic approach to research transfer

A systematic approach is needed if the potential benefits of research are to be maximized. This will be facilitated if the health-care system and local health-care organizations value evidence-based approaches and quality improvement. There are three interrelated stages to promote research transfer:
- identifying and prioritizing problems for research transfer
- developing an implementation plan for research transfer
- monitoring the impact of research transfer.

Whilst these stages represent a logical, sequential approach, in practice they can overlap or occur contemporaneously.

Identifying and prioritizing problems for research transfer

Problems with research transfer become apparent in a number of ways:
- population health surveillance may reveal poor outcomes
- critical event analysis may reveal specific problems in health-care delivery
- stakeholder or professional opinion perceives a gap between evidence and current practice
- publication of new evidence, systematic reviews, or definitive guidelines may identify opportunities for improvement on current performance.

Problems with research transfer are likely to be multifactorial at any point in time. Typically, there are limited resources in health-care systems for interventions to promote research transfer and the problems need to be prioritized, preferably within an explicit process that considers the following issues:
- What is the extent of suboptimal variation in the population outcome?
- Could research transfer achieve better population outcomes?
- Where is maximal health gain most likely if research transfer is effective?
- How does the topic complement agreed local, regional, or national health priorities?
- Is there momentum for local initiatives to enhance research transfer?

The prioritization process should identify a limited and achievable number of manageable topics for research transfer at the local level. Once prioritized, a systematic approach to implementation can proceed.

Developing an implementation plan for research transfer

Creating local coalitions for action

Research transfer often requires coordinated action by a range of local organizations and health-care professionals at national and local levels. Creation of a local multidisciplinary coalition of stakeholders will support implementation efforts. Creative thinking with due attention to local politics, power-bases, and champions for innovation are critical.

Developing local evidence messages

Research evidence is usually not presented in a format that is easily accessible to professionals; it is usually necessary to develop, to synthesize, and to translate research findings into a concrete, easily understandable format (for example, an evidence-based guideline). Local health-care organizations and individual professionals are unlikely to have the necessary skills or resources required for rigorous development of guidelines. As a result, it is preferable to identify and adapt existing systematic reviews or methodologically valid guidelines. This local adaptation process should involve a multidisciplinary group (with adequate technical and administrative support) (Box 6.7.3).

Box 6.7.3 Example of a multidisciplinary group for microscopic hematuria referral guidelines

- general practitioners
- urologist
- nephrologist
- anaesthetist
- theatre nurse
- specialist nurse
- public health specialist
- manager
- patient representative

Identifying barriers and facilitators to change

It is important to identify local barriers and facilitators to inform the choice of implementation strategies. Within any individual setting there are likely to be a number of different barriers and facilitators operating at five different levels (Box 6.7.4). Individual professionals in any target group may vary in their preparedness for change and face different barriers and facilitators. Different 'segments' in the target group may be identified and may need different implementation approaches. A variety of methods can be used to elicit information about barriers to evidence-based practice, such as informal discussions with key professionals, purposeful qualitative research (focus groups), and representative surveys.[6] Rather than focusing on a specific practice, another recent approach has instead attempted to assess the capacity of practitioners to conceptualize and apply an evidence-based approach to any issue.[7]

Box 6.7.4 Possible barriers to evidence-based practice

These may occur:
- within the health-care system, for example if the method of reimbursement provides perverse incentives to professionals
- within the health-care organization, for example if there is an inappropriate skill mix or if the organizational culture does not embrace purposeful change
- within local professional peer groups, for example if the desired behaviour change is counter to prevailing norms and attitudes
- within individual professionals, for example if individuals lack knowledge about research findings, skills to perform a procedure, or awareness of referral pathways or others' roles and responsibilities
- within professional–patient consultations, for example within busy consultations, professionals may overlook important items of care.

Choosing strategies

An evidence base has emerged over the last two decades that, while incomplete, is an essential first reference point from which to consider strategies to promote research transfer. At the outset of planning, reference to systematic reviews within the discipline of research transfer is highly recommended. Continual updates of evidence of the effectiveness of various interventions is supported globally by the Cochrane Effective Practice and Organisation of Care Group[8] (Box 6.7.5).

There are no 'magic bullets'; most interventions can be effective under some circumstances, but none are effective under all circumstances. For example, a recent systematic review of strategies to disseminate and implement clinical practice guidelines included 235 studies.[9] Seventy-three per cent of comparisons evaluated multifaceted interventions, although the maximum number of replications of a specific multifaceted intervention was 11 comparisons. Overall the majority of comparisons reporting compliance with guidelines (86.6%) observed improvements in care; however, there was considerable variation in the observed effects, both within and across interventions. Commonly evaluated single interventions were reminders (38 comparisons), dissemination of educational materials (18 comparisons), and audit and feedback (12 comparisons). There were 23 comparisons of multifaceted interventions involving educational outreach. The majority of interventions observed modest to moderate improvements in care. For example, the median absolute improvement in performance across interventions ranged from 14.1% in 14 cluster randomized comparisons of reminders, 8.1% in four cluster randomized comparisons of dissemination of educational materials, 7.0% in five cluster randomized comparisons of audit and feedback, and 6.0% in 13 cluster randomized comparisons of multifaceted interventions involving educational outreach. No relationship was found between the number of component interventions and the effects of multifaceted interventions.

At present there is little empirical evidence linking the effectiveness of different interventions in overcoming the influence of specific facilitators and barriers. In general, the choice of strategy should reflect the perceived barriers at whatever level (refer to Box 6.7.4), the evidence about the effectiveness of different strategies, available resources and practical considerations. For example:
● Political interventions resulting in macro health reform may be necessary if the barriers relate to the health-care system.
● Specific organizational interventions may be necessary if the barriers relate to the local health-care organization.

- Approaches involving social influence (local consensus processes, educational outreach, opinion leaders, marketing, etc.) may be useful when barriers relate to local professional peer groups.
- Audit and feedback may be useful when health-care professionals are unaware of suboptimal practice and to reinforce change.
- Educational approaches may be useful where barriers relate to health-care professionals' knowledge, skills, and attitudes; in general, interactive educational activities are more likely to lead to research transfer.
- Reminders and patient-mediated interventions when barriers relate to information processing within consultations.

Research transfer requires adequate resources for the development of local evidence messages and implementation activities. Decision makers should be transparent if implementation strategies are selected primarily on the basis of their affordability rather than proven or hypothesized impact (for example, interventions that will address only a limited number of barriers or targeting heterogeneous groups of professionals). Research transfer may not incur substantial additional costs if existing structures can be harnessed to support it. For example, quality improvement units or departments within hospitals may include individuals with appropriate technical skills to support development and implementation of local guidelines. Existing post-graduate educational mechanisms can be exploited to support dissemination and implementation activities. Performance management, even within large, complex organizations, can reinforce fundamental principles such as evidence-based practice.

Evaluating impact

Ultimately, it is changes in the population outcome of interest that will vindicate the planned approach to research transfer that is advocated here. For example, an equitable reduction in mortality rates from colorectal cancer at a population level requires effective transfer to the public of sound dietary advice (effective recommendations to prevent colorectal cancer) through to targeting of clinical services to ensure intensive treatment of individuals with diagnosed disease, recurrence, or metastases (surgery, oncology, nursing, and palliative care). To guide implementation decisions within service settings, each of these elements of a comprehensive colorectal cancer service plan, performance indicators (either process or outcome variables) should be developed to monitor progress accompanied by regular monitoring of these indicators against targets. Alternatively, strategies can be evaluated within formal research projects; implementation research (the scientific study of methods to promote the uptake of research findings) is an emergent focus of health services research.[9,10]

Key issues

As in any emerging discipline, the evidence base for research transfer remains patchy and often of uncertain generalizability. Public health practitioners are encouraged to apply the same critical processes to the appraisal of published research reporting successes and failures in research transfer as they do when deciding about clinical service initiatives or new public health *programmes*. Furthermore, greater demand for a more scientifically sound knowledge base in research transfer will accelerate development of the discipline. There is greater recognition that research transfer requires sophisticated, theoretically informed and phased designs.[11] Practitioners who seek to transfer evidence into practice must work with these epistemological deficits as best they can.

References

1 Grol R (1997). Beliefs and evidence in changing clinical practice. *BMJ*, **315**, 418–21.

2 Ketley D, Woods KL (1993). Impact of clinical trials on clinical practice: example of thrombolysis for acute myocardial infarction. *Lancet*, **342**, 891–4.

3 Woods KL, Ketley D, Lowy A et al. (1998). Beta-blockers and antithrombotic treatment for secondary prevention after acute myocardial infarction. Towards an understanding of factors influencing clinical practice. The European Secondary Prevention Study Group. *Eur Heart J*, **19**, 74–9.

4 Ward JE (1997). Reducing cervical cancer by two-thirds: a public health target within our reach? *Aust NZ J Public Health*, **21**, 248–9.

5 US Preventive Services Task Force (2003). *Counselling to prevent tobacco use and tobacco-caused disease: US*, publication no. 04–0526. Agency for Healthcare Research and Quality, Rockville, MD.

6 Wensing M, Grol R (2005). Methods to identify implementation problems. In: Grol R, Wensing M, Eccles M (eds) *Improving patient care. The implementation of change in clinical practice*. Elsevier, London.

7 Adily A, Ward JE (2004). Evidence-based practice in population health: a regional survey to inform workforce development and organisational change. *J Epidemiol Commun Health*, **58**, 455–60.

8 Cochrane Effective Clinical Practice and Organisation of Care Group. http://www.epoc.uottawa.ca (accessed 31 May 2005).

9 Grimshaw JG, Thomas RE, MacLennan G et al. (2004). Effectiveness and efficiency of guideline dissemination and implementation strategies. *Health Technol Assess*, **8**(6).

10 Grol R, Wensing M, Eccles M (eds) (2005). *Improving patient care. The implementation of change in clinical practice*. Elsevier, London.

11 Grol R, Baker R, Moss F (eds) (2004). *Quality improvement research: understanding the science of change in health care*. BMJ Publishing, London.

6.8 Using guidance and frameworks

Gene Feder and Chris Griffiths

Objectives

After reading this chapter you should be better able to:
- understand, appreciate, and identify issues where guidance and frameworks could help
- identify existing and relevant guidelines
- assess their validity
- adapt them to local circumstances
- support clinicians in their implementation.

Why is the implementation of clinical guidelines an important public health activity?

Clinicians and public health professionals are inundated by a tide of guidance and frameworks. These are often in the form of clinical guidelines, and come from government, national and international health agencies, professional colleges, health-care funders, and the pharmaceutical industry. Guidance on effective clinical practice is necessary because most clinicians do not have the time to go back to primary research or even systematic reviews for the majority of practice decisions or policy. Public health professionals have a vital role to play in helping clinical colleagues use guidance, both in day-to-day practice and in development of clinical policy. In this chapter we focus on the use of clinical guidelines as an example of the application of guidance or frameworks in practice. Guidelines themselves are only tools for clinicians or managers and need to be integrated into broader clinical or management systems.

What are clinical guidelines?

The principles of clinical guidelines (Box 6.8.1) can also be applied to health care policy guidelines. We do not address guidance linked to financial rewards (e.g. the new quality and outcomes framework for UK general practice) or obligatory frameworks (e.g. managed care requirements in the USA).

Box 6.8.1 **What are clinical guidelines?**

Clinical guidelines are: 'Systematically developed statements to assist practitioner and patient decisions about appropriate health care for specific clinical circumstances'.

Identifying specific skills needed to implement guidelines

In order to bring added value to the process of implementing guidelines there are six important competencies that you need to either have yourself (unlikely) or have in the team (more likely) (Box 6.8.2).

Box 6.8.2 **Competencies**

- collaborating with clinicians and other stakeholders to define policy issues
- searching for relevant guidelines
- appraisal of the validity of the guidelines and their applicability to the local context
- adaptation of guidelines
- analyzing and addressing obstacles to their implementation
- assessment of the impact of the guidelines

What are the stages in a guidelines implementation project?

Like any complex process involving different groups of people with different perspectives, it is important to manage the process of guideline implementation carefully. There are at least eight identifiable stages in the process. Some of these will overlap. It is important to appreciate the potential barriers that may occur at any of these stages in planning implementation.

Identifying a clinical issue

To justify devoting resources to guideline adaptation and implementation, a clinical issue must be important. Ideally at least three criteria should be fulfilled:

- the condition or issue should have a large impact on public health or health-care resources
- there should also be demonstrable and unjustified variation in its clinical management
- there should be some evidence for what constitutes good practice (Box 6.8.3).

Box 6.8.3 Example of a suitable issue for guideline implementation

In a local audit of survivors of a myocardial infarction it was found that although 92% were using aspirin 6 months later only 30% were using beta-blockers, with a range of 12 to 72% in different general practices. Secondary prevention of coronary heart disease is an obvious subject for guideline implementation, with a large health impact and unjustified variation in clinical management.

Although these are necessary conditions, they are not sufficient. Discussion with clinicians is crucial; they also need to think that the issue is important and so worth their commitment to an implementation project. The genuine involvement of opinion leaders (which increases the likelihood of implementation) is likely to be more successful if initiated at an early stage. Potential barriers to improvement should also be considered early. If these are judged to be insurmountable, then another issue should be prioritized.

Forming a local guidelines group

Choose no more than a dozen people. This should include three types of people:

- clinicians, managers, and others who will be implementing the guidelines on the ground
- 'content' experts (people who know the subject well)
- someone with the competence to identify, appraise, and summarize guidelines or systematic reviews.

The group will need to have a Chair, with all the usual management skills for guiding the process, and a timetable for meetings. The group's objectives must be clear and not too ambitious (see Box 6.8.4).

Identifying national or regional guidelines

National and regional guidelines are increasingly accessible via the Internet and may be identified on bibliographic databases, although they are not necessarily indexed in the commonly available databases. Some of the better-developed guideline websites include full text versions or abstracts (Box 6.8.5).

Box 6.8.4 Realistic and unrealistic objectives for development of local guidelines

Realistic objectives

- Develop local guidelines on use of beta-blockers after myocardial infarction.
- Identify national or international guidelines on use of beta-blockers after myocardial infarction.
- If none found, identify systematic reviews of use of beta-blockers after myocardial infarction.
- Appraise guidelines or systematic reviews and choose most valid one.
- Adapt to local context and circulate to target clinicians for comment.
- Develop implementation *programme* with general practitioner leaders and consultant physicians.

Unrealistic objectives

- Develop local guidelines on primary and secondary prevention of cardiovascular disease.
- Search for relevant randomized controlled trial evidence.
- Appraise individual trials and summarize.
- Formulate recommendations directly based on trial evidence.

Box 6.8.5 Identifying national or regional guidelines

Search terms for common bibliographic databases:

- Medline and Healthstar 'guideline' (publication type) and 'consensus development conference' (publication type). Healthstar includes journals not referenced in Medline and grey literature CINAHL 'practice guidelines' (publication type). Includes full text version of some guidelines.
- EMBASE 'practice guidelines' (subject heading). This is used for articles about guidelines and for those that contain practice guidelines; the term was introduced in 1994.

Useful websites:

- National Guideline Clearinghouse (http://www.guideline.gov/): the largest database of full text appraised guidelines in the world, sponsored by the Agency for Healthcare Quality and Research. Understandable bias towards US guidance, but includes guidelines from other countries (accessed 26 July 2005).
- National Institute for Health and Clinical Excellence (http://www.nice.org.uk/): growing number of full text national guidelines for England and Wales, as well as guidance on individual drugs and technologies (accessed 26 July 2005).
- Scottish Intercollegiate Guidelines Network (http://www.sign.ac.uk/guidelines/index.html): full text versions of guidelines and quick reference guides (accessed 1 August 2005).

Appraising the validity of guidelines

When you have identified relevant guidelines you need to appraise their validity before choosing which to adapt for your own use. Adopting recommendations from guidelines of questionable validity may harm patients or waste resources on ineffective interventions. Within the UK there are now well-established guidelines programmes (Scottish Intercollegiate Guidelines Network for Scotland and the National Institute for Health and Clinical Excellence for England and Wales) using rigorous methods and formal appraisal within the programmes. If appraised guidelines are not available, you can do your own appraisal using a validated appraisal tool (Box 6.8.6).

Box 6.8.6 UK guidelines appraisal tool

This is a 37-item instrument that has been validated to test the methodological quality of guidelines. It is not intended to give a 'pass/fail' assessment, but does allow a judgement of validity and comparison of different guidelines on the same clinical topic. See: http://www.agreecollaboration.org/ (accessed 26 July 2005).

Adapting guidelines to fit local circumstances

This is an essential part of the process. For example, if a guideline recommends a drug not licenced in your country or an investigation that is not available, then the recommendation of the guideline must be changed. Development of a local version also allows information about local services and referral pathways. If the 'source' guideline is more than a couple of years old you should update it by identifying recent systematic reviews from bibliographic databases and sources like the Cochrane Library. Lastly, there is the issue of local ownership. Although this may be exaggerated as an issue, there is no doubt that involvement of clinicians in adapting guidelines to local circumstances does increase knowledge about guidelines, although not necessarily adherence to them.

Piloting and identifying barriers to implementation

Once the development group has agreed on a draft guideline it is advisable to pilot the guidelines in real-life practice settings: recommendations may turn out to be impossible to implement, no matter how much thought the guidelines group has invested in them. This also gives an opportunity to identify barriers to implementation. These may relate to:

- people: target clinicians (skills, knowledge, attitudes, rules, or norms about roles)
- culture: the organizational context (e.g. style of management and willingness to change within clinical teams)
- structures: structural and resource issues can stall perfectly logical guidance for purely practical reasons (e.g. lack of resources for prescribing or extra staff).

Failure to clarify and specifically address these barriers with implementation strategies will result in failure or weakened impact.

Strategies for dissemination and implementation

The previous stages will be wasted if the guidelines are not used in practice. Research on the implementation of guidelines and other sources of evidence gives us a basis for designing strategy at this stage. Tailor your strategy to address the barriers identified. Passive methods of giving guidelines to clinicians (e.g. just through the post) are unlikely to be effective, unless there are other drivers for change. Multifaceted programmes, especially those that explicitly tackle obstacles to implementation, engage clinicians face to face, and build in reminders or prompts into the consultation are more likely to work. Recent research has cast some doubt over the need for multifaceted approaches for implementation of all guidance.

Monitoring the impact of guidelines

Set up some form of routine data collection to assess whether the guidelines are used in clinical practice. Where guidelines make prescribing and referral recommendations this is relatively straightforward when data are stored electronically. In the UK the introduction of clinical governance means that acute health-care trusts and primary care trusts have a statutory obligation to monitor performance through these methods. Linking performance measures back to evidence-based guidelines makes them more likely to seem credible to clinicians, particularly if they have been involved in the guidelines programme.

What is actually involved in getting something done?

The importance of managing the process

Implementing a guideline is like any other development work: it needs to be carefully designed and managed. Regular reviews of progress are vital, perhaps by a steering group consisting of the multidisciplinary panel that adapted the guidelines. The group needs to monitor the progress of the implementation (particularly when a labour-intensive approach such as outreach visits is being used), watch for new or unforeseen barriers, and check data on expected changes in practice. Like all monitoring and programme evaluation, it is important to decide early on the standards and criteria you are going to use, and at what level you will judge their fulfilment.

Embedding into organizational structures

Always take the opportunity to embed any process of change within a larger context. Implementation may be more easily achieved by including it within local organizational structures (e.g. clinical governance in UK primary care, or an integrated care pathway in secondary care).

Potential problems

Mismatch between guidance and available resources

Lack of resources will hinder implementation if recommendations require extensive new tasks outside clinicians' usual roles or prescription of medication where clinicians may be penalized for excessive spending. Barriers such as clinicians taking on new roles and prescribing resources should be addressed at the outset. Think carefully if resources are likely to be big problem.

Insufficient attention to implementation and review

Effective implementation will always demand time, enthusiasm, and resources; choosing implementation methods that are likely to give the best return on available investment is vital. Even when the guidance appears to be implemented, don't assume that change will follow automatically without review of progress and, if necessary, changes in strategy.

Myths

There are many myths associated with guideline development and implementation. Three of the most rehearsed are:

Clinicians do not use guidelines

Although clinical guidelines often get a bad press—for instance, because of suggestions that they limit clinical freedom—research shows that carefully chosen strategies do result in effective implementation of guidelines both in primary and secondary care settings.

Guidelines should always be developed locally from scratch to ensure local ownership

There is commonly held view that adaptations of national guidelines don't work. The validity of nationally and internationally generated guidance needs to be appraised before being adapted, but to start from scratch with guidance at a local level is grossly inefficient. Nationally developed guidelines do have sufficient credibility, especially if they are adapted to local circumstances by respected opinion leaders.

Guidelines lead to litigation

Although the legal status of guidelines varies between different countries, overall they have not been used to override expert opinion in courts of law. On the other hand, if clinicians implement faulty guidelines it is they, rather than the authors of such guidelines, who are likely to increase their liability in negligence. The relationship between guidelines and clinician liability will vary between countries and is likely to evolve over the next few years.

The increasing importance of governance means that every team, clinician, and policy maker needs to be able to justify their professional practice. An evidence base and a value base should underpin every decision and action. At an individual level there may be good reasons not to adhere to a particular recommendation in the guidance in relation to a specific patient. In this case, justification for significantly deviating from the guidance needs to be explicit, preferably in the medical record.

Pitfalls

Two randomized trials of guideline implementation in general practices in east London illustrate success and failure:

- Despite using a multifaceted strategy to implement diabetes and asthma guidelines (outreach visits, consultation prompts, and audit with feedback), it was found that general practices with poor organization (e.g. no practice manager) or with internal conflict between clinicians failed to implement guidelines. The lesson learned is that chaotic practices need organizational support before guidelines can take root.

- A trial tested the use of postal reminders concerning guidelines to patients discharged after a myocardial infarct and to their general practitioners. The results indicated that some general practitioners did not see it as their responsibility to address secondary prevention in patients discharged from hospital. Furthermore, whilst practice nurses could have played a larger part in providing secondary prevention, this part of their role was poorly encouraged. The lesson here is that the roles and responsibilities of target clinicians may need to be addressed before attempting to change clinician behaviour.

Key determinants of success

Six important actions are associated with successful development and implementation of guidelines:

- setting priorities clearly
- setting clear and attainable objectives
- collaborating early with stakeholders
- identifying and targeting barriers to change
- choosing the most powerful implementation strategy that resources will allow
- ensuring that a rigorous project management approach is used.

Further resources

Feder G, Eccles M, Grol R, Griffiths C, Grimshaw J (1999). Using clinical guidelines. *BMJ*, **318**, 728–30.

Grimshaw JM, Thomas RE, MacClennan C et al. (2004). Effectiveness and efficiency of guideline dissemination and implementation strategies. [review] *Health Technol Assess*, **8**(6), iii–iv, 1–72.

Grol R (1997). Personal paper. Beliefs and evidence in changing clinical practice. *BMJ*, **315**, 418–21.

Hurwitz B (2004). How does evidence based guidance influence determinations of medical negligence? [review] *BMJ*, **329**(7473), 1024–8.

Hutchinson A, Baker MR (1999). *Making use of guidelines in clinical practice*. Radcliffe, Oxford.

Sheldon TA, Cullum N, Dawson D et al. (2004). What's the evidence that NICE guidance has been implemented? Results from a national evaluation using time series analysis, audit of patients' notes, and interviews. *BMJ*, **329**(7473), 999.

6.9 Evaluating health-care systems

Nick Hicks

Objectives

The objectives of this chapter are to help you to:
- identify and understand the key issues likely to be involved in the evaluation of a health-care system and
- design and undertake an evaluation of a health-care system.

Definition

A health-care system comprises the organization or organizations that together finance and provide health care to a defined population. Typically, health-care systems are defined by sources of finance, e.g. at the level of country or state, or by membership of a defined organization, e.g. a managed care organization such as Kaiser Permanente in the US.

Why is this an important public health issue?

Health-care systems are a significant direct determinant of health (Bunker[1]):
- they can reduce mortality for major conditions, e.g. coronary heart disease, appendicitis, pneumonia
- they can help eliminate and prevent infectious diseases, e.g. polio, smallpox, mumps, measles, etc
- they can reduce morbidity, e.g. hip arthritis, cataract repair.

More recently, as the links between health and poverty have become better understood and the economic impact of health-care systems has increased, it has been recognized that health-care systems also have indirect effects on health. In developed countries health-care systems:
- create a sense of security, safety, and well-being (Churchill[2]) among those who have secure and convenient access to high-quality health services
- create a market for goods and services, spending about 9% of a county's wealth as measured by gross domestic product (OECD range 6–14%)

- create employment—about 9% of the population in the UK are employed in health and social care
- may contribute to wealth redistribution (when the poor pay less for health care yet consume more than the wealthy) or may exacerbate inequalities (if the poor have inferior access to health services or contribute a greater percentage of their wealth to pay for access to care).

The vast majority of the public place a high value on having (or being able to believe they have) ready access to high-quality health care. The importance the public attach to health care and the major costs of providing health care mean that the impact and consequences of health-care systems extend beyond the health sector. As a consequence:

- the public's perceptions of the functioning of health-care systems can influence the public's electoral choices
- the funding, organization, and functioning of health-care systems can be subjects through which political debate is conducted.

What are the approaches to take?

The section above illustrates that health-care systems produce a wide range of direct and indirect outcomes that are of significance to a wide range of potential stakeholders—ranging from politicians and taxpayers to those who work in and use health-care services.

Before beginning to design any evaluation of a health-care system it is essential to ask:

- Why is this evaluation being undertaken?
- Who wants (and is paying for) the evaluation?
- What dimensions of outcome are relevant to those commissioning the evaluation?
- Are there other significant outcomes that it is important to incorporate into the study?
- What is/are the question/s that this evaluation is trying to answer?
- Is the study meant to describe the impact and outcomes of a health-care system and/or explain why those outcomes have arisen?
- How much time is there to undertake the evaluation?
- How much resource is required and what is available?
- What skill sets are required?

Evaluations of health-care systems are often undertaken to inform policy decisions about funding, organization, and management of health services or to evaluate policy decisions already made. Many individuals and groups—including perhaps even yourself, your profession, and your team—may have a vested interest in the results.

Be aware that the choice of outcomes to be studied can often reflect the values and preferences of those undertaking and commissioning the research. It is helpful if you are aware of your own values and prejudices.

What is the order in which to do things?

Planning and undertaking an evaluation of a health-care system is, in many respects, no different from planning and undertaking an evaluation of a treatment, a health-care pathway, or a health-care institution.

Once you have answered as many of the questions listed above as possible you will have a good idea of what is expected of evaluation and the likely use to which it will be put. You need to design an evaluation that is 'fit for purpose'.

The next stage is to clarify the specific questions the evaluation will address, the outcome measures you will use, and the date by which the results and report are required (this is particularly important if the evaluation is to be used to support a decision-making process which already has a defined timetable).

When evaluating a health-care system it is rare for a single outcome measure to suffice. Typically, several types of outcome measures must be obtained in an attempt to build up as complete a picture as possible of the relevant aspects of the health-care system being evaluated. Much of the skill of the evaluator is in the selection of the relevant outcomes and the ability to see and understand the possible explanatory links between them. Dimensions of system outcome that may be of interest include:

- measures of access, e.g. by time (how long do people wait), geography (e.g. rural versus urban)
- measures of equity, e.g. by race, by socio-economic group, by gender, by age
- measures of patient experience
- measures of public opinion
- measures of quality of care—often using process as well as outcome measures
- measures of patient and system safety, e.g. rates of adverse events, nosocomial infection rates
- measures of activity, e.g. admission rates, occupied bed days/1000 population
- measures of cost, e.g. £/1000 people , £/unit activity, %GDP
- measures of work-force numbers and skill-mix
- measures of efficiency, often expressed as a ratio of an output to an input (e.g. number of operations/surgeon, operations/£)
- measures of effectiveness, e.g. age–sex standardized mortality rates and case fatality rates
- measures of population health status—morbidity, mortality, and well-being; but beware that there are many factors other than health-care systems that influence population health status.

Further information about how to collect and interpret each of these can be found elsewhere in this book.

Interpretation of the results of an evaluation of a health-care system often requires reference to and comparison with the results for similar dimensions of health system outcome produced by other health-care systems. If this is the case, then ideally the relevant data would be collected as part of the study, i.e. a comparative evaluation. However, this is frequently not possible, so a literature search is required. In addition to the usual biomedical literature it is worth asking your librarian to help you with a search of the health and policy and economic literature. It may also be worth looking at the websites of organizations such as:

- The World Health Organization (http://who.dk and http://www.euro.who.int/cindi/20020319_1/)
- The OECD (http://www.oecd.org/)
- The Institute of Medicine (http://www.iom.edu/)
- CDC (http://www.cdc.gov/eval/)
- Agency for Health Care Research and Quality (http://www.ahrq.gov/clinic/outcomix.htm)
- The King's Fund (http://www.kingsfund.org.uk/)
- The Commonwealth Fund of New York (http://www.cmwf.org/)
- The Nuffield Trust (http://www.nuffieldtrust.org.uk/) (all accessed 15 June 2005).

Frequently an evaluation is expected to go beyond mere description of the outcomes that a health-care system produces; an explanation of why the system produces the results that it does is also often wanted. This is likely to require a detailed qualitative approach, especially if the answer is thought to lie in the detail of the way work is organized or managed, or if such 'soft' issues as organizational culture are thought to be important explanatory factors.

Although the evaluation is more likely to concentrate on the direct consequences of the health-care system, there will also be times when there is interest in the indirect effects of the health-care system in question which are important—such as the economic impact of the health-care system and the impact of the health-care system on transport and the environment (which are issues of increasing concern to the public, politicians, and planners). If this is case, then it may be appropriate to incorporate and use the methods of health impact assessment (see Chapter 1.5) into the design of your evaluation.

What are the skills and competencies?

The sections above illustrate the wide range of outcomes that you may want to incorporate into your evaluation. The precise skills and competencies required will depend on what it is you want to measure. But it is important to realize that it is unlikely that any one individual will possess all the necessary skills to undertake the evaluation by themselves. Typically, you (or whoever is leading the evaluation) will need to put together, or draw upon the expertise of, a multiprofessional and multidisciplinary team. Alternatively, especially if you are inexperienced in the evaluation of health-care systems (and if you have a budget to spend), it may be more efficient to commission the study from an expert group that regularly undertakes evaluations of the sort that you want done.

You are likely to want to include people with skills and experience in at least some of the following:

- health services research
- health economics

- statistics
- health and public policy
- workforce
- public health
- academic health service management
- qualitative researcher
- opinion researchers
- organizational psychology
- health and patient-derived outcomes
- report writing
- politics and health.

Who else needs to be involved?

It is often wise to make sure that whoever has asked for the evaluation is aware of how you intend to undertake the evaluation, when it will be completed, and the extent to which you think it is or isn't likely to answer the questions they want answered.

Not all the data you require will necessarily be in the public domain. You may need to negotiate access to the data.

You may also need to seek advice about whether the data to which you have access can be used for the purposes for which you want to use it. For example, if the data you have access to have been collected from patients in the course of routine clinical practice you may be restricted in the secondary uses to which the data can be put. The rules and the interpretation of the rules are changing and being debated—so rather than setting out the current understanding here it would be wise to seek advice at the time.

Should you need to approach patients and/or members or the public, and if you work in a health-care organization, you are likely to need to seek ethical committee approval for your study. If in doubt, seek the advice of your local research ethics committee or of your local research governance team.

The results of evaluations of health-care systems can be of great significance and potentially very sensitive. You should agree in advance how the results will be presented, to whom, in what format, and who will own the data. You should also establish the extent to which you will be able to publish your work and conduct further analysis of the raw data.

Potential pitfalls

Health-care systems are usually large, complicated, and expensive. They have multiple consequences, some intended, others unintended. The unintended consequences can be as significant as those that were intended. It is important to recognize this complexity and avoid too narrow a conceptualization of the impact of health-care systems. And, in as much as the explicit aim of many health-care systems is to improve health, a key pitfall to avoid is over-attribution of the link between health-care systems and population health status.

But perhaps the two key pitfalls to avoid are:
- The risk of being or appearing naïve. Do not be naïve and present your findings as though the outcomes you measure are the only ones that matter; do not forget that people have vested interests that lead them to ask for evaluations that focus on particular outcomes, or evaluations that specifically avoid examination of other outcomes, because they have a specific agenda to pursue.
- Failing to create a team with the necessary diverse range of skills and resources required for the evaluation you want to undertake.

Dogma, myths, and fallacies

It's a myth to think that health system evaluation is any of the following:
- Easy—it's not. It's difficult
- Produces unequivocal, simple results: the best evaluations demonstrate a range of consequences caused by a health-care system and illustrate the trade-offs that need to be considered when devising and implementing policy aimed at improving one or more dimensions of outcome
- Value neutral. Every stage of the evaluation including design, selection of outcome measures, interpretation and presentation of the results reflects value judgements.

Examples

For an interesting example of health-care system evaluation, the controversies that it can cause, and the different interpretations that can arise, see the comparative study of the Kaiser Permanente system in the US and the UK NHS undertaken by Feachem and colleagues,[3] and the subsequent online debate that it generated (see http://bmj.bmjjournals.com/cgi/content/full/324/7330/135 (accessed 22 July 2005)).

A good example of interpretation based on integration of quantitative and qualitative data, again based on comparison of the same health-care systems Kaiser and the NHS, can be found in the paper by Ham.[4]

Further reading
Bunker JP, Frazier HS, Mosteller F (1994). Improving health: measuring effects of medical care. *Milbank Q*, **72**, 225–58.
World Health Organization (2000). *The World Health Report 2000: health systems—improving performance*. World Health Organization, Geneva.

References
1 Bunker JP (1995). Medicine matters after all. *J R Coll Physicians*, **29**, 105–12.
2 Churchill LR (1994). *Self interest and universal healthcare: why well insured Americans should support coverage for everyone*. Harvard University Press, Cambridge, MA.
3 Feachem RGA, Sekhri N, White KL (2002). Getting more for their dollar: a comparison of the NHS with California's Kaiser Permanente. *BMJ*, **324**, 135–43.
4 Ham C (2005). Lost in translation? Health systems in the US and the UK. *Soc Policy Admin*, **39**, 192–209.

6.10 Evaluating patient experience and health-care process data

Edmund Jessop

Objective

The objective of this chapter is to help you to analyze health-care processes as two separate elements:
- Patient experience—did the patient feel well cared for?
- Effective process—was their health improved?

Patient experience

The first question is best answered by direct survey. You can devise your own survey or use standard instruments such as the Picker patient experience questionnaire.[1] Nothing very complicated here, just do it!

The National Health Service in England now runs regular patient experience surveys (see the website[2] for the survey questionnaire and report and read this for suggestions about aspects of care which patients find important).

Don't get complacent when you analyze the results—patients are very vulnerable and give praise readily. In England nearly three-quarters (74%) of respondents rated the hospital care they received as excellent (38%) or very good (36%), so 74% 'very good' or 'excellent' is an *average* result (in England at least).

Effective process—a clue to outcome

For patient experience, direct survey is best; but for outcome, direct survey is difficult and expensive. So we are forced to use data which are imperfect but cheap and readily available—process data.

When you use process data, remember that many health-care processes do nothing to improve or safeguard health. So focus on processes that you know to be *effective*.

For instance, immunization for diphtheria is highly effective, and so the number of immunizations given is a good (though not perfect) measure of population immunity. So:

- immunisation coverage (process) for diphtheria vaccine predicts freedom from diphtheria (outcome)

but

- number of grommets inserted (ineffective process) gives no information about reduction in disability from hearing loss (outcome).

Box 6.10.1

An effective process predicts outcome. An ineffective process predicts nothing.

When is a process effective?

How can we tell if a process is effective? If asked to evaluate a specific treatment such as drug-eluting stents you will probably have to find and appraise research evidence (see chapter 2.11). But for common services such as cancer services, screening programmes, or tuberculosis control, you can look for published summaries. It's best to use publications from your own country—this gives your findings greater impact if they imply a need for change. Good collections are available at the Centre for Reviews and Dissemination (http://www.york.ac.uk/inst/crd/ehcb.htm (accessed 25 July 2005)) and the Agency for Healthcare Research and Quality (http://www.ahcpr.gov/clinic/epcix.htm (accessed 25 July 2005)).

You should also find out if a professional society has published guidelines. For example, in the UK, tuberculosis control programmes would be evaluated against guidelines from the British Thoracic Society. I find that the quickest route to contact details for professional societies is Google (http://google.com (accessed 25 July 2005)).

Remember that in public health we are interested in population coverage, so try to relate the process to your population: age, sex, ethnic group, location, and so on.

Health-care process evaluation— examples

Here are some examples to get you thinking.

Preventive medicine

Immunization *coverage* is a basic process measure: because the effectiveness of vaccines is known, coverage predicts outcome. With measles, for example, vaccine coverage of 95% or more will eradicate the disease, while coverage or 70% or less will result in epidemics.

Relate information on clinic *attendance* to what you know about your population. Many teenagers are sexually active by the age of 16, so your sexual health clinics should be seeing some children aged 16 or younger.

No attendance by people from ethnic minority groups may indicate that the service is inaccessible or unfriendly. (But, as we said above, the process of attending a clinic does not ensure the desired outcome of people using contraception correctly and avoiding unwanted pregnancy.)

Screening process (see Chapter 3.6)

The aim of screening for, say, breast cancer is to avert death from breast cancer. The outcome—reduction in death from breast cancer—is almost undetectable in routine statistics.

But process measures can help (Table 6.10.1). Population coverage is the obvious first essential. Another measure is the number of unnecessary operations, i.e. biopsies which turned out to be benign. The ratio of benign:malignant is therefore a useful process measure. The number of cancers detected can be a useful measure if the number expected in the screened population is known accurately: too few implies cancers are being missed, too many implies over-diagnosis.

Table 6.10.1 Process measures of the UK breast screening programme

Objective	Criteria	Minimum standard
To maximize uptake	Percentage of eligible women who attend	More than 70%
To achieve optimum image quality in mammograms	Minimum detectable contrast 5–6 mm detail	Less than 1%
To minimize anxiety in women awaiting results of screening	Percentage of women who are sent their result within 2 weeks	More than 90%

Source: UK NHS Breast Screening Programme October 1998.[3]

Primary care process (see Chapter 3.9)

The common measures of primary care process are:
- consultations or attendances
- prescriptions.

The *quality* of consultations is not easy to monitor, though looking at the number and variety of complaints may give some clue. Most people prefer prompt treatment, so waiting times for appointments, or for response to emergencies, should be important process data for primary care. These data are not, however, widely used.

Effective prescribing includes the use of preventive medication for asthma and aspirin for people who have had an acute myocardial infarction. Ineffective prescribing includes using appetite suppressants for obesity instead of advice on diet and exercise. This can form a basis for using pharmacy or prescribing data to judge quality: for example one could count the total number of prescriptions for appetite suppressants, and the ratio of preventer to reliever for asthma drugs.

Process data on referrals from primary care to secondary or specialist care are widely used but are largely unhelpful because no one knows what constitutes good practice. Are high or low referral rates good, bad, or just random variation?

Good primary care should avert severe asthma or diabetic coma. Hospital admission rates for asthma or diabetic coma have been used to indicate poor primary care.

Acute hospital process

For specialist care, *time spent waiting* is an important process measure.
Surgical operations can be classified into three categories:

- category 1: life saving (e.g. cardiac surgery)
- category 2: highly effective (e.g. cataract removal, cochlear implant)
- category 3: outdated or ineffective in a high proportion of patients (e.g. inserting grommets, diagnostic curettage in young women, radical mastectomy).

This simple scheme allows one, with some caveats, to use process data on operations to form judgements on health care for a population. For example, a very low rate of cochlear implants (less than 1 per million population) implies failure to provide a highly effective procedure.

You need to be sure of data coverage for this work: many country-wide health-care data systems (e.g. in the UK) do not capture operations in the private sector, and often miss operations done in the clinic.

Medical specialties are much more difficult than surgical specialties to evaluate through process data. Mental health services are even worse. There are two key problems:

- *lifelong illness*: surgery is often associated with a cure; medical treatment, however, is often one episode in lifelong illness
- *variation in severity*: major surgery indicates a patient with more disability than minor surgery, but a diagnosis such as bronchitis or depression may conceal disability ranging from trivial to total.

Both of these problems apply even more to mental illness.

Summary

- Survey patient experience directly—just do it!
- Health care *process* often tells you little about health or health status.
- Effective process may predict outcome, ineffective process predicts nothing.
- A huge number of process data are generated by most health services. Process data come cheap.
- How closely people adhere to guidance can give an indication of quality of process (see Chapter 6.8).
- Being able to show that your process meets defined standards in certain criteria is the basis not only of audit but also of clinical governance (see Chapter 6.11).

Further resources

A good introduction to UK data on hospital inpatients:
Goldacre MJ (1981). Hospital inpatient statistics: some aspects of interpretation. *Commun Med*, **3**, 60–8.

Two cautionary examples:
Black N (1985). Glue ear: the new dyslexia? *BMJ*, **290**,1963–5.

Hill A (1989). Trends in paediatric medical admissions. *BMJ*, **298**, 1479–83.

Use of GP attendance data (short but very good):
Fry J, Dillane JB, Fry L (1962). Smog: 1962 v 1952. *Lancet*, **ii**, 1326.

Process data for needs assessment:
Roderick PJ, Jones I, Raleigh VS, McGeown M, Mallick N (1994). Population need for renal replacement therapy in Thames regions: ethnic dimension. *BMJ*, **309**, 1111–14.

Smith P, Sheldon TA, Martin S (1996). An index of need for psychiatric services based on in-patient utilisation. *Br J Psychiat*, **169**, 308–16.

Comprehensive use of process and other data to evaluate performance:
Healthcare Commission. *NHS Performance Ratings 2005*. Available at: http://ratings2005.healthcarecommission.org.uk/ (accessed 20 January 2006).

References

1 Jenkinson C, Coulter A, Bruster S (2002). The Picker patient experience questionnaire: development and validation using data from in-patient surveys in five countries. *Int J Qual Health Care*, **14**(5), 353–8.
2 Department of Health. *National survey of NHS patients*. Available at: http://www.dh.gov.uk/PublicationsAndStatistics/PublishedSurvey/NationalSurveyOfNHSPatients/fs/en (accessed 20 January 2006).
3 NHS (1998). *National Health Service breast screening programme. Guidelines on quality assurance visits*. NHS BSP (Breast Screening Programme) publication no 40, appendix 2. NHS BSP Publications, Sheffield.

6.11 Clinical quality, governance, and accountability

Pamela Hall and Gabriel Scally

This chapter is based on Chapter 6.8 of the first edition of this book by Dr Cameron Bowie.

Objectives

After reading this chapter you will have a better understanding of:
- the concepts of individual and organizational accountability
- how health organizations can use clinical governance to safeguard and demonstrate the quality of the services that they provide
- how public health professionals can contribute to improvement in the quality of health-care services by using these tools.

Definitions and concepts

The generally accepted definition of clinical governance (in the UK) is that proposed by Scally and Donaldson in 1999: 'Clinical governance is a system through which NHS [and other health-care] organizations are accountable for continuously improving the quality of their services and safeguarding high standards of care by creating an environment in which excellence in clinical care will flourish'.[1] A more compact definition of clinical governance is 'a framework that helps NHS [and other health-care] organizations provide safe and high quality care'.[2]

The most important elements of clinical governance are clarity of purpose and clear lines of accountability. Accountability is all about being demonstrably responsible for one's actions. In the context of clinical governance, the essence of accountability is the identification and acceptance of the role and responsibility of each clinician and manager.

Development of clinical governance

The development of clinical governance in the UK in the late 1990s was driven by a series of high-profile failures in the quality of clinical services, resulting in serious harm to patients. Earlier in that decade, concerns about the way in which private corporations conducted their business had lead to a landmark report on corporate governance, the Cadbury Report.[3] As had happened in the 1980s with clinical audit, public health (because of its organizational base being within the NHS) quickly adopted and adapted the concept and started to use the term 'public health governance'. Consequently, there are two aspects of governance which are relevant to public health practitioners:

- The contribution that public health practitioners can and do make to the assessment and improvement of the quality of clinical services.
- The necessary incorporation of the principles of governance within public health practice even when it is not engaged in issues of personal health service provision.

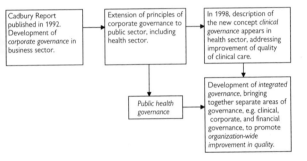

Why is clinical governance a public health issue?

Although improvement of the health of populations and communities is much more reliant on broad determinants of health, access to high-quality personal health services is a significant component of health improvement. The Pan-American Health Organization has identified a very useful list of 11 essential public health functions. The ninth of these is 'Quality assurance in personal and population-based health services'. Assurance is one of the three key public health tasks identified by the Institute of Medicine.[4] Because of their skill base, public health practitioners are well placed to develop a clear understanding of the interactions between individual health professionals and health organizations in the pursuit of delivering high-quality care to patients (see Chapter 6.9).

Who is responsible for clinical governance?

In health care, individuals and organizations have separate but complementary responsibilities for ensuring the quality of clinical care. Clinical governance should embrace all of the individual and collective activity involved in delivering clinical services to patients.[2] Clinicians, technical staff, ancillary workers, and managers should be able to demonstrate to patient and employers (and external agencies with responsibility for monitoring and regulating health care) that their individual and team contribution to a service is of consistently high quality (see Chapter 7.8).

In England, all NHS organizations have a statutory duty not only to maintain quality but to have in place adequate processes for improving it; this is known as the *duty of quality*.[5]

Components and domains of clinical governance

The concept of clinical governance is a feature of health-care systems in many countries, although it is defined in different ways in different settings. The Table 6.11.1 outlines some of the features that are common to systems for delivering high-quality health care, and broadly corresponds to a model for clinical governance arrangements.

Table 6.11.1 From clinical governance to integrated governance. An example of how components of clinical governance can fit with other quality improvement mechanisms (developed from[6-8] and work undertaken in NHS Executive North Thames Regional Office in 1998).

1. **Setting evidence-based standards**			
2. **Delivering services: Clinical governance**			
	2a. Clinical effectiveness	Service planning based on the best evidence of effective treatment, within resource constraints	Lifelong learning
	2b. Clinical audit	Comparing actual practice with 'best practice' or another standard; identifying areas for improvement; implementing change.	Based on patients' needs
	2c. Risk management	Appreciating the potential risks and benefits of each decision, in terms of patient and staff safety.	Open and transparent
	2d. Quality assurance	Being explicit about standards, and having in place systems to respond to errors.	
	2e. Organizational and staff development	Ensuring that staff and organization are equipped for changes in technology, patients' expectation etc.	Professional regulation
3. **Monitoring performance against standards**			

Other models of clinical governance have been proposed and are being used. For example, the Western Australia Department of Health model of clinical governance is based on four 'pillars'; consumer value, clinical performance and evaluation, clinical risk and professional development, and management.[9]

Individuals and organizations should consider whether a particular area of service delivery is so important as to warrant specific consideration of the arrangements for clinical governance, for example if patient safety is involved. The prominence given to clinical governance systems will vary depending on the other pressures faced by the organization and may well be heavily influenced by the priorities of those with political responsibility for the health service. The concept of quality has many important (and often competing) dimensions, and different health-care services may end up having very different priorities in terms of the promotion of quality (see Chapter 6.1).

Box 6.11.1 Integrated governance

Traditionally, different domains of governance within health-care organizations have been organized almost independently of each other. Integrated governance has been defined as 'Systems and processes by which [health-care organizations] lead, direct and control their functions in order to achieve organisational objectives, safety, and quality of services, and in which they relate to the wider community and partner organisations'.[10] This approach attempts to bring together clinical, corporate, financial and other areas of governance to promote a shared organizational approach to improving the quality of health services.

The challenges of promoting accountability, responsibility, and governance

Delivering clinical care is complex. There are at least five specific challenges that must be addressed to create a system with the necessary mechanisms and incentives to maintain quality. Public health professionals working with or for health-care organizations have a role in all of these challenges:
1. applying population-based evidence to individual patients
2. managing the multidisciplinary nature of modern clinical care
3. empowering clinicians in a receptive environment
4. coping with the changing nature of professional practice
5. maintaining openness.

The professional application of population-based evidence to individuals within a limited budget

Clinical care has unique features which distinguish it from financial and other service industries. The organization of such care demands a particular approach to governance:

- each patient is different, often with multiple needs requiring individual professional assessment and intervention. Although good evidence must come from populations, it ultimately has to be applied to individuals
- the genetic make-up and socio-economic background of each patient contribute to variable and often unpredictable outcomes
- technology and medical science are changing rapidly. Clinicians need to be up-to-date, and their teams need to be highly responsive to new evidence and new approaches to service provision
- resources are limited, requiring decisions to be made about their most effective and efficient use.

The consequence of these features, with respect to quality and accountability, is that professionals at the point of service delivery are best placed to define what standards are realistic, how they can be monitored, and what changes in practice are possible to make improvements. Indeed, top-down standard setting does not seem to work in health care without strenuous efforts made to persuade clinicians of their appropriateness.[11] Bottom-up standard setting *within a broad and consistent quality framework* and addressing local priorities, is more likely to encourage ownership.[12]

The multidisciplinary nature of modern clinical care

It is rare for one individual clinician to meet all of the health needs of a patient. The growth in the proportion of elderly people and the presence of multiple conditions means that the care patients require is frequently complex. A wide range of professionals and services is usually required if patients' needs are to be met. Every clinician is therefore responsible for contributing to high-quality teamwork.[13] This will mean that most audit activities will need to be genuinely multidisciplinary. However, medical subspecialization is so developed that, for some aspects of care, clinicians can only assess themselves by comparing their performance with that of colleagues from other institutions. The arrangements for participation in audit will inevitably be highly varied, but public health professionals with a responsibility for commissioning personal health services will wish to be satisfied that all clinicians providing care are engaged in meaningful audit programmes.[14] The move which is taking place in some countries from a managed health service to a regulated health service places substantial responsibility on external regulators and inspectorates. They will wish to have access to skills (e.g. from public health professionals) to assist in this area of their activities.

Empowering clinicians in a receptive environment

Empowering clinicians to adopt an approach which emphasizes the continuous improvement of quality of care is a key task in health services management. An important component of this is the promotion of a supportive culture where clinical errors are acknowledged and learnt from. Such errors need to be regarded as an opportunity to improve patient safety rather than an occasion for the 'naming, blaming, and shaming' of those involved in what are almost always multiple systemic problems rather than individual acts of omission or commission. In adopting this approach, the role of management changes from a passive to an active partner in the delivery of the quality component of care. Managers must be as interested in *quality* of care as they are in the *quantity and cost.*[1] (See Chapter 6.9.)

The changing nature of professional practice

The social environment in which health professionals work is changing, with profound effects on the nature of clinical practice.[15–17] Many patients rightly demand more involvement in decisions about their own care and have their own perceptions of priorities and quality. They have access to an enormous amount of information, of varying accuracy, via the media and the Internet. Staff, many of whom will have trained and begun practice in a different era, must be encouraged to address these issues through their continuing professional development programmes. Professional autonomy and clinical freedom are in retreat, as patients demand empowerment, not paternalism.

Maintaining openness

The public is also demanding more openness. When something goes wrong, most patients and their carers want to be told three things: they want to be told what went wrong; what can be done to put it right or reduce the ill-effects; and what is being done to ensure it never happens again. Professional organizations are responding, sometimes hesitantly, as complaints about health care are increasingly frequent, and are often publicised in local and national media. Health-care workers and managers sometimes have a tendency to adopt defensive postures in response to criticism. To address this, involvement of patients and carers in the planning and governance of personal health services is vital. From the perspective of public health professionals, involvement in the task of developing public engagement is clearly an area of growing importance and where new skills are needed.

Promoting an environment in which quality can flourish

The key to clinical governance is trust; individuals and teams must be able to trust the organizational systems in which they work, confident that other individuals and teams are making their stated contribution to patient care. Trust does not exist by right, it is earned by demonstrating a commitment to quality in practice every day, by everyone. To promote governance, organizations will need to:

- ensure that systems are in place for recognizing, managing, and learning from both good and poor practice
- facilitate genuine multidisciplinary team working, and communication between teams

- encourage joint working between clinicians and managers, with a clear statement of responsibilities
- develop shared information to monitor standards
- ensure that appropriate professional training and development is available and accessible when needed.

The role of the public health practitioner

The skill set of public health professionals can contribute to good clinical governance in various ways.

Much of the assessment of health-care quality relies upon a high level of data analysis and interpretation. An epidemiologic perspective and approach can be extremely helpful and can often be delivered by public health professionals with a high degree of objectivity because of their separation from, but understanding of, the direct care process.

The second key area is in the realm of public engagement, where they can bring a population perspective to issues that might otherwise be considered within a narrow scope.

Finally, the planning role is one where the population-based approach is particularly important and where there is often a high level of public interest.

Further reading

Allen P (2000). Clinical governance in primary care: accountability for clinical governance: developing collective responsibility for quality in primary care. *BMJ*, **321**, 608–11.

Black N (1998). Clinical governance: fine words or action? *BMJ*, **316**, 297–8.

Dawson S, Garside P, Moss F (ed.) (1998). Organisational change: the key to quality improvement. *Qual Health Care*, **7**(Supplement).

Donaldson LJ (1998). Clinical governance: a statutory duty for quality improvement. *J. Epidemiol. Commun Health*, **52**, 73–4.

Huntington J, Gillam S, Rosen R (2000). Clinical governance in primary care: organisational development for clinical governance. *BMJ*, **321**, 679–82.

Institute for Healthcare Improvement. http://www.ihi.org/IHI (accessed 25 April 2005).

Lugon M (ed.) (2000–5). *Clinical Governance Bulletin*. Royal Society of Medicine Press, London. Available at: http://www.rsmpress.co.uk/cgb.htm (accessed 25 April 2005).

McColl A, Roland M (2000). Clinical governance in primary care: knowledge and information for clinical governance. *BMJ*, **321**, 871–4.

Millenson ML (1997). *Demanding medical excellence doctors and accountability in the information age*. Chicago University Press, Chicago, IL.

NHS Clinical Governance Support Team. http://www.cgsupport.nhs.uk/ (accessed 25 April 2005).

Pringle M (2000). Clinical governance in primary care: participating in clinical governance. *BMJ*, **321**, 737–40.

Scally G, Donaldson LJ (1998). The NHS's 50 anniversary. Clinical governance and the drive for quality improvement in the new NHS in England. *BMJ*, **317**, 61–5.

South Essex Health Authority Clinical Governance Group (2002). *A framework for assuring clinical governance in public health practice.* South Essex Health Authority, Brentwood. Available at: http://www.fph.org.uk/prof_standards/downloads/general_standards/St andards_SEssex_HA_doc.pdf (accessed 3 January 2006).

United Kingdom Central Council (UKCC) (1992). *The scope of professional practice.* UKCC, London.

References

1 Scally G, Donaldson LJ (1999). Clinical governance and the drive for quality improvement in the new NHS in England. *BMJ*, **317**, 61–5.

2 NHS Appointments Commission (2003). *Governing the NHS: a guide for NHS boards.* NHS Appointments Commission, London.

3 *Report of the Committee on the Financial Aspects of Corporate Governance* [Cadbury Report] (1992). Gee, London. Available at: http://rru.worldbank.org/Documents/PapersLinks/1253.pdf (accessed 29 September 2005).

4 Institute of Medicine. *The future of public health* (1988) and *Health communities: new partnerships for the future of public health* (1996). Institute of Medicine, Washington, DC. Both available at: http://www.nap.edu/books/0309038308/html/ and http://www.nap.edu/books/030905625X/html respectively. (accessed 20 January 2006).

5 HMSO (2003). *Health and Social Care (Community Health and Standards) Act 2003.* HMSO, London.

6 NHS Executive (1999). *Clinical governance. Quality in the new NHS*, HSC 1999/065. Department of Health, London.

7 Donaldson L (2001). The first 500 days: renewal, reform, reflection. *J Epidemol Community Health*, **55**, 371–2.

8 Wright J, Hill P (2003). *Clinical governance.* Churchill Livingstone, London.

9 Western Australia Department of Health (2005). *Western Australia clinical governance guidelines*, Information Series no 1.2, 2nd edn. Western Australia Department of Health, Perth.

10 NHS Confederation (2004). The development of integrated governance. *Debate* **3**.

11 Dyke G (1998). *The new NHS charter—a different approach; report on the new NHS charter.* Department of Health, London. Available at: http://www.dh.gov.uk/assetRoot/04/10/60/95/04106095.PDF (accessed 25 April 2005).

12 Department of Health (2004). *Standards for better health.* Department of Health, London. Available at: http://www.dh.gov.uk/assetRoot/04/08/66/66/04086666.pdf (accessed 25 April 2005).

13 General Medical Council (2001). *Good medical practice.* General Medical Council, London. Available at: http://www.gmc-uk.org/standards/default.htm (accessed 25 April 2005).

14 Treasure T (1998). Lessons from the Bristol case. *BMJ*, **316**, 1685–6.

15 Freidson E (1989). *Medical work in America (essays on health care)*. Yale University Press, New Haven, CT.

16 Krause E (1996). *Death of the guilds: professions, states, and the advance of capitalism, 1930 to the present*. Yale University Press, New Haven, CT.

17 Policy Commission on Public Services (2004). *Making public services personal: a new compact for public services. The independent Policy Commission on Public Services report to the National Consumer Council*. National Consumer Council, London. Available at: http://www.ncc.org.uk/ publicservices/policy_commission.pdf (accessed 25 April 2005).

Personal effectiveness

Introduction

The whole of this handbook is aimed at increasing your effectiveness. Sometimes that means careful self-examination of your personal effectiveness. That is the focus of this part.

Leadership and management are critical for effective public health practice. These attributes can and should be distinguished, although both are needed for effective collaboration. Developing relationships is the key to managing change with people and groups as diverse as colleagues, vulnerable communities, or the minister's office. These settings are explored in chapters that apply particularly to your work as an individual public health practitioner. The appeal of Chapters 7.1–7.6 will vary according to the stage of your career, but all of us have a responsibility for continual improvement of our own professional practice (Chapter 7.8).

Professional isolation is a hazard that takes many forms. Consider yourself, for example, as the report writer, or as an expert working on a consultancy contract (Chapters 7.3 and 7.6). All authors in this section suggest ways to connect, communicate, and collaborate with colleagues more productively.

Public health sometimes has a reputation for being well intentioned but meddlesome. Giving unsolicited advice can fall into this category. If you are providing advice, please follow Horace (Roman poet, 65–8 B.C.) and at least remember to be brief.

CSG

7.1 Public health leadership

Fiona Sim

Objectives

This chapter should equip you with many of the complementary skills which are necessary to turn excellent public health technical practice into *effective* public health practice.

Definitions

Leadership

Great leaders are usually characterized as highly charismatic, high-profile individuals—Churchill, Mandela, Thatcher, Hitler—some we may wish to emulate, others not. They shared attributes of immense power to influence, communication of a clear vision which would be attractive to their followers, and the ability to deliver that vision.

In your workplace or community you could probably identify someone, not necessarily charismatic or extrovert, or even very senior, who has been the architect of a substantial change and made it happen.

Public health leadership

Public health leadership is the application of such leadership characteristics to the cause of improving the health of a given population or community.[1–3]

A former Chief Medical Officer for England[4] has described leadership as:
- knowing where you want to go and setting the direction of travel
- taking people with you on the journey in spite of their differences in views and methods, working background, and rates of travel
- giving sufficient time and energy to the process of changing things for the better—learning to do things in a different way.

Aims of public health leadership

The aims of public health leadership may include:
- attributable improvement in the health of a population or community
- better collaboration at organizational and individual levels
- a higher profile for public health
- greater efficiency in health decision-making

Is leadership different from management?

Leadership complements and differs from management in some important respects. Whilst an effective manager requires planning and problem-solving

Table 7.1.1 Distinctions between managers and leaders (after Kotter[5])

Manager	Leader
Coping with complexity	Coping with change
Ensuring order and consistency	Delivering change
Planning and budgeting	Setting direction—developing a vision
Organizing and staffing to accomplish objectives	Aligning people
Problem solving	Motivating and inspiring

skills to produce largely predictable, desirable results, a leader will go further *to establish the vision* and take it forward, usually by motivating and developing others, to produce significant, sometimes dramatic, change. Table 7.1.1 illustrates these distinctions.

Why is leadership an important public health attribute?

For a public health practitioner to be effective technical skills and knowledge are essential but not sufficient. Imagine absorbing all the information in this handbook and yet being unable, in the face of opposing views, to articulate and implement your sound professional, evidence-based advice?

Every public health practitioner must to be able to exercise leadership skills, even if his/her role is not explicitly a 'leading' one. For instance, it may at some time be appropriate for the public health member of any team to take the lead, with the agreement of the team.

A programme of work around public health leadership

Virtually any piece of work in public health lends itself to scrutiny of the public health leadership element. For example, if you were expected to implement a local screening programme you would set yourself objectives, based on your professional competence and integrity.

Review of this task will reveal aspects that required competent public health leadership:

- having a clear vision of what you were trying to achieve and why
- working across organisational boundaries by communicating appropriately and effectively
- understanding and gaining the trust of service users
- persevering in the task through to implementation and evaluation
- demonstrating professional integrity—and thereby moral courage.

Competencies for leadership

It is easy to see that technical knowledge and skills lead to technical competence; for public health leadership, however, whilst acquisition of relevant competencies *should* lead to competence, the evidence to date is largely circumstantial. This is due in part to a lack of research in this area and partly because the competencies comprise skills and attitudes, some of which we may acquire at an early age while others can be learned later.

> Box 7.1.1 Competencies usually associated with effective public health leadership include:
>
> Knowledge
> - Good grasp of the core knowledge base required for public health practice
>
> Skills
> - Ability to define and articulate a clear vision
> - Ability to share the vision so that others are influenced to adopt it
> - Resilience and perseverance towards the vision despite difficulties
> - Maintenance of professional integrity
>
> Attitudes
> - Self-esteem combined with critical self-appraisal
> - A degree of humility to allow one to acknowledge that someone else is right
> - An understanding and respect of others' beliefs and perceptions, which may differ from one's own
> - Personal values including a 'passion' for public health

Orientation and execution of leadership tasks

Public health leadership requires the participation and commitment of other people.

Many public health practitioners have little formal power in the traditional sense, such as control of substantial budgets or a large directly employed workforce. It is essential, therefore, that they are able to achieve commitment to their vision by others. A 'command and control' model of leadership becomes redundant.

Leadership is important at different levels in public health practice:
- Personal: for effective leadership, the public health practitioner should have a clear understanding of his/her own strengths and weaknesses, personality type, and preferred leadership styles.
- Organizational: to be an effective public health leader within an organization, the practitioner must understand fully the organization's structure, its culture, key players to be influenced, financial position, and decision-making processes.

- Community: for public health leadership to be effective within a community, the practitioner must understand its culture and history and be able to identify and engage its key members, who may include community leaders, politicians, and journalists, for instance. He/she must work *with and through* leaders of other relevant organizations in order to effect changes that will improve the health of the community.

The public health vision *and* the role of the public health leader must be clearly articulated. In an established public health system these may be obvious. But in developing systems, the practitioner will need to deploy the appropriate leadership skills and demonstrate the attitudes most likely to result in success. We can be inspired by pioneer public health leaders, including Snow, Chadwick, and Simon, who created their own vision and persevered to achieve their societal goals.[6]

Potential pitfalls

- Recognizing a public health challenge and producing a technically competent project plan to address it is necessary, but not sufficient.
- Neither vision nor professional expertise alone will lead to change—political skills including diplomacy, communication. and timing are just as important.
- Leadership may not always be from the front. Exercising different styles of leadership in different circumstances is necessary—in leading an outbreak investigation, getting local industry to take seriously your vision for workplace health, or introducing changes in clinical practice.
- Avoid appearing pious in your enthusiasm to do good. Understand that others may not share the vision unless it is explained explicitly in terms of the evidence upon which it is based.

Unpicking dogma

- 'Leaders are born and not made.' This assertion is not based upon fact or evidence. It appears from the evidence that there are few inherent attributes of leadership other than intelligence and aptitude. Much of the research on this subject has been based on military leadership, so aptitude has been found to comprise features such as the ability to respond rapidly in warfare. In public health, a quick mind to respond to debate and challenge under pressure, and a willingness to learn continually and from every situation are more clearly important.
- It has been suggested that physical height lends itself to leadership: history refutes that assertion.
- That a particular personality type is likely to make a better leader is often discussed. It is the case that when leaders have been studied, the majority have 'extrovert' personalities, according to widely used personality type inventories. So some people may have a natural potential for leadership. This does not, however, rule out the possibility of other people becoming effective leaders, and many do so.

- 'What is your leadership style?' is a commonly asked question at interviews. The effective leader may well have a preferred style, but will have a whole battery of styles to suit different situations.[7]
- Leadership is just a fancy term for management. Well, it is neither fancy nor the same, as described earlier.

Determinants of success

Clarity of vision and the perseverance to ensure its implementation by engaging all relevant parties is most likely to lead to success. There will often need to be flexibility in the vision—the world is a dynamic place and what is clearly appropriate today may need some amendment in the near future.

Successful leadership requires imagination and plenty of energy and perseverance, in addition to sound technical skills and a commitment to professional integrity and respect for the views of others.

How will I know if I have been successful?

Success may take several years. If the vision is based on evidence, it should be possible to monitor progress towards objectives. This will serve to support the vision as well as to encourage those involved with implementation that the direction of travel is correct. Objectives set at the outset might include qualitative as well as quantitative measures of success, the latter including the extent of involvement of partner organizations, amount of positive media coverage, or knowledge of the initiative among the local community.

The practicalities of acquiring leadership skills

Consider the following in your personal plans for continuing professional development:

- Understand your personality type, the way you operate, your personal and professional strengths and weaknesses. You will gain a clearer understanding of how you operate, how others see you, and how they operate or could be developed. Of the well-known tools, the Myers Briggs Type Inventory (MBTI)[8] may be helpful. Whilst the theory provides an interesting and informative read, consult a personal development consultant or your human resources department for expertise in interpretation of your personal profile.
- Make better use of the mass media. The media are very effective at conveying to the public either positive or negative health messages. Most people can benefit from media training, which is available from many sources. Your organization's press office would usually be a good

starting point. And establish a rapport with the local reporters, so that next time a public health issue is about to hit the headlines, existing trust will help counter any tendency to inflate or bias a story.
- Know and respect your partners, both within and outside your organization. Remember, it may be just as important to engage a major budget holder within your organization as to form an alliance with a chief executive of another body, or a community leader, so remember partnership working 'inside and out'.
- Be confident about your public health skills, competencies, and attitudes and your understanding of the local scene, not only its demography and epidemiology but also its key players, culture, politics, and its priorities outside health. This means acquiring and maintaining a high standard of professional practice. The public health message is more likely to be understood and respected if articulated clearly and accurately, whilst using language suited to the audience. Different modes of communication are effective with different audiences, so it is worthwhile exploring and becoming familiar with techniques not often taught formally to professionals, like story telling. And a little humility is valuable: professional arrogance has no place in the specialist practice of public health.

Further resources

Adair J (1993). *Effective leadership*. Pan Books, London.
BAMM (British Association of Medical Managers). *'Fit to Lead' programme*. Available at: http://www.bamm2go.com/CMS/index.php (accessed 16 February 2005)
Barger N, Kirby L (1995). *The challenge of change in organizations*. Davies-Black, Palo Alto, CA.
Calman K (1998). Lessons from Whitehall. *BMJ*, **317**, 1718–20.
Department of Health (1997). *The new NHS: modern, dependable*, Cm 3807. The Stationery Office, London.
Department of Health (1999). *Saving lives: our healthier nation*, Cm 4386. Department of Health, London. Available at: http://www.archive.official-documents.co.uk/document/cm43/4386/4386.htm (accessed 30 September 2005).
Grainger C, Griffiths R (1998). For debate: public health leadership—do we have it? Do we need it? *Public Health Med*, **20**, 375–6.
Griffiths S, McPherson K (1997). We need strong public health leadership. *BMJ*, **314**, 685.
Hunter D, Rayner G (2004). Guest editorial: UKPHA and WFPHA Conference plenary presentations. *Public Health*, **118**, 461–87.
Kotter J (1996). *Leading change*. Harvard Business School Press, Boston, MA.
Leadership in Public Health (journal). Mid-American Regional Public Health Leadership Institute (MARPHLI), Chicago, IL.
Leape LL, Berwick DM (2000). Safe health care: are we up to it? *BMJ*, **320**, 725–6.
Mann JM (1997). Leadership is a global issue. *Lancet*, **350** (Suppl III), 23.

Novick LF, Woltring CS, Fox DM (ed.) (1997). *Public health leaders tell their stories.* Aspen, Gaithersburg, MD.

Pencheon D, Koh YM (2000). Leadership and motivation. *BMJ,* **321** (7256), S2.

US Centre for Health Leadership and Practice. http://www.cfhl.org/ (accessed 16 February 2005).

US National Public Health Leadership Institute. http://www.phli.org/ (accessed 16 February 2005).

Wright K, Rowitz L, Merkle A *et al.* (2000). Competency development in public health leadership. *Am J Public Health,* **90**(8), 1202–7.

References

1 Acheson D (1988). *Public health in England: the report of the Committee of Inquiry into the future development of the public health function,* Cm 289. HMSO, London.

2 Wanlesss D (2004). *Securing good health for the whole population.* HM Treasury, London. Available at: http://www.hm-treasury.gov.uk/consultations_and_legislation/wanless/consult_wanless04_final.cfm (accessed 30 September 2005).

3 Department of Health (2004). *Choosing health: making healthy choices easier.* HMSO, London. Available at: http://www.dh.gov.uk/PublicationsAndStatistics/Publications/PublicationsPolicyAndGuidance/PublicationsPolicyAndGuidanceArticle/fs/en?CONTENT_ID=4094550&chk=aN5Cor (accessed 30 September 2005).

4 Calman K (1998). Lessons from Whitehall. *BMJ,* **317**, 1718–20.

5 Kotter J (1990). *A force for change.* Harvard Business School Press, Boston, MA.

6 Holland WW, Stewart S (1997). *Public health the vision and the challenge,* Rock Carling Fellowship monograph. Nuffield Trust, Leeds.

7 Goleman D (2000). Leadership that gets results. *Harvard Business Rev,* **78**, 78–90.

8 Briggs Myers I, Myers P (1980). *Gifts differing, understanding personality type.* Davies-Black, Palo Alto, CA.

7.2 Effective meetings

Edmund Jessop

Introduction

All meetings are negotiations. Whether it is a 10-minute meeting with your boss, a regular meeting with colleagues or a 20-minute presentation to a committee, you are trying to change what someone else thinks. They start the meeting with one set of views: you want to move them nearer to your point of view.

So there are two essentials for any meeting:

- YOU—know what you want to achieve from the meeting
- THEM—find out as much as you can about them.

Before the meeting

Think about your aims

Public health is about changing the way other people think. The best way to do that is face to face. Most people hate meetings, but part of the reason for this is that they see meetings as a chore, not an opportunity. Of course some, even many, meetings are tedious and unproductive. But if you don't go into a meeting knowing what *you* want out of it, you certainly won't get it.

Like any negotiation, sort out in your own mind beforehand:

- what would be the best result for you (opening position) and
- what is the minimum acceptable (your fall-back position).

For example, your opening position is probably complete acceptance of your policy; but as your fall-back, would you rather have partial acceptance or decision deferred until later? What points are you willing to compromise on? How much you are prepared to change your views?

Research before the meeting

Find out as much as you can about the other people who will be there. It is especially important to find out:

- what other people believe
- what other people want to achieve.

Of course, you need to ask these questions of yourself first.

Even if the meeting is with someone you know well, what is he or she likely to think about the issue you want to raise with them at the time?

If you are attending an unfamiliar meeting, find out about the people who will be there. Do they like the big picture or the detail? Should you be thorough or quick? Will they be impressed by government policy or dismissive of it? Sometimes quoting the opinion of a medical academy or expert society will impress, sometimes it will antagonize. Use your friends and colleagues to get the inside information on the people who will be at your meeting.

A successful negotiation is one in which you get what you want and they get what they want—at least to some extent. Listen hard and long: find out as much as you can about what they want. You can't do that if you haven't questioned thoroughly and listened carefully.

Most people are reasonable, but people want different things in life. No one deliberately seeks (except in war) to damage other people's health by *commission* but many of us do it unwittingly by *omission*. So if it seems to you that other people are not working for public heath, there must be a reason. This reason is important to them. Maybe it seems trivial, irrelevant, or outrageous to you: but it is stopping you from changing the way they think. So you need to find out what that reason is. Only then can you start to resolve the difference between you.

Sell the benefit not the proposal

Focus on how they will benefit, not what you want to do. And concentrate on benefits that are relevant to them. Of course you can only do this if you've already found out what they want.

Remember that differences exist in the mind, not in reality

To resolve a conflict of opinion, you need to address the other person's mind, not the 'objective facts'. Scientifically trained workers find it hard to understand why people don't respond to objective data. But if you lived next to a toxic waste dump, and your child developed leukemia, no amount of scientific evidence on exposure, doses, and latent periods would convince you that the waste dump was safe. The same is true in any meeting, from a discussion of where to put the coffee machine to agreeing on a multimillion pound budget.

Build the relationship

Public health work takes time. The people you are meeting today will be people you have to work with again in the future:

The relationship is more important than any one meeting.

So sometimes you need to lose gracefully and come back next time. As Dale Carnegie said 'no one ever wins an argument'. If you have an argument and 'win', the other person is left feeling bruised and battered. This is always damaging to a long-term relationship. You can't afford that kind of ill will in public health work. Your success depends on other people, so you need other people to be on your side.

Setting up your own meeting

When you set up a meeting, good administration is important. If people arrive flustered, or unprepared, or can't come at all, you won't achieve your aim.

Timing

Give people plenty of notice that you want to meet them. It is difficult to generalize but 4 weeks' notice for a half-day meeting and 6 weeks or more for an all day meeting is about right for senior people. People of national importance may need 6 months' notice or more.

Be aware of committee cycles: find out regular dates, for example budget-setting meetings. You may need to map a sequence of meetings (e.g. ethics committee before grant committee, or personnel committee before finance committee).

Venue

The venue is important, so get the best you can afford. People who are cold, sitting in uncomfortable chairs, and who have had a long, difficult journey will not be paying attention to you. Think about parking, wheel-chair access, and refreshments.

Should you invite other people to your office or go to visit them; or meet on neutral territory? For one-to-one meetings it is more polite to put yourself out by going to them; for big meetings you have to be the host. If conflict is severe, neutral territory is best.

If you are expecting conflict, don't sit people who are likely to disagree directly opposite each another. It reinforces the feeling that it's 'us' against 'them'. In public health everyone is facing a common problem: death and disease. Have everyone facing a screen or board on which the problem you have in common—an outbreak, an overspend, whatever—can be described. You can do this even in one-to-one meetings: never sit across a desk from someone.

Agenda

Send out an agenda so that everyone has the chance to prepare for the meeting. Most people *won't* prepare, but if you don't send an agenda they *can't*.

Help them to know which are the important items, perhaps by indicating on the agenda how long you expect to spend on each item. It is wise to allow 10–15 minutes for people to settle in with small or routine items before tackling the major topic.

During the meeting

Meetings are the live theatre of public health: exciting, exhilarating, and unpredictable! Actually, of course, most meetings are very boring, but if you have thought beforehand what you want out of the meeting, your time will not have been wasted completely. But remember:

Build the relationship: you'll be meeting again!

Listen: don't speak

Even if you've been invited just to give a presentation you need to listen first. So get there early to guage to mood of the meeting, and find out who is asking what.

If you're the first to speak on a topic, human nature ensures that the next two or three speakers will oppose what you've said, if only to show they can think for themselves. So bide your time and present your ideas towards the end of discussion on an item. Sometimes this will mean not revealing your own opinion in any briefing paper you have circulated before the meeting.

Words matter: use them carefully
You will not build the relationship by giving offense. If in doubt, find out beforehand from a colleague what terms are acceptable to your audience. Most people become disproportionately irritated by the use of certain words and phrases. If you know what these preferences are before meetings it can only help.

If you've achieved your objectives, stop arguing
After you've achieved your objectives, anything else you say can *only* make things worse, so shut up! Of course this means you need to be listening hard to know when you have won. But all too often people throw away victory by continuing to argue their case and alienating people who have already been won over.

Use summary statements
With more than five people in a meeting, normal conversation is impossible and special tactics are needed. If more than eight people are present, you will not get more than one chance to speak on any topic. Often a summary statement ('soundbite')—a single phrase or sentence which puts across a message or creates an image—will be more effective than a speech in helping other people to change their minds or modify their views.

Don't read or refer to papers in the meeting
If you are reading you are not listening. In the meeting, it is more important to concentrate hard on what is going on in the meeting than to read some point of detail. If someone asks a detailed query the correct response is to say, 'I'll get back to you after the meeting', and carry on with more important business of listening hard to the discussion. If you read the papers before hand (even if you only skim them), there will be much less need to read *during* the meeting.

After the meeting

- After the meeting always follow through.
- After formal meetings, send out notes of what was decided and who agreed to take what action.
- Even informal meetings are worth written follow-up to ensure no misunderstanding (and no reneging on agreements) (see Box 7.2.1).

Box 7.2.1 A 'follow-up' letter

Dear Jim

This is to confirm that you, Fred and I agreed yesterday to write a 1500-word paper together entitled 'Waiting list solutions that work' within the next 2 weeks. I will let you have the statistics by Thursday, and you will do the first draft within 5 working days. We agreed to meet next on Wednesday 30th March at 3 pm in your room

Julie.

cc Fred

Further resources

Fisher R, Ury W, Patton B (1999). *Getting to Yes. Negotiating agreement without giving in.* Random House, London.

McNamara C (1999). *Basic guide to conducting effective meetings.* Available at: http://www.mapnp.org/library/misc/mtgmgmnt.htm (accessed 28 April 2005).

7.3 Effective writing

Edmund Jessop

Introduction

The most important thing to remember when you write is that no one *has* to read what you write. Never think that because what you write is important people will read it: they won't. Consider for a moment how much material you have not read in the past 2 weeks.

If what you write is difficult to read, people will simply give up. So you must do everything in your power to make it easy for your readers. In essence, you can't force people to read: you have to tempt them.

Objectives

This chapter should help you make your writing more enjoyable to create and to read. Consequently, it should be more effective in initiating and sustaining appropriate change in others.

Writing has three stages: before, during, and after. The most important stage is before.

Before you write

Know who you are writing for

Are you writing for:

- Your boss?
- Co-workers?
- A committee?
- The general public?

This seems obvious, but it is the key to success. If you are going to tempt people to read, you must know who they are and what they like. Always keep the reader in mind. It is sometimes easier to think of some person you know rather than a whole group: if writing for old people, write for your aunt. If writing a committee paper, think of one typical member of the committee and write for him or her.

Give them what *they* want to *read*—not what *you* want to *write*

Never fall into the trap of thinking people *must* read what you write; they won't. Even if it is telling them about their own pay rise, there will always be some people who won't read it. So give them your message in the form they want it—make it easy for them.

Most people don't want scientific methodology: so don't give it to them. If you do, they'll probably just give up and move on to something easier. And if *they* have stopped reading, *you* have stopped persuading.

If your readers (e.g. a grant-giving committee) have asked you to complete a form, *complete the form*. Don't leave items out. Don't add pages of extra material. If it says do it in 12-point type, don't try to cram more in by using a smaller font. Your aim is to help them to your way of thinking; and failing to heed their instructions will not achieve that aim.

Be active in finding out what your readership wants: if writing for a committee ask to see previous committee papers. Speak to the secretary of the committee.

Give it to them on time

Hit the deadline—even if it means your paper isn't perfect: 'You want it good or you want it Thursday?' being the classic response of the newspaper reporter. A report or paper which arrives after the decision is made is worthless. So find out when decisions will be made. And never 'table' a paper, i.e. give the paper out for the first time at the meeting at which you want it discussed. No one can read it properly so the only correct course of action for a chairperson if you do this is to ignore your paper completely.

Allow time for all stages of writing, review, and distribution to hit the deadline.

And remember that the formal meeting at which, say, budgets are agreed is often a formality: all details may have been sorted out long before. So you need to check if minds will be made up *before* the formal decision.

Be aware of their constraints

The usual constraints are:
- people's attitudes, prejudices, way of life
- local regulations, law, or policy
- precedent
- available funding.

Think what each may mean for your readers. You may be able to alter constraints, but if not you must at least show awareness of them.

Think before you write

If your thoughts are woolly your writing will be woolly. Each piece of writing should have a single aim, and the whole structure of your piece should lead to this aim. Spend time thinking this out.

Write down your aim. Make it short and clear, for example
- to persuade this school to adopt a no smoking policy
- to persuade this committee to give me a research grant.

The next stage is to decide what are the individual messages that are most likely to sell your idea. This may need further thought. For a school smoking policy it could be:
1. smoking causes cancer in non-smokers or
2. smoking is a fire hazard.

Message 1 may seem more important to public health workers but message 2 was what got the ban on smoking throughout the London underground transport system. Choose the message which will achieve your aim, not the one you most want to put.

Do all your homework before you put pen to paper (or finger to keyboard)

This usually means:

- key statistics
- research literature
- law and government policy
- local precedents (what have they done before on this or similar issues?).

Make sure you can prove every assertion you make. You may not want to fill the text with scientific references, but truth matters: don't rely on memory! Readers will increasingly want to check references online, so give Internet website references (URLs) when you can. Ensure you make the date of access clear, as the internet is a very dynamic medium.

Write a framework

When you have all the facts in your head, write a framework for your piece. This needs to give:

- a major heading for each two or three pages (2000–3000 words)
- minor headings per half page (500–1000 words)
- a main point for each paragraph (100–200 words).

Start with the major headings, then fill in the minor headings, and finally the points for each paragraph. You now have a clear line of thought for your piece, be it a one-page memo or a 10,000 word report. Without a framework, your reader will find it hard to follow your line of thought and will probably give up trying.

Make a word budget

Make a word budget for each section. For example:

- introduction, 300 words
- evidence base, 500 words
- local situation, 500 words
- recommendations, 250 words.

When you are writing

Don't write anything until you have the shape of your entire piece clear in your mind and/or sketched out on paper. Cut and paste is easy with computers but it is lazy and destroys the clarity of thought both you and your readers need. A pencil and paper can encourage structure in a way that computers often do not.

Use short words

Think what you would say in conversation: 'he had a stroke' not 'he had a cerebrovascular accident'. Sometimes the short word loses precision—'heart attack' may mean acute myocardial infarct or ventricular fibrillation; but think, does this distinction matter to my readers? If not use the short word.

There is one exception to this rule: don't give offense. More on this below.

Use short sentences

Whenever you are about to use a comma don't. Put a full stop and start a new sentence.

Don't give offense

Words such as leper and cretin have technical meanings but they give offense and have been replaced by 'person with Hansen's disease' and 'person with congenital hypothyroidism'. This is an exception to the 'use short words' rule. It may look odd, but if you give offense people will stop reading and your writing will not achieve its aim (quite apart from common decency).

Don't use abbreviations

People read word groups, not individual letters or words, so in reading (unlike speaking) readers don't get slowed up by a lack of abbreviations. Abbreviations, because they are all capitals, *are* difficult to read. If you must abbreviate, spell it out in full the first time, e.g. acquired immune deficiency disease (AIDS).

Use headings and subheadings

Most people don't read: they skim. So help them to skim. Headings can be extremely useful in telling the reader something.

If there is a house style use it; readers are familiar with it and anything different is a distraction. Even if you think your style is better it isn't because you must give your readers what they are used to. If there is no house style, keep to a standard format for the font size, underlining, and so on.

Structure your piece

A good general structure for a briefing paper is as follows:

1. table of contents (if more than 10 pages long)
2. summary
3. purpose or aim
4. background
5. precedent or local/national policy
6. current issues (i.e. why now?)
7. options including implementation
8. cost
9. politics
10. recommended option and why
11. document control—authorship, reason (for info, action…) sent to whom, date, version….

You should number the paragraphs of a document—this can help readers refer to particular passages in meetings or correspondence.

Use lists

Lists are easy to skim. More than three of anything demands a list. Use bullets for up to four items, but for more than that use numbers.

Use graphics

Try to put a chart, graph, or picture in to break up the text. Newspapers do it to attract readers—so should you. It is easy enough to insert graphics into text with modern software, though considerable effort may be needed to generate a good graphic.

Electronic mail

With email the message header may be the *only* thing people read, so use the header for your message not the topic. Try this sample:

- 'Read your papers before tomorrow's meeting' versus 're: Tomorrow's meeting'
- 'Home called: no dinner tonight' versus 'Telephone message for you'
- 'Teenage pregnancy rate lowest ever' vs. 'Latest health statistics'

Remember that some people never read their email. If they want it as paper, send it as paper.

Advertising

Advertising copy is a special form of writing not used by most public health workers. However, advertising techniques can be extremely useful. Techniques include slogans, phrases, and campaign titles. Advertisers and public health practitioners have much in common. They are in the business of using data effectively to change behaviour and action—usually via a response that has an emotional or subjective element. The power of phrases to change thought and action can be profound. 'Add life to years, as well as years to life' is a good example.

Advertisers are often heard to say 'If you to have explain your policy, you're dead'.

After you write

Don't send it off

Once your paper is written, mull it over. Never send a paper out as soon as it is written: even with the most urgent deadline walk away for an hour or so. Better still leave it overnight or over a weekend. Then come back with a fresh eye and reread your work. At this point you will always see something that could have been said better!

Get some feedback

Always ask a colleague to read it for content. Specify that you want comments on content or some colleagues will merely try to improve your grammar and miss the big points. Ask them specifically to look for:

- material that just looks wrong (e.g. statistics for circumcisions that exceed the number of male births in your locality)
- important issues that have been missed (e.g. abortion clinics as well as maternity units in a study of conception).

If possible, though this is often difficult, ask someone like the intended reader to review it for clarity. Don't get defensive when people point out errors and inconsistencies. Be grateful.

Consider the distribution list carefully

Send it to your intended readership, but also think 'Who else should see this?' This is particularly important for correspondence. Do a mental check of people in your own organization and in other agencies. Other organizations won't distribute it internally to everyone you think should see it, so mail them directly. In general anyone who will be affected by what you write should see it.

Offer to meet the individual or group you have sent it to

Offering your time shows your commitment to the cause, as well as giving an opportunity to lobby, and clarify any issues.

Summary

These rules may seem daunting, but as with so much in life they become much easier with practice. Writing well can be one of easiest ways of improving your personal effectiveness. Moreover, reading well can be a good way of writing well—improving your ability and experience in both spheres is an enjoyable art form in itself.

Further resources

Easy reading

Bryson B (1987). *Troublesome words*, 2nd edn. Penguin, Harmondsworth.

Truss L (2003). *Eats, shoots and leaves*. Profile Press, London.

Tim Albert Training. Effective written communications. http://www.timalbert.co.uk/ (accessed 13 July 2004).

Reference works

Burchfield RW (ed.) (1999). *Fowler's modern English usage*, revised 3rd edn. Clarendon Press, Oxford.

Economist style guide. Profile Books, London, 1999 (see http://www.economist.com/research/StyleGuide/)

Strunk W, White EB (1979). *The elements of style*, 3rd edn. Allyn and Bacon, Boston, MA. Full text available at http://www.bartleby.com/141/ (accessed 13 July 2004).

Writing for publication in the medical literature

Albert T (1996). Publish and prosper. *BMJ*, **313**(7070), classified supplement.

Albert T (2000). *A–Z of medical writing*. BMJ Books, London.

Albert T (2000). *Winning the publications game*, 2nd edn. Radcliffe Medical Press, Oxford.

How to do graphics

Tufte E (1983). *Visual display of quantitative information*. Graphics Press, Cheshire, CT.

7.4 Working with the media

Alan Maryon-Davis

Objectives

After reading this chapter you should be able to:
- develop a strategy for working with the media, both as an individual practitioner and as a representative of your department
- review and strengthen your strategy, if you already have one in place
- undertake simple media tasks, such as writing a press release or being interviewed by a journalist, with more confidence.

This chapter addresses the basics of working with the print and broadcast media. More provocative engagement with the media is described elsewhere in this handbook (see Chapter 4.7).

Working with confidence

As health professionals we tend to be rather wary of working with the media. Like fire, publicity can be a great source of light—but can also be erratic and risky. Besides, it often takes an awful lot of matches just to get it started. Yet the media's influence and reach are invaluable to us. We need to engage large numbers of people and convey information, change attitudes, and trigger actions for health improvement. We must therefore learn how to make the most of this potential with a few basic skills and a coherent approach.

We talk of 'the media' as a single entity. In reality of course it is very plural, not only in terms of its various modalities, like print, radio, or television, but also because it comprises a diverse collection of individual journalists and programme makers, all trying to attract readers, listeners, or viewers. Fortunately for us, health issues make good copy, and media professionals need us as much as we need them. This makes our task a little easier.

Developing a media strategy

There are generic and specific elements to a media strategy.
Generic elements comprise:
- knowing and cultivating your media—print, broadcast, or web-based, understanding how they can help you in your work across the board, how they operate, who they reach, what their constraints and limitations are, and what risks are attached.

- developing media skills—learning how to frame a story, write a press release, how to use the different media in combination (media mix), how to be interviewed, how to take part in a studio discussion, and building a team of people who can do these things with confidence.
- providing media back-up—anticipating the information or materials that might be needed by your media journalists, researchers, and producers, and being prepared to provide this at short notice.

Specific elements concern the issue you are planning to promote. This involves being clear about what you're trying to achieve and asking yourself:

- What am I trying to say? (messages)
- Who am I trying to say it to? (target audience)
- How best can I get it across to them? (media mix).

To which should be added:

- What support or follow-up should I provide?
- What parallel approaches should I adopt?
- How will I know if I've succeeded?

Simple clear messages, tailored to your target group, delivered through an appropriate media mix, is the recipe for success. If you can back that up with support, for example by providing a helpline or an information leaflet, and ensure that the relevant services are primed and ready to respond to increased demand, your intervention is likely to be even more effective.

Be clear about your messages

The fewer key messages the better—a maximum of five, preferably no more than three. These should be:

- topical and newsworthy (the 'hook')
- meaningful and relevant to the target audience (the 'angle')
- informative or motivating
- in plain language and jargon-free
- accurate, valid, and backed up by reliable evidence
- agreed by your partners or managers.

Understand your target audience

Be clear who you're trying to reach and what their needs and interests are likely to be. This is crucial for framing your story and finding the right angle. If possible, meet and talk to service users themselves to gain an understanding of how they receive messages through the media—what issues they are interested in, what papers they read, radio programmes they listen to, TV programmes they watch. You need to understand how to 'grab' their interest and enthusiasm, what is the best mix of media to use, and at what level to pitch your messages.

Cultivate the media

Be familiar with their output and look for opportunities. Talk to, and if possible meet with, reporters and producers. Focus on those who usually cover health stories. Explain what you're trying to do and what you can do for them. Try to be available if they need instant public health advice or information. By and large they want to get it right.

For each issue, event, or campaign write a well-constructed press release (see below) and follow this up with a phone call to 'sell' your story to the appropriate editor—news editor, health editor, features editor, or programme editor. Be clear and succinct about the hook, angle, and messages. Mention any launch event or photo opportunity. Whenever possible, try to tie the story to something happening locally or nationally.

Make use of available help

Use your organization's press officer or communications manager. They can advise you on how to *frame* your messages and which media are best for reaching the target group (see Chapter 4.7). More importantly, if you *don't* use your organization's press officer, not only will you not be availing yourself of quality advice but your messages may be out of step with your organization's current policy. Always be clear, to the press and to others, on whose behalf you are speaking. Even if you claim you are speaking as an individual, it may be thought more newsworthy by journalists if they forget this.

Your organization's press officer will usually have a working relationship with key journalists and producers, and perhaps a budget which can be used to set up a press conference, or pay for an 'advertorial' in the local paper. If you don't have this level of support, try to link in with a partner organization that does.

Using spokespeople and case studies

People bring news stories and features to life. The audience can identify with them and they help 'sell' your story to the editors.

The spokesperson may be yourself, a colleague, or someone working for the initiative, project, or service you're promoting. You may need more than one spokesperson if there are many media slots to cover, in which case it is important to make sure they convey the same key messages. They might also benefit from the practical interview guidance below.

The case study might be a member of the general public or particular community group, or a patient, client, or other representative of the target group you're trying to reach. They too should be clear about the key messages and must have given their permission to be interviewed or featured.

In lining up your spokesperson or case study:
- brief them thoroughly on the purpose of the exercise
- agree what their particular contribution should be
- check their availability against the media slots you're trying to fill
- give them copies of any fact-sheets, campaign, or follow-up materials
- note their phone number in case of last-minute snags
- but *do not* give this to the media without permission—instead ask your spokesperson or case study either to make contact with the journalist/researcher/producer themselves or agree to be contacted by them.

Photo opportunities

Newspapers and magazines often prefer to run a 'picture-story'—a picture with a brief caption containing the essential information. This can be a good way of raising awareness of an issue, campaign, or service and can often be followed up later with more in-depth coverage. The trick is to come up with an idea that will grab the picture editor's attention—something visually interesting or amusing involving 'real' people. Using a well-known celebrity is a device that often pays off.

Staging a press event

A tried and tested approach is to set up an event such as a press briefing or campaign launch which combines a few speakers to provide different perspectives on the issue, a press pack to give the essential information (background, fact-sheet, key messages, contacts) and a photo opportunity. To carry this off successfully requires skill and experience and careful attention to organizational detail. Wherever possible, seek the assistance of any communications staff you may have access to.

Writing a press release

Unlike a paid-for advertisement or advertorial, a press release doesn't guarantee your story will be covered. News desks are buried under mountains of press releases. How can you make yours stand out?

Ten important guidelines
1. Keep it short and simple—preferably one side of A4 maximum.
2. Devise a 'catchy' headline based on the main angle of the story.
3. Use short sentences and only a few statistics.
4. The introductory paragraph should summarize the whole story in a few lines—what, why, who, where, when, and how.
5. The second paragraph fleshes out the detail—fuller background can be given in a 'notes for editors' section at the end.
6. The third paragraph can give a direct quote from the spokesperson and a plug for any action you want taken.

7. Editors are more inclined to use the story if they can lift text direct from the press release.
8. Always give a contact name with daytime and evening phone numbers.
9. Follow up with a phone call offering information booklets, photographs, or photo opportunities.
10. Consider putting on a formal press conference with a panel of speakers and convivial hospitality.

It should be possible to cut a press release at any word count and for it still to make sense.

Responding to press enquiries

If you are rung up by a journalist:

- make a note of their name and their publication or programme
- be open, fair, and honest. Don't try to bluster and pretend you know what you don't
- if they ask a question you are not sure about say you'll check it out and call them back—and make sure you do
- avoid saying 'no comment'. Explain why you can't answer that particular question—perhaps because of confidentiality or because the matter is *sub judice*.
- avoid making 'off the record' comments—they have a habit of finding their way onto the record.

Being interviewed on radio or television

Approach each programme separately via the producer or researcher. Whether you call them or they call you, you are likely to find yourself being assessed not only on the merit of your story but also on how well you put it across. If you seem to be saying the right things in the right way, you may be invited to take part.

Before committing yourself to being interviewed, try to find out:

- What is the programme's format and style?
- What sort of audience does it have?
- How are they pitching the item?—what is the topical hook?
- In what capacity are you appearing?—personal or representative?
- Is it a one-to-one interview, or a studio discussion? If so, with whom, and what's *their* angle?
- Is it live or pre-recorded?
- How long will your item be? (you need to know how to pace yourself)
- What are the likely questions?
- Will it be in the studio, or will they come to you? (you may need to obtain permission for the recording to take place).

When deciding what your messages should be:

- decide on a few key messages and get them clear in your head—you can use brief notes for radio, but not for TV. Make sure they're jargon-free

- one or two real examples may add color, but avoid using names unless you have been given permission to do so
- quote statistics very broadly: rather than '34.7%' say 'about a third' or 'about one in three'
- get your points across *early*—you never quite know when the item will be over
- a light touch of humor *may* help, but only if appropriate. If in doubt, don't
- make sure that any resource you're promoting, such as a leaflet or a service, is in plentiful supply and someone is primed to provide it.

Radio interviews or phone-ins

Radio is a cosy, intimate medium so just talk naturally with the interviewer. Remember that the listeners are usually doing something else at the same time, so be upbeat, friendly, and plain speaking.

If you find yourself taking part in a phone-in, here are a few more points to bear in mind:

- agree the ground you want to cover with the anchor-person so that callers are kept to the subject
- write each caller's name down so that you can personalize your answers
- talk directly to the caller as if you were giving one-to-one advice
- don't ramble on too long with each call, keep moving on to the next.

Television interviews

Dress simply and plainly. No glinting jewellery or jarring patterns. Avoid white, bright red, green or blue, which can 'flare' on the screen. Go for gentle, muted colors instead.

When you are in front of the camera:

- sit up—don't slouch. Look alert and engaging
- if your mouth is dry have a sip from the water on the table
- maintain eye contact with the interviewer, otherwise you'll look shifty
- don't fidget.

Measuring success

Individual feedback

At the individual level you can guage how well you did in a radio or TV appearance by asking a few people to listen to or watch the programme and give you some honest feedback. This will be more useful if they are fairly representative of the target audience you are trying to reach. If possible, record the programme so that you can learn how to do better next time.

Media coverage

A broader assessment of the effectiveness of a press release or campaign can be obtained by auditing the coverage achieved, for example the number and reach of newspapers carrying the story or slots gained on radio and TV.

Public response

Ultimately, the key measure is the practical response achieved in terms of take-up of whatever support materials, service, or behaviour change you are trying to promote. Requests for support materials or an increase in service use are usually easy to count and can often be directly attributed to the media coverage, but behaviour change is likely to be much more difficult to assess or attribute.

Media training

As with most things, you learn best by doing. But you can help to avoid the pitfalls by having media training. A number of educational bodies and commercial organizations offer courses to develop basic media skills. Check to see if your organization can arrange this for you and your colleagues.

Further resources

Albert T (2000). *A–Z of medical writing*. BMJ Books, London. (A practical guide to communicating medical and health messages to various audiences in a clear and engaging way.)

BBC Training and Development website http://www.bbctraining.com/index.asp (This excellent website leads to a feast of online courses covering a wide range of media skills including radio, television, journalism, and web authoring. Accessed on 15 April 2005.)

Chapman S, Lupton D (1994). *The fight for public health: principles and practice of media advocacy*. BMJ Books, London.

Easton G (2004). Working in the media 3: Getting your message across. *StudentBMJ*, **12**, 265–308. (A basic guide to the nuts and bolts of writing and broadcasting for a general audience. Also available at www.studentbmj.com/issues/04/07/careers/284.php (accessed 15 April 2005)).

Gabbay J, Porter J (ed.) (1995). *Communication skills*. Faculty of Public Health Medicine, London.

7.5 Communicating risk

Nick Steel and Charles Guest

Learn what people already believe, tailor the communication to this knowledge and to the decisions people face and then subject the resulting message to careful evaluation.

Morgan[1]

Objective

By reading this chapter you will be able to use an understanding of risk perception to communicate about risk more effectively.

Why is this an important public health issue?

Policy makers, scientists, clinicians, and the public do not always share a common understanding of risks to public health in many areas. Examples are the safety of food or medicines, control of infectious diseases, risks from pollutants or natural hazards, or the dangers of a poor diet. Public perceptions of the risks can be very different from 'expert' perceptions. However, there are some predictable patterns. Risk communication is relevant to all staff dealing with potential public health risks. There is an increasing moral and legal requirement for the public sector and private industry to inform populations about the health hazards to which they might be exposed.

Definitions

Risk

Risk is the probability that a particular adverse event occurs during a stated period of time, or results from a particular challenge.[2] It can never be reduced to zero.

Absolute risk is the probability of an event in a population, as contrasted with *relative risk*, which is the ratio of the risk of an event among the exposed to the risk among the unexposed.

Attributable risk is the rate of an event in exposed individuals that can be attributed to the exposure. Some people find the number needed to harm (NNH) more comprehensible than the attributable risk. The NNH is the number of people exposed that would result in one *additional* person being harmed over and above the background risk in the general population.

Risk assessment

Risk assessment is the qualitative and quantitative assessment of the likelihood of adverse effects that may result from exposure to specified health hazards (or from the absence of beneficial influences). It has two components, risk estimation and risk evaluation.

Risk estimation relies on scientific activity and judgement. Statistics about past harmful events can be used to predict both the size and the likelihood of future harmful events, including estimates of uncertainty. It involves identifying the health problem and the hazard responsible, and quantifying exposure in a specified population.

Risk evaluation relies on social and political judgement. It is the process of determining the importance of the identified hazards and estimated risks from the point of view of those individuals or communities who face the risk. It includes the study of risk perception and the trade off between perceived risks and benefits. The term 'outrage' has been used to describe the things that the public are worried about that experts traditionally ignore.[3]

Risk communication

Risk communication is the way in which information about risk is communicated to various audiences. It is a two-way process that needs to be considered at all stages of risk management (Figure 7.5.1).

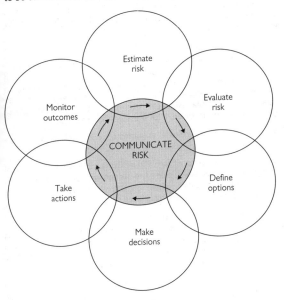

Figure 7.5.1 The risk management cycle[4]

Tasks for effective risk communication

Identify and involve relevant stakeholders

The first step is to identify all those within the organization who will be involved, in order to:
- agree a line to take to avoid sending contradictory messages
- identify who will lead the communication process
- involve public affairs or a press office if available
- consider legal advice
- consider the timescale.

Involving external stakeholders early will improve trust and generate useful information. Accept and involve the public, media, professional groups, experts, special interest groups, the local community, patients, politicians, manufacturers, environmentalists, and health officials as partners in risk communication.

Clarify objectives

Who are you trying to communicate with? Do you want to warn, reassure, or inform? You are unlikely to resolve all conflict over a controversial issue, but may clarify disagreements, minimize conflict, and improve decision-making. Extra care is needed when you wish to both reassure (the risk is tolerable) and at the same time to warn (but if, in the unlikely event that the situation changes, the following emergency action will be necessary). If behaviour change is desired, consider the wider influences on behaviour.

Anticipate potential pitfalls

Check the source of your information. Is it consistent with other knowledge? Is it peer reviewed? Expert overconfidence is a common cause of failure in risk communication. It can be countered by explicitly seeking to uncover uncertainties, and by seeking different views to expose assumptions about your scientific evidence. Listen to the language and signs of concern of all persons involved. Pilot messages before release:

> One should no more release an untested communication than an untested product.[5]

> Resist the temptation to offer bland reassurance where there is real uncertainty. If the news is bad, share the burden with other stakeholders. Distinguish between scientific knowledge and value judgement, and recognize that emotion is an appropriate force for policy change.

Consider the target audience's risk perceptions

Analyze the different perspectives of, for example, politicians, the media, and scientists. What relative weights should be given to the results from different domains, such as the health and environment sectors? Produce written materials and other information sources if needed.

Monitor and review each communication routinely

Keep records of decisions taken and the resulting outcomes, and identify learning points.

What are the competencies needed to achieve these tasks?

Effective risk communication requires:
- commitment to openness and acceptance of the need to share uncertainty
- familiarity with the language of risk
- understanding of risk perception
- recognition of the benefit of continual learning from experience.

Commitment to openness

Early, on-going, open, and honest interaction is a pre-requisite to effective and ethical risk communication.[6] Uncertainties should be openly addressed, if only because subsequent events may show that a risk prediction was flawed, or result in a contradictory message. These will reduce trust, which is easy to lose but hard to gain. If we do not trust the source, we will not trust the message. People find it difficult to judge between experts when they disagree.

The language of risk

Table 7.5.1 Risk scales (from Calman and Royston[7])

Risk	Risk magnitude	Unit in which one adverse event would be expected ('community risk scale')	Distance containing one 'risk stick' 1 m long ('distance analogue risk scale')	Example (based on number of deaths in Britain per year)
1 in 1	10	Person	1 m	
1 in 10	9	Family	10 m	
1 in 100	8	Street	100 m	Any cause
1 in 1000	7	Village	1 km	Any cause, age 40
1 in 10,000	6	Small town	10 km	Road accident
1 in 100,000	5	Large town	100 km	Murder
1 in 1,000,000	4	City	1000 km	Oral contraceptives
1 in 10,000,000	3	Province or country	10,000 km	Lightning
1 in 100,000,000	2	Large country	100,000 km	Measles
1 in 1,000,000,000	1	Continent	1,000,000 km	
1 in 10,000,000,000	0	World	10,000,000 km	

The range of magnitudes of risk that we face is so wide that the extremes can be hard to grasp. A logarithmic scale can span this wide range and provide a basis for describing risk. Such a scale can be anchored to the size of human communities, or use the analogy of a 1 m 'risk stick' in a certain distance (Table 7.5.1). A potential problem of using risk comparisons is that people tend to over-estimate the risk of death from dramatic causes such as lightning, and under-estimate the risk from common problems such as stroke.

Risk perception

Risk perception involves people's beliefs and feelings within their social and cultural context. A particular risk or hazard means different things to different people, and different things in different contexts. An understanding of risk perception underpins all effective risk communication.

Framing

The way information about risk is presented affects the choices that will be made. For example, both patients and doctors prefer treatment with a 90% *survival* rate to treatment with a 10% *mortality* rate, although the measures are equivalent.[8]

Absolute and relative risk

It is important to distinguish between absolute and relative risk. The anxiety generated in the UK over the doubling of the relative risk of venous thrombosis with third-generation oral contraceptives compared with second-generation ones obscured the message that the absolute risk was minimal.[9] Estimated reduction in relative risk gives a more favourable impression of the benefits of medical treatment than reduction in absolute risk.

Acceptability

It cannot be assumed that a risk is acceptable just because it is smaller than another risk that people already take. The qualitative aspect is more important than the quantitative aspect in risk perception. Risks are usually considered less acceptable if they:
- are involuntary (e.g. genetically modified food or pollution) rather than voluntary (e.g. skiing or smoking)
- arise from a novel or human-made source
- cause hidden damage, perhaps through onset of illness many years after exposure
- pose a danger to small children or pregnant women
- are poorly understood by science
- damage identifiable rather than anonymous victims
- are close—concern diminishes with distance
- threaten a form of illness arousing particular dread (e.g. death from cancer rather than a sudden heart attack).[10]

Working with the media

Journalists are constrained by the nature of their work to convey complex information about health risks simply, unambiguously, and dramatically. Public health practitioners need to acknowledge the uncertainty of many health risks.

In a fight between 'terribly dangerous' and 'perfectly safe', the winner will be 'terribly dangerous'. But 'modestly dangerous' is a contender. Activists can afford to exaggerate, but industry and government cannot. Move to the middle of the see-saw.[3]

The following are indicators of potential media interest:

- questions of blame
- secrets and 'cover-ups'
- conflict (between experts or experts versus public)
- links to sex or crime
- human interest through identifiable heroes or villains
- links with existing high-profile issues or personalities
- strong visual impact
- signal value, or suggestion that the story is a sign of further problems.[10]

Continual learning from experience

Routine and honest review of experiences and dissemination of learning points improves future risk communication.

Examples of success and failure in risk communication

Success

Singapore showed good risk communication during the outbreak of severe acute respiratory syndrome (SARS) in 2003, when the Prime Minister acknowledged that it made sense for other countries to restrict travel to Singapore until SARS was under control. In contrast, China urged people not to cancel trips to Guangdong Province, Hong Kong asserted that Hong Kong was absolutely safe and did not have an outbreak, and Toronto was slow to take action. Singapore also communicated well over the decision to close schools, which a minister explained was not on medical grounds but because teachers and doctors reported that parents were concerned about risks to their children.[11,12]

Failure

The complex saga of bovine spongiform encephalopathy (BSE) in cattle and its possible links with a new variant of the human disease Creutzfeldt–Jakob disease (vCJD) has aroused considerable public concern (Box 7.5.1).

Box 7.5.1 Communicating the BSE–CJD epidemic in the United Kingdom and Australia

United Kingdom

The Ministry of Agriculture was perceived to be secretive, and was criticised for denying the possibility of a link between BSE in cattle and nvCJD in humans. The Minister for Agriculture denied risks of human infection from BSE, but later a group of 'eminent scientists' reported that they had stopped eating British beef. Articles in the press contained estimations of wildly differing numbers of people who may have contracted nvCJD.

Australia

The government provided easy access to information via the media and a telephone information line to prevent the release of contradictory information and to acknowledge that there were risks involved, although small. Coordinated media liaison between government agencies helped to promote balanced reporting by the Australian media. It is not possible to say whether the government's media strategy would have been as effective if BSE had been discovered in Australia.

Key points

Avoid secrecy, the denial of risk, and contradictory messages. Acknowledge uncertainty promptly.

Adapted from Banwell and Guest[13]

How will you know if your communication about risk has been successful?

Success means reaching a shared understanding of risk with the relevant target audience. This can be assessed in terms of how close you have come to fully meeting your objectives about the purpose of the communication. Absence of outrage is usually the desirable outcome, and, as usual, this attracts little attention or gratitude!

Further resources

Dibb S (2003). *Winning the risk game: a three point action plan for managing risks that affect consumers*. National Consumer Council, London. Available at: http://www.ncc.org.uk/risk/risk_game.pdf (accessed 3 January 2006).

Strategy Unit (2002). *Risk: Improving government's capability to handle risk and uncertainty*, summary report. Strategy Unit, Cabinet Office, London. Available at: http://www.strategy.gov.uk/downloads/su/RISK/REPORT/downloads/ su-risk-summary.pdf (accessed 3 January 2006).

Sunstein CR (2002). *Risk and reason: safety, law, and the environment*. Cambridge University Press, Cambridge.

Zeckhauser R, Kip Viscusi W (2000). Risk within reason. In: Connolly T et al. (eds) *Judgement and decision making: an interdisciplinary reader*. Cambridge University Press, Cambridge.

The United Kingdom Parliament (2000). *House of Lords Select Committee on Science and Technology London, Third Report* [session 1999–2000 science and society]. Available at http://www.parliament.the-stationery-office.co.uk/pa/ld199900/ldselect/ldsctech/38/3801.htm (accessed 3 January 2006).

References

1 Morgan MG (1993). Risk analysis and management. *Sci Am*, July, 24–30.
2 Royal Society Study Group (1992). *Risk: analysis, perception and management*. Royal Society, London.
3 Sandman PM (1993). *Responding to community outrage: strategies for effective risk communication*. American Industrial Hygiene Association, Fairfax, VA.
4 The Presidential/Congressional Commission on Risk Assessment and Risk Management (1997). *Framework for environmental health risk management*, Final report volume 1. Washington, DC.
5 Morgan MG, Fischhoff B, Bostrom A, Lave L, Atman C (1992). Communicating risk to the public. *Environ Sci Technol*, **26**, 2048–56.
6 National Research Council (1989). *Improving risk communication*. National Academy Press, Washington, DC.
7 Calman KC, Royston GH (1997). Risk language and dialects. *BMJ*, **315**, 939–42.
8 McNeil BJ, Pauker SG, Sox HC, Tversky A (1982). On the elicitation of preferences for alternative therapies. *N Engl J Med*, **306**, 1259–62.
9 Calman KC (1996). Cancer: science and society and the communication of risk. *BMJ*, **313**, 799–802.
10 Department of Health (1997). *Communicating about risks to public health: pointers to good practice*. Department of Health, London.
11 Sandman PM, Lanard J (2003). Fear is spreading faster than SARS—and so it should! http://www.psandman.com/col/SARS-1.htm (accessed 3 January 2006).
12 Fung A (2003). SARS: how Singapore outmanaged the others. *Asia Times*, 9 April. Available at: http://www.atimes.com/atimes/china/ED09Ad03.html (accessed 3 January 2006).
13 Banwell C, Guest CS (1998). Carnivores, cannibals, consumption and unnatural boundaries: the BSE-CJD epidemic in the Australian press. In: McCalman I, Penny B, Cook M (eds) *Mad cows and modernity: cross-disciplinary reflections on the crisis of Creutzfeldt-Jakob disease*, pp. 3–36. National Academies Forum, Canberra.

'We overreact to some risks and virtually ignore others. Often too much weight is placed on risks of low probability but high salience (such as those posed by trace carcinogens or terrorist action); risks of commission rather than omission; and risks, such as those associated with frontier technologies, whose magnitude is difficult to estimate. Too little effort is placed on ameliorating voluntary risks, such as those involving automobiles and diet... We need to acknowledge that risks to life and limb are inherent in modern society—indeed in life itself—and that systematic strategies for assessing and responding to risks are overdue.'

R. Zeckhauser and W. Kip Viscusi

7.6 Consultancy in a national strategy

Charles Guest

Objectives

This chapter introduces the steps for developing a public health strategy. It should assist you to play a constructive role as a public health consultant (see definition below), working closely with government officials, policy advisers, and other stakeholders in the creation of a major strategy.

You will consider:

- the definition of a public health problem and the development of a strategy as a response to it
- the need to create and clarify objectives
- the need to collect and analyze relevant information
- the development of proposals and options, with appropriate balance between brevity and comprehensive detail
- the importance of a detailed study of options, which should include the case against, as well as for, the options favoured by the consultant
- consultation, one activity for improving a draft of the strategy.

Implementation and evaluation of the strategy are addressed only briefly.

Definitions

In this chapter, the word *consultant* is used in a general sense to indicate a provider of independent professional advice or services, on a contractual basis. An independent consultant working alongside government agencies will have a quite distinct role from that played by employees of those agencies (public servants). Also, distinguish the role played by medical specialists as salaried officers of a health service (e.g. consultants in public health medicine).

A public health strategy is an organized programme for public health activity at a local, regional, or national level. In this chapter 'strategy' comprises the development and documentation of a specific agenda in public health. 'Policy', a more general term, refers to a course of action, expedient or prudent, that may be less adequately documented than a specific public health strategy (see Part 4).

Development of a strategy should include many of the same evidence-based steps that apply to the development of guidelines. This chapter assumes some familiarity with the latter process and addresses additional steps and departures from the more circumscribed activity of developing guidelines.

Why is this an important public health activity?

Strategies represent tangible public health activities that often have large associated budgets. Most people are affected by a number of public health strategies. At some time, most practitioners will participate in the development or implementation of a public health strategy.

Methods, stages, and tasks of developing a public health strategy

Initial clarification

Whether or not to develop a major public health strategy is usually a decision taken at a high level in a government department after politicians, special interest groups, or journalists have moved an issue onto the national agenda. People in the public health field may have participated in that process, or their influence may have been slight. As the consultant, you should appreciate the circumstances that produced the requirement for a strategy, such as changes in:

- population health status
- health services
- perspectives in sectors other than health (e.g. environment or transport)
- financing
- economic and performance pressures
- alliances.

A potential for improvement in at least some of these variables may justify the development of a strategy. If you are contributing to early decisions about the possible development of a public health strategy, your advice should:

- provide structure to promote systematic thought and action about a major problem that has been poorly understood
- gather the minimum necessary information, with appropriate analysis
- indicate a range of options for public health action
- communicate results of this work to the client in a timely and understandable way.

Other stages may then follow:

Defining the scope of the public health problem

A more formal definition will usually be required, in consultation with a reference group of senior officials and stakeholders, referred to in this chapter as the steering committee. A review of the relevant epidemiology and potentially effective interventions is usually required, with reference to the current position. Public opinion survey data may be available: they should be considered early in the strategy process. (Alternatively, surveys may be planned as a research activity, noted below.)

Establishing the policy framework

This includes identification of guiding principles (including, but not restricted to, 'government policy') and appropriate key partners, and then, according to the circumstances, contributing to the:
- establishment of priorities
- definition of roles and responsibilities
- planning of research and development
- scope of intervention—tools for the strategy, e.g. guidelines, standards, regulation, legislation, grants, subsidies, tax credits
- development of a work plan for some or all of these tasks (implementation)
- planning of the evaluation (measurable achievements and other outcomes).

Consultation

You may play a role in the conduct of consultations, of possible relevance at several phases in the development of a strategy. These may serve to obtain critical information and to foster a receptive attitude among stakeholders to the development of a strategy. The methodology for consultation should be developed to include views from a wide range of individuals and organizations by such methods as focus groups, interviews, and written submissions.

Drafting the strategy

This will be then be informed by:
- views of the government (the client) and the steering committee
- results of the consultations
- review of the literature
- your own observations.

The draft strategy is then usually subject to further consultation and revision before approval at senior levels.

Managing the strategy's development

Assemble essential resources

Influence with policy makers, peers, and the public, for any activity in public health, has to be earned and cannot be granted by fiat. You will have earned at least some influence if you play a major role in the development of the strategy. If you do not also have it, ensure that your contract[1] enables you to obtain the necessary:
- legal authority
- convening power
- information
- scientific and technical expertise (e.g. for community health assessments, epidemiology, health education campaigns, or detailed policy analysis (see below))
- advocacy, lobbying, and public relations skills.

The development of many strategies requires simultaneous attention to inputs and process.[2]

Inputs

Management

Good management is essential for the development of a strategy, including:

- competent leadership and senior management
- effective communication of objectives and priorities by the executive to all staff
- openness that seeks positive external linkages
- performance guidelines that adequately define success and failure, with due reference to integrity and ethical standards.

Staff

Appropriately qualified and motivated staff may need to be recruited and retained. Time must be allowed for this. Training may be relevant to the development of staff in major national policy activity, but you may not have time for this during the more constrained schedule for developing a new strategy.

Information technology

Is your equipment adequate? For example, do you have enough storage and processing power and software to perform tasks efficiently in the field?

Process assessment

The public health consultant needs to rapidly identify and use networks in government (within and between portfolios) and outside it. The views of those likely to be affected should be sought actively and carefully incorporated in the development of the strategy.

Detailed analysis should establish:

- the successes and failures of previous and related programmes
- possible consequences, intended and unintended, of options for the strategy
- the institution's capacity to implement the strategy, including the support at middle and lower levels necessary for the achievement of objectives.

Outputs

An immediate output of a strategy's development is represented by its publication. The published strategy may be accompanied by other background or technical reports.

The publication should specify:

- the problem to be addressed, with adequate analysis
- the scientific basis on which the strategy was developed
- who will do what, when.

Desirable features include:

- creative approaches to options and their implications
- coherence with other programmes and strategies
- practicality
- cogent advocacy of the preferred options.

A background report[3] could specify:

- how the need for the strategy was identified
- how the strategy was developed

- how strategy development has been funded, and the resources available for implementation
- who was responsible for development of the strategy
- who was consulted
- possible—as well as probable—outcomes of the strategy
- cost-effectiveness of solutions identified
- the time-frame for evaluation.

Dissemination and implementation require much greater attention than previously accorded to many major strategies. Approaches now include:
- summaries on the Internet and elsewhere
- mass media
- professional and consumer organizations
- incentives.

Engaging people in the importance of a strategy

The whole spectrum of public interests, government, and management must be engaged if a public health strategy is to achieve its goals. You should promote the development of goals that all health and other sectors can share.

As with any collaborative venture:
- seek the early involvement of partners
- identify reasons (additional to the public health concerns) for others, including representatives of industry or the private sector, to become actively involved
- expect and listen to a wide range of opinions about the development of the strategy
- obtain influential endorsements.

Potential pitfalls

Under-estimating complexity
Public health strategies may cross conventional governmental portfolios, or require new intergovernmental relations. Consider institutional constraints early. Avoid too large a task with too few resources.

Inadequate communication
For example, lack of awareness and understanding of the strategy among the target population or failure to legitimate the approach among professionals of all affected sectors may lead to people ignoring or undermining the new approach.

'We have the minister's full support'
Continued support from within government should not be assumed, even if the development of a public health strategy was the minister's

initiative. Choosing not to decide about possible government projects is sometimes the preferred option for politicians and their advisers. They will sometimes go to extremes to avoid association with an initiative that could fail.

The development of a strategy distorts the political process, while the real questions remain undebated

This is perhaps the worst pitfall, from the citizen's perspective. Technical issues should not be allowed to obscure political questions, while the public health consultant cannot and should not assume the responsibilities of the elected representative.

Particular problems for the independent consultant

Avoid:
- arrogance
- self-censorship (tell clients what they need to know, not what you think they want to hear)
- creating problems rather than solving them
- neglect of current clients while chasing new ones.[4]

What are the key determinants of success?

- Political support
- Committed, adequate financial resources
- Collaboration across sectors
- Community participation.

How will you know when/if you have been successful?

Development of the strategy

Desirable qualities of the process and outputs of the strategy include:
- comprehensiveness
- timeliness
- responsiveness (e.g. evidence of adequate consultation with interested parties)
- clarity
- practicality
- relevance
- fairness (e.g. recommendations are balanced and equitable, as well as objective)
- cost-effectiveness (comparative costs for various solutions should be provided).

Subsequent evaluation
- Were the objectives of the strategy met?
- Did the original objectives remain in place?
- What has actually been implemented?[5]
- Has the public health problem itself changed?
- What relevance does the strategy now have?
- What were the outcomes? Were they anticipated or not?

Your role as consultant
- Was your analysis of the problem accurate?
- If the strategy was developed according to your plans, did you predict the outcome?

Also assess your efficiency, e.g. the timeliness of preparation and real costs of your input to the strategy. The measurement of effectiveness assumes a causal link between your role as a consultant and the outcome of the strategy. This will probably remain a matter only for speculation.

Conclusion

Like any project in public health, a strategy requires:
- collaboration that may be broad, while retaining sufficient focus for effectiveness
- adaptability to local and regional needs
- careful attention to the allocation and use of resources, including government and other infrastructure.

This chapter has addressed strategy as a product, in contrast to part 5 of this book. A parting thought for all of us:

> No matter how beautiful a strategy might be, it is wise, occasionally, to see what it achieves.
>
> Attributed to Winston Churchill, 1874–1965

Further resources
Harvard Business School (2004). *Harvard business essentials. Manager's toolkit.* Harvard Business School Press, Boston, MA.

Walt G (1994). *Health policy.* Zed Books and Witwatersrand University Press, London.

Swayne LE, Ginter PM, Duncan WJ (1996). *The physician strategist.* Irwin, Chicago, IL.

References
1 Lasker RD and the Committee on Medicine and Public Health (1997). *Medicine and public health: the power of collaboration.* New York Academy of Medicine, New York.
2 Uhr J, Mackay K (ed.) (1996). *Evaluating policy advice: learning from Commonwealth experience.* Federalism Research Centre, Australian National University and Commonwealth Department of Finance, Canberra.

3 National Health and Medical Research Council (Australia) (1999). *A guide to the development, implementation and evaluation of clinical practice guidelines*. National Health and Medical Research Council (NHMRC), Canberra.
4 Nelson B, Economy P (1997). *Consulting for dummies*. IDG Publications, Foster City, CA.
5 Rist RC (1994). Influencing the policy process with qualitative research. In: Denzin NK, Lincoln YS (eds) *Handbook of qualitative research*, pp. 545–57. Sage, Thousand Oaks, CA.

7.7 Being a political activist

J. A. Muir Gray

One person is a crank, two people are a pressure group, three people are public opinion

Objectives

After reading this chapter, you should be clearer as to how action can be initiated by raising the profile of a public health issue through lobbying and direct action.

Case study

The first report of The Royal Commission on Environmental Pollution was published in the UK in 1971. It had highlighted the problems of the illicit dumping of toxic waste—known as 'fly tipping'—at sites, such as waste ground, not registered to receive it. Although the problem had first been identified in 1963, the government had not acted. Throughout 1971, the Royal Commission lobbied the government to act on this matter, because of the potential danger to water supplies and the risk to public health, but to no avail. Until one day a Midlands lorry driver called Lonnie Downes took the matter into his own hands. He had discovered that fellow drivers were being given a bonus of £20 a week to dump toxic waste (which was described as 'suds oil'). After complaining to the management, he was threatened with dismissal. Several weeks later, he was offered a promotion; Lonnie declined. Lastly, he was offered £300 to leave the firm; again Lonnie declined. Instead, he went to the local branch of the Conservation Society, which then sent a detailed report to the Secretary of State for the Environment. Despite this, the government still decided not to act.

The Conservation Society then sent its findings to the press. The story was published in the Birmingham *Sunday Mercury* on 10 January 1972. On 24 February that same year, 36 drums of sodium cyanide were found on a derelict piece of ground near Nuneaton where children were known to play. The government finally acted. A Bill was drafted and passed into law by 30 March 1972.

On this occasion, the evidence alone, even that from a scientifically respectable government report, was not enough to determine policy. Decisions taken by policy makers and managers can be made either in response to public pressure or from an ideological position in which the scientific evidence may play only a negligible part.

Making and amending laws

The process by which law is made or amended is sometimes weird and wonderful, but the public health professional can make an impact by doing one or more of the following:

- raising the public awareness of an issue
- lobbying politicians personally
- lobbying politicians through pressure groups
- becoming a politician
- breaking the law.

Political action can be very exciting and seductive, so it is wise to pause before suddenly embarking on the campaign, and reflect on the following questions.

> **Box 7.7.1 Five points to ponder before getting politically active**
>
> - could present legislation be enforced more effectively?
> - what do the public think about this problem and the proposed legislation?
> - what is the current best evidence about the need for, and benefits of, legislative change?
> - what else should I stop doing to create time for political action?
> - what will my boss and my employer think about my getting involved?

Raising the issue with the public

This is the first step. The fact that some change is required, and the reason for that change, needs to be raised within the consciousness of the electorate, either as a new idea or as an issue that is more important than they previously considered. It may be sufficient to say something must be done but it is more effective to describe what should be done.

Issues can be raised by press releases and other means of getting coverage in the media (see Chapters 4.7 and 7.4). However, as in so many aspects of life, it is insufficient by itself and other steps must be taken to change the law.

Lobbying politicians personally

A lobby is an open space in a house of legislature, open in architecture and open in style, for politicians and the public to meet. Lobbying is the process of influencing the members of a legislature and it is the right of every citizen to influence their representative. Lobbying is an art, not a science, and there is no evidence on which to base guidelines other than experience, but it is possible to identify ways of lobbying that appear to be more effective.

Box 7.7.2 Guidelines for effective lobbying

- Focus: don't lobby politicians on everything but let them know you are willing to give information on any public health issue
- Aim at the right level—start locally and work up
- Don't rely on letters alone—make an appointment for an interview
- In an interview, listen, and leave a note of your main points
- Don't embarrass your employer—keep people informed about your political activities.

It is essential to lobby the representative of the population concerned even though they appear to be powerless or even though they are known to be opposed to the desired course of action. Even if lobbying does not change the politician's mind, it has an impact on the vehemence of their feelings and this may be very important.

Lobbying politicians through pressure groups

In the United States the word 'lobby' has come to mean the pressure group itself. For example, the gun lobby works with highly paid consultants running sophisticated campaigns to influence politicians by a wide variety of methods, usually stopping just short of corruption by money.

Corruption need not be money alone, for it is defined as 'the perversion of integrity by money or favours', and in many countries favours are used by those promoting goods or services hostile to the public health.

There have been pressure groups for health for many years but it was in the 1960s that consumer pressure groups blossomed, as attitudes changed and leaders emerged. Ralph Nader, who took on the American car industry on the issue of safety, became an icon of this activity in this period.

There are now hosts of health pressure groups. Public health professionals who wish to influence policy should ask the questions presented in Figure 7.7.1.

ASH (Action on Smoking and Health), Greenpeace, and Amnesty International are all examples of pressure groups who are powerful forces for health improvement. They usually have highly skilled and committed staff who may have some reservations concerning the public health professional who wants to get involved. Pressure group workers are usually on low pay and shorter contracts, so it is wise to approach with humility and an eagerness to learn from very effective operators.

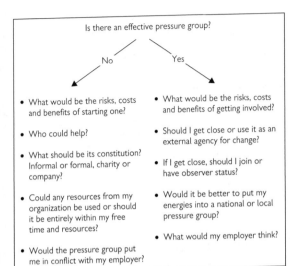

Is there an effective pressure group?

No | Yes

No
- What would be the risks, costs and benefits of starting one?
- Who could help?
- What should be its constitution? Informal or formal, charity or company?
- Could any resources from my organization be used or should it be entirely within my free time and resources?
- Would the pressure group put me in conflict with my employer?

Yes
- What would be the risks, costs and benefits of getting involved?
- Should I get close or use it as an external agency for change?
- If I get close, should I join or have observer status?
- Would it be better to put my energies into a national or local pressure group?
- What would my employer think?

Figure 7.7.1 Pressure groups

Becoming a politician

If many of the causes of ill-health can be tackled effectively by political action, it could be argued that every public health professional should become a politician; if some do, then why not all?

There is no formal study of this issue with a single conclusion, but possible reasons why not all public health practitioners are politicians are set out below:

- a politician has to sign up to a broad range of party policies, some of which require the individual to compromise
- policies are often based on ideology not evidence, because politics is based on values: the person who likes evidence-based decision-making may find this unsatisfactory
- politicians in power have power; those who are not may have less power than the public health professional managing a budget
- the politician has to cover many issues other than those which directly affect health; the public health professional can focus on health issues.

Even the public health professionals who become successful politicians may find that they are steered away from health jobs for fear they will fail to do what politicians are there to do: bring values to decision making and challenge the professionals. The politician's role has been most eloquently described by Enoch Powell in his book *A new look at medicine and politics*, in which he argued not only that doctors were not necessarily better Ministers of Health than generalists (and could be less effective) but also that any politician in a post for more than 2 years started using the jargon of their officials and had lost the edge they contributed to a department before they became institutionalized.

Breaking the law

Most public health professionals break the law frequently, but usually in a way that endangers the public health rather than protecting it. Speeding is one of the most common offences and has a significant effect on mortality. However, the type of law-breaking that might protect the public health—an environmental protest that triggers police action, for example—is less commonly committed by public health professionals, particularly if they are employed, directly or indirectly, by a government. Law-breaking may be necessary to improve the public health, but law-making and enforcement has had an even greater impact and the skills of the public health professional are best used in this activity.

Personal survival amongst organizational change

Structural change in government and health-care organizations is frequent. In times of structural change in an organization, the job of the orthopaedic surgeon is relatively secure. The public health practitioner, however, is more exposed, often because of our inability to describe what we do quickly and clearly and concisely.

The following experience-based survival skills tips I pass on, gleaned from those people who have survived a series of organizational changes:

- never try to guess the future; always do the job you are currently paid to do to the best of your ability
- never put your faith in institutions, only in individuals
- make sure you can describe public health and your own contribution to the service in one minute if someone asks you to do so
- keep fit, constantly attend training courses, and keep a good record of the training and the professional development that you have done, and plan to do.

Further resources

Machiavelli N (1998). *The Prince*. Penguin, Harmondsworth.

References

1. Powell JE (1976). *Medicine and politics; 1975 and after*. Pitman Medical, London. (The best guide to how to work with full-time politicians and senior civil servants.)

7.8 Improving professional practice

Caron Grainger

Overview

Many aspects of daily work provide opportunities for improving practice, most of which will come under the broad heading of governance, including:

- appraisal, assessment, and continuing professional development (CPD)
- audit
- complaints management and risk management.

This chapter focuses on the process loosely termed 'performance review' (including appraisal and assessment) and CPD, enabling you to:

- understand the role of performance review in improving performance
- understand the principles of setting, and recording, a personal development plan (PDP)
- understand the principles of mentorship.

Why is this an important public health area?

Public health practitioners work in a rapidly changing environment. Practitioners must be able to constantly update skills, recognize opportunities for development in their professional portfolios, and know how to access training and development to meet these needs. This area of practice is likely to become more important, particularly for public health doctors, as professional regulation continues to be tightened up, and demonstration of both competence to practice and of continuing professional development is required.

Definitions

Performance review is a formal process, usually between employee and their line manager, of assessing performance against agreed objectives, identifying training and development needs, and setting objectives for the next work period. It encompasses elements of both:

- *Appraisal*: a non-threatening two-way dialog exploring and agreeing objectives to be attained, or progress in attaining agreed objectives, and the individual development needs of the appraisee, enabling them to maximize their experience.
- *Assessment*: a formal one-way process, assessing performance against pre-set competencies, standards, or objectives.

A *personal development plan* (PDP) is a method of identifying gaps in professional knowledge, skills, or attributes and planning how to address these deficits, often performed with another professional, e.g. boss, mentor, colleague. The aim should be to identify training needs for individual development and to support the individual in the role they play in meeting the organization's requirements. It may also be known as a personal learning plan.

A *learning need* is the gap between your current and your desired or optimal level of competence required to undertake a task.

Continuing professional development (CPD) is a purposeful, systematic activity by individuals, teams, and organizations to maintain and expand their knowledge, skills and attributes required to fulfil their potential to:

- work towards improving the health of the population
- meet the needs of patients and health-care priorities of the population served.

The process of performance review

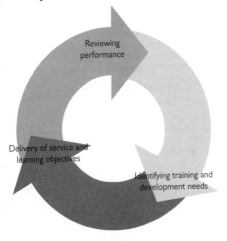

Figure 7.8.1 The process of performance review

Any system of performance review (Figure 7.8.1) should be focused on motivating staff through unbiased, objective feedback in *both* directions between manager and staff member. Successful performance review is a cyclical activity, which takes a joint problem-solving approach, reviewing personal, career, and organizational goals through:[1]

- assessing performance against agreed objectives and standards of competence

- a two-way appraisal reviewing and reflecting upon personal, educational, and job-related achievements and training/development needs
- recognition of the contribution of an individual towards organizational goals, including the collaborative setting of standards for future work in the context of the local business plan.

All organizations have differing systems for performance review, often very simplistic. Work with your system but adapt it to meet your needs. It can be particularly helpful to reflect on the following types of questions before your appraisal:

- How good a public health practitioner am I?
- How well do I perform? (How do I know this? How do I compare? If you want develop a portfolio approach to your appraisal, look at Form 3 of elements of doctors' appraisal below)
- How up to date am I?
- How well do I work in a team?
- What resources and support do I need?
- How well am I meeting my service objectives?
- What are my development needs?

It is important to recognize that good performance review includes consideration of the wider development needs of an individual beyond the immediate job, for example developing them for a new job, or within their wider professional activities. Similarly, there must be recognition that duties and responsibilities, and the environment in which we work, and therefore learning needs, change over time. These elements should all be considered as parts of performance review.

The process of developing PDPs

Personal development plans (PDPs) should provide the blueprint for continuing professional development. Developing a PDP requires:

- identifying learning needs—often as part of performance review
- designing learning experiences and locating resources for learning
- evaluating the outcome of learning
- recording learning objectives.

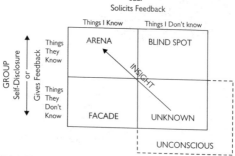

Figure 7.8.2 The Johari Window

This process requires critical awareness, an appreciation of the context in which knowledge and skills will be applied, an understanding of a practitioner's personal learning style, and reflection. Many individuals find it helpful to review their learning needs, and identify means of meeting them, with another practitioner, e.g. boss or mentor, who provides an external, balanced view of both strengths and weaknesses.

Identifying learning needs

These are often carried out in three parts:
- A self-assessment of learning needs, reviewing your development needs in four main areas:
  - to fulfil the duties of your current role
  - to meet the requirements of a change in duties or role, e.g. a new job
  - general keeping up to date
  - specialist interest or personal development needs.
- Reviewing your self-identified development needs with another practitioner or mentor. The Johari window[2] (Table 7.8.1) can help with this process, encouraging you and your mentor to look at your skills and competencies. Through disclosure and feedback, and subsequent development, the unknown area is reduced and the arena (known to self and other) increased.
- Prioritizing learning needs, by considering:
  - corporate versus departmental versus personal work objectives
  - how big the learning need is
  - how urgent the need to close this gap is
  - whether resources are available
  - the commitment of the individual/department/organization to meeting the need.

Designing learning experiences and locating resources for learning

To identify the most appropriate learning experience, consider your learning style (see list below) and the settings in which learning can take place. Kolb identifies four main learning styles:[3]
- *Activist*: learns best from 'having a go', often in adverse or pressured situations
- *Pragmatist*: learns best from practical/real life situations, often following a role model. Takes a 'common sense' approach
- *Reflector*: learns best from assimilating information prior to action, and having the opportunity to review what they observe without the pressure to perform
- *Theorist*: needs to understand the theoretical framework before participating in complex situations. Requires structured situations, logical frameworks, and clear purpose.

Matching the learning setting to the learning preference of an individual will enable them to process new information as quickly as possible. There are four main settings for learning (Table 7.8.2), planned and unplanned, on the job (internal CPD) and off the job (external CPD). Within these four main categories are a variety of learning opportunities, e.g. didactic lectures, learning sets, one-to-one training, self-directed learning, distance learning, etc.

Table 7.8.1 Learning settings

	Planned		
External	For example, attend a 1-day course on improving chairmanship skills	For example, have someone assess your chairmanship skills at the beginning and end of a learning process	Internal
	For example, noting styles of chairmanship on a TV documentary	For example, observe chairmanship skills in others	
	Unplanned		

Evaluating the outcome of learning

As part of setting learning objectives it is important to recognize how you will evaluate the impact of your learning. Evaluation criteria can be either:

- qualitative, e.g. your perception of change, your insight as a result of learning
- quantitative, e.g. the use of an objective assessment tool, such as an examination, or external assessment of performance.

It is worth noting the difference between output, i.e. the knowledge or skill that has been acquired, and outcome, or how you're applying this knowledge and skill to greater effect. A simple way of assessing outcome is to ask whether what you have learned has resulted in change in practice.

Table 7.8.2 A template for a PDP

What development needs do I have?	Expected outcome	How will I address them?	Timescale completed?
Explain the need	How will your practice change as a result of the development activity?	Explain how you will take action, and what resources you will need?	
To improve chairmanship skills (specific)	All meetings have a clearly defined agenda, adequate time for discussion involving all parties, and clearly agreed decisions/actions which are appropriately recorded (achievable, measurable)	Observe chairmanship skills in three others. Read a book on chairing meetings. Attend a 1-day course on improving chairmanship skills. Have someone assess my chairmanship skills at the beginning and end of the 6 months' learning	6 months period (timed, realistic)

Recording learning objectives

Having identified learning needs and potential outcome indicators, it is possible to set a learning objective according to SMART criteria:

- Specific
- Measurable
- Achievable
- Realistic/Relevant
- Timed.

A template for recording your PDP is given in Table 7.8.3.

Learning portfolios[4]

These can be helpful to demonstrate learning to date (often from a mix of work based and learning from outside work that has contributed to your development) and identified learning needs. A good portfolio will comprise:

- evidence of learning
- reflection and commentary on the learning, including how learning has been applied to your everyday practice.

Your portfolio should eventually build into an inventory of your skills and achievements, together with future aspirations. Items to include in a learning portfolio are shown in Box 7.8.1. If you want a paperless version of a learning portfolio, look at The Faculty of Public Health website which includes an electronic register for recording your learning (http://www.fph.org.uk/)

Box 7.8.1 Items to include in a learning portfolio

- examination certificates, registration certificates etc.
- CV
- summary of posts to date, and learning from those posts
- appraisal forms
- objectives of current post
- (adverse) incidents and reflection upon them
- audit projects
- teaching experience
- research experience and aspirations, publications
- career intentions
- personal learning plan
- anything else that you feel is relevant, which demonstrates learning from an event.

Mentors[5]

A mentor (literally 'wise one') can be a useful source of support in identifying and planning personal development. A good mentor will help you consider your roles and responsibilities 'in the round', i.e. the balance of work and home, development needed in the current job and for future jobs, and will play a variety of roles (see Box 7.8.2). Key issues for managing a mentoring relationship include:

- Agree a mentoring contract i.e. how long the relationship will last for, how often the meetings will be held, confidentiality, boundaries.
- Give thought to who you approach as a mentor. Whilst they are not necessarily friends, they must be a trusted and respected individual you can relate to easily.
- Look for someone who can translate his or her personal experience into generic 'how to's'.
- Your learning needs will vary over time. One individual may not be able to provide all the help you need, but should be able to direct you to others as appropriate. Similarly, consider whether one individual should be used on an ongoing basis, or should be picked for particular skills to help resolve a short-term training need, or a mixture of the two.
- Mentors are usually senior to you and usually work in a different organization. Mentors may come from the same organization, although this can be sensitive, particularly if they are your boss's boss and you are seen to be going above your boss's head!

Box 7.8.2 **Roles in mentoring**

- sounding board
- joint problem solver
- ratifier
- mirror
- coach
- repository
- referee
- flaw finder
- connector and networker
- empathizer
- guide

A brief word for doctors working in the UK—appraisal and revalidation

Medical consultants in the UK are required to have an annual professional appraisal, supplementary to any organizational performance review. There is a plethora of forms which need to be completed prior to and during the appraisal process (summarized below in Table 7.8.4).[6] The most detailed information is that contained in Form 3, where you should cross-reference your day-to-day work against a series of headings, including the 10 key areas of good public health practice. In reality many of the categories are interrelated, and one piece of work will often illustrate good practice in multiple areas. I personally find that the easiest way of doing this is to set aside a couple of hours in front of

Table 7.8.3 Medical appraisal forms in the UK

Form 1	Background details
Form 2	Details of your current public health activities, including clinical practice, subspecialist skills, on-call responsibilities, teaching/academic work, management activities, research, examining, work for regional, national or international organizations etc.
Form 3	Record of reference documentation supporting the appraisal and report on development action in the past year, covering the following areas: good public health practice, as defined by the 10 key areas of good public health practice[7] maintaining good public health practice—your CPD activities, including a summary progress against your current PDP teaching and training relations with individuals and communities working with colleagues probity health management activity research (if you undertake any)
Form 4	Summary of appraisal discussion (this bit is returned to your employer) and PDP
Form 5	Personal and organizational effectiveness including the development of services, delivery of service outcomes, workload, how the organization can support you better
Form 6	Detailed confidential account of appraisal interview if required

my work computer, and identify written papers to slot into each section, and then edit it down and cross-reference as necessary. Remember that we are here to do jobs, and therefore not all sections will necessarily be relevant to all people all of the time—my appraisal folder currently has nothing against research, but lots about management. Equally, it may not be possible (or indeed necessary) to cover all areas within a year.

At the time of writing, the Chief Medical Officer for England is reviewing revalidation for doctors, to ensure that it is 'fit for purpose'.

Further resources

Two websites are useful for professional development:

The Faculty of Public Health website (http://www.fph.org.uk/) includes information about professional standards, appraisal for medical consultants, and information for CPD, including an electronic register for recording your learning.

The British Medical Association also runs a learning resource, more focused on General Practitioners and those with a clinical background. However, it does include a good many management topics, which are useful if you are working in a Primary Care Trust (http://www.bmjlearning.com/planrecord/index.jsp).

There are many resources for professional and personal development on the web. Search and you will find! However, the resource is so vast that you need to formulate your search strategy carefully, and don't forget it is all very variable in quality, so don't forget those critical appraisal skills. It is also worth searching both professional and personal development terms. Try www.google.co.uk

References

1 Standing Committee on Postgraduate Medical Education (SCOPME) (1999). *Doctors and dentists. The need for a process of review*, a working paper. SCOPME, London.
2 Luft J, Ingham H (1955). *The Johari-window: a graphic model for interpersonal relations*. University of California, Western Training Laboratory, Los Angeles, CA.
3 Kolb DA (1984). *Experiential learning: experience as the source of learning and development*. Prentice-Hall, Englewood Cliffs, NJ.
4 Brigden D (1999) Constructing a learning portfolio. Career focus articles. *BMJ Classified*, 3 July, 2–3. Available at: http://bmj.bmjjournals.com/cgi/content/full/319/7201/S2a-7201 (accessed 1 October 2005).
5 Grainger C (2002). Mentoring—supporting doctors at work and play. *BMJ Career Focus*, **324**, S203. Available at: http://careerfocus.bmjjournals.com/cgi/content/full/324/7353/S203 (accessed 1 October 2005).
6 UK Faculty of Public Health. *Guidance on NHS Appraisal for Public Health Consultants*. Available at: http://www.fph.org.uk/prof_standards/downloads/appraisal_form_public_health_consultants.pdf (accessed 30 January 2006)
7 UK Faculty of Public Health. *Good Public Health Practice – General Professional Expectations of Public Health Physicians and Specialists in Public Health*. Available at: http://www.fph.org.uk/prof_standards/downloads/appraisals/B_GPHP.pdf (accessed 30 January 2006)

Organizational development

Introduction

Give us grace to accept with serenity the things that cannot be changed,
courage to change the things which should be changed, and the wisdom
to distinguish the one from the other.

Reinhold Niehbuhr (1892–1971)

We live with too much change in too short a time. Some changes are
deliberate, planned, and purposeful, some appear random and chaotic,
and others are merely fashions. To survive requires a careful examination
of ourselves, dealt with in Part 7. Part 8 is about examination of our
surroundings: the organizations and relationships that are integral to the
role of the public health practitioner.

Many approaches are required to cope in a changing environment, to
develop public health as a constant learning activity. Being prepared
to study the process of change from perspectives that include psychology
and management need not lead to an eclectic free-for-all.

This part contains two chapters about people: working with others engaged in the public health endeavour (teams), and working with those we
purport to serve ('consumers'); and three chapters on development
techniques: project planning, business planning, and assessing good public
health action.

Assessing our effectiveness is a critical element for collaboration in
public health. Working with consumers should now be considered critical
for all of us. We are all consumers, although we now recognize that
the commercial connotations of that term can sometimes be unhelpful in
the public health endeavour.

CSG

8.1 Working in teams

Annabelle Mark and Mike Jones

Team working is important in areas such as public health because issues are often bureaucratic, political, and multidisciplinary.

Objectives

This chapter should help you to understand:
- what a team is
- how to make it work
- problems in team work and
- managing these problems.

Definition

- Teams are groups of people working together towards *common goals*
- 'The whole is greater than the sum of its parts'
- Teams provide a sense of belonging, a source of help and support, a sense of shared purpose.

Why is this an important public health issue?

No individual in public health knows all the answers, or can represent all the *issues and opinions*—so teams are more likely than individuals to be effective.

What are the defined tasks?

There are important tasks that any team member must understand if the team is going to work:
- appreciating individual roles and behaviour
- sharing the development process
- identifying problems
- improving team activity and effectiveness.

When joining a team, ask yourself what you will gain:
- I will look important = *status*
- I will feel important = *self-esteem*
- I like to mix with others = *affiliation*

- I like to have influence = *power*
- I achieve my goals more quickly with others = *goal achievement.*

Once you have assembled your team you need to think about how it works. Remember that teams thrive on variety. Teams of clever people or people with similar personalities are often *not* as effective.

Key competencies

It is necessary to recognize the different behaviours of team members and use them to the team's advantage in achieving its objectives. Three types of behaviour are important to a team: task-focused, team-maintenance, and self-orientated behaviours.

Example: self-orientated behaviour and the development of hierarchies

Hierarchies develop in any group (although genuine teams are often characterized by their lack of formal hierarchy). We can see this by observing the pattern of interruption—more interrupting often equates to desire for more influence, so for example look to see if doctors interrupt more than nurses or men interrupt more than women.

Effective team working depends on every person:

- knowing what the team is there to do
- taking full advantage of how the team can help each person to do it
- minimizing the ways in which the team may hinder any individual contributing fully
- acknowledging individual development needs.

Developing the team

Teams contain both roles and norms. *Roles* can be categorized as:

- functional roles—what I do as a doctor, nurse, accountant, or community representative (often professionally defined)
- team roles—how I like to behave and contribute, by for example leading the team or collecting information, or contributing ideas (often personally defined).

While most people know their functional role, identifying your team role is critical to success. Belbin[1] originally described eight essential team roles which should be allocated within the team:

- coordinator = chairing role
- resource investigator = external liaison
- shaper = goal setter
- implementer = translates ideas to action plans
- plant = the ideas person
- monitor evaluator = analyst of ideas and action
- team worker = develops team spirit
- completer finisher = minds details and targets.

(The Belbin Self-Perception Inventory[1] will assist in identifying these roles for each team member.)

Team members can have more than one preferred team role, but all roles must be covered, *even if the team is fewer than eight in number.*

Knowing which are the least favoured roles shows where a weakness in the team may appear—ask team members which roles they most and least wish to fulfil.

Norms are often summarized as 'the way we do things around here' and operationalize the team culture.

How do teams in public health work?

Teams in public health involve professionals and members of the community. The way each one works will vary according to the *task* and *timescale*. They are usually one of three types:
- a crisis team
- a project team
- a planning team.

Examples

A *crisis team* must move fast to achieve its task, unhelpful behaviours may be reinforced, for example failing to listen to others (see Chapter 3.1).

A *project team* will have specific goals and timescales but need help in developing ideas and a shared view, especially if members rely only on their representative or professional roles to guide them (e.g. re-engineering the emergency admissions system for a busy hospital).

A *planning team* will have more time. This is not always an advantage as individuals lose the motivation and pressure to contribute. Remember, the less time the team has to do something, the more it will focus on the task, rather than the team. To avoid poor team-working good team leadership is essential. Good leaders share mutual trust and respect with their followers—leaders are thus best chosen by the team but can change according to the task or roles required.

The context of team working is also critical to its success (see Box 8.1.1).

Potential pitfalls in teams

These include:
- poor listening
- domination by individuals or subgroups
- negative (destructive) criticism
- hidden conflicts
- divisive arguments
- absenteeism.

In addition specialists must not exclude others by their use of jargon. Agreeing on a common language is about a shared culture within the team.

Beware of stereotypes

Get each member of the team to express their attitudes to other roles like doctors or managers or the public. The group then shares this information to see how they see others and how others see them. This activity is an essential part of team building. Time spent on such activities is rarely wasted; it breaks down barriers and increases trust.

Engaging people in team building

Like individuals, teams have recognizable development paths and life-cycles, and like life, some stages of this development can be uncomfortable (see Box 8.1.1).

Box 8.1.1 Team development in extreme conditions

Developing capacity in the Ministry of Health in Afghanistan presents major challenges. The country has, over the last 25 years, suffered from a series of military incursions, seemingly uninhibited internal violent strife, unstable structures and systems, an insecure environment, extraordinary poverty, and economic weakness. Ethnic, tribal, geographic, and language differences set the scene for a population which experiences extreme health disadvantage, particularly featuring communicable diseases, maternal and child morbidity and mortality and, of course, trauma. Internal communications are poor.

Trust does not thrive under these conditions. Team development for leadership in the Ministry of Health is blocked. In particular:

- 'Forming' is undertaken, but many individuals stop in 'storming' mode, possibly because any sense of future is so weak. The concept of deferred gratification is alien to many.
- The system is beset by 'groupthink'. Historically, individuals have learned to become risk averse in terms of organization. Conformity or the groupthink effect retards efforts to reform service planning and delivery.
- Leadership has become either mechanical (with too much focus on job specification, titles, and administrative structures) or aggressive. The prevailing, practical leadership style tends to be very directive.
- The capacity to deliver resource investigator, plant, and company worker (implementer) roles is limited. Low risk roles—monitor evaluator, completer-finisher and chair (coordinator) —are more readily identified.

The Ministry of Health is confronting these challenges to team development. The concept of 'deconcentration' from the Ministry to the provinces is being tried. Deconcentration differs from decentralization or devolution, aiming to enable provincial health managers to plan and manage local services in a locally sensitive, specific, and focused way, but within the protection of the Ministry of Health. As provincial teams mature, gain confidence, and gain skills, they are expected to achieve independence from the Ministry, as they expose themselves to measured risk. Incentives to promote team work, crossing cultural, political, and professional divides, will be identified in a long-term process requiring a high degree of patience and trust.

Stages of development

The most frequently used model developed by Tuckman[2] to describe the team development process consists of these phases:

* *forming*: the testing phase—information gathering
* *storming*: infighting and demotivation—barrier recognition
* *norming*: sharing ideas and tasks—developing shared interdependence
* *performing*: achieving together—group maturity and task progress.

These stages represent a circular process which may stop, get stuck, or begin again, especially when there are changes in:

* team membership
* task
* environment
* team norms or roles.

Avoidance of any of these stages damages the development of trust and team effectiveness.

To summarize, team-building involves:

* setting shared goals
* shared understanding of each other's roles and personalities
* understanding of the team process.

Conflict, conformity, and team work

Conflict between personalities can have very negative effects *but* conflict over ideas enhances team development. Conflict therefore has both a negative and positive role. Conflict in teams usually appears as either disputes about what to do (objectives), or who should do it (boundaries).

Public health professionals find themselves in conflict with others because their concern is with the health of the community as whole, rather than specific individuals within it.

Conflict can also indicate failures of communication—don't assume everyone understands your role, even if it seems obvious. If in doubt, check by asking for feedback.

Is conformity better? (see Box 8.1.1)

In team terms, a lack of conflict can cause *groupthink*;[3] the group becomes more important than the tasks it has to perform. This can have disastrous results, because the team risks developing any or all of the following characteristics:

* a sense of invulnerability
* unquestioning belief in its own morality
* pressures to conform, suppressing opposition
* rationalization of the unacceptable to achieve consensus
* an illusion of unanimity
* self-censorship of any deviation from the group.

Some tensions are both healthy and productive, especially where teams are unreceptive to ideas that come from elsewhere.

How do you recognize poor team working?

There are 10 warning signs of poor team working[4] (this list can be used as formal exercise within a team):

1. People are often late or miss meetings.
2. Positions are entrenched by professional roles ('it's not my job')
3. Too much time is spent going over the same ground.
4. Individuals are doing complete projects in their own right.
5. Too much work is changed or has to be redone.
6. Some people seem to have their own hidden agenda.
7. People accept tasks but never get them done on time.
8. Deadlines are OK, but there are too few detailed plans.
9. Teams seem to produce long reports but are short on real output.
10. Priorities keep being changed as problems arise.

(List adapted with permission of the publisher, Kogan Page.)

Agreement with more than three of these statements suggests there may be a significant problem. Agreement with more than five indicates that you have a serious problem causing stress to team members.

Characteristics of effective teams

Effective teams know how to:

- make decisions and
- develop new ideas and ways of achieving specific objectives

. . . by using and developing all available skills and resources.

Make decisions

Decision-making in a team should include:

- presentation of the problem
- seeking information
- not accepting the first solution
- looking for alternatives
- avoidance of conflict-reducing techniques such as majority voting
- encouragement of difference and risk-taking
- establishing agreement/consensus.

Develop new ideas and ways of achieving specific objectives

Developing creativity can be essential to effective team working by, for example, 'brainstorming'. This method separates generation of ideas from critical examination, as the latter inhibits the need for spontaneity and creativity.

For *effective* brainstorming:

- a team member notes ideas on a board that everyone can see
- members contribute ideas for a fixed period, e.g. 10 minutes
- each new idea is displayed separately and clearly

- do not criticize or make any evaluations at this point
- once the time limit is up, proceed to evaluation, keeping the best for further work.

Brainstorming allows group members to participate fully in the creative process, because no critical barriers are allowed to develop. In any creative exercise, the team leader should:

- avoid competing with the team
- be a good listener
- not allow others to be put on the defensive
- keep the energy level high
- use every member
- avoid manipulating the team.

Summary

Successful teams comprise members who:

- share norms and goals
- understand their environment
- appreciate each other's different roles
- welcome innovation and new ideas
- value each other
- are exciting to work with
- constantly review and renew
- achieve their objectives.

Further resources

Deeks M (2004). Cross-cultural teamworking within the Cochrane Collaboration. Available at: www.cochrane.org/docs/crossculturalteamwork. doc (accessed 5 May 2005).

West MA, Tjosvold D, Smith KG (eds) (2005). *The essentials of teamworking: international perspectives.* Wiley, London.

References

1 Belbin RM (1996). *Management teams—why they succeed or fail*, p. 74. Butterworth Heinemann, London. Available at: http://www.belbin.com/ (accessed 5 May 2005).

2 Tuckman BC (1965). Development sequence in small groups. *Psychol Bull*, **63**(6), 384–99.

3 Janis JL (1982). *Groupthink*, 2nd edn. Houghton Mifflin, Boston, MA.

4 Davis J, Milburn P, Murphy T, Woodhouse M (1992). *Successful team building*, p.182. Kogan Page, London.

8.2 Managing projects

Gabriel Scally

Objectives

After reading this chapter you should understand the general principles of project management and what it might contribute to your effectiveness as a public health professional.

Definition

Project management is the skill of successfully balancing time, quality, and resources in order to produce a particular change or product.

Why is this an important public health skill?

There are many factors connected to modern public health practice that make the set of skills and approaches used in project management very useful.[1] The timescales of delivery of public health work, whether it be a health impact assessment or an acute service review in the health service, do not allow the luxury of a prolonged, sequential approach to undertaking tasks. Indeed the computer jargon phrase 'multitasking' can be said to apply to much of public health work. Similarly, the complexity of relationships between all those involved has grown, as partnership working across organizational boundaries is central to the achievement of public health goals.[2]

The planning skills that have been part of public health practice for many years are still important, but an emphasis on 'delivery' has accompanied the introduction of general management into health systems worldwide. The ability to see a project all the way through to successful completion is as important as the initial research and professional opinion about what needs to be done.

What is a project?

Consider projects as one-off tasks with a definite outcome or product. The task will never have been done before and there is not usually an opportunity to try again and perhaps get better each time. They therefore carry a higher than usual risk of failure; using a project management approach is an attempt to reduce those risks and achieve a successful outcome. Project management is used very frequently in the construction industry and in the world of information technology. In both these sectors timescales are short, the price of failure can be extremely high, the processes are highly complex, often involving many different participants, and, crucially, it may not be possible to have a second chance.

In public health, tasks such as the production of a complex report, the development of a health strategy, or the reorganization of a hospital or community service all lend themselves to project management.

What is involved in getting started?

Building commitment

Sometimes the decision to proceed with a project is obvious to all concerned. It may be, however, that different contributors have different perspectives on what needs to be done, or even if it needs to be done at all. It is usually impossible to get widespread commitment to a project without those whose involvement in it is essential being aware of the work or resources required of them. It is therefore necessary to try to develop a shared vision of the goals of the project. This can then be built on to construct a clear and unambiguous definition of the task. Of particular interest to participants, or their managers, will be the resources that the project will consume and the timescales predicted for the various stages. The engagement of proposed participants or supporters can be achieved by consultation on a written proposal or by means of a developmental workshop where they can be actively engaged in creating the vision and defining the goals. The importance of community involvement, and even leadership, is stressed in much of public health work, and gaining trust and respect amongst community leaders may take time.

Feasibility

The issue of feasibility is a central feature at this point. A review of the steadily growing literature on the effectiveness of interventions may provide clear evidence as to whether what is being suggested is likely to be beneficial or not. The absence of a strong evidence base does not necessarily invalidate a proposed course of action, but it may indicate that a pilot stage might be appropriate. It might also argue for the project to take the form of a research study, with implications for the design, funding, and objective of what is being proposed.

Build the team

There are many situations where an individual may work on a complex task unaided, but increasingly public health professionals work in teams. Of all the serious constraints to successfully negotiating the 'start-up' phase, the difficulty of identifying and building the team that is necessary to achieve overall success may be the most serious. Almost inevitably, high-performing individuals will have a host of tasks awaiting their attention and this may make it difficult to gain their commitment. The nature of multi-agency or cross-directorate working means that individuals may never have worked together before, and may have loyalties to their own organization or professional group which need to coped with. Team building is a particular skill which is important in any work setting but particularly so in project work (see Chapter 8.1).

What are the key components in planning the project?

If and when the go-ahead for a project is given, the process of detailed planning begins. A crucial part of the planning process is to use every opportunity to gain commitment from all those important to the success of the project. Effective communication is therefore vital. The essence of the planning phase is to break down the project into a series of tasks that can be allocated an appropriate amount of resource in terms of time or money. The allocation of time will of course depend on the nature of the project and the input, but should be quantified, whether it is in hours, days, or weeks. The sequence of these tasks is identified and detailed timescales given to each task so that they are scheduled to flow one from another. The usual way of illustrating this is using a Gantt chart; that is a bar chart, or timeline, of greater or lesser complexity. The interrelation between the subtasks determines the timing and allows the identification of milestones.

Quality control

Those most engaged in the work of the project might well be too deeply involved to be able to provide objective analysis of the quality of what is being done. This is overcome by a checking of the quality by an identified individual or group at pre-determined points along the schedule. This may be by someone who is the main 'customer' or by external advisers.

Identification of risk

Risk may take many forms, for example the policy may change from on high during the course of the project, new research may discredit an intervention, or an important contributor may leave for a new job. The important thing is to identify potential risks and what impact they might have on the project. Then, if they are deemed to be significant, an assessment can be made of what can be done to avoid the risk or lessen its potential impact if it does come about.

Approvals

It may be necessary to get further approvals before implementation commences. A major project will consume substantial resources and may well be critical to the work of several organizations, so getting high-level approval may well be a wise course.

How is the project executed?

The most important person in the course of a project is the project manager. This individual has to have the confidence of her or his seniors and be able to command a response from the individual team members when the time is right for them to make their contribution. The choice of project manager is therefore vital. The tasks during this phase include the monitoring of progress against the plan, dealing with conflicts and delays, and defining and agreeing any deviations from the plan. The project manager should be highly visible during all this activity, particularly if many organizations are involved and there may be variability in the levels of commitment.

Controlling progress in a complex project will rarely be easy, as things will inevitably go off-schedule or be seen to be more difficult than envisaged at the planning stage. The ability to think creatively to overcome problems will be an important skill for the team to exercise. Should the obstacles become insuperable, a decision-making process will need to be constructed in order to redefine the project, perhaps by making it less ambitious, or perhaps even to agree its abandonment.

How will you know if you have been successful?

If the task definition has been a precise and collectively owned one then it should be obvious when the end point has been achieved. The most rewarding part of any successful project is completing it and standing back to admire the results whilst accepting all the praise that is given. However, it is easy to lose the attention of team members as minds inevitably drift into thinking about what their next assignment is or how they will cope with the backlog of work that has built up in their absence. Getting the last little effort in order to finish the project may take a disproportionate amount of effort on behalf of the project manager, but achieving completion is important if the project is not to drag on needlessly. Similarly you should try to have a definite finishing point at which the product, whatever that might be, is handed over and accepted by those who gave it the go-ahead. Planning the party for the team is a way of drawing things to a close as well as letting off steam.

Some projects may have to be repeated in the future, even if not in exactly the same form, so it is useful to conduct a brief evaluation of how the project went. A particular public health report may have to be produced annually for example, and the next person who is assigned responsibility may be very grateful for details of what exactly went wrong during the proof-reading stage. It is also a useful contribution to staff appraisal, as they may have been working outside their usual line management structure for the duration of the project. The identification of skills developed during the course of the project may identify some that are transferable to other areas of work. The documentation of successes and failures may seem like a pointless task when the main body of work is already over, but if the organization is to get better at doing what it does, then evaluation is vital.

Further resources

Turner RJ (1993). *The handbook of project-based management*. McGraw-Hill, Maidenhead.

Project Management Institute. http://www.pmi.org (accessed 5 June 2006).

References

1 McKinlay JB and Marceau LD (2000). To boldly go . . . *Am J Public Health*, **90**, 25–32.

2 UK Department of Health (1999). *Saving lives: our healthier nation.* Cm 4386. The Stationery Office, London.

8.3 Operational and business planning

Paul Watson and Peter Wightman

What is business planning?

Any organization (including public health organizations) has corporate plans. These describe what an organization as a whole will do over a specific time period. The focus is on the greater good, balancing different priorities. Corporate plans are made at two levels:
- *Strategic* planning: this process outlines the overall direction for a service area or organization over a long timescale, usually a minimum of 5 years.
- *Business* planning is one of the two ways in which corporate plans are put into action. Business plans usually cover a single financial year and are the main process for allocating resources within an organization.

Objectives

This chapter will help you
- understand the fundamentals of business planning
- understand the steps in using business planning to commission services
- develop an effective business case.

Why is business planning important in public health?

Failure to engage in an effective manner with your organization's planning process will severely limit your ability to effect change. For example you may have spent months or even years on developing a funding bid only to see it fail by missing a bidding deadline or being unaware of a key planning meeting. Public health practitioners need to be as central to the decision-making of the organization as possible. The business planning of any organization concentrates on :
- securing agreement about the main *priorities* for an organization
- allocating its *resources* (see Chapter 1.4)
- outlining how *strategies* will be implemented (see Chapters 5.2 and 7.6).

Using the business planning process to commission services

The corporate process could be run by a purchaser with its service providers or within a provider with its budget-holders.

Step 1: clarify the strategic direction and ensure that the business planning relates to this

- What is the longer-term strategy of your organization?
- Is it realistic and credible, for example is it (likely to be) owned by constituencies (e.g. those from whom you may be commissioning services?).
- Is the way in which you plan to implement the strategic plan (through business planning) consistent with other priorities (e.g. national priorities, priorities of local partner agencies . . .?).

Step 2: identify pre-existing commitments and priorities outside your immediate control ('must dos')

The first call on any resources involves pre-existing agreements (e.g. commitments from previous years) and the 'must dos'. Must dos include:

- inevitable service pressures (e.g. a continuing rise in emergency admissions)
- national political imperatives such as the achievement of waiting time targets.

Defining 'must dos' are a key element of negotiations both between and within organizations.

Step 3: preliminary work with service providers/budget holders

There are three stages here:

- Aim to make a forecast early in the planning cycle regarding the funding that will be available (perhaps a minimum and maximum) and ensure the service providers/budget holders know these details.
- Establish if any funding is left for discretionary developments after commitments (see below).
- Invite service providers to prepare their own individual business cases (ensure these are likely to be realistic—hence the importance of providers knowing the resource limitations and avoiding wasted effort if resources are limited). You, as a commissioner of services, should provide an indication of your organization's priorities.

Step 4: prioritization of discretionary developments

- Priority-setting work takes place before and after funding is announced.
- A local, inclusive, and open process is needed.
- Aim to involve key local constituencies in the emerging plan (e.g. public watchdog organizations).
- Once funding is announced, the Board takes decision on priorities for consultation.

Step 5: consultation

It is essential to run a public consultation process if there are likely to be high-profile changes to the quantity or configuration of services available.

Step 6: implementation

Finalize service delivery agreements with the providers: financial resources, and the process of quality assessment on your part; activity levels, indicators of quality, change objectives, deliverables, on their part.

Developing a business case

When promoting a particular development you will need to prepare a *business case*. This outlines what you would like to develop and how. Remember, whatever you are proposing, you will be competing with other people with their own business cases. The focus should be on:

- planning the details of the way forward from the perspective of an individual service…
- usually within a known and agreed wider strategy and…
- presenting the case to funders.

The six steps are therefore the following.

Step 1: is there a strategy?

Ideally the business case is written in the context of an agreed strategy.

Step 2: reality check

It is important to assess if the case stands a realistic chance of success to avoid wasted effort:

- is it financially feasible? (what is likely to be the upper limit of resources available?)
- is it politically feasible?

Step 3: inclusive process

A standard structure for a business case:

- strategic context
- objectives
- costs: capital and revenue
- staffing
- timetable: what will be achieved by when
- wider impact: e.g. implications for support services of a new consultant appointment
- success criteria: enable evaluation
- source of funding: national bids, local authority, charities
- risk assessment (e.g. recruitment, sources of funding)

Appraisal of other options will be required if major investment is involved.

Step 4: prepare the case

If you forget to prepare, prepare to be forgotten!

The principles for preparing the case are:

- Define the problem to which you consider your case to be (part of) the solution. Carefully chosen data that are properly referenced, appraised, and presented can be very powerful at this stage.
- Genuinely consider the different options, particularly across professional boundaries (e.g. a health visitor versus a community development worker).
- Be inclusive: involve all interested parties. Backing from key opinion leaders is essential.
- Be clear which parts of the process are the responsibility of the funder and which are the responsibility of the provider.

Step 5: convincing decision makers

Use the *formal channels*. Ensure you meet the required deadlines in the required manner. Make specific links to the organization's strategy or identified priorities. Ideally you (or someone you know very well) should present the case directly instead of relying on others to present the case for you.

Use the *informal channels*: explain the case to key decision makers (clinical and managerial) and the key support officers who are involved with, and administer, the corporate process. Ensure clinical champions are involved early in the process, not forgetting to use *their* informal networks to present the case. Senior, direct sponsorship is highly desirable (by the Chief Executive or a Director). Avoid the over use of informal networks.

In presenting the case *your message* should be clear about what the health problem is and how the proposal addresses this.

Step 6: implementation

If the case is successful but less funding is available than desired, you may need to renegotiate priorities. If you have developed a realistic and mutually respectful relationship with the providers this need not be difficult. You will need to ensure careful management of change in implementation: never lose sight of the key objective(s) and maintain a close focus on the key success criteria.

Key determinants of success

- Genuine initiatives always cost more and take longer to implement than you think—add 50% to your initial estimates!
- Know all the deadlines—months of hard work can be wasted by missing a deadline.
- Always base your day to day activities on the formal processes—however, also use informal networks to build up a constituency for your case.

Box 8.3.1 Securing funding for diabetes services in a UK health authority responsible for commissioning health care

How were funds secured through the corporate planning process even without this problem having national priority? The successful business case included:

- *Senior sponsorship.* Two health authority directors and the trust medical director personally supported the case.
- *Inclusive development.* The strategy was developed through a process of interviews and group discussion of multidisciplinary groups and also a GP questionnaire.
- *Clear message.* Four key parts to the message: comparison showed lower levels of medical and nurse staffing; there were specific service problems illustrated by the complaints of patients and the written concerns of GPs; benchmark comparisons showed many service shortfalls; international trends for increasing incidence.
- *Pragmatism.* Shortage of public funding meant the start was delayed. However, firm commitment was gained to meet the full year effect the following year (i.e. a prior commitment). It can be easier to get people to agree to something if it can be deferred.
- *Realistic three-year investment plan* costed at an affordable level.

The lesson: there is no magic bullet to ensure that business planning is successful. However, there are many approaches and techniques that are likely to increase the chance of success. Combining approaches and techniques often helps.

Box 8.3.2 The service and financial framework in the UK NHS

Since 1991 the UK National Health Service (NHS) has been funded through a series of service agreements between purchasers and service providers. This process put hospitals and community services in competition with each other and encouraged a 'bidding up' mentality with each provider trying to secure the largest slice of purchasers' funds as possible. This often meant that both purchasers and providers overspent against available resources as the system became over-extended. Since 1998, each Health Authority has had to produce a Service and Financial Framework for its district. This includes an early, open declaration of cash limits for individual NHS organizations within the district. This helps give providers a sense of what its business plan can realistically contain and means that it is made clear that individual organizations can only increase their budget at the expense of another organization within the local NHS. This helps avoid an over-bidding culture in what is strictly a cash-limited system.

The lesson: be open, honest, and realistic, and warn colleagues that compromise may be necessary.

- It is possible to bring about change that defies the spirit of the times or existing political priorities. However, this takes much longer and needs far more work—be selective when you go against the flow!
- Always be on the look out for opportunities that can further your cause—luck is often about spotting and exploiting opportunities. Be ready and prepared to take advantage of any fortuitous changes in policy, people, or resources.
- Pay attention to shifts in the regulatory framework and political priorities; this will often be the making or breaking of your case.

Further resources

de Geus A (1997). *The living company*. Nicholas Brearley Publishing, London.

Flanagan N, Finger J (2003). Planning. In: *The management bible*. Plum Press, Toowong Queensland.

Gericke C, Kurowski C, Ranson MK, Mills A (2005). Intervention complexity—a conceptual framework to inform priority setting in health. *Bull World Health Org*, **83**, 4.

Handy C (1976). *Understanding organisations*. Penguin, London.

See also Chapters 7.2 and 7.3 in this handbook.

8.4 Involving the public

Vikki Entwistle and Bec Hanley

Objectives

After reading this chapter, you should:
- understand why it is important to involve the public in public health work
- be aware of a range of ways in which people can be involved
- be able to start planning appropriate public involvement in public health initiatives.

Definitions

We use the term 'the public' to refer broadly to members and representatives of the various groups with issues amenable to public health practice (see examples in Box 8.4.1). In the first edition of this handbook we used the term 'consumers' to cover these groups. There is no one overarching term that is acceptable to all the groups, but we have changed our terminology to reflect current trends[1] and a growing recognition that the commercial connotations of the term 'consumer' may be particularly problematic in public health contexts.

We use the term '*involvement*' to cover a range of methods that public health professionals can use to engage the public in their work. Our focus is on doing things *with* people rather than doing things *to* people.

Box 8.4.1 Examples of public health's 'publics'

- People living in a particular geographic area
- People of a particular age, gender, or sexual orientation
- People from a particular ethnic or religious group
- People who engage in particular behaviours (e.g. smokers, drivers who drink alcohol)
- People who may be exposed to an environmental health hazard
- People who have a particular health problem or risk factor
- People who use, or might use, a particular health service
- Carers and family members of people with health problems

Why is public involvement important?

There are two basic reasons for involving the public:
- to improve the quality of public health activities
- because we should, as a matter of principle, respect people's capacity for self-determination, and this generates a commitment to enable people to understand and influence matters that affect them (see Chapter 1.7).

Public involvement can improve the quality of public health activities

Professional education and training can equip public health practitioners with important knowledge and skills. They do not, however, provide all the insights that are needed to deliver public health activities in the most useful ways. Consider the questions in Box 8.4.2.

Box 8.4.2 Do you really know what it is like . . .

- to live with asthma, depression, diabetes (or other health problems or disabilities)?
- to live in poverty, in fear of violent crime?
- to be addicted to alcohol, or to try and then fail to give up smoking?
- to care for a severely disabled child, a spouse with cancer, or a parent with Alzheimer's disease?
- to be on the 'receiving end' of health services in your local area?

People who have these experiences often have insights that health-care providers do not have. They see behaviours, problems, and services from different perspectives.

Some public health projects are based on public health practitioners' assumptions about what the intended beneficiaries need, want, and will respond to. Your projects are more likely to be effective if you actively find out how the intended beneficiaries see their own needs and concerns and, where possible, work with them, using mutually acceptable approaches to achieve jointly agreed goals.

Greater awareness of peoples' views and concerns might affect:

- what you regard as a public health problem
- which public health problems you prioritize for action
- how you define and measure problems
- what interventions you think should be used to address problems
- how you judge the effectiveness of interventions.

Active involvement of members of the groups whose health you seek to benefit might also mobilize support for your goals and help ensure that any interventions you use are acceptable.

The case summaries in Boxes 8.4.3 and 8.4.4 illustrate how public involvement may contribute to public health activities.

Involvement as a matter of principle

A principled commitment to enable people to understand and influence matters that affect them requires those responsible for certain public health activities to involve relevant members of the public in their work. Such requirements are also emphasized by commitments to promote democratic participation, social equality, and the development of disadvantaged communities.

Box 8.4.3 Community involvement in the Watcombe Housing Project[2]

A family doctor raised concerns about a high call-out rate from people living in the most deprived areas covered by his practice. A local health authority manager organized a discussion about these areas with a number of local service providers and voluntary sector agencies, and a community development worker was funded to work on a 3-year health gain initiative.

The community development worker learned that residents of one housing estate were concerned about problems with damp and condensation in their homes, and the impact these were having on their health. She helped the residents conduct a survey to document the problems. The survey evidence helped to secure the formation of an interagency partnership (with resident representation) and a commitment from the local council to improve the heating, insulation, and ventilation in the homes on the estate.

The health authority and council were keen to evaluate the benefit of the housing upgrades on residents' health. They consulted with the residents, explained the rationale for using a randomized controlled trial design, and gained agreement that people would be allocated to have their homes upgraded in the first or second phase of the work according to the order that a local councillor drew addresses out of a bucket at a public meeting. A high proportion of residents participated in the trial, completing baseline and follow-up questionnaires, and participating in nurse-led health assessment interviews.

Local leaders reflected on the importance of community involvement for the success of the initiative and the evaluation. They noted that this was facilitated by the community development worker (subsequently the research assistant on the trial), who served as a trusted local advocate for the work, kept people informed, and gave them the support they needed to participate.

Box 8.4.4 A peer support project for people with learning disabilities[3]

Recognizing that health promotion campaigns were not reaching people with learning disabilities, a local group set up a programme to enable people with learning disabilities to share health promotion messages with their peers.

Two community nurses recruited 14 people with learning disabilities and trained them to teach others about healthy eating, looking after themselves, taking more exercise, and the health risks of alcohol and smoking. The training itself prompted two of the four smokers in the group to give up. Once it was complete, the group began to talk about health issues to groups of young people with learning disabilities and to staff of learning disability services. They developed a poster and short exercise video particularly for people with learning disabilities, and designed a T-shirt that helped give them an identity and feel more confident when talking to others. The group continued to practice their teaching skills, and went on to speak at several conferences.

Planning public involvement

A range of people might contribute to public health activities by various means. For any given activity some forms of involvement will be more appropriate than others, but there are no hard and fast rules about which forms of involvement are 'best'.

We suggest you think about four interlinked questions:

What do you want to achieve by involving people?

For example, you might want to:

- understand a group's views and concerns in order to ensure the appropriateness of interventions intended for their benefit
- work more closely with community members to help ensure they can access the services they most value
- ensure you are, and are seen to be, open with and accountable to the groups you aim to serve.

What constraints are you operating under?

- What time and resources can you allocate?
- How negotiable are the aims and approaches of the activity?
- Are there any regulations or policies (for example relating to confidentiality, payments) that might prevent certain forms of involvement?

Who should or could usefully be involved in shaping the activity?

- Who will be affected by the proposed activity?
- Who has insights, expertise, and opinions that might benefit your work?

In addition to the groups listed in Box 8.4.1, consider those who represent them, including leaders of local residents, ethnic, religious, or other social groups, and people who work or volunteer in organizations such as health consumer councils and patient support groups.

How might/should you engage them?

Box 8.4.5 lists some of the ways that can be used to identify the views of different groups and communities, and engage people in public health activities.

Box 8.4.5 How might you identify public views and engage with people?

- read community newsletters and reports of research exploring people's views
- consult key individuals in relevant community organizations
- hold focus group discussions
- conduct surveys
- hold open meetings
- run citizens juries or lay consensus conferences
- invite people to comment on drafts of proposals, campaign messages, information leaflets
- include people on project teams, working groups, or committees
- ask relevant groups and communities to lead or undertake projects themselves.

The approaches vary among other things in terms of:
- the extent to which they allow the public to influence agendas and activities
- the skills, time and resources that they require of public health staff and the people they involve.

Some approaches are more suitable for some groups than others. For example, experienced community representatives are usually more able to work with health professionals and health service managers around committee tables than are arbitrarily chosen individuals with experience of living in particular circumstances. Special interest groups can offer useful insights relating to particular issues, but it is not usually appropriate to expect them to provide *the* public perspective on general health matters.

What counts as good practice for involvement?

Many of the principles of good practice for involving community members in public health activities reflect the principles of good practice for any consultation exercise or multidisciplinary or multiagency effort. We suggest that the following points are particularly important:

Be willing to listen, discuss, and be influenced

If you are not prepared to take people's concerns and ideas seriously, then your efforts and their time and goodwill will be wasted. However, this does not mean that you should simply do whatever anyone you seek to involve first suggests—or that a person or group that wears a public hat and shouts loudly should always have their way. A respectful discussion in which all parties are open to being influenced by the others is likely to be more constructive.

Offer a clear invitation

When inviting people to get involved, be ready to tell them:
- about the project or activity you are asking them to contribute to
- why you have asked them to help
- what you are (and are not) expecting of them in terms of expertise, time, and effort
- what are the key constraints on what you may do or achieve
- what support you will provide to enable them to contribute effectively
- what (if anything) you hope that they (or their communities) will get out of it.

Accept that people may choose not to become involved.

Remove practical barriers to involvement

Make sure, for example, that:
- meeting places are accessible (e.g. that venues are served by public transport, that people in wheelchairs can get into and around buildings)
- communication media are appropriate (e.g. that there are facilities for people with hearing or sight impairments)
- participants' travel and childcare expenses are covered.

Take active steps to enable people to contribute
- Provide clear briefings about the aims and context of the task
- Avoid unnecessary jargon and explain necessary jargon
- Offer training and support if necessary.

Follow up!
- Thank people
- Ensure people can see that their contribution was valued
- Keep people informed about the ongoing progress and outcomes of the initiative to which they contributed.

Two possible distractors

The issue of representativeness

The claim that the people who tend to participate in public health projects as 'public' representatives are rarely typical is often raised as an objection to public involvement. This objection, however, usually misses the point. An articulate advocate might not look like the 'average' member of the group you are interested in but might well be able to contribute important insights from that group's perspectives and offer an important communication link to other members of the group.

The injunction to involve people 'at all stages'

This widely used recommendation reflects the point that the benefits of public involvement are more likely to materialize if the views of relevant people are considered at all (particularly early) stages of projects than if people are just brought in to comment on almost-completed tasks. It does not have to mean expecting members of the public to take on every task in a project.

What constitutes success in public involvement?

Public involvement can be undertaken with a variety of aims, and opinions differ about which criteria should be used to judge its success. You might ask:
- Was the process by which you involved people fair and appropriately inclusive?
- Did the people who were involved find the process acceptable?
- Did you and they feel their involvement was valuable and valued?
- Did public involvement (positively) influence what you did?
- Did it seem to make a (positive) difference to the outcome?

A recent review of patient and public involvement efforts in the UK argued that involvement should lead to change, but found that many involvement initiatives had made no tangible or significant impact.[4] It identified various possible reasons for this.

As you learn from your experiences of public involvement, share your insights with others. Many people are grappling with the practicalities (and sometimes difficulties) of involving people to benefit public health. Progress in this area will be faster if we can learn from each other.

Further resources

Chambers R, Drinkwater C, Boath E (2003). *Involving patients and the public: how to do it better.* Radcliffe Medical Press, Oxford.

Department of Health (2003). *Strengthening accountability. Involving patients and the public: practice guidance.* Stationery Office, London.

INVOLVE: Promoting public involvement in NHS, public health and social care research http://www.invo.org.uk/ (website offering information and resources relating to public involvement in public health research; accessed 15 February 2005).

Jakubowska D, Crossley P (1999). Developing skills in consulting with the public. *BMJ*, **319**, S2–3.

References

1 Hanley B, Bradburn J, Barnes M *et al.* (2004). *Involving the public in NHS, public health and social care research: briefing notes for researchers*, 2nd edn, p. ii. INVOLVE, Eastleigh.

2 Somerville M, Basham M, Foy C, *et al.* (2002). From local concern to randomised trial: the Watcombe Housing Project. *Health Expectations* **5**, 127–35.

3 Engaging Communities Learning Network and Natpact (2005). *Stories that can change your life: communities challenging health inequalities.* Department of Health, London.

4 Commission for Health Improvement. *Sharing the learning on patients and public involvement from CHI's work. Involvement to improvement.* Available at: http://www.healthcarecommission.org.uk/assetRoot/04/01/01/88/04010188.pdf (accessed 3 October 2005).

8.5 Criteria for assessing effective public health action

Chris Spencer Jones

Objective

This chapter should help you to measure your progress towards creative and sustainable public health practice. It is intended to address the absence of criteria and standards against which to audit much of the wide spectrum of public health work.[1]

Definition

'Effective public health action' is defined as the work that achieves the desired public health outcome. This must include some improvement in measurable health outcome, or a clear indication of likely possible benefit in terms of process. This handbook contains many useful and well-described tips on effective practice. Yet competent work that does not lead to health improvement or a better system of health protection may not add value.

Many of us are measured already: academics in terms of publications, civil servants in terms of policy development, and practitioners in local settings through changes in routine population measures.

The tools offered are generic, to help us to be effective in achieving health improvement. Though often well conceived they may lack a fully evidenced foundation and public health practitioners need to have a range of valid measures, making use of peer review and external assessment. For commissioners of public health, effective public health needs to have an impact on a perceived problem.

Understanding success criteria in public health will help us not just with evaluation of what we do but also help us to shift our collective efforts to where they are most beneficial. A useful question to ask ourselves and each other, when setting our agenda, is: 'If this endeavour were to be successful, how would we know?'

Deconstruct to reconstruct

Right task, right person, right time

It is your responsibility to ensure that any work you do is likely to improve health. Your relationship with the objectives of the organization is two-way. You need to *shape* the objectives in the longer term as well as *meeting* them in the shorter term (see Chapter 4.4). It is not unusual to be asked to take on ill-defined tasks that present a problem to somebody in a powerful position.

Table 8.5.1 Right task?

Consider	Essential	Desirable
Opportunity cost	The work is likely to bring health benefits	There are health benefits available that can and will be measured
Management support	The work is supported explicitly by the public health department you are associated with	The organization you work for requests a plan, agrees on the plan, and supervises the plan
Work programme	The task fits into a portfolio of work that offers job satisfaction	At completion you will meet both personal and organizational objectives
Allies	The people affected by the work expressed willingness to support the work	The people affected by the work are part of the commissioning process
Whether it can be done	There is an end-point that can be identified	The task is to change something specific—not the world!

Table 8.5.2 Right person?

Consider	Essential	Desirable
Your engagement	You were asked to become involved because you have competencies essential to progress the issue	You were consulted about the nature of the work from an early stage and are able to comment upon your contribution
Skill-mix	The work can only be done if you possess the required skills or can develop them effectively on the job	The task requires public health skills in proportion to the time you are requested to invest
Politics	Your involvement in this work strengthens your links with the people who make decisions affecting health	Your contribution is likely to be appreciated

Table 8.5.3 Right time?

Consider	Essential	Desirable
Timing	Your involvement is welcomed by key individuals	You don't have to push the door wide—somebody is holding it open for you
Timetable	Something is going to happen within an explicit timescale and this piece of work will influence events	A timetable is agreed at the start—that takes account of relevant external constraints
Timing of engagement	There is time to consider the value of your contribution	You can weigh up the benefits of involvement in the context of your own and your department's overall work programme
Product	The outcome of the work is anticipated by an audience	The product is of wide interest—perhaps it is publishable

You need to ensure that the right task is being performed (in the right way) by the right person at the right time. Use the check lists from Tables 8.5.1, 8.5.2 and 8.5.3.

The politics of effecting change is not something be avoided in public health. Part of the work of public health practitioners is to change people's understanding, attitudes, opinions, and actions in a way that improves health.

Organization for excellent execution

Table 8.5.4 Criteria for excellent execution

Steps	Essential	Desirable
Problem into tasks (see Chapter 1.2)	Definable blocks of achievable work	Every person relevant identified
Project planning (see Chapter 8.2)	A structured project plan endorsed by your department	Project plan endorsed by your organization
Engagement	Identify people who share common objectives	Share project planning with possible partners in action
Consultation	Project plan shared with key players following approval	Project plan agreed with key players in advance
Communication	Ensure everybody in your organization who acts in the same field is aware of developments	Define a network of key players and interested parties and keep them informed
Project monitoring	Regular reports on progress to your department	Supervision by trusted colleague or mentor
Time keeping	Complexity of task matches timetable	Other relevant timetables identified
Record keeping	Details of all work undertaken kept separately	Annual report on activity of individuals

Wherever they are working, the capable practitioner will work effectively in a wide diversity of environments, with a wide variety of people and organizations and always holding the public health objectives in mind, before any other objectives. This requires turning problems into tasks that are possible, that will create outcomes that are beneficial and definable (see Table 8.5.4).

Achieving positive change requires careful forethought and preparation. Whenever a piece of work seems set to last more than a few weeks or take more than a few hours it is useful to define the work in terms of a project. When we are 'consulted' a less formal approach will suffice. A project should have a project plan, and be managed accordingly (see Chapter 8.2).

Effective public health action is creative and proactive. Many of us work in a reactive environment, with pressures that bend us towards consultancy and away from defined projects. Whatever the circumstances we have to make the best of them, carrying a positive message and remaining firmly focused on our objectives.

What went wrong?

Table 8.5.5 Preventive action against pitfalls

Pitfall	Prevention
Under-estimation of complexity	Achieving change is complex. Detail the stages required to make change happen and the complexity soon emerges
Take too much on oneself	Remember: in public health the highest standard is to involve others fully, not to do well only what you can do. We will have optimal impact when we work to gain the understanding and commitment of others
Expectations too high	A clear project plan with agreed aims, objectives, and methods overcomes this if circulated to all key people. It will tell them something useful is going to happen—even if it will not do all they seek
Lack of focus	Talk over what you are trying to achieve with somebody else. If it still isn't clear then start from scratch. If it was somebody else's project then go back to them for clarity. If it still isn't clear then downgrade this work quietly, quickly
Undermining	Let facts, reason, and logic solve this one. Remain resolute!
Impossible	Look through the files and find out how many people have been involved in the recent past. If more than two other people have had a go already then assume you will do no better. Fresh soil is generally more fertile, though it may look harder to dig over!
Hurry and fudge	Difficult tasks can be done quickly, but complex tasks cannot. Differentiate and spell out complexity through a project plan. It is worth spending a couple of days to prevent taking on a complex task with inadequate time or resources
The boss mucks it up	It is his or her prerogative. Take it well and find a way of entering the event into the vocabulary of the department. It helps if you understand your boss! Do you always get it right? Use humour

Even with careful commissioning, precise and careful planning, and deployment of adequate personal skills a piece of work may be less than successful. The major pitfalls and their prevention are shown in Table 8.5.5.

All these pitfalls cause us strain and stress. They are all common and we need to have the humility to take responsibility for our contribution. When we feel stress we need to identify the source and apply a remedy. In particular, when we are away from our known competencies it is best to consider ourselves more as a trainee than as a practitioner, taking cautious steps and with a degree of supervision.

If things are not working well you need help:

- Tell somebody it's not working—but not just anybody. Tell somebody who is in a position to help.
- Start asking people about their success stories. Ask them for tips.
- Identify which criteria you are failing on, which competencies you are light on.
- Consider whether you would benefit from supervision (or different supervision!).
- Is it you? If you think everybody around you is OK then it probably isn't you, but if everybody else looks bad, well what about you?
  Consider finding a mentor or paying a professional listener to listen to your story (see also Chapter 7.8).

Formal public health audit, with other members of your department or within a looser affiliation, is helpful. Together with self-reflective learning it is the best way to increase your effectiveness.[2]

Competencies

To fulfil the criteria for successful public health action you need all the public health competencies. In particular you need to be able to:

- deconstruct and reconstruct an issue
- plan in detail
- work with others—and make them work with your agenda
- win over other people
- reflect on your own work with honesty.

Key determinants of success

What really matters is that we make ourselves useful. Ideally, indispensable. We have to take part in agendas that are shaped by and matter to the communities we serve. We must have a sense of responsibility for the work that we do; a sense not only that it matters but also a certainty that it will achieve health benefits.

Key determinants are:

- the right task at the right time
- planning and execution of plans avoiding pitfalls
- patience
- prioritization
- partnership working
- participation in the execution of one's own plans

• explicit goals
• reflection incorporated in action.

Personal effectiveness is very important, in particular leadership skills and complementary management abilities (see chapter 7.1).

How will you know when you have succeeded?

Public health outcomes are diverse. They can be 'hard', such as community action to address deprivation. They can be 'soft', such as clarifying what may need to be done to make specific improvements. They may be highly organized, such as instigation of a preventive programme. They may be *ad hoc*, such as clarifying evidence on effectiveness. They may be concerned with the wider public health agenda, such as advocacy on behalf of excluded communities. They may be concerned with the biomedical model, such as health service reviews. Table 8.5.6 summarizes the criteria of success.

It is helpful to hold regular reviews, discussing issues using an agreed, structured approach. The preparation and implementation of a public health annual report provides a good opportunity for reflection on successes and failures.

Table 8.5.6 Criteria of success

People indicators	Activity indicators
Commissioners increasingly ask for work that seeks to achieve public health goals	Information and ideas developed by you and your colleagues are adopted by other people or agencies
Partners from other agencies build public health into their work programmes	Measurable health gains are linked to your initiatives
Our colleagues and seniors feed back that we are working well, through a formal process of review	Acceptance by peer reviewed journals of reports of your work. Positive column inches in the media, successful input to radio or television

Further resources

Landrum L, Baker S (2004). Managing complex systems: performance management in public health. *J Public Health Manage Pract*, **10**, 13–18.

Wright K, Rowitz L, Merkle A *et al.* (2000). Competency development in public health leadership. *Am J Public Health*, **90**, 1202–7.

References

1 Richardson A, Jackson C, Sykes W (1992). *Audit guidelines in public health medicine: an introduction*. Nuffield Institute for Health Services Studies, University of Leeds, Leeds.

2 Jacobs R, Gabbay J (1994). *An action research report on audit in public health departments*. Faculty of Public Health Medicine of the Royal College of Physicians of the United Kingdom, London.

A chronology of public health practice

Charles Guest and Katherine Mackay

This book has sought to identify effective methods for modern public health practice, building not only on past success but also learning from failure. Some past highlights are gathered here. Any historical summary has an unavoidable arbitrariness: selection criteria for the following list cannot be precise. The items included are, or were, clearly significant for practice, rather than the possibly simpler documentation of scientific advance. Some dates are approximate: we have tried to avoid spurious precision. We hope to reduce the bias of a First World/Western perspective in the next edition; epidemiological history may also be over-represented here at present. Please send us your suggestions on the evaluation card.

?1500 BC: Old Testament (Leviticus): religious practices of the Hebrews, including cleanliness, disinfection, food and water protection, hygiene of maternity.

c.460–375 BC: Hippocrates, Greek physician (descendant of a hereditary guild of magicians), insisted on scientific methods, including clinical observation; prolific author whose *Aphorisms* and *Airs, Waters and Places* recognize the importance of climate, environment, and diet. The Hippocratic Oath still provides a widely observed ethical code.

c.430 BC: First European account of a widely fatal epidemic (in Athens). Resignation and stoicism was the contemporary response, although the role of contagion was recognized.

AD c.60: Pliny the Elder proposes, in his *Natural History*, the use of respirators to avoid dust inhalation (a hazard as ancient as the manufacture of stone tools).

Medieval: Lepers (probably including many without true leprosy) isolated from the general population, with uncertain public health effect.

900s: Hospitals established in the East.

1215: Magna Carta provides the foundations of human rights.

1347–51: The Black Death spreads across Europe, with high mortality and social disruption.

1377: Initiated by Ragusa, Italian city-states are the first to develop practical methods to reduce contagion, including quarantine, isolation of the sick, and waste disposal.

1500s: Syphilis spreads rapidly through Europe. Sexual nature of transmission recognized; control measures include the examination of prostitutes and social exclusion of sufferers. Rubbish collectors employed to clear away rubbish on the streets in a number of municipal authorities, a strategy that spreads across Europe by 1700.

1546: Fracastoro publishes his treatise *On Contagion*, clearly presenting the notion of infection as caused by minute infective agents.

1600s: Filtration of water in France in households and the army. Variolation (the induction of mild smallpox to reduce mortality, an ancient practice in Asia), spreads to Africa, Europe, the Ottoman Empire, and the Americas.

1662: John Graunt analyzes population data, publishing *Natural and Political Observations...on the Bills of Mortality*.

1691: William Petty publishes *Political Arithmetic*, including calculations of regional needs for hospitals and physicians.

1700: Ramazzini publishes the first comprehensive treatise on the health of workers.

1717: Giovanni Maria Lancisi links malaria with exposure to swamps, and particularly to mosquitoes.

1742: John Pringle claimed that disease was caused by the chemical emanations from decaying human wastes (miasma) and advocated the 'Sanitary Idea'.

1753: Naval surgeon James Lind publishes *Treatise on Scurvy*, describing citrus fruit as effective prevention, based on empirical work.

1765: Manchester forbade the practice of drowning cats and dogs and washing dirty linen in its Shute Hill water reservoir.

1775: Percival Pott describes scrotal cancer in chimney sweeps, probably the first cancer associated specifically with an occupational exposure.

1787: Association for the Abolition of the Slave Trade formed.

1796: Jenner immunises James Phipps with cowpox virus, demonstrating protection against smallpox, thus initiating vaccination.

1830s: Cholera arrives in Europe.

1839–42: First Opium War in China, ending with the treaty of Nanjing. Western domination of China's treaty ports begins.

1844: Royal Commission on Health in Towns.

1847: Semmelweiss shows that child-birth fever is preventable by medical attendants washing their hands with chloride of lime, confirming the observations of Oliver Wendell Holmes and others.

1847: Edwin Chadwick's sanitary campaign results in the English Public Health Act.

1851: First International Sanitary Conference, Paris. European countries attempt consensus on international quarantine regulations.

1854: John Snow shows that cholera spreads through contaminated drinking water, developing theories from Thomas Shapter and others.

1854: Florence Nightingale's reform of nursing practice during the Crimean War reduces the death rates of wounded soldiers.

1864: Henri Dunant founds the Red Cross; first Geneva Convention.

1870: Pasteur devises the process for killing bacteria in milk.

1882: Koch discovers the bacillus causing tuberculosis. Subsequently, Koch, Pasteur, and others identify bacterial causes of many diseases, including cholera, diphtheria, and pneumonia.

1899: London School of Tropical Medicine founded, later expanded to include 'Hygiene' in all climates. Many schools of public health established during the twentieth century.

1914: Goldberger begins studies of pellagra in Alabama, eventually showing the disease is caused by nutritional deficiency.

1918–19: Spanish influenza pandemic.

1921: Marie Stopes establishes a birth control clinic.

1928: Fleming discovered the antibacterial effect of penicillin.

1930s: Eugenic extremism of the Nazi party in Germany.

1939: Publication of the first major medical paper proposing a link between cigarette smoking and lung cancer in Germany by Dr F. H. Muller.

1940: Florey, Chain, and Heatley purify penicillin and demonstrate its clinical effect.

1940s: USA and Britain fortify foods such as margarine and flour with various vitamins and minerals, including vitamins A and D, calcium, thiamine, iron, riboflavin, and niacin.

1945: Intervention trial, fluoridation of water to reduce dental caries.

1946: 61 countries approve the constitution of the World Health Organization, becoming a branch of the United Nations in 1948.

1946: United States Public Health Service establishes the Communicable Disease Centre, later the Centres for Disease Control and Prevention.

1948: National Health Service begins in Britain. Later many other European and Commonwealth countries institute state-provided assistance for medical care. Universal Declaration of Human Rights

1949: Framingham Study—probably the best known cohort study of heart disease—begins, focusing attention on risk factors and prevention of chronic disease.

1950s: Mass spraying of DDT in many countries initially proves a dramatic success in reducing malaria rates.

1953: Watson and Crick discover the structure of DNA.

1954: Polio vaccine introduced.

1958: WHO launches the Eradication of Smallpox Program.

Mid-20th century: Spread of hepatitis associated with the reuse of syringes.

1960s: Developments in injury control, including seatbelts for motor vehicle occupants.

1961: Cholera strain *eltor* appeared in Indonesia, eventually leading to crises in Asia, Africa, and the Americas.

1962: *Silent Spring* by Rachel Carson, an early influence on public understanding of environmental degradation.

1964: US Surgeon General's report *Smoking and Health*.

1965: Bradford Hill publishes criteria for epidemiological assessment of the causes of disease, developing postulates from David Hume, John Stuart Mill, Robert Koch and others

1970s: Yaws (*Framboesia tropicana*) largely eliminated by massive treatment programs with penicillin.

1974: Lalonde Report, *A New Perspective on the Health of Canadians*, launches a worldwide effort for health promotion.

1974: WHO launches the Expanded Program of Immunisation to protect all children of the world from six diseases.

1976: Swine flu outbreak (with only one confirmed death) in the United States of America. President Ford launches a national immunization campaign, which allegedly had adverse effects on many recipients.

1977: WHO declares the worldwide eradication of smallpox—last indigenous case in Somalia. WHO resolution 'Health For all by the Year 2000'.

1978: Alma Ata declaration for health-care workers, governments, and the world community to protect and promote the health of all the people of the world through primary health care.

1983: Isolation then culture of the human immunodeficiency virus.

1986: The Ottawa Charter for Health Promotion.

1988: Californian voters pass Proposition 99 (Tobacco Tax and Health Promotion Act 1988), for a comprehensive tobacco control program. By 2004 this is credited with reducing California's smoking rates to among the lowest in the United States at 15.4% (from 22.8% in 1988).

1990s: Decline in sudden infant death syndrome, following educational campaigns about unsafe sleeping position.

1992: HIV epidemic in China caused by unsafe needle practices while taking blood donations.

1993: Foundation of the Centre Francois Xavier Bagnoud, Harvard School of Public Health, an academic centre to focus exclusively on health and human rights.

1993: Program of Universal Salt Iodization established. Cochrane Collaboration established to undertake systematic reviews of all aspects of health care.

1998: Following the Jakarta Declaration, reaffirming principles and practice of health promotion, the World Health Assembly passes its first resolution on health promotion, with strategies to: build healthy public policy, create supportive environments, strengthen community action, develop personal skills, and reorient health services.

1999: WHO launches global tobacco-free initiative.

2000: WHO announces elimination of polio from the Western Pacific Region. United Nations Millennium Goals, for improvements in health, education, environmental sustainability, and reduced poverty.

2001: Human Genome Project completed. Anthrax apparently deliberately spread through US mail system, following the attacks on the World Trade Centre, New York City, provoking global concerns about bioterrorism not seen since the Cold War.

2003: Severe Acute Respiratory Syndrome(SARS).

2005: Preparations for pandemic influenza accelerate.

Further resources

Bal D, Kizer K, Felten P, Mozar H, Niemeyer D (1990). Reducing tobacco consumption in California. Development of a state-wide anti-tobacco use campaign. *J Am Med Assoc*, **264**, 12.

Detels R, McEwen J, Beaglehole R, Tanaka H (ed.) (2004) *Oxford Textbook of Public Health*, 4th edn. Oxford University Press, New York.

Gray S, Pilkington P, Pencheon D, Jewell, T (2006). Public health in the UK: success or failure? *J R Soc Med*, **99**, 107–11.

Hetzel B (2002). Eliminating iodine deficiency disorders—the role of the International Council in global partnership. *Bull World Health Org*, **80**, 410–17.

Porter R (1997). *The greatest benefit to mankind. A medical history of humanity from antiquity to the present.* HarperCollins Publishers, London.

Rosen G (1993). *A history of public health*. Johns Hopkins University Press, New York.

Stoto M (2002). The precautionary principle and emerging biological risks: lessons from swine flu and HIV in blood products. *Public Health Rep*, **117**, 546–52. Available at: http://www.publichealthreports.org/userfiles/117_6/117546.pdf (accessed 5 October 2005).

The United Nations (2000). *UN millennium development goals*. Available at: http://www.un.org/millenniumgoals/ (accessed 5 October 2005).

The US National Library of Medicine (2002). *Smallpox, the great and terrible scourge*. Available at: http://www.nlm.nih.gov/exhibition/smallpox/sp_variolation.html (accessed 5 October 2005).

World Health Organization (2003). SARS: lessons from a new disease. In: *The World Health Report 2003*. World Health Organization, Geneva. Available at: http://www.who.int/whr/2003/chapter5/en/index.html (accessed 5 October 2005).

Golden rules of public health practice

Professor John Wilkinson and
Sir Kenneth Calman

Public health is described as being concerned with improving the health of the population, rather than treating the diseases of individual patients.[1] This chapter tries to deal with the more practical and pragmatic side of public health practice, and in it we offer 10 rules of thumb for those in public health trying to make a difference. Others will have their own 10 golden rules—these are ours!

1. Stick to the facts—evidence, numbers, etc.

Public health should be an evidence-based specialty. Good public health practice is based on hard science. It is dependent on collecting, analyzing, interpreting, and making use of good quantitative and qualitative evidence. Good public health practitioners know their territory backwards. It is surprising how little some people involved in health use evidence regularly. This might just involve a quick call to the information department for a search of the latest key journals on a particular area, or the latest routine data. The National Library for Health (http://www.library.nhs.uk/) publishes a regular summary of clinical evidence which is distributed to all doctors.[2] This is complemented by many similar electronic resources (see p. 629) to support public health practice. With increasing access to the Internet, it is no longer necessary to visit the library—it's on your desktop!

2. Work with anyone—seek out allies

Allies may come from all areas. Allies in public health can often come from the most surprising of sources. The public health agenda is very populist.

Be wary of prejudice. Public health suffered greatly at the hands of *Dr Finlay's Casebook*, a 1960s television series based on characters created by A. J.Cronin in which Dr Finlay was often involved in heroic battles against the pedantic bureaucrat Dr Snoddy, the medical officer of health for Tannochbrae. Public health is not the most glamorous of specialties. It is not brain surgery or a specialty that is very often the feature of TV soap operas. However, it has the potential to improve the quality of life of the many and so its impact can be immense. You only have to look back over the centuries at where the major improvements in health have come from (food, clean water, housing, sanitation are but a few examples). (See *A chronology of public health practice*, p. 617.) Despite this, public health is often at the butt of insults 'drain doctors', 'people that can't hack it in the clinical world'. You have to take these insults on the chin—don't rise to the bait! You need to get around—have a good pair of boots to understand your patch and meet everyone. Be helpful and show humility!

3. Always prepare

Preparation is crucial. Alwyn Smith famously said that the public health practitioners' operating theatre is the meeting room. He got much ridicule for this, but there is a much truth in it. It is no good turning up to meetings without ever having read the papers, never mind actually applying some thought to the issues under discussion. It is important to consider not only the content of any pre-circulated material, but to think what you want to achieve and how you will be best placed to do so with those present.

4. Look long term, but remember short term

Public health practitioners achieve their objectives over the longer time period. It is one of the difficulties that public health practitioners often face. Governments and leaders are reluctant to think further ahead than the normal 4- or 5-year term of parliament or their presidency. There are some exceptions to this, but you can't get away from the fact that governments (in whatever country) have the simple desire to get re-elected. Any public body, such as public health organizations will also have this timescale. Although gaining support for achieving the long-term goals in public health is possible *it is essential* to have some very readily identifiable strategies to demonstrate progress toward these goals. 'Early wins' is a term often used in this context.

5. Know the politics

Politics is everything if you are trying to achieve
Most public health practitioners in the UK work within an organization which involves hierarchies and management in a way that is not quite so familiar to clinicians (though of course this is now also changing). There is a noticeable difference when working with public health practitioners in other countries—they are continually talking about ways of influencing 'policy makers'. Public health practitioners in all the home countries of

the UK are an intimate part of the decision-making process by being members of boards. It is an immensely privileged position and should be used. This means getting to know your chief executive and what makes him or her tick, and how he or she works. The first thing to do in a new senior management post is to get to know what will hit the buttons of your boss.

Negotiation is a key part of public health. Skills acquired in negotiation training will have great use. Often you are trying to move people closer to your positions—you will need to know how to make deals, when to compromise and when not.

Read widely, it broadens the mind and you never know when it is going to come in handy!

Don't worry too much about structures—there will be another one along in a minute

Within the past 20 years, it is possible to count around 20 structural changes to the NHS in the UK. The pace of change is becoming faster by the year. On average structural change occurs within the NHS every 3 years. Some organizations have been known to be abolished before they have come into existence. Of those that made it into the world some have not lasted a year, such as the four DHSCs (Departments of Health and Social Care) created in 2002 in England. However, most people working in public health are relatively fixed in geography and will not move. It is surprising how robust individuals are to such changes and how individuals regularly re-emerge in new guises. It always pays to have good relationships with colleagues, as you don't know when you might be interviewed by them.

Politics is everything if you are trying to achieve change in any organization. The political climate that an individual working in public health needs to be aware of may extend from the international to the very local, even the politics of the office (perhaps especially the politics of the office!). It is essential in public health to have good political 'antennae'. The same action undertaken at different times can have profoundly different effects depending on the political climate.

Understand the power politics

In any organization—and most of public health at a strategic level is undertaken in quite heavily managed organizations—it is essential to understand who wealds the power. This might not just be the chief executive (it might not even be the chief executive). In many instance the directors of finance hold a great deal of sway. Money is a very measurable indicator of both process and outcome, it is a unit that everyone will understand.

6. Don't take on too much

Know your own limitations

Failure to deliver is one of the biggest potential risks for public health, and with an almost limitless agenda the likelihood of this happening in an undisciplined individual is high. You sometimes just have to say 'no'—or if it's something that needs to be done, agree what is going to drop off your agenda. Don't assume that if you aren't chased up for a given piece of work that it has been forgotten—it probably hasn't and will resurface when you least expect it.

Always deliver what you say you will deliver

The current British Prime Minister, Tony Blair, said the second term of his Labour government was about 'delivery, delivery, delivery'. Unlike clinical medicine, where your problems often have a voice, public health problems often do not. Sometimes problems will rebound unexpectedly and will assume a disproportionately high media profile. You need to make promises you can keep—deliver!

7. Develop your staff

This is true in any organization, but in public health is particularly important given the sparse nature of key skills. Increasingly, to maintain formal registration, it is necessary to demonstrate a portfolio of CPD (continuing professional development). In earlier days in public health this only related to those with a medical qualification. This has now been extended to all public health specialists (although it is only doctors who at the moment need to demonstrate such activity to maintain registration). With the creation of a register for all those working in the public health field, staff development will no longer be an option. Look at the promotion of your staff to more senior positions as a reflection of your ability to develop your staff and not as a reason for remorse about losing a key member of staff.

8. Always know someone who can

The breadth of public health will inevitably mean you will not have the ability to retain all the necessary skills at any one time. Therefore maintaining networks of skills and expertise is vital. Always know someone who can, even if you can't. Examples include good statisticians. Many of us have trained in statistics, some of us even understood the subject as we did it. However, unless skills such as these are being used regularly they are likely to deteriorate.

9. Turn up

'The world is run by people who turn up.' The first rule of politics is to be there! Woody Allen said that 80% of the success of his career could be put down to just turning up. It is surprising how little attention is paid to this very simple maxim. In public health as much is achieved inside the meeting as outside, and so you sometimes need to weigh up whether even if the agenda doesn't look very stimulating there will be people present with whom you can do business.

10. Learn from your mistakes

Everyone will have their own list of 10 dos and don'ts; these are just a few. They will change throughout a career and you will add your own. Always be prepared to learn and to make mistakes (but not too many and not particularly big ones!) and be humble!

References
1 Faculty of Public Health of the Royal College of Physicians of the United Kingdom. *What is public health?* Available at: http://www.fph.org.uk/about_faculty/what_public_health/default.asp (accessed 29 June 2005).
2 *National Library for Health. Clinical Evidence Concise* 13. BMJ Publishing, London. Available at: http://www.clinicalevidence.com (accessed 29 June 2005).

Sources of reference

This list is highly selective, and, due to the highly volatile nature of the Internet, highly susceptible to change. Send us your favourites for inclusion in the next edition on the evaluation card.

Research and evidence

Bandolier: http://www.jr2.ox.ac.uk/bandolier/
BMJ Public Health: via http://bmj.bmjjournals.com/cgi/collection
BioMed Central Public Health: http://www.biomedcentral.com/bmcpublichealth/
Centre of Reviews and Dissemination: http://www.york.ac.uk/inst/crd/
Cochrane Collaboration: http://www.cochrane.org/index0.htm
Guide to Clinical Preventive Services: http://cpmcnet.columbia.edu/texts/gcps/gcps0000.html
How to Read a Paper: http://bmj.bmjjournals.com/collections/read.shtml
Netting the Evidence: Introduction to Evidence Based Medicine on the Internet: http://www.shef.ac.uk/scharr/ir/netting/
Oxford Centre for Evidence Based Medicine: http://www.cebm.net/index.asp
PubMed: http://www.ncbi.nlm.nih.gov/entrez/query.fcgi
UK Department of Health R&D: http://www.dh.gov.uk/PolicyAndGuidance/ResearchAndDevelopment/fs/en
UK National electronic Library for Health: http://www.nelh.nhs.uk/

Clinical guidelines

National Guideline Clearinghouse of the Agency for Healthcare Research and Quality (AHRQ): http://www.guideline.gov/
New Zealand Guidelines Group: http://www.nzgg.org.nz
Scottish Intercollegiate Guidelines Network: http://www.sign.ac.uk/

Public health guidance

Public health excellence at NICE: http://www.publichealth.nice.org.uk/

Inequalities

Acheson on inequalities:
http://www.archive.official-documents.co.uk/document/doh/ih/contents.htm
UK Department of Health: http://www.dh.gov.uk/PolicyAndGuidance/
HealthAndSocialCareTopics/HealthInequalities/fs/en

Training and education

Association of Schools of Public Health: http://www.asph.org/
Public Health Resource Unit, Oxford, UK: http://www.phru.nhs.uk/

Statistical software

StatsDirect statistical software: http://www.public-health.com/

Collections of public health Internet resources

Public Health Informatics at The University of Manchester: http://www.
ukph.org/

Determinants of health

WHO. Social determinants of health. The solid facts: http://www.who.
dk/document/e59555.pdf

Public health in the media

BBC www.bbc.co.uk news health site: http://news.bbc.co.uk/hi/english/
health/default.stm
Quackwatch: http://www.quackwatch.com/index.html

Other agencies and organizations

American Public Health Association: http://www.apha.org/
Association of Public Health Observatories: http://www.apho.org.uk
Australasian Faculty of Public Health Medicine: http://www.medeserv.
com.au/racp/afphm/index.htm
Faculty of Public Health of the Royal Colleges of Physicians of the United
Kingdom: http://www.fph.org.uk/
Healthcare Commission for Health Improvement: http://www.healthcare
commission.org.uk

Royal Institute of Public Health: http://www.riphh.org.uk/
Royal Statistical Society: http://www.rss.org.uk
UK National Institute for Health and Clinical Excellence (NICE): http://www.nice.org.uk/
UK Public Health Association: http://www.ukpha.org.uk/

Public health agencies in the UK

The UK Health Protection Agency

The Health Protection Agency (HPA) (http://www.hpa.org.uk/) is an independent body that protects the health and well-being of everyone in England and Wales.

The agency plays a critical role in protecting people from infectious diseases and in preventing harm when hazards involving chemicals, poisons, or radiation occur. It also prepares for new and emerging threats, such as a bioterrorist attack or virulent new strains of disease.

The HPA runs the Centre for Infections (http://www.hpa.org.uk/cfi). This unit undertakes national surveillance of communicable disease and provides epidemiological assistance and coordination in the investigation and control of infection in England and Wales.

The UK Health Protection Agency: work on response to chemical incidents

The Health Protection Agency runs a surveillance service of chemical incidents throughout England and Wales (http://www.hpa.org.uk/chemicals/default.htm). It also provides a link between the Regional Service Provider Units for Chemical Incidents (RSPUs) and government, and liaises between RSPUs in incidents involving more than one region. RSPUs are organizations which provide support to subscribing health authorities in responding to and managing chemical incidents. They provide a 24-hour a day, 365-day a year toxicologic, environmental, epidemiologic, and chemical emergency management service. There are five RSPUs covering the UK. For example, the RSPU for the West Midlands region is The Chemical Hazards Management and Research Centre (CHMRC) based at the University of Birmingham (http://www.publichealth.bham.ac.uk/chapd/index.htm). The CHMRC can be contacted via its hotline on 020 7394 5112.

National Poisons Information Service

The National Poisons Information Service (NPIS) comprises six poisons centres (Belfast, Birmingham, Cardiff, Edinburgh, London and Newcastle). They provide a year-round, 24-hour a day service for health-care staff on the clinical aspects of patients who may have been poisoned.

The NPIS can be contacted on 0870 600 6266. Enquiries are routed to the nearest regional unit.

UK Environment Agency

The Environment Agency (http://www.environment-agency.gov.uk/) is responsible for all environmental issues in the UK. It is responsible for the implementation of integrated pollution prevention control (IPPC) which involves protecting public health from the effects of industrial pollution. It is also responsible, in conjunction with the Health and Safety Executive (HSE), for implementing the emergency planning legislation for major industrial processes.

The Environment Agency runs regional control centres to deal with environmental pollution incidents. These can be contacted via the Environment Agency's hotline (0800 807060). They also operate a 'floodline' (0845 988 1188) to handle enquiries about problems caused by flooding. General enquiries can be made by calling 0845 133111.

UK Health and Safety Executive (HSE)

Responsible for implementation of health and safety legislation in most major activities and businesses. The HSE (http://www.hse.gov.uk/) is involved in emergency planning for industrial complexes and has access to considerable expertise in the fields of toxicology and emergency planning.

Drinking Water Inspectorate

The Drinking Water Inspectorate (http://www.dwi.gov.uk/) ensures that the water companies in England and Wales supply water that is safe to drink and meets the standards set in the Water Quality Regulations. It also investigates complaints from consumers, and incidents that affect or could affect drinking water quality.

It can be contacted on 020 7944 5956 or via the website (above)

UK Food Standards Agency (FSA)

The Food Standards Agency (http://www.foodstandards.gov.uk/) provides advice and information to the public and to the government on food safety, in addition to enforcement and monitoring of food standards.

It can be contacted on 020 7276 8829 (helpline) or by E-mail at helpline@foodstandards.gsi.gov.uk.

Environmental Health Departments (EHDs)

EHDs have responsibility for a range of issues that impact upon public health including air, water, food, and housing quality. They also have an important role in emergency situations. Each EHD will have its own emergency contact arrangements with which the local professionals should be familiar.

National Chemical Emergency Centre (NCEC)

The National Chemical Emergency Centre (http://www.the-ncec.com/) operates a national 24-hour chemical incident response centre, supported by the UK Department of Environment, Food and Rural Affairs (DEFRA) and the Chemical Industries Association (CIA). The service is by subscription only.

The NCEC can be contacted on 01235 463060 or by E-mail at ncec@aeat.co.uk

Public health genetics

Public Health Genetics Unit: http://www.phgu.org.uk/index.php

Agencies outside the United Kingdom

United States Environmental Protection Agency (USEPA)

The USEPA (http://www.epa.gov/) is responsible for all environmental issues in the USA. Its website provides databases, newsletters, and other information concerning environmental protection.

Centres for Disease Control and Prevention (CDC) (USA)

The US Centres for Disease Control and Prevention (http://www.cdc.gov/) provides information on many aspects of public health, such as infectious disease, environmental health, and health promotion, and serves as the national focus for public health issues in the United States.

Agency for Toxic Substances and Disease Registry (ATSDR) (USA)

The ATSDR (http://www.atsdr.cdc.gov/) is concerned with the public health implications of hazardous substances. The website provides a number of services including databases of hazardous chemicals and toxicity standards.

US Chemical Safety and Hazard Investigation Board

The Chemical Safety and Hazard Investigation Board (http://chemsafety.gov/) is an independent federal agency that investigates chemical incidents and provides information on the prevention of such incidents. This agency is also mandated to provide assistance to agencies outside the USA.

The Board can be contacted at info@csb.gov.

The National Institute for Occupational Safety and Health (NIOSH) (USA)

The NIOSH (http://www.cdc.gov/niosh/homepage.html) is responsible for conducting research and making recommendations for the prevention of work-related disease and injury. A number of databases related to occupational health and safety, including occupational standards for chemicals, are available from their website.

The US Food and Drug Administration (FDA)

The FDA (*http://www.fda.gov/*) provides information on a number of subjects ranging from food and drug safety and disease, to devices that emit radiation (cellular phones etc.).

Other sites relating to food and environmental health

UK sites

Public Health Institute of Scotland: http://www.phis.org.uk/
Scottish Public Health Observatory: http://scotpho.org.uk/
UK Department of Environment, Food and Rural Affairs (DEFRA): http://www.defra.gov.uk/
Wales Centre for Health: http://www.wch.wales.nhs.uk

Other European sites

European Health Portal: http://ec.europa.eu/health-eu/index_en.htm
Health and Consumer Protection DG (European Commission):
   http://europa.eu.int/comm/dgs/health_consumer/index_en.htm
The Institute of Public Health in Ireland: http://www.publichealth.ie/
Ireland and Northern Ireland's Population Health Observatory: http://
   www.inispho.org
Food safety—from the farm to the fork (European Commission):
   http://europa.eu.int/comm/dg24/health/sc/scf/index_en.html
The European Food Information Council: http://www.eufic.org/

Other global sites

Centre for Nutrition Policy and Promotion (USA): http://www.usda.gov/cnpp/
Food and Agriculture Organization of the United Nations (FAO):
   http://www.fao.org/
United States Department of Agriculture (USDA): http://www.usda.gov/
US Environmental Protection Agency (EPA): http://www.epa.gov/
US Food and Drug Administration (FDA): http://www.fda.gov/

Law and public health

Centre for Law and the Public's Health at Georgetown and Johns Hopkins
    Universities: http://www.publichealthlaw.net/

International sites

Canadian Public Health Association: http://www.cpha.ca/
European Public Health Alliance: http://www.epha.org/
Harvard School of Public Health: http://www.hsph.harvard.edu/
Public Health Foundation, Washington, DC: http://www.phf.org/
School of Public Health at Johns Hopkins: http://www.jhsph.edu/
United States Department of Health and Human Services: http://www.os.
    dhhs.gov/
World Health Organization (WHO): http://www.who.int/en/
Yale School of Public Health: http://info.med.yale.edu/eph/

and finally...

If you have been looking for information on zoonoses, go to
http://www.dh.gov.uk/PolicyAndGuidance/HealthAndSocialCareTopics/fs/
en#5587068 and, if all else fails, try the Boy Scouts' *Public Health Badge
Handbook* (unfortunately, now out of print, but it's very good, if you can
find it!)

Abbreviations and glossary

This list aims to standardize some of the more frequently used terms in this book. The glossary is restricted to words or phrases with a technical meaning in the broad field of public health practice. Selected resources follow the list below, including a recommended general dictionary, a guide to usage, and, of primary importance, the latest edition of Last's *Dictionary of Epidemiology*. Many terms below are defined at greater length in the latter. While we have intended to provide a sufficient list here, the annotation '(see Last)' indicates either that we have closely followed the *Dictionary of Epidemiology* or that it contains a more elaborate description that may be particularly helpful.

AHRQ: Agency for Healthcare Research and Quality (http://www.ahrq.gov/ accessed 28 June 2005)

AIDS: Acquired immune deficiency syndrome

BSE: Bovine spongiform encephalopathy

Case mix: An index of the type of illnesses managed in a health-care facility

CDSR: Cochrane Database of Systematic Reviews, part of the Cochrane Library coordinated by the International Cochrane Collaboration (see chapter 2.11 and http://www.cochrane.org/index0.htm accessed 28 June 2005)

CHD: Coronary heart disease

Clinical governance: A framework for continuous quality improvement (see Chapter 6.11)

Clinical indicators: Measurements of aspects of clinical care related to quality

CME: Continuing medical education

Cochrane Collaboration: The international organization that prepares and disseminates systematic reviews of the effects of health-care interventions (http://www.cochrane.org/index0.htm accessed 28 June 2005)

Co-morbidity: The simultaneous presence of two or more health disorders

Cost–benefit analysis: An analysis in which the economic and social costs of medical care and the benefits of reduced loss of net earnings due to preventing premature death or disability are considered (see Last)

CPD: Continuing professional development

CRD: Centre for Reviews and Dissemination, York, UK (http://www.york.ac.uk/inst/crd/ accessed 28 June 2005)

DALY: see Disability-adjusted life year

Diagnosis-related group (DRG): Classification of hospital patients according to diagnosis and intensity of care required, used by insurance companies to set reimbursement scales (see Last)

Disability: Temporary or long-term reduction of a person's capacity to function (see Last)

Disability-adjusted life year: Measure adopted by the World Bank to estimate the burden of disease by combining premature mortality and disability (see Last)

Dose: The stated quantity of a substance to which an organism is exposed

DRG: see Diagnosis-related group

ECG: Electrocardiogram

EIA: Environmental impact assessment

EMBASE: An European electronic database of health-related scientific references (see Chapter 2.11). This database has a significant (~40%) overlap with Medline, but has a more European and pharmacological emphasis

ESD: Ecologically sustainable development

EU: European Union

Evaluation: A process that attempts to determine as systematically and objectively as possible the relevance, effectiveness, and impact of activities in the light of their objectives (see Last)

Evidence-based health care/medicine/public health: Systematic use of evidence derived from published research and other sources for management and practice

Exposure: A measure of the actual contact with an agent (usually chemical, physical, or biological)

Expressed needs: Needs expressed by action, e.g. visiting a doctor

FAO: Food and Agriculture Organization (of the United Nations) (http://www.fao.org/ accessed 28 June 2005)

Felt needs: What people consider and/or say they need when asked

Focus group: Small, convenient sample of people brought together to discuss a topic or issue with the aim of ascertaining the range and intensity of their views, rather than arriving at a consensus (see Last)

GDP: Gross domestic product

Goal: A general statement of direction and intent (usually measurable)

GP: General practitioner (family doctor)

Handicap: Reduction in a person's capacity to fulfil a social role as a consequence of an impairment or disability, or other circumstances (see Last)

Hazard: The intrinsic capacity of an agent, a condition, or a situation to produce an adverse health or environmental effect

Health: The extent to which an individual or a group is able to realize aspirations and satisfy needs, and to change or cope with the environment. Health is a resource for everyday life, not the objective of living; it is a positive concept, emphasizing social and personal resources as well as physical capabilities. Your health is related to how much you feel your potential, to be a meaningful part of the society in which you find yourself, is adequately realized (see Last)

Healthcare Commission (UK): A UK body that assures, monitors and helps improve the quality of patient care (http://www.healthcare commission.org.uk accessed 28 June 2005)

Healthcare resource groups: Classification of patients according to severity and intensity of care required, used by insurance carriers (or equivalent) to compare resource use throughout a health system

Health impact assessment: An assessment process to look at the impact on health of government policies or other actions, completed or projected (see Chapter 1.5)

Health outcome: Health status, sometimes related to the effects of health care or other interventions

HeaLy: Healthy life years. A composite indicator that incorporates morbidity and mortality into a single number (see Last)

HIA: see Health impact assessment

HRG: see Healthcare resource groups

IARC: International Agency for Research on Cancer

ICD-10: International Classification of Disease, edition 10

ICD-9 (CM): International Classification of Disease, edition 9 (clinical modification)

Impairment: A physical or mental defect at the level of a body system or organ. Contrast with Disability and Handicap (see Last)

Medline: An electronic database that provides citations, sometimes including abstracts, from the biomedical literature (beginning 1966)

National Institute for Health and Clinical Excellence (NICE): NICE is the UK independent organization responsible for providing national guidance on the promotion of good health and the prevention and treatment of ill-health. (http://www.nice.org.uk/ accessed 28 June 2005)

National service framework (UK): National service frameworks set national standards and define service models for a specific service or care group, put in place programs to support implementation, and establish performance measures against which progress within an agreed timescale will be measured

NeLH (UK): National electronic Library for Health (http://www.nelh.nhs.uk/ accessed 28 June 2005)

NGO: Non-governmental organization

NHS: National Health Service (UK)

NICE: see National Institute for Health and Clinical Excellence

Normative needs: Needs as defined by a health professional

OECD: Organization for Economic Cooperation and Development

PCT: Primary Care Trust

PDP: Personal development plan

Prevention paradox: a measure whose effect is considerable at a population level, but minimal at an individual level (see Last)

Public health: The science and art of preventing disease, prolonging life, and promoting health through the organized efforts and informed choices of society, organizations, public and private, communities and individuals. Public health practice is the emphasis in this book, while public health may also be considered as a discipline or a social institution

Public health practitioner: In this book, includes anyone working in the broad field of public health, neither defined by formal qualifications nor restricted to a professional group.

PubMed: A service of the National Library of Medicine, provides access to over 11 million citations from Medline and additional life science journals. PubMed includes links to many sites providing full text articles and other related resources. (http://www.ncbi.nlm.nih.gov/PubMed/ accessed 28 June 2005)

QALY: Quality-adjusted life year

RCT: Randomized controlled trial

Risk: The probability that a particular adverse event occurs during a stated period of time, or results from a particular challenge. It can never be reduced to zero

Screening: The systematic application of a test or inquiry to identify individuals at sufficient risk of a specific disorder to benefit from further investigation or direct preventive action among persons who have not sought medical attention on account of symptoms of that disorder

SIDS: Sudden infant death syndrome

SMR: Standardized mortality ratio

Stakeholders: Persons or organizations with an interest that may affect the outcome of an activity. Responses to stakeholders may include collaboration, involvement, monitoring, or defense

STD: Sexually transmitted disease

Surveillance: The ongoing, systematic collection, collation, and analysis of data and the prompt dissemination of the resulting information to those who need to know so that an action can result

SWOT: (Analysis of) strengths, weaknesses, opportunities, and threats

Target: A specific change, intended within a given time period

UNESCO: United Nations Economic, Social and Cultural Organization

UNICEF: United Nations Children's Fund

URL: Uniform resource locator (technical name for a Web address)

WHO: World Health Organization

Further resources

Burchfield RW (ed.) (1999). *Fowler's modern English usage*, revised 3rd edn. Clarendon Press, Oxford.

Last JM (ed.) (2001). *A dictionary of epidemiology*, 4th edn. Oxford University Press, Oxford.

New Oxford dictionary of English (1998). Oxford University Press, Oxford.

When a word causes more confusion than clarity, it is time to stop using it.

Wittgenstein, 1889–1951

Bibliography

Abdel Aziz MI, Radford J, McCabe J (2000). *Health impact assessment, Finningley Airport.* Doncaster Health Authority. Available at: http://www.phel. nice.org.uk/ hiadocs/79_finningley_airport_hiareport.pdf (accessed 15 June 2005).

Abelson J, Eyles J, McLeod CB, Collins P, McMullan C, Forest-Pierre G (2003). Does deliberation make a difference? Results from a citizens panel study on health goals priority setting. *Health Policy*, **66**(1), 95–106.

Abrahams D (2002). *Foresight Vehicle Initiative comprehensive health impact assessment. Executive summary.* IMPACT—International Health Impact Assessment Consortium, University of Liverpool. Available at: www.ihia. org.uk/ document/impacthiareports/FVI.pdf (accessed 15 June 2005).

Abrahams D, den Broeder L, Doyle C et al. (2004). *EPHIA—European policy health impact assessment: a guide.* IMPACT, University of Liverpool. Available at: http://www.ihia.org.uk/document/ephia.pdf (accessed 15 June 2005).

Abubakar I (2005). Investigating outliers. *INphoRM*, issue 5. ERPHO, Cambridge Available at: http://www.erpho.org.uk/download.asp?id=11454& typeID=2 and http://www.phi.man.ac.uk/default.aspx.

Acheson D (1988). *Public health in England: the report of the Committee of Inquiry into the future development of the public health function,* Cm 289. HMSO, London.

Acheson D (1998). *Report on the inquiry into health inequalities.* The Stationery Office, London.

Acheson ED (1988). *Public health in England. Report of the Committee of Inquiry into the future development of the public health function.* HMSO, London.

Adams L, Pintus S (1994). A challenge to prevailing theory and practice. *Crit Public Health*, **5**, 17–29.

Adams P, Baxter PA, Aw TC, Cockcroft A, Harrington JM (ed.) (2000). *Hunter's diseases of occupations,* 9th edn. Edward Arnold, London.

Adily A, Ward JE (2004). Evidence-based practice in population health: a regional survey to inform workforce development and organisational change. *J Epidemiol Commun Health*, **58**, 455–60.

Agency for Toxic Substances and Disease Registry (1996). *Guidance for ATSDR health studies.* US Department of Health and Human Services, Washington, DC. Available at: www.atsdr.cdc.gov/HS/gd1.html (accessed 14 March 2005).

Agency for Toxic Substances and Disease Registry. *A primer on health risk communication principles and practices.* Available at: http://www.atsdr. cdc.gov/HEC/primer.html.

Alexander FE, Boyle P (1996). *Methods for investigating localised clustering of disease,* IARC Scientific Publication No. 135. International Agency for Research on Cancer, Lyon.

Alexander FE, Cuzick J (1996). Methods for the assessment of disease clusters. In: Eliott P, Cuzick J, English D, Stern R (eds) *Geographical and environmental epidemiology methods for small-area studies*, pp. 238–50. Oxford University Press, Oxford.

Allardyce J, Morrison G, Van Os J, Kelly J, Murray RM, McCreadie RG (2000). Schizophrenia is not disappearing in south-west Scotland. *Br J Psychiat*, **177**, 38–41.

American Heart Association (22 October 2003). *New York city restaurant survey supports smoking ban*. Available at: www.americanheart.org/presenter.jhtml?identifier=3016321 (accessed: 22 June 2005).

Anthony D, Milne R (1997). *Growth hormone for growth hormone deficient adults* (Development and Evaluation Committee Report No 47). Wessex Institute for Health Research and Development, Southampton.

Arblaster L, Entwistle V, Lambert M, Forster M, Sheldon T, Watt I (1995). *Review of the research on the effectiveness of health service interventions to reduce variations in health*, CRD Report 3. NHS Centre for Reviews and Dissemination, York.

Arblaster L, Lambert M, Entwistle V et al. (1996). A systematic review of the effectiveness of health service interventions aimed at reducing inequalities in health. *J Health Serv Res Policy*, **1**, 93–103.

Ardern K (2003). *Rapid health impact assessment of the private finance initiative proposal: a whole system approach in St Helens and Knowsley*. South Liverpool Primary Care Trust, Liverpool. Available at: http://www.phel.nice.org.uk/hiadocs/Rapid_HIA_of_PFI_Proposal.pdf (accessed 15 June 2005).

Ashenden R, Silagy C, Weller D (1997). A systematic review of the effectiveness of promoting lifestyle change in general practice. *Fam Pract*, **14**(2), 160–75.

Aspinall PJ, Jacobson B (2005). *Health equity audit: a baseline survey of Primary Care Trusts in England*. London Health Observatory, London. Available at: http://www.hda-online.org.uk/Documents/health_equity_audit.pdf.

Atkinson P (1981). *The clinical experience*. Gower, Farnborough.

Australian Government NHMRC/NRMMC (2004). *Australian drinking water guidelines*. National Health and Medical Research Council, Natural Resource Management Ministerial Council 2004. Available at: http://www.nhmrc.gov.au/publications/synopses/eh19syn.htm (accessed 13 March 2005).

Australian Hospital Association (1996). *Green health care. Environmental assessment manual*. Australian Hospital Association, Canberra.

Ayer AJ (1936). *Language, truth and logic*. Penguin, London.

Badamgarav E, Weingarten SR, Henning JM et al. (2003). Effectiveness of disease management programs in depression: a systematic review. *Am J Psychiatry*, **160**, 2080–90.

Bailit M, Dyer MB (2004). *Beyond bankable dollars; establishing a business case for improving healthcare*, Commonwealth Fund publication no 754. Available at: http://www.cmwf.org/usr_doc/Bailit_beyond_bankable_dollars_business_case.pdf (accessed 20 January 2005).

Bajekal M (2005). Healthy life expectancy by area deprivation: magnitude and trends in England, 1994–1999. *Health Statist Q*, **25**, 18–27.

Banwell C, Guest CS (1998). Carnivores, cannibals, consumption and unnatural boundaries: the BSE-CJD epidemic in the Australian press. In McCalman I (ed) *Mad Cows and Modernity: the crisis of Creutzfeldt-Jakob disease.* National Acadamies Forum, Canberra.

Barnes R (2004). HIA and urban regeneration: the Ferrier Estate, England. In: Kemm J, Parry J, Palmer S (eds) *Health impact assessment. Concepts, theory, techniques and applications*, pp. 299–307. Oxford University Press, Oxford.

Barratt A, Trevena L, Davey HM, McCaffery K (2004). Use of decision aids to support informed choices about screening. *BMJ,* **329**, 507–10.

Barry MJ, Fowler FJ Jr, Mulley AG Jr, Henderson JV Jr, Wennberg JE (1995). Patient reactions to a program designed to facilitate patient participation in treatment decisions for benign prostatic hyperplasia. *Med Care,* **33**(8), 771–82.

Bartley M, Blane D, Montgomery S (1997). Education and debate. Socio-economic determinants of health: health and the life course: why safety nets matter. *BMJ,* **314**, 1194.

Battersby J, Flowers J, Harvey I (2004). An alternative approach to quantifying and addressing inequity in healthcare provision: access to surgery for lung cancer in the east of England. *J Epidemiol Commun Health,* **58**(7), 623–5.

Baum F (1995). Researching public health: behind the qualitative-quantitative methodological debate. *Soc Sci Med,* **40**, 459–68.

Baxter PJ, Anthony PP, MacSween RNM, Scheuer PJ (1997). Angiosarcoma of the liver in Great Britain 1963–73. *BMJ,* **2**, 919–21.

BBC News (31 May 2004). *Ireland smoking ban a success.* Available at: http://news.bbc.co.uk/1/hi/business/3763471.stm (accessed 22 June 2005).

Beaglehole R, Bonita R (1997). *Public health at the crossroads.* Cambridge University Press, Cambridge.

Beauchamp T, Childress J (2001). *Principles of biomedical ethics,* 5th edn. Oxford University Press, Oxford.

Belbin RM (1996). *Management teams—why they succeed or fail,* p. 74. Butterworth Heinemann, London. Available at: http://www.belbin.com/ (accessed 5 May 2005).

Benedict R (1935). *Patterns of culture.* Routledge and Kegan Paul, London.

Benneyan JC, Lloyd RC, Plsek PE (2003). Statistical process control as a tool for research and healthcare improvement. *Qual Saf Health Care,* **12**(6), 458–64.

Benton T (1977). *Philosophical foundations of the three sociologies.* Routledge Kegan Paul, London.

Benzeval M, Judge K (1996). Access to health care in England: continuing inequalities in the distribution of GPs. *J Publ Health Med,* **18**, 33–44.

Berger PL, Luckman T (1967). *The social construction of reality.* Anchor Books, New York.

Berrino F, Gatta G, Chessa E, Valente F, Capocaccia R (1998). The EUROCARE II study. *Eur J Cancer,* **34**, 2139–53.

Berry G, Newhouse ML (1982). Mortality of workers manufacturing friction materials using asbestos. *Br J Ind Med,* **39**, 344–8.

Berwick DM (1991). Controlling variation in health care: a consultation from Walter Shewhart. *Medical Care,* **29**(12),1212–25.

Berwick DM (1996). A primer on leading the improvement of systems. *BMJ*, **312**(7031), 619–22.

Berwick DM (1998). The NHS's 50 anniversary. Looking forward. The NHS: feeling well and thriving at 75. *BMJ*, **317**, 57–61.

Berwick DM, Leape LL (1999). Reducing errors in medicine. *BMJ*, **319**,136–7.

Berwick DM, Nolan TW (1998). Physicians as leaders in improving health care: a new series in *Annals of Internal Medicine*. *Ann Intern Med*, **128**(4), 289–92.

Beveridge W (1942). *Social insurance and allied services*. HMSO, London.

Bhopal RS (1991). A framework for investigating geographical variation in diseases, based on a study of Legionnaires' disease. *J Public Health Med*, **13**(4), 281–9.

Bhopal RS (1995). Public health medicine and primary health care: convergent, divergent, or parallel paths? *J Epidemiol Commun Health*, **49**, 113–16.

Birley MH (1995). *The health impact assessment of development projects*. HMSO, London.

Black D, Morris JN, Smith C, Townsend P (1992). *Inequalities in health: the Black report*. Pelican, Harmondsworth.

Black N (1992). Research, audit, and education. *BMJ*, **304**, 698–700.

Black N (2001). Evidence-based policy: proceed with care. *BMJ*, **323**, 275–9.

Black N, Barker M, Payne M (2004). Cross sectional survey of multi-centre clinical database in the United Kingdom. *BMJ*, **328**, 1478–81.

Blaxter L, Hughes C, Tight M (1996). *How to research*. Open University Press, Buckingham.

Blumenthal D, Ferris T (2004). *The business case for quality: ending business as usual in American health care*. Available at: http://www.cmwf.org/usr_doc/715_Blumenthal_business_case.pdf (accessed 20 January 2005).

Bodenheimer T (2000). Disease management in the American market. *BMJ*, **320**, 563–6.

Bodenheimer T, Wagner EH, Grumbach K (2002). Improving primary care for patients with chronic illness. *J Am Med Assoc* **288**, 1775–9.

Bolsin S, Colson M (2000). The use of the Cusum technique in the assessment of trainee competence in new procedures. *Int J Qual Health Care*, **12**(5), 433–8.

Bouchier I (1998). *The third report of the expert group on cryptosporidium in water supplies*. DEFRA and Department of Health, London.

Bowen T, and Forte P (1997). Activity and capacity planning in an acute hospital. In: Cropper S, Forte P (eds) *Enhancing health services management*, pp. 86–102. Open University Press, Buckingham.

Bowling A (1997). *Measuring health: a review of quality of life measurement scales*, 2nd edn. Open University Press, Buckingham.

Boyle P, Maisonneuve P, Napalkov P (1995). Geographical and temporal patterns of incidence and mortality from prostate cancer. *Urology*, **46**(3, Suppl. A), 47–55.

Boynton PM, Greenhalgh T (2004). Selecting, designing and developing your questionnaire. *BMJ*, **328**, 1312–15. Available at: http://bmj.bmjjournals.com/cgi/content/full/328/7451/1312 (accessed December 2004).

Brewster D (1999). Environmental management for vector control. Is it worth a dam if it worsens malaria? *BMJ* **319**, 651–2.

Brigden D (1999) Constructing a learning portfolio. Career focus articles. *BMJ Classified*, 3 July, 2–3. Available at http://bmj.bmjjournals.com/cgi/content/full/319/7201/S2a-7201 (accessed 1 October 2005).

Briggs Myers I, Myers P (1980). Gifts differing, understanding personality type. Davies-Black, Palo Alto, CA.

Bronnum-Hansen H (2005). Health expectancy in Denmark, 1987–2000. *Eur J Public Health*, **15**(1), 20–5.

Brook RH, Ware JE Jr, Rogers WH, *et al.* (1983). Does free care improve adults' health? Results from a randomized controlled trial. *N Engl J Med*, **309**,1426–34.

Brown S, Lumley J (1993). Antenatal care: a case of the inverse care law? *Aust J Public Health*, **17**(2), 95–103.

Brownson RC, Baker EA, Leet TL, Gillespie KN (2003). *Evidence based public health*. Oxford University Press, New York.

Brundtland GH, Frenk J, Murray CJ (2003). WHO assessment of health systems performance. *Lancet*, **361**(9375), 2155.

Bryant J, Loveman E, Chase D *et al.* (2002). Clinical effectiveness and cost-effectiveness of growth hormone in adults in relation to impact on quality of life: a systematic review and economic evaluation. *Health Technol Assess*, **6**(19), 1-106.

Bryman A (1998). Quantitative and qualitative research strategies in knowing the social world. In: May T, Williams M (eds) *Knowing the social world*. Open University Press, Buckingham.

Bryman A (2004). *Social research methods*, 2nd edn. Oxford University Press, Oxford.

Bullas S, Ariotti D (2002). *Information for managing healthcare resources*. Radcliffe Medical Press, Abingdon.

Burke W, Zimmern R (2004). Ensuring the appropriate use of genetic tests. *Nat Rev Genet*, **5**, 955–9.

Bush JW, Chen MM, Zaremba J (1971). Estimating health program outcomes using a Markov equilibrium analysis of disease development. *Am J Public Health*, **61**(12), 2362–75.

Cabinet Office (1999). *Professional policy making for the 21st century*. Cabinet Office, London.

Caldwell J (1986). Routes to low mortality in poor countries. In: *Population and development review 12*. Centre for Population Studies of the Population Council, New York.

Calman K (1998). Lessons from Whitehall. *BMJ*, **317**, 1718–20.

Calman KC (1996). Cancer: science and society and the communication of risk. *BMJ*, **313**, 799–802.

Calman KC, Royston GH (1997). Risk language and dialects. *BMJ*, **315**, 939–42.

Cambois E, Robine J-M, Brouard N (1999). Life expectancies applied to specific statuses: a history of the indicators and the methods of calculation. *Population: an English Selection*, **11**, 7–34.

Carey V, Chapman S, Gaffney D (1994). Children's lives or garden aesthetics? A case study in public health advocacy. *Aust J Public Health*, **18**, 25–32.

Carr-Hill R, Chalmers-Dixon P (2003). *A review of methods for monitoring and measuring social inequality, deprivation and health inequality*. South East Public Health Observatory, Oxford.

Casebeer A (1993). Application of SWOT analysis. *Br J Hosp Med*, **49**, 430–1.

Casemore DP (1992). A pseudo-outbreak of cryptosporidiosis. *Commun Dis Rep CDR Rev* **2**(6), R66–R67.

CASPfew. *Sources of evidence*. Available at: http://www.phru.nhs.uk/casp/sources.htm (accessed 26 June 2005).

Centres for Disease Control (1990). Guidelines for investigating clusters of health events. *Morbidity and Mortality Weekly Report*, **39**(RR-11), 1–23.

Centres for Disease Control and Prevention (1999). Ten great public health achievements—United States, 1900–1999 (1999). *Morb Mortal Wkly Rep*, **48**(12), 241–8.

Centres for Disease Control and Prevention (2001). Updated guidelines for evaluating public health surveillance systems: recommendations from the guidelines working group. *Morbidity and Mortality Weekly Report*, **50**(RR-13), 1–35. Available at: http://www.cdc.gov/mmwr/preview/mmwrhtml/rr5013a1.htm.

Centres for Disease Control and Prevention (2004). Framework for evaluating public health surveillance systems for early detection of outbreaks; recommendations from the CDC Working Group. *Morbidity and Mortality Weekly Report*, **53**(RR-5), 1–13. Available at: http://www.cdc.gov/mmwr/preview/mmwrhtml/rr5305a1.htm.

Centres for Medicare and Medicaid Services. *Medicare provider analysis and review (MEDPAR) of short-stay hospitals*. Available at: http://www.cms. hhs.gov/statistics/medpar/default.asp (accessed 20 March 2005).

Centre for Reviews and Dissemination, University of York. *Health technology assessment database*. Available at: http://www.york.ac.uk/inst/crd/htahp.htm (accessed 28 December 2004).

Chapman S (1998). *Over our dead bodies: Port Arthur and Australia's fight for gun control*. Pluto, Sydney.

Chapman S (2004). Advocacy for public health: a primer. *J Epidemiol Commun Health*, **58**(5), 361–5.

Chapman S, Lupton D (1994). *The fight for public health: principles and practice of media advocacy*. BMJ Books, London.

Charmaz K (2004). Grounded theory. In: Bryman A, Liao TF (eds) The Sage encyclopedia of social science methods, Vols 1–3. Sage, Thousand Oaks, CA.

Chenet L, McKee M, Fulop N et al. (1996). Changing life expectancy in central Europe: is there a single reason? *J Publ Health Med*, **18**, 329–36.

Chenet L, McKee M, Leon D, Shkolnikov V, Vassin S (1998). Alcohol and cardiovascular mortality in Moscow, new evidence of a causal association. *J Epidemiol Comm Health*, **52**, 772–4.

Chenet L, Osler M, McKee M, Krasnik A (1996). Changing life expectancy in the 1980s: why was Denmark different from Sweden? *J Epidemiol Comm Health*, **50**, 404–7.

Christophides N, Dominello A, Chapman S (1999). The new pariahs: how the tobacco industry are depicted in the Australian press. *Aust NZ J Public Health*, **23**, 233–9.

Church J, Saunders D, Wanke M, Pong R, Spooner C, Dorgan M (2002). Citizen participation in health decision-making: past experience and future prospects *J Public Health Pol*, **23**(1), 12–32.

Churchill LR (1994). *Self interest and universal healthcare: why well insured Americans should support coverage for everyone.* Harvard University Press, Cambridge, MA.

Clark NM (2003). Management of chronic disease by patients. *Ann Rev Public Health*, **24**, 289–313.

Clinical Standards Advisory Group (1998). *Cleft lip and/or palate: report of the CSAG Committee.* The Stationery Office, London.

Cochrane Effective Clinical Practice and Organisation of Care Group. http://www.epoc.uottawa.ca (accessed 31 May 2005).

Cochrane Library. http://www.cochrane.org/index0.htm (accessed 30 June 2005).

Commission for Health Improvement. *Sharing the learning on patients and public involvement from CHI's work. Involvement to improvement.* Available at: http://www.healthcarecommission.org.uk/assetRoot/04/01/01/88/04010188.pdf (accessed 3 October 2005).

Commission of the European Communities (2000). White Paper on food safety. Brussels 12 January 2000, COM(1999) 719 final. Commission of the European Communities, Brussels.

Commission of the European Communities (2002). *Communication from the Commission on impact assessment,* COM(2002) 276 final. CEC, Brussels.

Committee on the Quality of Health Care in America, Institute of Medicine (2001). *Crossing the quality chasm: a new health system for the 21st century.* National Academy Press, Washington, DC.

Commonwealth Department of Health and Aged Care (2001). *Public health outcome funding agreement 1999/2000–2003/2004 between the Commonwealth of Australia and New South Wales.* Australian Government Publishing Service, Canberra.

Commonwealth Department of Health and Aged Care and Australian Institute of Health and Welfare (1999). *National health priority areas report: diabetes mellitus 1998* (AIHW cat. No PHE 10). AusInfo, Canberra.

Commonwealth Department of Health and Ageing (for enHealth Council) (2002). *Environmental health risk assessment: guidelines for assessing human health risks from environmental hazards: June 2002.* Available at: http://www.health.gov.au/internet/wcms/Publishing.nsf/Content/health-pubhlth-publicat-document-metadata-env_hra.htm (accessed 14 March 2005).

Commonwealth Department of Human Services and Health (1994). *Better health outcomes for Australians. national goals, targets and strategies for better health outcomes into the next century.* Australian Government Publishing Service, Canberra.

Conceicao P, Ferreira P (2000). *The young person's guide to the Theil index: suggesting interpretations and exploring analytical applications,* Report no 14. UTIP.

Congressional Budget Office (2004). *An analysis of the literature on disease management programs.* Congressional Budget Office, Washington, DC. Available at: http://www.cbo.gov/showdoc.cfm?index=5909 (accessed 10 June 2005).

Coote A (ed.) (2002). *Claiming the health dividend.* King's Fund, London.

Costello A, Osrin D, Manandhar D (2004). Reducing maternal and neonatal mortality in the poorest communities. *BMJ*, **329**, 1166–8.

Coughlin SJ (1999). The intersection of genetics, public health and preventive medicine. *Am J Prev Med*, **16**, 89–90.

Cox RAF, Edwards FC, Palmer K (ed.) (2000). *Fitness for work: the medical aspects*, 3rd edn. Oxford University Press, Oxford.

Cretin S, Shortell SM, Keeler EB (2004). An evaluation of collaborative interventions to improve chronic illness care: framework and study design. *Eval Rev*, **28**(1), 28–51.

Crimmins EM, Saito Y, Hayward MD (1993). Sullivan and multi-state methods of estimating active life expectancy: two methods, two answers. In: Robine J-M, Mathers CD, Bone MR, Romieu I (eds) *Calculation of health expectancies: harmonization, consensus achieved and future perspectives/Calcul des espérances de vie en santé : harmonisation, acquis et perspectives*, pp. 155–160. John Libbey Eurotext, Montrouge.

Critchley JA, Capewell S (2002). Why model coronary heart disease? *Eur Heart J*, **23**, 110–16.

Crowley C, Harré R, Tagg C (2002). Qualitative research and computing: methodological issues and practices in using QSR NVivo and NUD*IST. *Int J Soc Res Methodol*, **5**(3), 193–7.

Cullinan P, Acquilla S, Ramana Dhara V (1997). Respiratory morbidity 10 years after the Union Carbide gas leak at Bhopal: a cross-sectional survey. *Br Med J*, **314**, 338–42.

Danesh J, Gault S, Semmence J, Appleby P, Peto R (1999). Postcodes as useful markers of social class: population based study in 26000 British households. *BMJ*, **318**, 843–5.

Daniels N, Kennedy B, Kawachi I (2000). Justice is good for our health. *Boston Rev*, **25**(1), 6–15.

Davies HTO, Nutley S, Smith PC (2000). *What works? Evidence-based policy and practice in public services.* The Policy Press, Bristol.

Davies PL (2004). *Is evidence based government possible? Jerry Lee Lecture 2004*, presented at the 4th Annual Campbell Collaboration Colloquium, Washington, DC, 19 February 2004. Government Chief Social Researcher's Office, Prime Minister Strategy Unit, Cabinet Office, London.

Davis DA, Thomson MA, Oxman AD, Haynes RB (1982). Evidence for the effectiveness of CME. A review of 50 randomized controlled trials. *JAMA*, 268(9), 1111–7.

Davis J, Milburn P, Murphy T, Woodhouse M (1992). *Successful team building*, p.182. Kogan Page, London.

Dawson A (2004). Vaccination and the prevention problem. *Bioethics*, **18**(6), 515–30.

Dawson A, Verweij M (eds). *Ethics, prevention and public health.* Oxford University Press, Oxford. (In press.)

Dawson A (2005). Risk perceptions and ethical public health policy: MMR in the UK. *Poiesis and Praxis*, **3**(4), 229–41.

de Bono E (1971). *Lateral thinking for management*. McGraw-Hill, Maidenhead.

de Bono E (1990). *Lateral thinking*. Penguin Books, London.

de Bono E (1994). Creativity and quality. *Qual Manag Health Care*, **2**(3), 1–4.

de Lepper MJC, Scholetn HJ, Stern RM (eds) (1995). The added value of *geographical information systems in public and environmental health*. Kluwer, Dordrecht (on behalf of the World Health Organization for Europe).

de Lorgeril M, Renaud S, Mamelle N et al. (1996). Mediterranean alpha-linolenic acid-rich diet in secondary prevention of coronary heart disease. *Lancet*, **343**, 1454–9.

Defoe D (1991). A journal of the plague year. (First published 1722). Penguin, Harmondsworth.

DeFriese GH, Fielding JE (1990). Health risk appraisal in the 1990s: opportunities, challenges, and expectations. *Ann Rev Public Health*, **11**, 401–18.

Denver Summit of the Eight (1997). *Final communique*.

Department for International Development (1997). *Eliminating world poverty: a challenge for the 21st century*. HMSO, London.

Department for International Development (1999). *International development strategy, better health for poor people: target strategy paper* (consultation document). Department for International Development, London.

Department for International Development (2000). *Department report 2000*. The Stationary Office, London.

Department for International Development (2000). *International development strategy paper, poverty eradication and the empowerment of women people: target strategy paper* (consultation document). Department for International Development, London.

Department of Health (1997). *Communicating about risks to public health pointers to good practice*. EOR Division, Department of Health, London.

Department of Health (1997). *Communicating about risks to public health: pointers to good practice*. Department of Health, London.

Department of Health (1998). *Smoking kills: a White Paper on tobacco*. The Stationary Office, London.

Department of Health (2000). *Good practice guidelines for investigating the health impact of local industrial emissions*. Department of Health, London.

Department of Health (2003). *Delivering investment in general practice: implementing the new GMS contract*. Department of Health, London.

Department of Health (2003). *Health equity audit: a guide for the NHS*. Department of Health, London.

Department of Health (2003). *Tackling health inequalities. A programme for action*. Department of Health, London.

Department of Health (2004). *Choosing health: making healthy choices easier*. The Stationary Office, London.

Department of Health (2004). *National standards, local action health and social care standards and planning framework*. Department of Health, London.

Department of Health (2004). *Standards for better health*. Department of Health, London. Available at: http://www.dh.gov.uk/assetRoot/04/08/66/66/04086666.pdf (accessed 25 April 2005).

Department of Health. *Communicating about risks to public health: pointers to good practice.* Available at: http://www.dh.gov.uk/assetRoot/04/03/96/70/04039670.pdf (accessed December 2004).

Department of Health. *Health Survey for England.* Available at: http://www.dh.gov.uk/ PublicationsAndStatistics/PublishedSurvey/HealthSurveyForEngland/fs/en (accessed 20 March 2005).

Department of Trade and Industry (1991). *Home and leisure accident research: twelfth annual report, 1988 data.* Department of Trade and Industry, Consumer Safety Unit, London.

Deperment of Health. *National survey of NHS patients.* Available at: http://www.dh.gov.uk/PublicationsAndStatistics/PublishedSurvey/NationalSurveyOfNHSPatients/fs/en (accessed 21 September 2004).

Detels R, McEwen J, Beaglehole R, Tanaka H (eds) (2002). *Oxford textbook of public health.* Oxford University Press, New York.

Devine F (1995). Qualitative analysis. In: Marsh D, Stoler G (eds) *Theory and methods in political science.* Macmillan, London.

Disease Management Association of America (2005). *Definition of disease management.* Disease Management Association of America, Washington, DC. Available at: http://www.dmaa.org/definition.html (accessed 31 May 2005).

Dixon A, Le Grand J, Henderson J, Murray R, Poteliakhoff E (2005). Is the NHS equitable? A review of the evidence. *J Health Serv Res Policy,*

Doll R, Peto R (1976). Mortality in relation to smoking: 20 years' observations on male British doctors. *BMJ,* **2**(6051), 1525–36.

Donabedian A (1980). The definition of quality: a conceptual exploration. In: *Explorations in quality assessment and monitoring. Volume I: The definition of quality and approaches to its assessment.* Health Administration Press, Ann Arbor, MI.

Donabedian A (2003). *An introduction to quality assurance in health care.* Oxford University Press, Oxford.

Donaldson C, Mooney G (1991). Needs assessment, priority setting, and contracts for healthcare: an economic view. *BMJ,* **303**, 1529–30.

Dowie R (1983). General practitioners and consultants: a study of outpatient referrals. King Edward's Hospital Fund for London, London.

Doyal L (1995). Rights and equity: moral quality in healthcare rationing. *Quality in Health Care,* **4**, 273–83.

Drever F, Whitehead M (ed.) (1997). *Health Inequalities,* Decennial Supplement, series DS No. 15. HMSO, London.

Drummond MF, O'Brien BJ, Stoddard GL Torrance GW (1997). *Methods for the economic evaluation of health care programmes,* 2nd edn. Oxford University Press, Oxford.

Dubois RW, Brook RH (1998). Preventable deaths: who, how often, and why?. RAND Corporation, Los Angeles, California. *Annuals of Internal Medicine,* **109**(7), 582–9.

Duhl L, Hancock T (1988). *A guide to assessing healthy cities.* WHO Healthy Cities, Paper No 3. FADL Publishers, Copenhagen.

Dyke G (1998). *The new NHS charter—a different approach; report on the new NHS charter.* Department of Health, London. Available at http://www.dh.gov.uk/assetRoot/04/10/60/95/04106095.PDF (accessed 25 April 2005).

Eastern Region Public Health Observatory (2004). Presenting performance indicators: alternative approaches. *INphoRM*, issue 4. Available at: http://www.erpho.org.uk/download.asp?id=7518&typeID=2.

Ebrahim S, Davey Smith G (2001). Multiple risk factor interventions for primary prevention of coronary heart disease (Cochrane review). In: *The Cochrane library*, issue 1. Update Software, Oxford.

Eddy DM (1990). Clinical decision making: from theory to practice. Designing a practice policy. Standards, guidelines, and options. *JAMA*, **263**, 3077–84.

Eddy DM (1990). Clinical decision making: from theory to practice. Resolving conflicts in practice policies. *JAMA*, **264**, 389–91.

Eddy DM (1991). What care is 'essential'? What services are 'basic'? *JAMA*, **265**, 782, 786–8.

Eddy DM (1994). Principles for making difficult decisions in difficult times. *JAMA*, **271**, 1792–8.

Editorial (1994). Population health looking upstream. *Lancet*, **343**, 429–30.

Egolf B, Lasker J, Wolf S, Potvin L. (1992). The Roseto effect: a 50-year comparison of mortality rates. *Am J Pub Health*, **82**, 1089–92.

Eliot G (1999). *Middlemarch*. Oxford University Press, Oxford.

Elliott P, Wakefield JC, Best NG, Briggs BJ (2000). *Spatial epidemiology—methods and applications*. Oxford University Press, Oxford.

Engaging Communities Learning Network and Natpact (2005). *Stories that can change your life: communities challenging health inequalities*. Department of Health, London.

Enkin M, Keirse MJN, Chalmers I (1989). A guide to effective care in pregnancy and childbirth. Oxford University Press, Oxford.

Enthoven A (1999). *Rock Carling Fellowship 1999. In pursuit of an improving National Health Service*. The Nuffield Trust, London.

European Commission: Public Health (2005). *Healthy life years in the core of the Lisbon strategy*. Available at: http://www.europa.eu.int/comm/health/ph_information/indicators/lifeyears_en.htm (accessed 25 June 2005).

Evans DA (1996). Stakeholder analysis of developments at the primary and secondary care interface. *Br J Gen Pract*, **46**, 675–7.

Fanshel S, Bush JW (1970). A health-status index and its application to health-services outcomes. *Operations Res*, **18**(6), 1021–66.

Farrant W (1994). Addressing the contradictions: health promotion and community health action in the United Kingdom. *Crit Public Health*, **5**, 5–17.

Feachem RGA, Sekhri NK, White KL (2002). Getting more for their dollar: a comparison of the NHS with California's Kaiser Permanente. *BMJ*, **324**(7330), 135–41.

Feinberg J (1973). *Social philosophy*. Prentice-Hall, Englewood Cliffs, NJ.

Fidler DP (2002). Global health governance: overview of the role of *international law in protecting and promoting global public health*, discussion paper No. 3. World Health Organization/London School of Hygiene and Tropical Medicine, Geneva/London. Available at: http://www.lshtm.ac.uk/cgch/Reports.htm (accessed 27 October 2004).

Fitch K, Bernstein SJ, Aguilar MD et al. (2001). *The RAND/UCLA appropriateness method user's manual*. RAND, Santa Monica, CA.

Fitzpatrick M (2001). *The tyranny of health—doctors and the regulation of lifestyle*. Routledge, London.

Fletcher SW (1997). Whither scientific deliberation in health policy recommendation? Alice in the wonderland of breast-cancer screening. *New Engl J Med*, **336**, 1180–3.

Flood RL and Jackson MC (1991). *Creative problem solving: total systems intervention*. Wiley, Chichester.

Florey CD (1993). Sample size for beginners. *BMJ*, **306**(6886), 1181–4.

Florin D, Coulter A (2001). Partnership in the primary care consultation. In: Gillam S, Brooks F (eds) *New beginnings—towards patient and public involvement in primary health care*. King's Fund, London.

Flowers J, Pencheon D (2002). *Introduction to health equity audit*. Eastern Region Public Health Observatory, Cambridge. Available at: http://www.erpho.org.uk/viewResource.aspx?id=6282 (accessed 22 January 2006).

Food and Agriculture Organization/World Health Organization (1992). *International conference on nutrition*. Food and Agriculture Organization, Rome.

Ford HL, Gerry EM (1999). Needs based services for people with MS. *Multiple Sclerosis*, **5**, S48.

Forrest C (2003). Primary care in the United States. Primary care gatekeeping and referrals: effective filter or failed experiment? *BMJ*, **326**, 692–5.

Forte P, Bowen T (1997). Improving the balance of elderly care services. In: Cropper S, Forte P (eds) *Enhancing health services management*, pp. 71–85. Open University Press, Buckingham.

Frankel S, Davey Smith G, Donovan J, Neal D (2003). Screening for prostate cancer. *Lancet*, **361**, 1122–8.

Frankel S, Eachus J, Pearson N et al. (1999). Population requirement for primary hip-replacement surgery: a cross-sectional study. *Lancet*, **353**(9161), 1304–9.

Freeman R (2000). *The politics of health in Europe*. Manchester University Press, New York.

Freidson E (1989). *Medical work in America (essays on health care)*. Yale University Press, New Haven, CT.

Freiman JA, Chalmers TC, Smith H Jr, Kuebler RR (1978). The importance of beta, the type II error and sample size in the design and interpretation of the randomized control trial. Survey of 71 'negative' trials. *N Engl J Med*, **299**(13), 690–4.

Fries JF (1980). Aging, natural death, and the compression of morbidity. *N Engl J Med*, **303**(3), 130–5.

Fung A (2003). SARS: how Singapore outmanaged the others. *Asia Times*, 9 April. Available at: http://www.atimes.com/atimes/china/ED09Ad03.html (accessed 30 September 2005).

Gabbay J (1999). The socially constructed dilemmas of academic public health. In: Griffiths S, Hunter DJ (eds) *Perspectives in public health*. Radcliffe Medical Press, Oxford.

Gakidou E, King G (2002). Measuring total health inequality: adding individual variation to group-level differences. *Int J Equity Health*, **1**(1), 3.

Gamm L (1998). Advancing community health through community health partnerships. *J Healthc Manag*, **43**, 51–67.

General Medical Council (2001). *Good medical practice*. General Medical Council, London. Available at: http://www.gmc-uk.org/standards/default.htm (accessed 25 April 2005).

General Practitioners Committee BMA (2003), *The NHS Confederation. Investing in General Practice. The New General Medical Services Contract*. The NHS Confederation, London.

Gigerenzer G (2003). Reckoning with risk: learning to live with uncertainty. Penguin, London.

Gill R (2000). Discourse analysis. In: Bauer MW, Gaskell G (eds) Qualitative researching with text, image and sound. Sage, London.

Gillam S (2004). What can we learn about quality of care from US health maintenance organisations? *Qual Primary Care*, **12**, 3–4.

Gillam S, Meads G (2001). *Modernisation and the future of general practice*. King's Fund, London.

Glaser BG, Strauss AL (1967). The discovery of grounded theory: strategies for qualitative research. Aldine, Chicago, IL.

Goddard M, Smith P (1998). *Equity of access to health care*. University of York, Centre for Health Economics, York.

Goddard M, Smith P (2001). Equity of access to health care services: theory and evidence from the UK. *Soc Sci Med*, **53**, 1149–62.

Gold RL (1958). Roles in sociological fieldwork. *Social Forces*, **36**, 217–23.

Goleman D (2000). Leadership that gets results. *Harvard Business Rev*, **78**, 78–90.

Goodman C (1996). A basic methodology toolkit. In: Szczepura A, Kankaapaa J (eds) Assessment of health care technologies. Wiley, Chichester.

Gostin LO (2004). International infectious disease law: revision of the World Health Organization's International Health Regulations. *J Am Med Assoc*, **291**, 2623–7.

Gostin LO (2004). Law and ethics in population health. *Aust NZ J Public Health*, **28**, 7–12.

Gostin LO, Sapsin JW, Teret SP et al. (2002). The Model State Emergency Health Powers Act: planning and response to bioterrorism and naturally occurring infectious diseases. *J Am Med Assoc*, **288**, 622–8.

Gould SJ (1998). The median isn't the message. In: Greenhalgh T, Hurwitz B (eds) Narrative based medicine, pp. 29–33. BMJ Books, London.

Grad FP (1990). *Public health law manual*. American Public Health Association, Washington, DC.

Grainger C (2002). Mentoring—supporting doctors at work and play. BMJ *Career Focus*, **324**, S203. Available at: http://careerfocus.bmjjournals.com/cgi/content/full/324/7353/S203 (accessed 1 October 2005).

Gray JA (1999) Post-modern medicine. *Lancet*, **354**, 1550–30.

Gray JAM (1997) *Evidence-based healthcare – how to make health policy and management decisions*. Churchill Livingstone, London.

Gray S, Pilkington P, Pencheon D, Jewell T (2006). Public health in the UK: success or failure? *J R Soc Med*, **99**, 107–11.

Greco PJ, Eisenberg JM (1993). Changing physicians' practices. University of Pennsylvania School of Medicine, Philadelphia 19104. *N Engl J Med*, **329**(17), 1271–3.

Green A (1999). *An introduction to health planning in developing countries*. Oxford University Press, Oxford.

Greenhalgh T(1997). *How to read a paper – the basics of evidence based medicine.* BMJ Books, London.

Greenhalgh T, Roberts G, Macfarland F, *et al.* (2004). Diffusion of innovations in service organizations: systematic review and recommendations. *Milbank Q*, **82**(4), 581–629.

Greenhalgh T, Herxheimer A, Isaacs AJ, Beaman M, Morris J, Farrow S (2000). Commercial partnerships in chronic disease management: proceeding with caution. *BMJ*, **320**, 566–8.

Grimshaw JG, Thomas RE, MacLennan G *et al.* (2004). Effectiveness and efficiency of guideline dissemination and implementation strategies. *Health Technol Assess*, **8**(6).

Grol R (1997). Beliefs and evidence in changing clinical practice. *BMJ*, **315**, 418–21.

Grol R, Baker R, Moss F (2002). Quality improvement research: understanding the science of change in health care. *Qual Saf Health Care*, **11**(2), 110–11.

Grol R, Baker R, Moss F (ed.) (2004). *Quality improvement research: understanding the science of change in health care.* BMJ Publishing, London.

Grol R, Wensing M, Eccles M (ed.) (2005). *Improving patient care. The implementation of change in clinical practice.* Elsevier, London.

Gruenberg EM (1977). The failures of success. *Milbank Memorial Fund Q*, **55**(1), 3–24.

Guy M (2001). Diabetes: developing a local strategy. In: Pencheon D, Guest C, Melzer D, Muir Gray JA (eds) *Oxford handbook of public health practice*, 1st edn, p. 559. Oxford University Press, Oxford.

Gwatkin DR, Guillot M, Heuveline P (1999). The burden of disease among the global poor. *Lancet*, **354**, 586–9.

Haegebaert S, Duche L, Desenclos JC (2003). The use of the case-crossover design in a continuous common source food-borne outbreak. *Epidemiol Infect*, **131**(2), 809–13.

Haga SB, Khoury MJ, Burke W (2003). Genomic profiling to promote a health lifestyle: not ready for prime time. *Nat Genet*, **34**, 347–50.

Hahn RA (1999). *Anthropology in public health.* Oxford University Press, Oxford.

Halliday JL, Collins VR, Aitken MA, Richards MPM, Olsson CA (2004). Genetics and public health—evolution, or revolution? *J Epidemiol Commun Health*, **58**, 894–9.

Ham C (2005). Lost in translation? Health systems in the US and the UK. *Soc Policy Admin*, **39**, 192–209.

Ham C, Hunter DJ, Robinson R (1995). Evidence based policy making. *BMJ*, **310**, 71–2.

Ham C, York N, Sutch S, Shaw R (2003). Hospital bed utilisation in the NHS, Kaiser Permanente, and the US Medicare programme: analysis of routine data. *BMJ*, **327**(7426), 1257.

Hamer L, Jacobson B, Flowers J, Johnstone F (January 2003). *Health equity audit made simple: a briefing for Primary Care Trusts and local strategic partnerships working document.* Available at: www.phel.gov.uk/knowledge/equityauditfina121.1.3.pdf (accessed 30 June 2005).

Hamlin C, Sheard S (1998). Revolutions in public health: 1848 and 1998? *BMJ*, **317**, 587–91.

Hanley B, Bradburn J, Barnes M et al. (2004). In: Steel R (ed) *Involving the public in NHS, public health and social care research: briefing notes for researchers*, 2nd edn, p. ii. INVOLVE, Eastleigh.

Harrington JM, Gill FS, Aw TC, Gardiner K (1998). *Pocket consultant: occupational health*, 4th edn. Blackwell Science, Oxford.

Harrington JM, Stein GF, Rivera RO, de Morales AV (1978). Occupational hazards of formulating oral contraceptives—a survey of plant employees. *Arch Environ Health*, **33**, 12–15.

Hart JT (1971). The inverse care law. *Lancet*, **1**(7696), 405–12.

Harvard University Gazette (2004). *Six new sustainability principles adopted*. Available at: http://www.news.harvard.edu/gazette/2004/10.14/09-sustain.html (accessed 13 December 2004).

Harvey I (1994). How can we determine if living close to industry harms your health?. *BMJ*, **309**, 425–6.

Hauck K, Shaw R, Smith PC (2002). Reducing avoidable inequalities in health: a new criterion for setting health care capitation payments. *Health Econ*, **II**, 667–77.

Health Evidence Network, World Health Organization Regional Office for Europe (2003). *Are disease management programmes (DMPs) effective in improving quality of care for people with chronic conditions?* WHO Regional Office for Europe, Copenhagen. Available at: http://www.euro.who.int/eprise/main/WHO/Progs/HEN/Syntheses/DMP/20030820_1 (accessed 10 June 2005).

Health Policy (1995) **33**. Special issue devoted to programme budgeting and marginal analysis.

Heath I (1995). *The mystery of general practice*, pp. 5–14. Nuffield Provincial Hospitals Trust, London.

Hemingway H, Crook AM, Banerjee S et al. (2001). Hypothetical ratings of coronary angiography appropriateness: are they associated with actual angiographic findings, mortality, and revascularisation rate? The ACRE study. *Heart*, **85**(6), 672–9.

Hemingway H, Marmot MG (1999). Evidence based cardiology: psychosocial factors in the aetiology and prognosis of coronary heart disease: systematic review of prospective cohort studies. *BMJ*, **318**, 1460–7.

Hicks NR (1994). Some observations on attempts to measure appropriateness of care. *BMJ*, **309**(6956), 730–3.

Hills M (1996). Some comments on methods for investigating disease risk around a point source. In: Eliott P, Cuzick J, English D, Stern R (eds) *Geographical and environmental epidemiology methods for small-area studies*, pp. 231–7. Oxford University Press, Oxford.

HMSO (2003). *Health and Social Care (Community Health and Standards) Act 2003*. HMSO, London.

Holland WW, Stewart S (1997). *Public health the vision and the challenge, Rock Carling Fellowship monograph*. Nuffield Trust, London.

Horton R (1998). The *new* new public health of risk and radical engagement. *Lancet*, **352**, 251–2.

Hrudey SE, Hrudey EJ (2004). *Safe drinking water—lessons from recent outbreaks in affluent nations*. IWA Publishing, London.

Hulscher MEJL, Wensing M, van der Weijden T, Grol R (2001). Interventions to implement prevention in primary care (Cochrane review). In: *The Cochrane library*, Issue 1. Update Software, Oxford.

Hunter D (2002). Management and public health. In: *Oxford textbook of public health*. Oxford University Press, Oxford.

Hurwitz B (1999). Legal and polical considerations of clinical practice guidelines. *BMJ*, **318**, 661–4.

Independent inquiry into inequalities in health (The Acheson report). The Stationery Office, London, 1998.

Institute for Healthcare Improvement (2003). *The Breakthrough Series: IHI's collaborative model for achieving breakthrough improvement*, IHI Innovation Series. Institute for Healthcare Improvement, Boston, MA.

Institute of Medicine (2003). *The future of the public's health in the 21st century*. National Academies Press, Washington, DC.

Institute of Medicine. *The future of public health* (1988) and *Health communities: new partnerships for the future of public health* (1996). Institute of Medicine, Washington, DC. Both available from http://www.nap.edu/ (accessed 25 April 2005).

International Agency for Research on Cancer (2004). *Tobacco smoking and involuntary smoking*, IARC Monographs on the Evaluation of Carcinogenic Risks to Humans Vol. 83. IARC, Lyon.

Ison E (2002). *Rapid appraisal tool for health impact assessment. A task-based approach*. Available at: http://www.phel.nice.org.uk/hiadocs/rapidappraisal%20tool_full_document.pdf (accessed 15 June 2005).

Jacobs R, Gabbay J (1994). *An action research report on audit in public health departments*. Faculty of Public Health Medicine of the Royal College of Physicians of the United Kingdom, London.

Jacobson B (2002). Delaying tactics. *Health Service J*, **112**(5793), 22.

Jain A, Ogden J (1999). General practitioners' experiences of patients' complaints: qualitative study. *BMJ*, **318**, 1596–9.

Janis JL (1982). *Groupthink*, 2nd edn. Houghton Mifflin, Boston, MA.

Jenkin R, Frommer M (2005). *A framework for developing or analyzing health policy*. The University of Sydney, Australia.

Jenkinson C, Coulter A, Bruster S (2002). The Picker patient experience questionnaire: development and validation using data from in-patient surveys in five countries. *Int J Qual Health Care*, **14**(5), 353–8.

Jewell D (1992). Setting standards: from passing fashion to essential clinical activity. *Qual Health Care*, **1**(4), 217–18.

Jones M (2000). Walk-in primary care centres: lessons from Canada. *BMJ*, **321**, 928–31.

Jordan J, Dowswell T, Harrison S, Lilford R, Mort M (1998). Whose priorities? Listening to users and the public. *BMJ*, **316**(7145), 1668–70.

Kaeferstein FK, Motarjemi Y, Bettcher DW (1997). Foodborne disease control: a transnational challenge. *Emerg Infect Dis*, **3**, 503–10.

Kahan JP, Park RE, Leape LL et al. (1996). Variations by specialty in physician ratings of the appropriateness and necessity of indications for procedures. *Med Care*, **34**(6), 512–23.

Kanavos PG, McKee M (2000). Cross-border issues in the provision of health services: Are we moving towards a European Health Policy? *J Health Serv Res Policy*, **5**, 231–6.

Kassirer JP (1993). The quality of care and the quality of measuring it. *N Engl J Med*, **329**(17), 1263–5.

Kassirer JP (1994). Incorporating patients' preferences into medical decisions. *N Engl J Med*, **330**, 1895–6.

Kemm J, Ballard S, Harmer M (2001). *Health impact assessment of the new home energy efficiency scheme*. National Assembly for Wales, Cardiff.

Ketley D, Woods KL (1993). Impact of clinical trials on clinical practice: example of thrombolysis for acute myocardial infarction. *Lancet*, **342**, 891–4.

Khaw K (1994). Genetics and environment: Geoffrey Rose revisited. *Lancet*, **343**, 838–9.

Khoury MJ, Little J, Burke W (2004). *Human genome epidemiology*. Oxford University Press, Oxford.

Khoury MJ, Thomson E (eds) (2000). *Genetics and public health in the 21st century*. Oxford University Press, Oxford.

Khoury MJ, Yang Q, Gwinn M, Little J, Dana Flanders W (2004). An epidemiologic assessment of genomic profiling for measuring susceptibility to common diseases and targeting interventions. *Genet Med*, **6**, 38–47.

Kibble A, Dyer J, Wheeldon C, Saunders PJ (2003). Public-health surveillance for chemical incidents. *Lancet*, **357**(9265), 1365.

Kindshauer MK (ed.) (2003). *Communicable diseases 2002—global defence against the infectious disease threat*, WHO/CDS/2003.15. World Health Organization, Geneva. Available at: http://www.who.int/infectious-disease-news/cds2002/intro.pdf.

King M (1990). Health is a sustainable state. *Lancet*, **336**, 664–7.

King's Fund (2004). *Public attitudes to public health policy*. Kings Fund Publications, London.

Kinmonth A-L, Marteau T (2002). Screening for cardiovascular risk: public health imperative or matter for individual informed choice? *BMJ*, **325**, 78–80.

Kirkwood BR (1997). *Measures of mortality and morbidity. Essentials of medical statistics*, pp. 106–17 Blackwell Scientific Publications, Oxford.

Klein R (1991). Risk and benefits of comparative studies: notes from another shore. *Milbank Q*, **69**(2), 275–91.

Knight K, Badamgarav E, Henning JM et al. (2005). A systematic review of diabetes disease management programs. *Am J Managed Care*, **11**, 242–50.

Kolb DA (1984). *Experiential learning: experience as the source of learning and development*. Prentice-Hall, Englewood Cliffs, NJ.

Kotter J (1990). *A force for change*. Harvard Business School Press, Boston, MA.

Kramer M (1980). The rising pandemic of mental disorders and associated chronic diseases and disabilities. *Acta Psychiatr Scand*, **62**(Suppl. 285), 382–97.

Krause E (1996). *Death of the guilds: professions, states, and the advance of capitalism, 1930 to the present*. Yale University Press, New Haven, CT.

Kravitz RL, Laouri M, Kahan JP et al. (1995). Validity of criteria used for detecting underuse of coronary revascularization. J Am Med Assoc, **274**(8), 632–8.

Krieger N, Northridge M, Gruskin S et al. (2003). Assessing health impact assessment: multidisciplinary and international perspectives. J Epidemiol Commun Health, **57**, 659–62.

Kunst AE, Groenhof F, Borgan JK et al. Socio-economic inequalities in mortality. Methodological problems illustrated with three examples from Europe. Rev Epidemiol Sante Publique, **46**(6), 467–79.

Kvale S (1996). Interviews: an introduction to qualitative research interviewing. Sage, Thousand Oaks, CA.

Labonte R (1993). Community development and partnerships. Can J Public Health, **84**, 237–40.

Laditka SB, Wolf DA (1998). New methods for analysing active life expectancy. J. Aging Health, **10**(2), 214–41.

Land KL, Guralnik JM, Blazer DG (1994). Estimating increment-decrement life tables with multiple covariates from panel data: the case of active life expectancy. Demography, **31**(2), 297–319.

Langham S, Basnett I, McCartney P et al. (2003). Addressing the inverse care law in cardiac services. J Public Health Med, **25**(3), 202–7.

Langley GJ et al. (1996). The improvement guide: a practical approach to enhancing organizational performance, 1st edn. Jossey-Bass, San Francisco, CA.

Lasker RD and the Committee on Medicine and Public Health (1997). Medicine and public health: the power of collaboration. New York Academy of Medicine, New York.

Last JM (1983). A dictionary of epidemiology. Oxford University Press, New York.

Le Grand J (1984). Equity as an economic objective. J Appl Phil, **1**, 39–51.

Le Grand J (1993). Can we afford the welfare state? BMJ, **307**, 1018–9.

Leape LL (2000). Institute of Medicine medical error figures are not exaggerated. J Am Med Assoc, **284**(1), 95–7.

Leask J, Chapman S (1998). 'An attempt to swindle nature': press reportage of anti immunisation, Australia 1993–97. Aust NZ J Public Health, **22**, 17–26.

LeBlanc R (1997). Definitions of oppression. Nurs Inq, **4**, 257–61.

Lee-Treweek G (2000). The insight of emotional danger: research experiences in a home for the elderly. In: Lee-Treweek G, Linkogle S (eds) Danger in the field: risk and ethics in social research. Routledge, London.

Leichter HM (1979). A comparative approach to policy analysis: health care policy in four nations. Cambridge University Press, Cambridge.

Leon DA, Morton S, Cannegieter S, McKee M (2003). Understanding the health of Scotland's population in an international context. London School of Hygiene and Tropical Medicine, London.

Leukaemia Research Fund (1997). Handbook and guide to the investigation of clusters of disease. Leukaemia Research Fund Centre for Clinical Epidemiology, University of Leeds.

Lewis R, Gillam S (eds) (1999). Transforming primary care. Personal medical services in the new NHS. King's Fund, London.

Liberati A, Sheldon T, Banta HD (1997). Eurassess project subgroup report on methodology—methodological guidance for the conduct of health technology assessment. *Int J Technol Assess Health Care*, **13**(2), 186–219.

Lilford RJ, Pauker SG, Braunholtz DA, Chard J (1998). Decision analysis and the implementation of research findings. *BMJ*, **317**, 405–9.

Lilford RJ, Pauker SG, Braunholtz DA, Chard J (1998). Getting research findings into practice: decision analysis and the implementation of research findings. *BMJ*, **317**, 405–9.

Lilienfeld AM, Lilienfeld DE (1980). *Foundations of epidemiology*. Oxford University Press, New York.

Lindberg W, McMorland J. From grassroots to business suits: the gay community response to AIDS. In: Davis P (ed.) *Intimate details and vital statistics. Aids, sexuality and the social order in New Zealand*. Auckland University Press, Auckland.

Livelihoods Connect. Creating sustainable livelihood to eliminate poverty. Available at: http://www.livelihoods.org/ (accessed 29 June 2005).

Lloyd EL (1999). The role of cold in ischaemic heart disease: a review. *Public Health*, **105**, 205–15.

Logie D (1992). The great exterminator of children. *BMJ*, **304**, 1423–6.

Lohr KN (1990). *Medicare: a strategy for quality assurance*. National Academy Press, Washington, DC.

Lomas J (1993). Making clinical policy explicit. Legislative policy making and lessons for developing practice guidelines. *International Journal of Technology Assessment in Health Care*, **9**(1), 11–25.

Lomas J, Sisk JE, Stocking B (1993). From evidence to practice in the United States, the United Kingdom, and Canada. *Milbank Quarterly*, **71**, 405–10.

Longhurst R (1987). Rapid rural appraisal: an improved means of information-gathering for rural development and nutrition projects. *Food Nutr*, **13**, 44–7.

Long SH, Marquis MS (1999). Geographic variation in physician visits for uninsured children. *J Am Med Assoc*, **281**, 2035–40.

Luft J, Ingham H (1955). The Johari-window: a graphic model for *interpersonal relations*. University of California, Western Training Laboratory, Los Angeles, CA.

Mackenbach J, Stronks K (2002). A strategy for tackling health inequalities in the Netherlands. *BMJ*, **325**, 1029–32.

Mackenbach JP, Kunst AE (1997). Measuring the magnitude of socio-economic inequalities in health: an overview of available measures illustrated with two examples from Europe. *Soc Sci Med*, **44**(6), 757–71.

MacLehose L, McKee M, Weinberg J (2002). Responding to the challenge of communicable disease in Europe. *Science*, **295**, 2047–50.

Mahoney M, Simpson S, Harris E, Aldrich R, Stewart Williams J (2004). *Equity focused health impact assessment framework*. Australasian Collaboration for Health Equity Impact Assessment, Newcastle, NSW. Available at: http://chetre.med.unsw.edu.au/files/EFHIA_Framework.pdf (accessed 15 June 2005).

Mannheim JB, Rich RC (1995). *Empirical political analysis: research methods in political science*, 4th edn. Longman, New York.

Manor O, Matthews S, Power C (1997). Comparing measures of health inequality. *Soc Sci Med*, **45**(5), 761–71.

Mant D, Fowler G (1990). Mass screening: theory and ethics. *BMJ*, **300**(6729), 916–8.

Mant J, Hicks N (1995). Detecting differences in quality of care: the sensitivity of measures of process and outcome in treating acute myocardial infarction. *BMJ*, **311**(7008), 793–6.

Manton KG (1982). Changing concepts of morbidity and mortality in the elderly population. *Milbank Memorial Fund Q*, **60**, 183–244.

Margo CE (2004). Quality care and practice variation: the roles of practice guidelines and public profiles. *Surv Ophthalmol*, **49**, 359–71.

Marmot M (2004). Status syndrome: how your social standing affects your health and life expectancy. Bloomsbury, London.

Marmot M, Wilkinson RG (eds) (1999). *Social determinants of health*. Oxford University Press, Oxford.

Marmot MG, Davey Smith G, Stansfeld S, Patel C, North F, Head J (1991). Health inequalities among British civil servants: the Whitehall II study. *Lancet*, **337**, 1387–93.

Marshall EC, Spiegelhalter DJ (1998). Reliability of league tables of in vitro fertilisation clinics: retrospective analysis of live birth rates. *BMJ*, **316**, 1701–5.

Marshall MN, Shekelle PG, Leatherman S, Brook RH (2000). The public release of performance data: what do we expect to gain? A review of the evidence. *J Am Med Assoc*, **283**(14), 1866–74.

Marshall MN, Shekelle PG, McGlynn EA, Campbell S, Brook RH, Roland MO (2003). Can health care quality indicators be transferred between countries? *Qual Saf Health Care*, **12**(1), 8–12.

Mathers CD, Robine J-M (1997). How good is Sullivan's method for monitoring changes in population health expectancies. *J Epidemiol Commun Health*, **51**, 80–6.

Mathers N, Hodgkin P (1989). The gatekeeper and the wizard: a fairy tale. *BMJ*, **298**, 172–4.

Maxwell RJ (1984). Quality assessment in health. *BMJ*, **288**, 1470–2.

Maxwell RJ (1992). Dimensions of quality revisited: from thought to action. *Qual Health Care*, **1**, 171–7.

McAlister FA, Lawson FME, Teo KK, Armstrong PW (2001). A systematic review of randomized trials of disease management programs in heart failure. *Am J Med*, **110**, 378–84.

McCallion G (1993). Planning care for elderly people. *Health Serv Manage Sci*, **6**(4), 218–28.

McCarthy N, Giesecke J (1999). Case-case comparisons to study causation of common infectious diseases. *Int J Epidemiol*, **28**(4), 764–8.

McClellan M, Brook RH (1992). Appropriateness of care. A comparison of global and outcome methods to set standards. *Med Care*, **30**(7), 565–86.

McGlynn EA, Asch SM, Adams J et al. (2003). The quality of health care delivered to adults in the United States. *N Engl J Med*, **348**(26), 2635–45.

McGuire A, Henderson J, Mooney G (1988). *The economics of health care: an introductory text*. Routledge, London.

McKee M, Healy J (eds) (2002). *Hospitals in a changing Europe*. European Observatory on Health Care Systems, Open University Press, Buckingham.

McKee M, Mossialos E, Baeten R (eds) (2002). The impact of EU law on health care systems. Peter Lang, Brussels.

McKee M, Rechel B, Schwalbe N (2004). Health and the wider European neighbourhood. EuroHealth, **10**, (3–4), 7–9.

McKinlay JB (1993). The promotion of health through planned sociopolitical change: challenges for research and policy. Soc Sci Med, **36**(2), 109–17.

McMichael AJ (1993). Planetary overload: global environmental change and the health of the human species. Cambridge University Press, Cambridge.

McMichael AJ, Campbell-Lendrum DH, Corvalán CF et al. (2003). Climate change and human health—risks and responses. World Health Organization, Geneva.

McNeil BJ, Pauker SG, Sox HC, Tversky A (1982). On the elicitation of preferences for alternative therapies. N Engl J Med, **306**, 1259–62.

McWhinnie JR (1981). Disability assessment in population surveys: results of the OECD common development effort. Rev Epidémiol Santé Publique, **29**, 413–19.

Médecins sans Frontières (1999). 1999:year in review. Médecins sans Frontières, Brussels.

Melville B (1993). Rapid rural appraisal: its role in health planning in developing countries. Trop Doct, **23**, 55–8.

Metz CE (1978). Basic principles of ROC analysis. Seminars in Nuclear Medicine, **8**(4), 283–98.

Midgley G (2000). Systemic intervention: philosophy, methodology, and practice. Kluwer Academic/Plenum, New York.

Milio N (1987). Making healthy public policy: developing the science by learning the art. Health Promotion Int, **2**, 263–74.

Mills PD, Weeks WB (2004). Characteristics of successful quality improvement teams: lessons from five collaborative projects in the VHA. Jt Comm J Qual Saf, **30**(3), 152–62.

Milne R, Clegg A, Stevens A (2003). HTA responses and the classic HTA report. J Public Health Med, **25**(2), 102–6.

Milner S, Bailey C, Deans J, Pettigrew D (2003). Integrated impact assessment: UK mapping project report. Northumbria University, Newcastle. Available at: http://www.phel.nice.org.uk/hiadocs/Integrated_impact_assessment_report_final.pdf (accessed 15 June 2005).

Milner SJ, Bailey C, Deans J (2003). 'Fit for purpose' health impact assessment: a realistic way forward. Public Health, **117**, 295–300.

Mitchell E, Scragg R, Stewart A et al. (1991). Results from the first year of the New Zealand Cot Death Study. NZ Med J, **104**, 71–6.

Moeller DW (2005). Environmental health, 3rd edn. Harvard University Press, Cambridge, MA.

Mohammed MA, Cheng KK, Rouse A, Marshall T (2001). Use of Shewhart's technique. Lancet, **358**(9280), 512.

Molla MT, Madans JH, Wagener DK, Crimmins EM (2003). Summary measures of population health: report of findings on methodological and data issues. Publication No. 2004–1258. US DHHS, Hyattsville, MD.

Molla MT, Wagener DK, Madans JH (2001). Summary measures of population health: methods for calculating healthy life expectancy. Statistical notes no. 21, pp. 1–21. National Centre for Health Statistics, Hyattsville, MD.

Monk R (1991). Ludwig Wittgenstein: the duty of genius. Vintage, London.

Montgomery AA, Fahey T (2001). How do patients' treatment preferences compare with those of clinicians? *Qual Health Care*, **10**(Suppl I), i39–i43.

Mooney G, Gerard K, Donaldson C, Farrar S (1992). *Priority setting in purchasing: some practical guidelines*, Research Paper 6. National Association of Health Authorities and Trusts (NAHAT), Birmingham.

Moore G (2000). *Managing to do better. General practice for the twenty-first century*. Office of Health Economics, London.

Morgan MG (1993). Risk analysis and management. *Sci Am*, July, 24–30.

Morgan MG, Fischhoff B, Bostrom A, Lave L, Atman C (1992). Communicating risk to the public. *Environ Sci Technol*, **26**, 2048–56.

Morrow RH, Hyder AA, Murray CJ, Lopez AD (1998). Measuring the burden of disease. *Lancet*, **352**(9143), 1859–61.

Moss SM (1991). Case-control studies of screening. *Int J Epidemiol*, **20**, 1–6.

Mossialos E, Dixon A, Figueras J et al. (eds) (2002). *Funding health care: options for Europe*. European Observatory on Health Care Systems, Open University Press, Buckingham.

Mossialos E, McKee M (2002). *EU law and the social character of health care*. Peter Lang, Brussels.

Mossialos E, McKee M (2002). Health care and the European Union. *BMJ*, **324**(7344), 991–2.

Muir CS, Fraumeni JF Jr, Doll R (1994). The interpretation of time trends. *Cancer Surv*, **19–20**, 5–21.

Mullan F, Epstein L (2002). Community-oriented primary care: new relevance in a changing world. *Am J Public Health*, **92**, 1748–55.

Mulley AG, Eagle KA (1988). What is inappropriate care? *JAMA*, **260**, 540–1.

Mulley AG, Mendoza G, Rockefeller R, Staker L (1996). Involving patients in medical decision making. *Quality Connection*, **5**, 5–7.

Murray C, Lopez AD (1997). Mortality by cause for eight regions of the world: Global Burden of Disease Study. *Lancet*, **349**, 1269–76.

Murray CJ, Lopez AD (1997). Global mortality, disability, and the contribution of risk factors: Global Burden of Disease Study. *Lancet*, **349**(9063), 1436–42.

Murray CJL, Salomon JA, Mathers C (1999). *A critical examination of summary measures of population health*. World Health Organization, Geneva (GPE discussion paper No. 12, quoted in *WHO World Health Report 2000*).

Murray CJL, Salomon JA, Mathers CD, Lopez AD (eds) (2002). *Summary measures of population health*. World Health Organization, Geneva.

National Centre for Health Statistics. *National Health Interview Survey (NHIS)*. Available at: www.cdc.gov/nchs/nhis.htm (accessed 20 March 2005).

National Committee for Quality Assurance (2005). *The Health Plan Employer Data and Information Set (HEDIS®)*. National Committee for Quality Assurance, Washington, DC. Available at: http://www.ncqa.org/Programs/HEDIS/ (accessed 6 June 2005).

National Guidelines Clearinghouse. www.guideline.gov/index.asp (accessed 27 July 2000).

National Health and Medical Research Council (Australia) (1999). *A guide to the development, implementation and evaluation of clinical practice guidelines.* National Health and Medical Research Council (NHMRC), Canberra.

National Healthcare Disparities Report. Available at: http://www.ahrq.gov/qual/nhdr02/prenhdr.htm (accessed 28 June 2005).

National Institute for Health and Clinical Excellence (2005). *Social value judgements: guidelines for the Institute and its advisory bodies. Draft for consultation.* National Institute for Health and Clinical Excellence, London.

National Public Health Partnership (2000). *A planning framework for public health practice.* National Public Health Partnership, Melbourne, Australia.

National Public Health Partnership (2000). *Deciding and specifying an intervention portfolio.* National Public Health Partnership, Melbourne.

National Public Health Partnership (2000). *Public health practice in Australia today: a statement of core functions.* National Public Health Partnership, Melbourne.

National Research Council (1989). *Improving risk communication.* National Academy Press, Washington, DC.

National screening programme for sight-threatening retinopathy. Available at: http://www.nscretinopathy.org.uk/pages/nsc.asp?ModT=A&Sec=16 (accessed 20 September 2005).

National Statistics, Official UK statistics. www.statistics.gov.uk (accessed 20 March 2005); Statistics Canada, Canadian statistics. http://www40.statcan.ca/z01/cs0002_e.htm (accessed 8 September 2005); National Centre for Health Statistics, US statistics. http://www.cdc.gov/nchs/ (accessed 21 March 2005).

Navarro V (1999). Health and equity in the world in the era of 'globalisation'. *Int J Health Serv*, **29**(2), 215–26.

Nelson B, Economy P (1997). *Consulting for dummies.* IDG Publications, Foster City, CA.

Nemery B, Fischler B, Boogaerts M, Lison D (1999). Dioxins, Coca-Cola, and mass sociogenic illness in Belgium. *Lancet*, **354**, 77.

Neuhauser D, Lweicki AM (1975). What do we gain from the sixth stool guaiac? *N Engl J Med*, **293**(5), 226–8.

Neutra R, Swan S, Mack T (1992). Clusters galore: insights about environmental clusters from probability theory. *Sci Total Environ*, **127**(1–2), 187–200.

New South Wales Department of Health (2000). *Strategic directions for health.* NSW Health Department, Sydney, Australia.

New York University School of Medicine (2005). *Literature, arts and medicine database.* Available at: http://endeavour.med.nyu.edu/lit-med/lit-med-db/ index.html (accessed 8 September 2005).

New Zealand Ministry of Health (2002). *Reducing inequalities intervention framework in reducing inequalities in health.* Ministry of Health, Wellington.

Newton J, Garner S (2002). Disease registers in England. Report for the Department of Health policy research programme. Available from www.erpho.org.uk (accessed 25 June 2005).

NHS (1998). *National Health Service breast screening programme. Guidelines on quality assurance visits.* NHS BSP (Breast Screening Programme) publication no 40, appendix 2. NHSBSP Publications, Sheffield.

NHS Appointments Commission (2003). *Governing the NHS: a guide for NHS boards.* NHS Appointments Commission, London.

NHS Centre for Reviews and Dissemination (1996). *Undertaking systematic reviews of research on effectiveness,* CRD Report no 4. University of York, York.

NHS Centre for Reviews and Dissemination (2000). *Evidence from systematic reviews of the research relevant to implementing the 'wider public health' agenda.* NHS Centre for Reviews and Dissemination, University of York, York.

NHS Confederation (2004). The development of integrated governance. *Debate* **3**.

NHS Executive (1999). *Clinical governance. Quality in the new NHS,* HSC 1999/065. Department of Health, London.

NHS Executive North Thames Region (1998). *Clinical Governance in North Thames: a paper for discussion and consultation.* NHS North Thames Region Office, London.

NHS Management Executive (1993). *Health Service Guidelines HSG(93)38: arrangements to deal with health aspects of chemical contamination incidents.* Department of Health, Health Aspects of the Environment and Food Division, London.

NHS Management Executive (1993). *Health Service Guidelines HSG(93)56: public health:responsiblities of the NHS and the roles of others.* Department of Health, Health Aspects of the Environment and Food Division, London.

NHS Modernisation Agency (2002). *Improvement leaders guide to setting up a collaborative programme.* Department of Health, London.

NHS National electronic Library for Health. http://www.nelh.nhs.uk/ (accessed 28 December 2004).

NICE (2003). *Full guidance on human growth hormone (somatropin) in adults with growth hormone deficiency,* no 64. National Institute for Clinical Excellence, London. Available at http://www.nice.org.uk/ page.aspx?o=83428 (accessed 28 December 2004).

NICE (2004). *Guide to the methods of technology appraisal.* National Institute for Clinical Excellence, London. Available at: http://www. nice.org.uk/pdf/TAP_Methods.pdf (accessed 28 December 2004).

Noji E (ed.) (1997). *The public health consequences of disasters.* Oxford University Press, New York.

Normand ST, Landrum MB, Guadagnoli E et al. (2001). Validating recommendations for coronary angiography following acute myocardial infarction in the elderly: a matched analysis using propensity scores. *J Clin Epidemiol,* **54**(4), 387–98.

Nutbeam D (2003). How does evidence influence public health policy? Tackling health inequalities in England. *Health Promotion J Aust,* **14**(3), 154–8.

O'Dea JF, Kilham RJ (2002). The inverse care law is alive and well in general practice. *Med J Aust* **177**(2), 78–9.

O'Carroll PW, Yasnoff WA, Ward ME, Ripp LH, Martin EL (eds) (2003). *Public health informatics and information systems.* Springer-Verlag, New York.

O'Connor AM, Stacey D, Rovner D et al. (2001). Decision aids for people facing health treatment or screening decisions. *Cochrane Database Syst Rev*, **3**, CD001431.

O'Keefe E, Scott-Samuel A (2002). Human rights and wrongs: could health impact assessment help? *J Law Med Ethics*, **30**, 734–8.

O'Keefe E, Scott-Samuel A. Health impact assessment: towards globalization as if people mattered. In: Kawachi I, Wamala S. (eds) *Globalization and health*. Oxford University Press, Oxford. (In press.)

Office of National Statistics (2004). Healthy life expectancy in Great Britain. *Health Statist Q*, **22**, 2.

Otten AL (1992). The influence of the mass media on health policy. *Health Affairs*, winter, 111–18.

Oxfam (1999). *Annual review 1998–9*. Oxfam, London.

Oxford English Dictionary (2000). OED Online, 2nd edn. Oxford University Press, Oxford.

Oxman AD, Sackett DL, Guyatt G (1993). Users' guides to the medical literature. I. How to get started. The Evidence-Based Medicine Working Group. *J Am Med Assoc*, **270**, 2093–5.

Oxman AD, Thomson MA, Davis DA, Haynes RB (1995). No magic bullets: a systematic review of 102 trials of interventions to improve professional practice. *Can Med Assoc J*, **153**, 1423–31.

Palmer CR (1993). Probablity of recurrence of extreme data: an aid to decision-making. *Lancet*, **342**(8875), 845–7.

Palmer G (1993). *The politics of breast-feeding*. Pandora, London.

Parkin DM, Whelan SL, Ferlay J, Teppo L, Thomas DB (2003). Cancer incidence in five continents, Vol. VIII. IARC, Lyon.

Patterson J (2004). *Health impact assessment of the North Huyton New Deal for Communities programme*. North Huyton NDC and Knowsley Primary Care Trust, Huyton.

Paul B (1955). *Health, culture and community*. The Sage Foundation, New York.

Paxton A (2001). The food miles report. Sustainable Agriculture, Food and Environment (SAFE) Alliance, London.

Payne N, Saul C (1997). Variations in use of cardiology services in a health authority: comparison of coronary artery revascularisation rates with prevalence of angina and coronary mortality. *BMJ*, **314**, 256–61.

Pencheon D (1998). Matching demand and supply fairly and efficiently. *BMJ*, **316**, 1665–7.

Peto R, Lopez AD, Boreham J, Thun M, Heath C Jr (1992). Mortality from tobacco in developed countries: indirect estimation from national vital statistics. *Lancet*, **339**(8804), 1268–78.

Petts J, Wheeley S, Homan J, Niemeyer S (2003). *Risk literacy and the public MMR, air pollution and mobile phones*. Department of Health, London. Available at: http://www.dh.gov.uk/PublicationsAndStatistics/Publications/Publi cationsPolicyAndGuidance/PublicationsPolicyAndGuidanceArticle/fs/ en?CONTENT_ID=4074013&chk=gkORsY (accessed 15 June 2005).

Phelps CE (1993). The methodological foundations of studies of the appropriateness of medical care. *N Engl J Med*, **329**(17), 1241–5.

Pierce J, Jameton A (2004). *The ethics of environmentally responsible health care*. Oxford University Press, New York.

Pirsig RM (1991). *Zen and the art of motorcycle maintenance.* Vintage Press, New York.

Plsek PE (1994). Tutorial: directed creativity. *Qual Manag Health Care*, **2**(3), 62–76.

Policy Commission on Public Services (2004). *Making public services personal: a new compact for public services. The independent Policy Commission on Public Services report to the National Consumer Council.* National Consumer Council, London. Available at: http://www.ncc.org.uk/ publicservices/policy_commission.pdf (accessed 25 April 2005).

Popay J, Williams G (1998). Partnership in health: beyond the rhetoric. *J Epidemiol Commun Health*, **52**, 410–11.

Potter J (2004). Discourse analysis. In: Hardy M, Bryman A (eds) Handbook of data analysis. Sage, London.

Powell JE (1976). *Medicine and politics; 1975 and after.* Pitman Medical, London. (The best guide to how to work with full-time politicians and senior civil servants.)

Pratt J (1995). *Practitioners and practices. A conflict of values?* Radcliffe Medical Press, Oxford.

Pratt J, Plamping D, Gordon P (1999). *Working whole systems.* King's Fund, London.

Preker AS, Harding A (2003). *Innovations in health service delivery: the corporatization of public hospitals.* World Bank, Washington, DC.

Public Health Advisory Committee (2004). *A guide to health impact assessment: a policy tool for New Zealand.* Public Health Advisory Committee, National Advisory Committee on Health and Disability, Wellington. Available at: http://www.nhc.govt.nz/PHAC/publications/ GuideToHIA.pdf (accessed 15 June 2005).

Public Health Classifications Project, National Public Health Partnership of Australia. Available at: http://www.nphp.gov.au/workprog/phi/ (accessed 29 June 2005).

Public Health Information Tagging Standard. http://www.phits.org/ (accessed 29 June 2005).

Quigley R, Cavanagh S, Harrison D, Taylor L (2004). Clarifying health impact assessment, integrated impact assessment and health needs assessment. Available at: http://www.publichealth.nice.org.uk/page.aspx? o=502661 (accessed 7 September 2005).

Rabinowitz HK, Diamond JJ, Markham FW, Hazelwood CE (1999). A program to increase the number of family physicians in rural and underserved areas. *J Am Med Assoc*, **281**, 255–60.

Raffle AE, Alden B, Quinn M, Babb PJ, Brett MT (2003). Outcomes of screening to prevent cancer: analysis of cumulative incidence of cervical abnormality and modelling of cases and deaths prevented. *BMJ*, **326**, 901–4.

Raine R, Hutchings A, Black N (2003). Is publicly funded health care really distributed according to need? The example of cardiac rehabilitation in the UK. *Health Policy*, **63**, 63–72.

Ramachandran A (1998). Epidemiology of non-insulin-dependent diabetes mellitus in India. In: Shetty P, Gopalan C (eds) *Nutrition and chronic disease: an Asian perspective*, pp. 38–41. Smith-Gordon, London.

Rawaf S, Bahl V (1998). *Assessing health needs of people from minority ethnic groups.* Royal College of Physicians, London.

Rawls J (1971). *A theory of justice.* Harvard University Press, Boston, MA.

Rechel B, Schwalbe N, McKee M (2004). Health in South Eastern Europe: a troubled past, an uncertain future. *Bull WHO,* **82**, 539–46.

Regidor E (2004). Measures of health inequalities: part 1. *J Epidemiol Commun Health,* **58**(10), 858–61.

Regidor E (2004). Measures of health inequalities: part 2. *J Epidemiol Commun Health,* **58**(11), 900–3.

Rennie D Flanagin A (1992). Publication bias the triumph of hope over experience. *JAMA,* 267(3), 411–2.

Report of the Committee on the Financial Aspects of Corporate Governance [Cadbury Report] (1992). Gee, London. Available at http://rru. worldbank.org/Documents/PapersLinks/1253.pdf (accessed 29 September 2005).

Resource Allocation Working Party (1976). *Sharing resources for health in England.* HMSO, London.

Reuben DB, Keeler E, Seeman TE, Sewall A, Hirsch SH, Guralnik JM (2003). Identification of risk for high hospital use: cost comparisons of four strategies and performance across subgroups. *J Am Geriatric Soc,* **51**(5), 615–20.

Rice N, Smith PC (2001). Capitation and risk adjustment in health care financing: an international progress report. *Milbank Q,* **79**, 81–113, IV.

Richards L (1999). Data alive! The thinking behind NVivo. *Qual Health Res,* **9**(3), 412–28. Available at: http://www.qualitative-research.net/fqs-texte/2–02/2–02welsh-e.pdf (accessed 24 June 2005).

Richardson A, Jackson C, Sykes W (1992). *Audit guidelines in public health medicine: an introduction.* Nuffield Institute for Health Services Studies, University of Leeds, Leeds.

Rist RC (1994). Influencing the policy process with qualitative research. In: Denzin NK, Lincoln YS (eds) *Handbook of qualitative research,* pp. 545–57. Sage, Thousand Oaks, CA.

Robert Wood Johnson Foundation and the Group Health Cooperative's MacColl Institute for Healthcare Innovation. *The chronic care model.* Robert Wood Johnson Foundation, Princeton, NJ. Available at: http://www.improvingchroniccare.org/change/index.html (accessed 5 June 2005).

Robine JM, Romieu I, Cambois E (1999). Health expectancy indicators. *Bull World Health Org,* **77**(2), 181–5.

Robinson R (1993). Economic evaluation and health care (a series of six articles in the *BMJ*). What does it mean? *BMJ,* **307**, 670–3. Costs and cost minimisation analysis. *BMJ,* **307**, 726–8. Cost effectiveness analysis. *BMJ,* **307**, 793–5. Cost utility analysis. *BMJ,* **307**, 859–62. Cost benefit analysis. *BMJ,* **307**, 924–6. The policy context. *BMJ,* **307**, 994–6.

Roland M (2004). Linking physicians' pay to the quality of care—a major experiment in the United Kingdom. *N Engl J Med,* **351**(14), 1448–54.

Rose G (1985). Sick individuals and sick populations. *International Journal of Epidemiology,* **14**(1), 32–8.

Rose G (1986). Epidemiology and health care planning: their place in medical education. *J R Soc Med,* **79**, 631–3.

Rose G (1990). The population mean predicts the number of deviant individuals. *BMJ*, **301**, 1031–4.

Rose G (1992). *The strategy of preventive medicine.* Oxford University Press, Oxford.

Rosen R (1993). *A history of public health.* Johns Hopkins, Baltimore MA.

Rothenberg RB, Thacker SB (1996). Guidelines for the investigation of clusters of adverse health events. In: Eliott P, Cuzick J, English D, Stern R (eds) *Geographical and environmental epidemiology methods for small-area studies,* pp. 264–77. Oxford University Press, Oxford.

Rothman KJ (1990). A sobering start for the cluster busters' conference. *Am J Epidemiol,* **132**(1, Suppl.), S6–S13.

Rothman KJ, Greenland S (1998). *Modern epidemiology* (2nd edn). Lippin-cott–Raven, Philadelphia.

Rouse A, Adab P (2001). Is population coronary heart disease risk screening justified? A discussion of the national service framework for coronary heart disease (standard 4). *Br J Gen Pract,* **51**, 834–7.

Royal Society of Medicine Press. *Effective health care bulletins.* http://www.york.ac.uk/inst/crd/ehcb.htm (accessed 30 June 2005).

Royal Society Study Group (1992). *Risk: analysis, perception and management.* Royal Society, London.

Ruberman W, Weinblatt E, Goldberg J et al. (1977). Ventricular premature beats and mortality after myocardial infarction. N Engl J Med, **297**, 750–7. (Cited in Sackett DL, Richardson WS, Rosenberg WMC, Haynes RB (1997). Evidence-based medicine: how to practice and teach EBM. Churchill Livingstone, New York.)

Ruwaard D, Kramers PGN, van den Berg Jeths A, Achterberg PW (1994). *Public health status and forecasts: the health status of the Dutch population over the period 1950–2010.* National Institute of Public Health and Environmental Protection, Bilthoven, The Netherlands. Sdu Uitgeverij, The Hague.

Ryan C (1991). *Prime time activism.* South End Press, Boston, MA.

Rychetnik L, Frommer M (2002). *A schema for evaluating evidence on public health interventions,* version 4. National Public Health Partnership, Melbourne. Available at: http://www.nphp.gov.au/publications/phpractice/schemaV4.pdf (accessed 26 June 2005).

Sackett DL, Haynes RB, Guyatt G, Tugwell P (1991). *Clinical epidemiology; a basic science for clinical medicine.* (2nd edn). Little and Brown, Boston, MA.

Sadhra SS, Rampal KG (ed.) (1999). *Occupational health: risk assessment and management.* Blackwell Science, Oxford.

Sandman PM (1993). *Responding to community outrage: strategies for effective risk communication.* American Industrial Hygiene Association, Fairfax, VA.

Sandman PM, Lanard J (2003). Fear is spreading faster than SARS—and so it should! Available at: http://www.psandman.com/col/SARS-1.htm (accessed 30 September 2005).

Savage J (2000). Ethnography and health care. *BMJ*, **321**, 1400–2. Available at: http://bmj.bmjjournals.com/cgi/content/full/321/7273/1400 (accessed December 2004).

Scally G, Donaldson LJ (1999). Clinical governance and the drive for quality improvement in the new NHS in England. *BMJ*, **317**, 61–5.

Schall MW, Duffy T, Krishnamurthy A, et al. (2004). Improving patient access to the Veterans Health Administration's primary care and specialty clinics. Jt Comm J Qual Saf, **30**(8), 415–23.

Schön DA (1983). The reflective practitioner: how professionals think in action. Temple Smith, London.

School of Health and Related Research in Sheffield, UK (SCHARR). Seeking the evidence: a protocol. Available at: www.shef.ac.uk/uni/academic/R-Z/scharr/ir/proto.html (accessed 26 June 2005).

Schulman KA, Berlin JA, Harless W et al. (1999). The effect of race and sex on physicians' recommendations for cardiac catheterization. N Engl J Med, **340**, 618–26.

Schuster MA, McGlynn EA, Brook RH (1998). How good is the quality of health care in the United States? Milbank Q, **76**, 517–63.

Schwartz WB, Joskow PL (1978). Medical efficacy versus economic efficiency: a conflict of values. N Engl J Med, **299**, 1462–4.

Scott A, Donaldson C (1998). Clinical and cost effectiveness issues in health needs assessment. In: Wright , (ed) Health needs assessment in practice, pp. 84–94. BMJ Books, London.

Scott-Samuel A (1996). Health impact assessment—an idea whose time has come. BMJ, **313**, 183–4.

Seddon ME, Marshall MN, Campbell SM, Roland MO (2001). Systematic review of studies of quality of clinical care in general practice in the UK, Australia, and New Zealand. Qual Health Care, **10**, 152–8.

Selby JV, Fireman BH, Lundstrom RJ et al. (1996). Variation among hospitals in coronary-angiography practices and outcomes after myocardial infarction in a large health maintenance organization. N Engl J Med, **335**(25), 1888–96.

Shekelle PG, Kahan JP, Bernstein SJ, Leape LL, Kamberg CJ, Park RE (1998). The reproducibility of a method to identify the overuse and underuse of medical procedures. N Engl J Med, **338**(26), 1888–95.

Shekelle PG, MacLean CH, Morton SC, Wenger NS (2001). Acove quality indicators. Ann Intern Med, **135**(8, Pt 2), 653–67.

Shekelle PG, Park RE, Kahan JP, Leape LL, Kamberg CJ, Bernstein SJ (2001). Sensitivity and specificity of the RAND/UCLA Appropriateness Method to identify the overuse and underuse of coronary revascularization and hysterectomy. J Clin Epidemiol, **54**(10), 1004–10.

Shkolnikov V, McKee M, Leon DA (2001). Changes in life expectancy in Russia in the 1990s. Lancet, **357**, 917–21.

Silverman D (1994). Analysing naturally occurring date on AIDS counselling: some methodological and practical issues. In: Boulton M (ed) Challenge and innovation: methodological advances in social research on HIV/AIDS. Taylor and Francis, London.

Silverstein MD, Ballard DJ (1998). Expert panel assessment of appropriateness of abdominal aortic aneurysm surgery: global judgement versus probability estimation. J Health Serv Res Policy, **3**(3), 134–40.

Silvestri G, Pritchard R, Welch HG (1998). Preferences for chemotherapy in patients with advanced non-small cell lung cancer: descriptive study based on scripted interviews. BMJ, **317**, 771–5.

Smedley BD, Stith AY, Nelson AR (eds) (2003). *Unequal treatment: confronting racial and ethnic disparities in healthcare.* National Academies Press, Washington, DC.

Smith AFM (1996). Mad cows and ecstasy: chance and choice in an evidence–based society. *J R Statist Soc,* **159**, 367–83.

Smith CJ (1986). Equity in the distribution of health and welfare services: can we rely on the state to reverse the 'inverse care law?'. *Soc Sci Med,* **23**(10), 1067–78.

Smith R (1991). Where is the wisdom? (editorial). *BMJ,* **303**, 798–9.

Smith R (1994). Towards a knowledge based health service. *BMJ,* **309**, 217–8.

Smith R, Beaglehole R, Woodward D, Drager N (eds) (2003). *Global public goods for health—health economic and public health perspectives.* Oxford University Press, Oxford.

Socialist Health Association. *The Black Report 1980.* Available at: http://www.sochealth.co.uk/history/black.htm (accessed 25 JUne 2005).

Sociologies of Health and Illness ELearning Databank (SHIELD). *The Black Report and inequalities in health.* Available at: http://www.ucel.ac.uk/shield/black_report/ (accessed 25 June 2005).

Somerville M, Basham M, Foy C, Ballinger G, Gay T, Shute S, Barton AG (2002). From local concern to randomised trial: the Watcombe Housing Project. *Health Expectations* **5**, 127–35.

Sox H, Blatt MA, Higgins MC, Marton KI (1998). *Medical decision making.* Butterworths, London.

Spear S (1999). Decoding the DNA of the Toyota production system. *Harvard Business Rev,* Sept–Oct, 95–106.

Spiegelhalter D (2002). Funnel plots for institutional comparison [comment]. *Qual Saf Health Care,* **11**(4), 390–1.

Spiegelhalter DJ, Myles JP, Jones DR, Abrams KR (1999). Methods in health service research: an introduction to Bayesian methods in health technology assessment. *BMJ,* **319**, 508–12.

Sram I, Ashton J (1998). Millennium report to Sir Edwin Chadwick. *BMJ,* **317**, 592–5.

Standing Committee on Postgraduate Medical Education (SCOPME) (1999). *Doctors and dentists. The need for a process of review,* a working paper. SCOPME, London.

Stansfeld S, Marmot MG (ed.) (2000). *Stress and heart disease.* BMJ Publications, London.

Starfield B (1994). Is primary care essential? *Lancet,* **344**, 1129–33.

Steel N (2000). Thresholds for taking antihypertensive drugs in different professional and lay groups: questionnaire survey. *BMJ,* **320**, 1446–7.

Steel N, Melzer D, Shekelle PG, Wenger NS. Forsyth D, McWilliams BC (2004). Developing quality indicators for older adults: transfer from the USA to the UK is feasible. *Qual Saf Health Care,* **13**(4), 260–4.

Stevens A, Gabbay J (1991). Needs assessment needs assessment. *Health Trends,* **23**(1), 20.

Stevens A, Gillam S (1998). Needs assessment: from theory to practice. *BMJ,* **316**, 1448–52.

Stevens A, Milne R (2004). Health technology assessment in England and Wales. *Int J Technol Assess Health Care,* **20**(1), 11–24.

Stevens A, Milne R, Burls A (2003). Health technology assessment: history and demand. *J Public Health Med*, **25**(2), 98–101.

Stevens A, Raftery J (eds) (1997). *Health care needs assessment*, 2nd series. Radcliffe Medical Press, Oxford.

Stiglitz JE (1993). *Economics*. W.W. Norton and Co., New York.

Stimson G, Fitch C, Rhodes T, Ball A (1999). Rapid assessment and response: methods for developing public health responses to drug problems. *Drug Alcohol Rev*, **18**, 317–25.

Strauss A, Corbin JM (1990). Basics of qualitative research: grounded theory *procedures and techniques*. Sage, Newbury Park, CA.

Strauss AL, Corbin JM (1998). Basics of qualitative research: techniques and *procedures for developing grounded theory*. Sage, Thousand Oaks, CA.

Sullivan DF (1971). A single index of mortality and morbidity. *Health Services Mental Health Administration Health Reports* **86**, 347–54.

Summerfield D (2000). Conflict and health: war and mental health: a brief overview *BMJ*, **321**, 232–5.

Tarlov AR, Ware JE Jr, Greenfield S, Nelson EC, Perrin E, Zubkoff M (1989). The medical outcomes study. An application of methods for monitoring the results of medical care. *JAMA*, **262**(7), 925–30.

Taylor A (1993). *Women drug users: an ethnography of an injecting community*. Clarendon Press, Oxford.

Taylor AL, Bettcher DW, Fluss SS, Deland K, Yach D (2002). International health instruments: an overview. In: Detels R (ed) *Oxford textbook of public health*, 4th edn, pp. 359–86. Oxford University Press, Oxford.

Taylor L, Gowman N, Quigley R (2003). *Evaluating health impact assessment*. Health Development Agency, London. Available at: http://www.phel.nice.org.uk/hiadocs/Evaluating_HIA.pdf (accessed 15 June 2005).

Tejada de Rivero D (2003). Alma-Ata revisited. *Perspect Health*, **8**, 1–6.

Teutsch SM, Churchill RE (eds) (2000). *Principles and practice of public health surveillance*. Oxford University Press, New York.

The Cochrane Collaboration. http://www.cochrane.org/index0.htm (accessed 28 December 2004).

The Copenhagen Declaration on Reducing Social Inequalities in Health (2002). *Scand J Publ Health*, **30**(Suppl. 59), 78–9.

The National electronic Library of Infection (NeLI). *Bugs & drugs on the web, NeLI antimicrobial resistance website*. http://www.antibioticresistance.org.uk/ (accessed 14 September 2005).

The Presidential/Congressional Commission on Risk Assessment and Risk Management (1997). *Framework for environmental health risk management*, Final report volume 1. Washington, DC.

The United States Agency for Healthcare Research and Quality. http://www.ahrq.gov/ (accessed 30 June 2005).

The World Bank (1993). *World development report 1993*. Oxford University Press, New York.

Timmins N (1996). *The five giants – a biography of the welfare state*. Fontana Press, London.

Tobacman JK, Scott IU, Cyphert S, Zimmerman B (1999). Reproducibility of measures of overuse of cataract surgery by three physician panels. *Med Care*, **37**(9), 937–45.

Tobey TA (1926). *Public health law: a manual of law for sanitarians.* The Commonwealth Fund, New York.

Toth FL (1988). Policy exercises: procedures and implementation. *Simulat Games,* **19**, 256–76.

Treasure T (1998). Lessons from the Bristol case. *BMJ,* **316**, 1685–6.

Tuckman BC (1965). Development sequence in small groups. *Psychol Bull,* **63**(6), 384–99.

Tudor Hart J (1971). The inverse care law. *Lancet,* **696**, 405–12.

Tudor Hart J (1988). *A new kind of doctor.* Merlin Press, London.

Tufte E (1983). *Visual display of quantitative information.* Graphics Press, Connecticut.

Tufte E (1990). *Envisioning information.* Graphics Press, Connecticut.

Tufte E (1997). *Visual explanations.* Graphics Press, Connecticut.

Tukey JW (1962). The future of data analysis. *Ann Math Stat,* **33**, 1–67.

Turning Point Model State Public Health Act. Available at http://www.publichealthlaw.net/Resources/Modellaws.htm (accessed 27 October 2004).

Uhr J, Mackay K (ed.) (1996). *Evaluating policy advice: learning from Commonwealth experience.* Federalism Research Centre, Australian National University and Commonwealth Department of Finance, Canberra.

UK Association of Cancer Registries. Guidelines on the release of confidential data. Available at: http://www.ukacr.org/confidentiality/ (accessed 25 June 2005).

UK Cabinet Office (1999). *Professional policy-making for the 21st century.* The Cabinet Office, London. Available at: http://www.e-democracy.gov.uk/knowledgepool/default.htm?mode=1&pk_document=33 (accessed 27 June 2005).

United Nations Development Programme (1997). *Human development report 1997.* Oxford University Press, Oxford.

United Nations Development Programme (2000). *Human development report 2000.* Oxford University Press, Oxford.

United States Government (2000). *Healthy people 2010.* Available at: http://www.healthypeople.gov/ (accessed 26 June 2005).

United States Presidential Congressional Commission on Risk Management (1997). *A framework for environmental health risk management.* US Government, New York.

Unwin N, Alberti G, Aspray T et al. (1998). Economic globalisation and its effect on health. *BMJ,* **316**, 1401–2.

Urquhart J (1996). Studies of disease clustering: problems of interpretation. In: Eliott P, Cuzick J, English D, Stern R (eds) *Geographical and environmental epidemiology methods for small-area studies,* pp. 278–85. Oxford University Press, Oxford.

US Preventive Services Task Force (2003). *Counselling to prevent tobacco use and tobacco-caused disease: US,* publication no 04–0526. Agency for Healthcare Research and Quality, Rockville, MD.

Van Wyk G (2003). *A systems approach to social and organizational planning.* Trafford Publishing, Victoria, BC.

Vayda E (1973). A comparision of surgical rates in Canada and in England and Wales. *N Engl J Med,* **289**, 1224–9.

Verstappen WH, van der Weijden T, ter Riet G, *et al.* (2004). Block design allowed for control of the Hawthorne effect in a randomized controlled trial of test ordering. *J Clin Epidemiol*, **57**(11), 1119–23.

Voyle J, Simmons D (1999). Community development through partnership: promoting health in an urban indigenous community in New Zealand. *Soc Sci Med*, **49**, 1035–50.

Wagener DK, Molla MT, Crimmins EM, Pamuk ER, Madans JH (2001). Summary measures of population health: addressing the first goal of healthy people 2010, improving health expectancy. In: *Healthy people 2010*, National Centre for Health Statistics statistical notes no. 22, pp. 1–13. US Department of Health and Human Services, Washington, DC.

Wagner EH (2000). The role of patient care teams in chronic disease management. *BMJ*, **320**, 569–72.

Wagstaff A, Paci P, van Doorslaer E (1991). On the measurement of inequalities in health. *Soc Sci Med*, **33**(5), 545–57.

Wagstaff A, van Doorslaer E (2004). Overall versus socioeconomic health inequality: a measurement framework and two empirical illustrations. *Health Econ*, **13**(3), 297–301.

Walberg P, McKee M, Shkolnikov V, Chenet L, Leon DA (1998). Economic change, crime, and mortality crisis in Russia: regional analysis. *BMJ*, **317**, 312–18.

Wallack L, Dorfman L, Jernigan D, Themba M (1993). *Media advocacy and public health: power for prevention.* Sage, Newbury Park, CA.

Walt G (1994). *Health policy: an introduction to process and power.* Zed Books, London.

Wanless D (2001). *Securing our future health: taking a long-term view. An interim report.* HM Treasury, London.

Wanless D (2004). *Securing good health for the whole population. Final report.* UK Department of Health, London. Available at: http://www.dh.gov.uk/assetRoot/04/07/61/34/04076134.pdf (accessed 29 June 2005).

Ward JE (1997). Reducing cervical cancer by two-thirds: a public health target within our reach? *Aust NZ J Public Health*, **21**, 248–9.

Warsi A, Wang PS, LaValley MP, Avorn J, Solomon DH (2004). Self-management education programs in chronic disease: a systematic review and methodological critique of the literature. *Arch Intern Med*, **164**, 1641–9.

Webb E (1998). Children and the inverse care law. *BMJ*, **316**(7144), 1588–91.

Weinstein MC, Fineberg HV, Elstein AS *et al.* (1980). *Clinical decision analysis.* WB Saunders, Philadelphia, PA.

Weiss CH (1979). The many meanings of research utilisation. *Public Admin Rev*, **39**, 426–31.

Wenger NS, Shekelle PG (2001). Assessing care of vulnerable elders: ACOVE project overview. *Ann Intern Med*, **135**(8 Pt 2), 642–6.

Wenger NS, Solomon DH, Roth CP *et al.* (2003). The quality of medical care provided to vulnerable community-dwelling older patients. *Ann Intern Med*, **139**(9), 740–7.

Wennberg DE, Wennberg JE (2003). *Addressing variations: is there hope for the future. Health Affairs* web exclusive. Available at: http://content.healthaffairs.org/cgi/content/full/hlthaff.w3.614v1/DC1 (accessed 22 July 2005).

Wennberg J, Gittelsohn A (1973). Small area variations in health care delivery: a population-based health information system can guide planning and regulatory decision-making. *Science*, **182**, 1102–8.

Wennberg JE (2002). Unwarranted variations in healthcare delivery: implications for academic medical centres. *BMJ*, **325**(7370), 961–4.

Wennberg JE, Fisher ES, Skinner JS (2002). *Geography and the debate over medicare reform. Health Affairs* web exclusive. Available at: http://content.healthaffairs.org/cgi/content/full/hlthaff.w2.96v1/DC1 (accessed 22 July 2005).

Wensing M, Grol R (2005). Methods to identify implementation problems. In: Grol R, Wensing M, Eccles M (eds) *Improving patient care. The implementation of change in clinical practice.* Elsevier, London.

West R (1987). High death rates: more deaths or earlier deaths? *J R Coll Physicians Lond*, **21**, 73–6.

Western Australia Department of Health (2005). *Western Australia clinical governance guidelines*, Information Series no 1.2, 2nd edn. Western Australia Department of Health, Perth.

What do we mean by appropriate health care? Report of a working group prepared for the Director of Research and Development of the UK NHS Management Executive. *Qual Health Care*, June, **2**(2), 117–23 (1993).

Wheeler DJ, Chambers DS (1992). *Understanding statistical process control*, 2nd edn. SPC Press, Knoxville, TN.

White K (1994). *Healing the schism: epidemiology, medicine, and the public's health.* Springer–Verlag, New York.

White K, Connolly J (1992). *The medical school's mission and the population's health: medical education in Canada, the United Kingdom, the United States, and Australia.* Springer–Verlag, New York.

WHO European Centre for Health Policy (1999). *Health impact assessment: main concepts and suggested approach*, Gothenburg consensus paper. ECHP, Brussels.

Whorton D, Krauss RM, Marshall S, Milby TH (1977). Infertility in male pesticide workers. *Lancet*, **2**(8051), 1259–61.

Wilkin D, Hallam L, Dogget M (1992). *Measures of need and outcomes in primary health care.* Oxford Medical Publications, Oxford.

Wilkinson R (1996). *Unhealthy societies: the afflictions of inequality.* Routledge, London.

Wilkinson R, Marmot M (eds) (2003). *Social determinants of health: the solid facts*, 2nd edn. World Health Organization, Copenhagen.

Will S, Ardern K, Spencely M, Watkins S (1994). *A prospective health impact assessment of the proposed development of a second runway at Manchester International Airport.* Written submission to the public inquiry. Manchester and Stockport Health Commissions.

Wilson T, Berwick DM, Cleary PD (2003). What do collaborative improvement projects do? Experience from seven countries. *Jt Comm J Qual Saf*, **29**(2), 85–93.

Woods KL, Ketley D, Lowy A *et al.* (1998). Beta-blockers and antithrombotic treatment for secondary prevention after acute myocardial infarction. Towards an understanding of factors influencing clinical practice. The European Secondary Prevention Study Group. *Eur Heart J*, **19**, 74–9.

World Bank (1993). *World development report 1993: investing in health.* Oxford University Press, Oxford.

World Cancer Research Fund (1997). *Food, nutrition and the prevention of cancer.* World Cancer Research Fund/American Institute for Cancer Research, Washington DC.

World Health Organization (1946). WHO constitution. Available at: http://www.who.int/trade/glossary/story046/en/ (accessed 25 June 2005).

World Health Organization (1978). *Alma-Ata: primary health care, Health for All series No 1.* World Health Organization, Geneva.

World Health Organization (1978). *Primary health care. Report of the International Conference on Primary Health Care, Alma-Ata, USSR, 6–12 September 1978.* World Health Organization, Geneva.

World Health Organization (1984). The uses of epidemiology in the study of the elderly: report of a WHO scientific group on the epidemiology of aging. *World Health Org Tech Rep Ser,* **706**: 1–84.

World Health Organization (1986). *Ottawa Charter for Health Promotion.* WHO, Geneva.

World Health Organization (1996). *Health consequences of the Chernobyl accident. Scientific report.* WHO, Geneva.

World Health Organization (1998). *The new emergency health kit,* WHO document WHO/DAP/98.10. World Health Organization, Geneva.

World Health Organization (1998). *World health declaration,* paragraph 111. World Health Organization, Geneva.

World Health Organization (1999). *World Health Report 1998.* World Health Organization, Geneva.

World Health Organization (2000). *The world health report 2000: health systems: improving performance.* World Health Organization, Geneva.

World Health Organization (2001). *The world health report 2001: mental health: new understanding, new hope.* World Health Organization, Geneva.

World Health Organization (2002). *The world health report 2002: reducing risk: promoting healthy life.* World Health Organization, Geneva.

World Health Organization (2003). Special issue on HIA. *Bulletin of the World Health Organization,* **81**(6). Available at: http://www.who.int/bulletin/ volumes/81/6/en/ (accessed 16 June 2005).

World Health Organization (2003). *The world health report 2003: shaping the future.* World Health Organization, Geneva.

World Health Organization (2004). *Framework Convention on Tobacco Control,* WHO doc. A56/VR/4 (2003). Available at: http://www.who.int/gb/ebwha/pdf_files/WHA56/ea56r1.pdf (accessed 27 October 2004).

World Health Organization (2004). *Guidelines for drinking water quality,* 3rd edn, Vol. 1 Recommendations. World Health Organization, Geneva. Available at: http://www.who.int/water_sanitation_health/dwq/gdwq3/en/ (accessed 13 March 2005).

World Health Organization (2004). *International Health Regulations: working paper for regional consultations*, WHO doc. IGWG/IHR/Working paper/12.2003. Available at: http://www.who.int/csr/ihr/revisionprocess/working_paper/en/(accessed 27 October 2004).

World Health Organization (2005). *Preparing a workforce for the 21st century: the challenge of chronic conditions*. World Health Organization, Geneva. Available at: http://www.who.int/chronic_conditions/resources/workforce_report.pdf.

World Health Organization Regional Office for Europe (1998). *21 Targets for the 21st century—a public health guide to the targets to the Health for All policy for the European region*. World Health Organization, Copenhagen.

World Health Organization Regional Office for Europe (2005). *Healthy cities and urban governance*. http://www.euro.who.int/healthy-cities (accessed 14 March 2005).

World Health Organization. *Facts related to chronic diseases*. World Health Organization, Geneva. Available at: http://www.who.int/dietphysicalactivity/publications/facts/chronic/en/ (accessed 31 May 2005).

World Health Organization. *Health systems performance*. Available at: http://www.who.int/health-systems-performance/ (accessed 21 March 2005).

World Health Organization. *The WHO family of international classifications*. Available at: http://www.who.int/classifications/en/ (accessed 20 March 2005).

World Health Organization. *WHO Statistical Information System (WHOSIS)*. Available at: www.who.int/whosis/ (accessed 21 March 2005).

World Health Organization/UNICEF (1990). *Breastfeeding in the 1990s: a global initiative (The Innocenti Declaration)*. World Health Organization, Geneva.

Wright J, Hill P (2003). *Clinical governance*. Churchill Livingstone, London.

Wright J, Walley J, Philip A et al.(2004). Direct observation for tuberculosis: a randomised controlled trial of community health workers versus family members. *Trop Med Int Health* **9**, 559–65.

Wright J, Williams DRR, Wilkinson J (1998). The development of health needs assessment. In: *Health needs assessment in practice* (ed. J Wright), pp. 1–11. BMJ Books, London.

Zimmern R, Cook C (2000). *Genetics and health: policy issues for genetic science and their implications for health and health services*. The Stationery Office, London.

Zimmern RL (1999). Genetics. In: Griffiths S, Hunter DJ (eds) *Perspectives in public health*, pp. 131–40. Radcliffe Medical Press, Oxford.

Index